Nigel Paneth, MD, MPH
Director, Program in Epidemiology
A-206 East Fee
Michigan State University
East Lansing, MI 48824-1316

OXFORD MEDICAL PUBLICATIONS

Commission of the European Communities
Health Services Research Series
No. 6

EUROPEAN COMMUNITY ATLAS OF 'AVOIDABLE DEATH'

SECOND EDITION
Volume One

W.W. Holland

Project Director

EC Working Group on
Health Services and
'Avoidable Deaths'

E.A. Paul (Project Co-ordinator), J. Barry, G. Bevan, D. Borgers,
M.H. Bouvier-Colle, V. Carstairs, L. Cayolla da Motta, D. Hansen-Koenig,
F. Hatton, P. Hooft, P. Humblet, E. Jougla, K. Juel, K. Kern, R. Lagasse,
A. Lakhani, P. Lauriola, J.P. Mackenbach, M. Medrano, P.L. Morosini,
G. Papaevangelou, M.L. Sequeira, C. Tsimbos

Oxford New York Tokyo
OXFORD UNIVERSITY PRESS
1991

Oxford University Press, Walton Street, Oxford OX2 6DP

Oxford New York Toronto
Delhi Bombay Calcutta Madras Karachi
Petaling Jaya Singapore Hong Kong Tokyo
Nairobi Dar es Salaam Cape Town
Melbourne Auckland

and associated companies in
Berlin Ibadan

Oxford is a trade mark of Oxford University Press
First edition published 1988

©ECSC – EEC – EAEC, Brussels – Luxembourg, 1991

Publication No. EUR 11157 of the
Commission of the European Communities,
Directorate-General Communications,
Information Industries and Innovation,
Luxembourg.

British Library Cataloguing-in-Publication Data
European Community atlas of 'avoidable death'
Vol. 1
—(Commission of the European Communities
health services research series: no. 6).
1. Epidemiology—European Economic
Community countries
I. Holland, Walter W.II. Series
614,4 24   RA650.6.A1
ISBN 0-19-261952-7

Library of Congress Cataloging in Publication Data
Data is available
ISBN 0-19-261952-7

Maps generated using INFO-MAP software
© Claymore Services, Exeter, England
Maps generated and text typeset from data supplied by
Cotswold Press Ltd, Eynsham, Oxford, England
Printed in Malta by Interprint Ltd.

PREFACE

The first edition of the *European Community Atlas of 'Avoidable Death'* was published in 1988. It described mortality from 17 conditions in 10 countries in 1974–78. This second edition describes 'avoidable mortality' in the European Community in 1980–84 and changes in 'avoidable mortality' between 1974–78 and 1980–84. In the second edition, the 10 countries who originally collaborated on the project have been joined by Spain and Portugal.

There is growing interest in evaluating and monitoring the performance of health services. Much effort has centred on rationalizing the enormous volume of data collected to produce a manageable series of measures that reflect the various facets of a health care system. Progress in the development of indicators of the quality and outcome of health care services has lagged behind that of measures of process and efficiency. The atlas represents an important step towards establishing outcome indicators to monitor health service performance, that are applicable nationally and internationally.

There are now numerous atlases which provide detailed ecological analyses of the geographical variation in the incidence of diseases both within individual countries and within regions of the world. Notable among these are atlases of the geographical variation in the incidence of cancers. This atlas of 'avoidable death' is unique in that it attempts to look systematically at the use of mortality data as a means of asking questions about the adequacy of health services provision.

Historically, maternal and infant mortality have gained wide acceptance as monitors for the quality of obstetric and infant care. This atlas extends the concept to other conditions from which most deaths should be avoidable, given timely and appropriate medical intervention or public health action.

Doubtless the choice of diseases will be the subject of much debate. However, the final list of diseases included in the atlas results from extensive discussion among the collaborating researchers. The conditions chosen were considered to be relevant to all the EC member countries, and to reflect important aspects of health care provision.

The atlas dramatically illustrates the wide variation in mortality rates both within and between member countries. No attempt has been made in the atlas to interpret the patterns observed or draw conclusions. This is wise, because the explanations for the observed variation are likely to be complex and depend on a number of factors, some of which may be beyond the control of health services providers. The function of the atlas is to provide indicators of aspects of health service provision where a problem may exist, and where further investigation would be worthwhile.

It is hoped that the atlas will stimulate countries to initiate detailed inquiries into the functioning of their health services. To aid researchers in this, the atlas includes descriptions of those parts of the health service implicated in the treatment or prevention of the individual conditions, and information on variation in health service inputs and in social conditions. The atlas should not be used to fuel 'witch hunts' or to apportion blame, but constructively to improve services.

To compile an atlas of this kind is a major achievement in itself. The data presented are available in some form within each country. But to generate meaningful data in a standard and comparable form required major re-analysis in unique ways. This was only possible through the close co-operation and commitment of a number of researchers familiar with the data collection systems of their country. It constitutes a valuable product of the medical research programme of the EC and it is an excellent example of what can be achieved through tapping the available data sources within the EC countries.

The researchers are to be congratulated on their collaborative effort and their most dramatic findings. I hope that it will stimulate further research into the financing and organization of health services in the EC, and pave the way for future collaboration between health services researchers within the EC.

June 1990
Paolo Fasella
Director-General for Science, Research and Development

PREFACE

La première édition de l'Atlas de la Communauté Européenne sur les *'Morts Evitables'* fut publiée en 1988. Elle décrivait la mortalité due à dix-sept affections, dans dix pays, sur la période 1974–78. La seconde édition décrit la mortalité 'évitable', dans la Communauté Européenne, en 1980–84, ainsi que les évolutions de la mortalité intervenues entre 1974–78 et 1980–84. Dans cette seconde édition, l'Espagne et le Portugal ont rejoint les dix pays qui étaient à l'origine du projet initial.

L'intérêt porté à l'évaluation et au contrôle du fonctionnement des services de santé va croissant. L'effort a été concentré sur la rationalisation de l'importante quantité de données collectées, afin de produire des séries de mesures qui reflètent les différentes facettes du système de soins. Le développement des indicateurs de qualité et de rendement des services de santé est resté en retard par rapport à celui des mesures de technique et d'efficacité. L'atlas représente une étape importante vers la mise au point d'indices d'évaluation des services de santé, qui soient applicables nationalement et internationalement.

Il existe maintenant de nombreux atlas qui procurent des analyses détaillées des variations géographiques de l'incidence des maladies, aussi bien à l'intérieur des pays qu'entre les régions du monde, et en particulier, sont notables, les atlas des variations géographiques de l'incidence des cancers. L'atlas de la mortalité 'évitable' est unique car il tente d'utiliser systématiquement les données de mortalité comme instrument de réponse à la question de l'adaptation des services de santé.

Historiquement, les mortalités infantile et maternelle ont finalement été largement considérées comme des contrôles efficaces des soins obstétricaux et pédiatriques. Cet atlas étend le concept à d'autres états pathologiques qui ne devraient pas conduire au décès si une intervention médicale ou une action de santé publique appropriée était donnée à temps.

Sans aucun doute, le choix des maladies sera le sujet de nombreux débats. Néanmoins, la liste finale des affections incluses dans l'atlas résulte d'une discussion approfondie entre les chercheurs qui ont collaboré à ce travail. Les maladies choisies ont été jugées comme adaptées à tous les pays de la Communauté Européenne et reflétant des aspects importants de la délivrance des soins.

L'atlas illustre fort bien les larges variations de la mortalité à l'intérieur de chacun des pays et d'un pays membre à l'autre. Aucune tentative n'a été faite pour interpréter les configurations observées ou pour tirer des conclusions. Ceci est sage, parce que les explications des variations observées sont vraisemblablement complexes et dépendent de nombreux facteurs dont certains échappent au contrôle des services de santé. La fonction de l'atlas est d'indiquer où certains aspects de la délivrance des soins peuvent éventuellement poser problème et où des investigations supplémentaires doivent être entreprises.

Il est à espérer que l'atlas stimulera dans les Etats le déclenchement d'enquêtes sur le fonctionnement des services de santé. Pour y encourager les chercheurs, l'atlas comporte la description de certains secteurs des soins impliqués dans le traitement ou la prévention des maladies individuelles, ainsi que des informations sur l'investissement des services de santé et les conditions sociales. L'atlas ne devrait pas être utilisé pour alimenter 'la chasse aux sorcières' ou pour distribuer des blâmes, mais positivement pour améliorer les services.

Compiler un atlas de cette sorte est une réalisation majeure en elle-même. Les données présentées sont disponibles sous des formes diverses dans chaque pays. Mais établir des statistiques significatives, d'une manière standardisée et comparable, suppose de nombreuses analyses supplémentaires selon des méthodes uniformisées. Cela fut rendu possible grâce à la coopération étroite et permanente de chercheurs, familiers des systèmes de collecte de données de leur pays. Ceci constitue un résultat intéressant du programme de recherche médicale de la Communauté Européenne, et donne un excellent exemple de ce qu'il est possible d'accomplir à partir de données déjà disponibles dans les pays de la Communauté. Il faut féliciter les chercheurs de leur effort de collaboration et des résultats remarquables de leurs recherches. J'espère que cet ouvrage encouragera des recherches ultérieures sur le financement et l'organisation des services de santé dans la CEE, et qu'il ouvrira la voie à une collaboration future des chercheurs sur ce thème à l'intérieur de la Communauté.

Juin 1990
Paolo Fasella
Directeur Général de la Science, la Recherche et le Développement

VORWORT

Die erste Ausgabe des *Atlas der Europäischen Gemeinschaft über 'Vermeidbare Sterbefälle'* wurde 1988 veröffentlicht; er beschrieb die Mortalität an 17 Todesursachen in 10 Ländern für die Jahre 1974–78. Die zweite Ausgabe befasst sich mit der 'vermeidbaren' Mortalität für die Jahre 1980–84, und Änderungen dieser Mortalität zwischen den Zeitspannen 1974–78 und 1980–84. Bei der zweiten Ausgabe sind inzwischen, zu den ursprünglich 10 am Projekt beteiligten Ländern, Spanien und Portugal hinzugestossen.

Das Interesse an Auswertung und Kontrolle des Funktionierens der Gesundheitsdienste nimmt ständig zu. Die Bemühungen richteten sich vor allem auf die Rationalisierung der bedeutenden Menge von gesammelten Daten, in der Absicht, eine Reihe von Massnahmen ergreifen zu können, die die verschiedenen Facetten eines gesamten Gesundheitsversorgungssystems wiederspiegeln. Der Entwicklungsfortschritt von Qualitäts-und Wirksamkeitsindikatoren in der Gesundheitsversorgung, ist hinter den Massnahmen für Verfahren und Leistungsfähigkeit zurückgeblieben. Der Atlas stellt einen wichtigen Abschnitt auf dem Weg zur Findung von national und international gültigen Ergebnisindikatoren, zur Kontrolle der Leistungen des Gesundheitswesens dar.

Es bestehen bereits zahlreiche Atlanten, die detaillierte ökologische Analysen und geographische Abweichungen im Auftreten gewisser Erkrankungen in den einzelnen Ländern, sowie in ganzen Regionen der Welt aufzeigen; bemerkenswert unter diesen sind Atlanten geographischer Abweichungen im Auftreten von Krebserkrankungen. Der hier erarbeitete Atlas über 'Vermeidbare Sterbefälle' ist einzigartig in seinem Versuch, den Gebrauch von Sterblichkeitsdaten systematisch als ein Mittel der Fragestellung über das Ausreichen von Gesundheitsdienstbereitstellung anzusehen.

Mütter-und Säuglingssterblichkeit werden seit langem weltweit als Kriterien der Qualität der Geburtshilfe und der Säuglingspflege akzeptiert. Dieser Atlas dehnt den Begriff auf andere pathologische Zustände aus, bei denen die meisten Todesfälle durch rechtzeitige medizinische Behandlung, oder angemessenes Eingreifen des öffentlichen Gesundheitsdienstes vermieden werden könnten.

Die Auswahl der Krankheiten wird zweifellos Anlass zu heftigen Debatten geben; wie auch immer, die endgültige Liste der in diesem Atlas aufgenommenen Krankheiten ist das Ergebnis eingehender Beratungen unter den Forschern, die an diesem Projekt mitgearbeitet haben. Die Auswahl der Krankheiten wurde als für alle EG-Länder bezeichnend angesehen und scheint wesentliche Aspekte der Gesundheitsversorgung wiederzuspiegeln.

Der Atlas zeigt deutlich, dass in den Sterberaten grosse Unterschiede auftreten, und zwar sowohl innerhalb der einzelnen Länder als auch zwischen ihnen. Es wurde hier nicht versucht, die gefundenen Fakten zu interpretieren oder daraus Schlüsse zu ziehen. Dies ist klug gehandelt, da die Gründe der beobachteten Abweichungen wahrscheinlich komplex sind und von einer Reihe von Faktoren abhängen, die ausserhalb der Kontrolle der Ausstatter der Gesundheitsdienste liegen. Die Aufgabe dieses Atlas ist es, aufzuzeigen, wo gewisse Aspekte der gesundheitlichen Versorgung möglicherweise Probleme aufweisen, und inwiefern weitere Untersuchungen von Nutzen sein könnten.

Es ist zu hoffen, dass der Atlas in den einzelnen Ländern einen Anstoss geben möge, Untersuchungen über das Funktionieren ihrer Gesundheitsversorgung anzuregen. Um die Forscher dabei zu unterstützen, enthält der Atlas Beschreibungen jener Teile des Gesundheitsystems, die mit der Behandlung oder Vorbeugung einzelner Krankheiten zu tun haben, sowie Informationen über Unterschiede in der Ausstattung der Gesundheitsdienste und über soziale Umstände. Keinesfalls soll der Atlas dazu benützt werden, um Diffamierung oder Kritik freien Lauf zu lassen, sondern dazu beitragen, die Gesundheitsdienste konstruktiv zu verbessern.

Einen Atlas dieser Art zusammenzustellen, ist an und für sich schon eine bedeutende Leistung. Die Daten, die hier veröffentlicht werden, sind innerhalb der einzelnen Länder bereits verfügbar; doch setzte das Erstellen bezeichnender Statistiken in standardisierter und vergleichbarer Form, eine bedeutende, in ihrer Art völlig neue Analyse voraus. Diese war aber nur durch enge und ständig verpflichtende Zusammernarbeit einer Anzahl jener Wissenschaftler möglich, die mit dem System von Dateneinbringung der jeweiligen Länder vertraut waren. Er stellt ein wertvolles Ergebnis des medizinischen Forschungsprogrammes der EG dar und gibt ein ausgezeichnetes Beispiel dafür, was unter Ausnützung von verfügbaren Datenquellen der EG-Länder erreicht werden kann.

Den Wissenschaftlern ist zu ihren gemeinschaftlichen Bemühungen und höchst bemerkenswerten Ergebnissen ihrer Forchungsarbeit, zu gratulieren. Ich hoffe, dass dieses Werk ein Anstoss zu weiterer Untersuchungen über die Finanzierung und Organisation des Gesundheitswesens in der EG sein wird, und den Weg für eine zukünftige Zusammenarbeit der Forscher innerhalb der Gemeinschaft auf diesem Gebiet ebnen wird.

Juni 1990
Paolo Fasella
Generaldirektor für Wissenschaft, Forschung und Entwicklung

CONTENTS

Graphs   263

Each set of maps and graphs above are in the following
disease order — disease (age group in years)
Tuberculosis (5–64)
Malignant neoplasm of cervix uteri (15–64)
Malignant neoplasm of cervix and body of uterus (15–54)
Hodgkin's disease (5–64)
Chronic rheumatic heart disease (5–44)
All respiratory diseases (1–14)
Asthma (5–44)
Appendicitis (5–64)
Abdominal hernia (5–64)
Cholelithiasis and cholecystitis (5–64)
Hypertensive and cerebrovascular diseases (35–64)
Maternal mortality (all ages)
Perinatal mortality
All causes (5–64)
All causes (all ages)

9.   **Tables of changes between 1974–78 and 1980–84   267**
Data tables on population, age-specific death rates, observed

numbers of 'avoidable deaths' and age-standardized death
rates for 1974–78 and 1980–84.
Table 9.1.1(a)–(o). Observed numbers of 'avoidable
deaths', crude death rates (per 100 000) and
age-standardized death rates (per 100 000) for 1974–78 and
1980–84 by disease and country.
Table 9.1.2(a). Populations of countries in 1974–78 and
1980–84 by sex and 10 year age groups.
Table 9.1.2(b)–(l). Observed numbers of 'avoidable deaths'
and age-specific death rates (per 100 000) for 1974–78 and
1980–84, and changes in age-specific deaths rates (per 100
000) between 1974–78 and 1980–84 by disease and country.
Table 9.1.3(a)–(c). Age-standardized death rates (per 100
000) for 1974–78 and 1980–84 standardized to the EC
standard, by disease and small area.

LIST OF PARTICIPANTS

Belgium

Dr R. Lagasse, Laboratoire d'Epidémiologie, Université Libre de Bruxelles, Campus Erasme CP 590/5, 808 route de Lennik, 1070 Bruxelles.

Dr P. Hooft, School voor Maatschappelijke Gezondheidszorg, Afdeling Gezondheidsecologie, Katholieke Universiteit Leuven, Kapucynenvoer 35 niv 03, B-3000 Leuven.

Dr P. Humblet, Laboratoire d'Epidémiologie, Université Libre de Bruxelles, Campus Erasme CP 590/5, 808 route de Lennik, 1070 Bruxelles.

Luxembourg

Dr D. Hansen-Koenig, Directeur Général adjoint de la Santé, Direction de la Santé, Division de la Médicine Préventive et Sociale, 22 rue Goethe, 1637 Luxembourg,

Federal Republic of Germany

Dr K. Kern, Ministerium für Umwelt und Gesundheit, Rheinland — Pfalz, Kaiser — Friedrich — Strasse 7, 6500 Mainz.

Dr D. Borgers, Institut für Dokumentation und Information über Sozialmedizin und öffentliches Gesundheitswesen, Westerfeldstrasse 35/37, 4800 Bielfeld 1.

Denmark

Dr K. Juel, Danish Institute for Clinical Epidemiology, 25 Svanemollevej, DK — 2100 Copenhagen.

France

Madame M. H. Bouvier-Colle, INSERM U-149, 16 Av. P. Vaillant-Couturier, 94807 Villejuif Cedex.

Madame le Docteur F. Hatton, Service d'Information sur les Causes Médicales de Décès, 44 Chemin de Rohde, 78110 Le Vésinet.

Mr E. Jougla, Service d'Information sur les Causes Médicales de Décès, 44 Chemin de Rohde-BP 34, 78110 Le Vésinet.

Greece

Professor G. Papaevangelou, Professor of Epidemiology and Medical Statistics, Athens School of Hygiene, 196 Alexandras Avenue, PO Box 14085, 11521 Athens.

Dr C. Tsimbos, Department of Statistics and Actuarial Studies, University of Piraeus, 40 Karaoli and Dimitrion Street, Piraeus — Athens.

Italy

Prof. P. L. Morosini, Laboratorio di Epidemiologia e Biostatistica, Istituto Superiore di Sanita, Viale Regina Elena 299, 00161 Roma.

Dr P. Lauriola, Servizio Igiene Pubblica USL n16, Via Canaletto 15, 41100 Modena.

Dr E. Magliola, Osservatorio Epidemiologico, Regione Lazio, Via Carducci 4, 00187 Roma.

Dr G. Feola, ISTAT, Reparto Statistiche Sanitarie, Viale Liegi 1, 00198 Roma.

Ireland

Dr J. Barry, Department of Health, Hawkin's House, Dublin 2.

The Netherlands

Dr J. P. Mackenbach, Instituut Maatschappelijke Gezondheidszorg, Erasmus Universiteit, PO Box 1738, 3000 DR Rotterdam.

United Kingdom: England, Wales, and Northern Ireland

Project director and members of coordinating team from the Department of Public Health Medicine, United Medical and Dental Schools of Guy's and St Thomas's (UMDS), St Thomas's Hospital, London SE1 7EH.

Project Director: Professor W. W. Holland

Ms M. Aristidou—Statistical Assistant(from August 1984–October 1988)
Mr G. Bevan—Health Economist (from November 1983)
Mr J. Charlton—Statistician (from November 1983–January 1986)
Ms J. Evans—Research Assistant (from February 1986–September 1988)
Mr S. Hartley—Research Assistant (from March 1990)
Dr A. Lakhani—Epidemiologist(from November 1983)

Mr A. McDermott—Statistical Assistant (from January 1989–November 1989)
Ms K. Patel—Statistical Assistant (from October 1988–June 1989)
Ms E. Paul—Statistician (from March 1986–June 1990)
Mr S. Phillips—Assistant Statistician (from January 1990)
Dr C. Summerbell—Research Assistant (from November 1988–November 1989)
Mrs E. Tritton—Research Assistant(from November 1983)

Scotland

Mrs V. Carstairs, Department of Community Medicine, Edinburgh University, Teviot Place, Edinburgh EH8 9AG.

Portugal

Professor Cayolla da Motta, Escola Nacional de Saude Publica, Avenida Padre Cruz, 1699 Lisboa Cedex.

Dr M. L. Sequeira, Departmente de Estudos et Pleneamendo da Saude, Av Alvares Cabral 25–30, 1200 Lisbon.

Spain

Dr M. J. Medrano, Centro Nacional de Epidemiologia, C/ Sinesio Delgado, 6, 28029 Madrid.

Commission of the European Communities

Dr A. Baert, DG XII/F/3, Rue de la Loi 200, B-1049 Brussels, Belgium.

LIST OF MAPS FOR THE PERIOD 1980–84

LIST OF TABLES FOR THE PERIOD 1980–84

LIST OF MAPS OF CHANGES BETWEEN 1974–78 AND 1980–84

LIST OF GRAPHS OF CHANGES BETWEEN 1974–78 AND 1980–84

LIST OF TABLES OF CHANGES BETWEEN 1974–78 AND 1980–84

1. INTRODUCTION

In the absence of health services, mortality would be determined by social, environmental and genetic factors. Health services, through preventive and remedial activities, and governments, through legislative policy, modify the influence of some of these factors, with the objective of reducing mortality. For some diseases medical knowledge is sufficiently advanced to prevent almost all deaths in more resilient age groups. For such deaths to be prevented, however, timely action is necessary and the observation of an appreciable number of deaths suggests that such action is not taken. For example, even though effective means of early detection and effective treatment are available, in the period 1980–84 there were over 5000 deaths from cervical cancer and 1400 from tuberculosis amongst individuals aged 5–64 years in England and Wales, with wide variation between different parts of the country. The sequence of events leading up to 'avoidable' disease, death, or disability of an individual can, however, be complex. For example, a case of diphtheria or poliomyelitis may be the consequence of failure by: a government to introduce the necessary legislation to promote or fund immunization programmes; health service managers to implement such programmes; a doctor to immunize all his or her patients because he/she forgot; the mother to take her baby to a clinic because it is too far away or because of the family's religious views. Diseases may be identified in which health education, immunization practices, continuity of care, surgical care, as well as other particular aspects of the health care system are important in avoiding unnecessary deaths. Geographical comparison of these 'avoidable deaths' should pinpoint areas with particular health care delivery problems. Time series analyses show the effect over time of intervention in these areas. Comparison with areas where action has been effective in reducing mortality may enable other areas to improve their performance.

It is difficult to assess the efficacy of health care services. Defining the outcome of health service intervention is not simple, and there are few relevant data available. An imaginative proposal was put forward in the papers of the Preventable and Manageable Diseases Working Group (Rutstein *et al.* 1976,1980).They propose an apparently practical and inexpensive method of devising outcome measures for Health Services by counting cases of 'unnecessary disease and disability, and unnecessary untimely deaths' as measures of the quality of medical care. Here medical care is defined in its broadest sense, that is prevention, cure and care, including the application of all relevant medical knowledge, the services of all medical and allied personnel, the resources of governmental, voluntary, and social agencies, and the co–operation of the individual himself. An excessive number of such unnecessary events serves as a warning signal of possible shortcomings in the health care system, and should be investigated further.For certain diseases or disabilities even a single event should warrant attention.

This atlas, which examines a selection of unnecessary untimely deaths, is the second publication of the EC Concerted Action Project on Health Services and 'Avoidable Deaths'. It has been prepared by representatives from member countries of the EC (see' List of participants') who all chose to participate. The first atlas describes 'avoidable' mortality in the EC for the years 1974–78. This second atlas describes mortality for the years 1980–84, and changes in mortality between 1974–78 and 1980–84. The time period 1980–84 was chosen because it was the most recent 5-year period for which data were available from every country participating in the study.

A number of conditions and age groups by condition were agreed for which, in general, given modern medical care and other interventions, deaths ought not to occur, although some of these 'avoidable' deaths are bound to occur even under optimal conditions. However, a high mortality in any one of these conditions may serve as an indicator of some inadequacy or reason for investigation.

The aims of the project were:

(1) to produce a set of maps of 'avoidable' deaths from a number of selected conditions for specified age ranges;
(2) to make comparisons between and within the participating countries;
(3) to relate the resulting variation to differing levels or modes of delivery of health service inputs;
(4) to describe changes in 'avoidable' mortality over time.

The English representatives formed the co-ordinating centre based at the United Medical and Dental Schools of Guy's and St Thomas's Hospitals, London. The centre received and analysed data from all participating countries.

The project was financed by the Commission of the European Communities, Directorate-General for Science, Research and Development (XII).

This atlas contains the maps of standardized mortality ratios (SMRs — see definitions section), standardized to the average age-specific mortality rates of both the EC as a whole and the individual country. Data on health inputs and indicators of social conditions, are given. No attempt has been made to allow for these factors when producing the maps themselves. The interpretation of the relationship between health service inputs, indicators of social conditions, and 'avoidable' deaths is complex and requires further research; at this stage we are just making relevant data available to enable appropriate questions to be posed and to make people aware of problems.

1. INTRODUCTION

En l'absence de services de santé, la mortalité serait déterminée par des facteurs sociaux, des facteurs liés à l'environnement, et des facteurs génétiques. En s'efforçant de changer les formes de la mortalité, les services de santé, par le biais d'actions préventives et curatives, et les gouvernements par la règlementation, modifient l'influence de quelques uns de ces facteurs dans le but de réduire la mortalité.

Si un traitement est entrepris à temps, les connaissances médicales sur certaines maladies sont suffisamment avancées pour que la plupart des décès puissent être prévenus, dans les groupes d'âge les plus réceptifs. Néanmoins, pour que de tels décès soient prévenus, une action appropriée doit être menée à temps; l'observation d'un nombre non négligeable de décès suggère qu'une telle action n'a pas été menée. Par exemple, dans la période 1980–84 il y a eu en Angleterre-Galles plus de 5000 décès par cancer du col de l'utérus et 1400 décès par tuberculose parmi les sujets âgés de 5–64 ans, avec de larges variations entre les différentes régions du pays, alors même que les moyens réels d'un dépistage précoce et d'un traitement efficace sont censés être disponibles. La séquence des événements conduisant à la maladie évitable, le décès, ou l'incapacité d'un individu peut être complexe. Par exemple, un cas de diphtérie ou de poliomyélite peut être la conséquence des carences: du gouvernement dans l'introduction de la législation nécessaire à la promotion ou l'instauration des programmes de vaccination; des responsables des services de santé pour mettre en oeuvre ces programmes; d'un médecin n'ayant pas vacciné tous ses patients par oubli; de la mère de famille ne conduisant pas son bébé à la clinique parce que trop éloignée, ou en raison de convictions religieuses. Il est donc possible d'identifier certaines affections, dans lesquelles l'éducation sanitaire, les pratiques vaccinales, la continuité des soins, la chirurgie ainsi que d'autres aspects particuliers du système de soins, sont importants pour éviter les morts inutiles. La comparaison géographique de ces 'morts évitables' devrait permettre de signaler les zones à problèmes, tandis que l'analyse des séries chronologiques devrait indiquer l'effet, à moyen terme, des interventions pratiquées dans ces régions. La comparaison avec les régions où la réduction de la mortalité a pu être effectuée, par une action appropriée, devrait permettre aux autres régions d'améliorer leurs performances.

L'efficacité des services de santé est difficile à évaluer. Les résultats de leurs interventions ne sont pas simples à définir et peu de données sont disponibles. Une autre solution a été imaginée, qui fut proposée dans les articles du Preventable and Manageable Disease Working Group (Rutstein *et al.* 1976, 1980). Ces articles proposaient une méthode apparemment pratique, et peu coûteuse, au problème de l'évaluation des services de santé, en comptant les cas de maladie et incapacité inutiles et les décès inutiles et prématurés pour mesurer la qualité des soins médicaux. Ici, les soins médicaux sont définis au sens large, c'est-à-dire prevention, cure et soins, incluant l'application de toute connaissance médicale appropriée, les services du personnel médical et auxiliaire, les ressources administratives, les actions sociales et volontaires, et la coopération de l'individu lui-même. Un nombre excessif de ces événements, considérés comme inutiles, donnerait l'alerte sur d'éventuelles imperfections du système de santé et devrait conduire à des investigations supplémentaires. Pour certaines maladies ou incapacités, un seul événement justifierait l'attention.

Cet atlas, qui présente une sélection des décès inutiles et prématurés, est la deuxième publication d'une Action Concertée de la Communauté Européenne sur les Services de Santé et les Morts 'Evitables'. Il a été préparé par des représentants des pays membres de la CEE (voir la liste des participants) qui ont tous choisi de collaborer au projet. Le premier atlas décrivait la mortalité 'évitable' dans la Communauté Européenne pour les années 1974–78. Ce second atlas décrit la mortalité des années 1980–84 et les changements intervenus entre 1974–78 et 1980–84. Cette deuxième période a été retenue parce qu'elle réunissait les cinq plus récentes années pour lesquelles les données étaient disponibles dans la plupart des pays participants.

Un certain nombre de conditions pathologiques, et les groupes d'âge les concernant, ont été retenus dans les situations optimales. Compte tenu des capacités de la médecine moderne et des interventions possibles, ces conditions à ces âges ont été considérées comme ne devant pas conduire au décès; même si tous les décès évitables ne peuvent pas être complètement éliminés, la mortalité élevée due à l'une d'entre-elles peut signaler quelque inadéquation ou justifier une investigation particulière.

Les objectifs du project étaient:

(1) produire un ensemble de cartes des 'morts évitables' à partir d'états pathologiques sélectionnés pour des âges spécifiques;
(2) réaliser des comparaisons entre et à l'intérieur des pays participants;
(3) établir un rapport entre la variation des résultats et les services de santé, à différents niveaux, ou modes de délivrance;
(4) décrire les évolutions dans le temps.

Les représentants anglais constituèrent le centre coordinateur installé à l'Ecole de Médecine de Guy's et St Thomas's Hospital à Londres. Le centre reçut et analysa les données statistiques fournies par tous les pays participant au projet. Le projet a été financé par la Commission des Communautés Européennes, Direction Générale des Sciences, de la Recherche et du Développement (XII).

Cet atlas contient les cartes des indices de mortalité relative (SMR voir le chapitre des définitions). L'ajustement de la mortalité a été réalisé d'une part avec les taux spécifiques par âge de la CEE entière, et d'autre part avec ceux de chaque pays. Certaines données relatives aux services de soins, et aux indicateurs sociaux sont également publiées. On n'a pas essayé de tenir compte de ces facteurs en produisant les cartes elles-mêmes car l'interprétation des relations entre l'équipement des services de soins, les indicateurs sociaux, et les morts 'évitables' est complexe et suppose des recherches supplémentaires. A cette étape il s'agit uniquement de fournir des données permettant de se poser les questions appropriées, et d'alerter le lecteur sur les problèmes d'interprétation.

1. EINLEITUNG

Ohne effektive Gesundheitsdienste würde die Mortalität in einer Bevölkerung ausschliesslich durch soziale, andere umweltbezogene und genetische Bedingungen bestimmt sein. Regierungen und Gesundheitsdienste versuchen, durch gesetzliche Massnahmen sowie präventive und kurative Leistungen einige dieser Faktoren positiv zu beeinflussen, mit dem Ziel die Mortalität zu senken. In Bezug auf einige Krankheiten ist das medizinische Wissen weit genug entwickelt, um in den jüngeren Altersgruppen die meisten Sterbefälle vermeiden zu können. Um jedoch solche Sterbefälle zu verhindern ist rechtzeitige Behandlung notwendig; dagegen bedeutet das Auftreten einer nennenswerten Anzahl dieser Sterbefälle, dass solche Hilfe nicht gewährt wurde. So gab es beispielsweise, trotz wirkungsvoller Früherkennungs-und erfolgreicher Behandlungsmethoden, im Zeitraum 1980–84 über 5000 Sterbefälle an Cervix-Karzinom und 1400 Todesfälle an Tuberkulose bei den 5–64 jährigen in England und Wales, mit grossen Unterschieden in Bezug auf verschiedene Landesteile. Die Gründe und die Folge von Ereignissen welche zu einem 'vermeidbaren' Todesfall führen, sind oft komplex; z.B. kann ein Fall von Diphterie oder Poliomyelitis auf folgende Ursachen zurückzuführen sein: eine Regierung, welche es unterlässt, die notwendigen Mittel für Impfprogramme bereitzustellen; die Nachlässigkeit von Gesundheitsdiensten bei der Durchführung; ein Arzt, der es unterliess alle Patienten zu impfen; eine Mutter, die aus Gründen der Entfernung oder religiöser Überzeugung ihr Baby nicht zum Arzt brachte usw.

Für eine Studie sollten Krankheiten ausgewählt werden, für deren Vermeidung z.B. Gesundheitserziehung, Impfprogramme, laufende Versorgung, chirurgische Versorgung oder andere spezielle Dienste relevant sind, um 'vermeidbare' Todesfälle zu verhindern. Geographische Vergleiche in Bezug auf 'vermeidbare' Todesfälle sollten es ermöglichen, Regionen mit besonderen Gesundheitsversorgungsproblemen herauszufinden; zeitbezogene Analysen können den Erfolg von Massnahmen in diesen Regionen überprüfen. Ein Vergleich mit Regionen, in denen Anstrengungen zu einer Verringerung der Mortalität geführt haben, könnte andere befähigen ihre Leistung zu verbessern.

Die tatsächliche Wirksamkeit der medizinischen Versorgung ist schwer einzuschätzen: ihre Ergebnisse sind nicht leicht zu definieren, und sachdienliche Daten stehen wenig zur Verfügung. Ein erfolgversprechender Vorschlag wurde in den Beiträgen der Arbeitsgruppe 'Vermeidbare und heilbare Krankheiten' unterbreitet (Rutstein u. Mitarbeiter 1976, 1980). Sie empfehlen eine offensichtlich praktizierbare und nicht kostspielige Methode zur Messung von Wirksamkeit und Qualität der Gesundheitsversorgung durch Zählen der Fälle von 'vermeidbarer Krankheit und Behinderung, sowie unnötiger und vorzeitiger Todesfälle'. Unter medizinischer Versorgung ist dabei im weitesten Sinne gemeint: Prävention, Heilung und Betreuung, u.a. Anwendung des gesamten medizinischen Wissens, der Dienste aller medizinischen Berufe, der Mittel des Staates sowie der freiwilligen und sozialen Organisationen, einschliesslich der Beteiligung des Individuums. Eine erhöhte Zahl unnötiger Ereignisse ist ein Warnsignal für Defizite des medizinischen Versorgungssystems und sollte

eingehender untersucht werden. Für bestimmte Krankheiten und Behinderungen ist ein einziges Ereignis von Bedeutung.

Dieser Atlas, in dem eine Auswahl unnötiger, unzeitgemässer Sterbfälle dargestellt werden, ist die zweite Publikation des gemeinsamen EG-Projekts über Gesundheitsversorgung und 'vermeidbare' Mortalität. Es wurde von Mitgliedern der Staaten der EG die teilgenommen haben (siehe Teilnehmerliste), vorbereitet. Der erste Atlas beschreibt die 'vermeidbare' Mortalität in der EG für die Jahre 1974–78. Der zweite Atlas stellt die Mortalität für die Jahre 1980–84, und Änderungen zwischen den Zeiträumen 1974–78 und 1980–84 dar. Der Zeitraum 1980–84 wurde ausgewählt, weil für diese 5-Jahresspanne die aktuellsten Daten in allen an der Studie beteiligten Ländern, zur Verfügung standen.

Die Arbeitsgruppe einigte sich auf die Auswahl bestimmter Krankheiten und Altersgruppen. Todesfälle an diesen Krankheiten sollten bei moderner medizinischer Versorgung nicht auftreten, obwohl einige wenige Todesfälle selbst unter optimalen Bedingungen vorkommen können. Eine Häufung von Todesfällen ist aber auf jeden Fall ein Indikator einer inadäquaten Situation und Grund für eine Untersuchung. Die Ziele des Projektes lauteten wie folgt:

(1) Anfertigung eines Atlas von 'vermeidbaren' Sterbefällen in Bezug auf bestimmte Krankheiten und Altersgruppen;
(2) vergleichende Betrachtung zwischen den beteiligten Ländern und ihren Regionen;
(3) Herstellung eines Zusammenhangs zwischen den Abweichungen bei den Todesfällen und Unterschieden in der medizinischen Versorgung;
(4) Änderungen an 'vermeidbarer' Mortalität im Zeitvergleich zu beschreiben.

Die Mitglieder der englischen Arbeitsgruppe bildeten das Koordinierungszentrum an der United Medical and Dental Schools of Guy's and St. Thomas's Hospitals, London. Das Koordinierungszentrum sammelte und analysierte die Daten aller beteiligten Staaten.

Das Projekt wurde durch die Kommission der Europäischen Gemeinschaft, Generaldirektorat für Wissenschaft, Forschung und Entwicklung, finanziert.

Dieser Atlas enthält Karten mit standardisierten Mortalitätsquotienten (SMR, siehe Erläuterungen). Die Standardisierung bezieht sich sowohl auf die durchschnittlichen altersspezifischen Raten der EG, als auch auf die Raten der einzelnen beteiligten Länder. Es werden auch Angaben über Gesundheitsleistungen und soziale Indikatoren zusammengestellt. Es wurde nicht versucht, diese Bedingungen in den Karten zu berücksichtigen. Die Interpretation der Beziehung zwischen Gesundheitsleistungen und Indikatoren der sozialen Lage auf der einen Seite, und 'vermeidbaren' Todesfällen auf der anderen Seite, ist komplex und verlangt weitere Forschung. In diesem Stadium werden zunächst die Daten zur Verfügung gestellt, um auf die Probleme aufmerksam zu machen und entsprechende Fragestellungen zu ermöglichen.

2. METHODS

Selection of indicators for health care outcome

Indicators based on mortality from 17 disease groups are presented in this atlas. These indicators were designed to measure the outcome of primary and secondary prevention and curative aspects of health services on the residents of defined geographical areas. Three of these causes of mortality (lung cancer, cirrhosis of the liver, and motor vehicle accidents), however, may be amenable predominantly to primary prevention at a national level. For the other diseases (tuberculosis, cervical cancer, cancer of the cervix and uterus, Hodgkin's disease, chronic rheumatic heart disease, childhood respiratory disease, asthma, appendicitis, abdominal hernia, cholecystectomy, hypertension and stroke, maternal and perinatal mortality and a group of infectious diseases such as whooping cough), it is reasonably certain that effective treatment or primary or secondary prevention could be provided by health care services. The indicators, which are termed 'avoidable death indicators', are intended to provide warning signals of potential shortcomings in health care delivery, although there may be other explanations. Two uses were envisaged for the indicators in this atlas:

(1) to examine whether there is geographical equity of outcome for specific areas of health service activity;
(2) to provide warning signals to be investigated by local studies, which would aim to identify avoidable factors and other problems so that management of local health services could be improved.

The selection of causes of death to be included as indicators of health care outcome began with a modified list of the 14 disease groups used by Charlton *et al.* in 1983 in their study of geographical variations in England and Wales. This was drawn from the list of 'sentinel health events' compiled by a working party on preventable and manageable disease in the United States, referred to above (Rutstein *et al.* 1980).

At the first workshop of the study a list of disease groups was reviewed by participants from all the EC countries, since different member countries may rank the importance of different diseases in varying orders. After review, 17 disease groups were agreed as indicators of primary and secondary prevention and curative care. The general principles underlying the choice of each disease group were that each should have identifiable effective interventions and health care providers. The tables in Appendix A show, for each of the disease groups selected, the ICD codes, age groups, and diseases included as well as the reasons which led the project team to consider these deaths 'avoidable' (i.e. factors which may contribute to mortality), and the health service and other interventions which could reduce mortality. Important health care providers have been identified and selected and relevant references are quoted. Strict age limits were set for each disease group to enhance the validity of mortality as an indicator of health service outcome. These disease groups were intended to cover a range of different health services. They do not include all conditions for which death is avoidable by medical intervention, nor would every

death from certain of these causes be avoidable, although it is expected that a substantial proportion could be prevented.

Maps and tables were produced to show local geographical variations in mortality from the following: tuberculosis; cervical cancer; Hodgkin's disease; chronic rheumatic heart disease; hypertensive and cerebrovascular disease; childhood respiratory disease; asthma; abdominal hernia; appendicitis; cholelithiasis and cholecystitis; and maternal and perinatal mortality. In addition, tables showing the numbers and rates of death from the infectious diseases in each country are presented.

Owing to problems with certification and coding in certain countries, data for cancer of the cervix and body of uterus were combined. Within the age range 15–54 years almost all deaths thus classified are likely to be from cervical cancer. Maps are presented both for deaths from cervical cancer and for deaths from cancer of the cervix and body of uterus.

For the three primary prevention indicators (lung cancer, cirrhosis of the liver and motor vehicle accidents) tables are presented by country only, since deaths from these diseases are less likely than deaths from the other disease groups, to reflect the outcome of current local health service interventions. The avoidability of these deaths is probably more dependent on national policies and factors outside the direct control of local health services.

The data

The *European Community Atlas of 'Avoidable Death'* for 1974–78 included mortality data from Belgium, Luxembourg, the Federal Republic of Germany, Denmark, France, Greece, Italy, Ireland, the Netherlands, England and Wales, Northern Ireland and Scotland. This atlas, covering the years 1980–84, also includes data from Spain and Portugal.

Mortality data for each country were supplied for the period 1980–84, except for Greece which supplied data for 1980–82, Spain, where the data relate to 1979–83, and Italy, where the data relate to 1979–83. Data on asthma were not available for the administrative areas of Greece or Portugal.

Population data from each country were supplied for the 5-year period 1980–84, with five exceptions: Italy, where the data was for 1979–83; and four countries which were only able to obtain regional population census data for one of the five years. The population data from France is for 1982; that from Greece, Ireland, and Spain relates to 1981. The assumption was made that these data represented the whole period 1980–84 for France, Ireland, and Spain and 1980–82 for Greece.

The data originate from the official agencies, and population data, for example, are based on censuses, using official estimates of changes between censuses if available. The sources are listed in Appendix B. The participants from each country are responsible for the accuracy of their own country's data, which were supplied to the co-ordinating centre classified by age, sex, and administrative area. The aim was to have administrative areas with approximately 500 000 population but, since existing administrative units had to be employed, areas vary in size. There were 451 administrative areas in the EC in 1980–84 for the purposes of this study, whereas in 1974–78 there were 360 areas. The inclusion of Spain and Portugal added another 70 areas. The data from the Federal Republic of Germany for 1974–78 was classified into 11 geographical areas. The population of these areas was disproportionately large (averaging 5 594 000 population). For the 1980–84 study the Federal Republic of Germany was able to provide data classified into 31 areas, with an average population of 1 984 000, closer to the population size of the administrative areas in other EC countries. In the Netherlands one administrative district in 1974–78 was divided into two in 1980–84.

The ninth revision of the International Classification of Diseases (ICD) was introduced in 1979. ICD8 codes were used to classify causes of death in the 1974–78 *EC Atlas of 'Avoidable Death'*; ICD9 codes have been used in the 1980–84 atlas. The possible effect of the change in ICD was examined using OPCS 'bridge coding' results where a 25 per cent sample of the deaths occurring in England and Wales in 1978 was coded according to both ICD8 and ICD9 (Table 2.1). The difference in deaths assigned to particular diseases was less than 10 per cent for each of the 'avoidable' causes except for chronic rheumatic heart disease.

The assumptions about the aetiology of chronic rheumatic heart disease changed between ICD8 and ICD9. In ICD8 it was assumed that diseases of the mitral or aortic valves (393–396) were rheumatic, unless stated to be non-rheumatic or the result of arteriosclerosis or hypertension.In ICD9 the only diseases of mitral or aortic valves assumed to be rheumatic in origin are mitral stenosis or obstruction, mitral disease, and mitral failure where no other indication is given. Other mitral conditions and conditions of the aortic valves are not assumed to be of rheumatic origin. However, if both the mitral and aortic valves are involved, rheumatic origin is assumed.

Death certificates that gave bronchitis, bronchiolitis or emphysema as the underlying causes of death but also mentioned asthma were classified as asthma in ICD9 but not in ICD8. This increased the total number of deaths classified as asthma in all age groups by 28 per cent, with 313 deaths classified as asthma using ICD8 and 401 deaths classified as asthma using ICD9. The difference between the two classifications was greater in the older age groups. In the age range 1–44 years, which includes the asthma deaths considered 'avoidable', the percentage change was 9 per cent. Analysis of SMRs for asthma in England and Wales for each year between 1974 and 1984 showed a continuing increase in mortality over time, even after allowance had been made for the change from ICD8 to ICD9 in 1979 (Burney, Lancet 1986).

Cholelithiasis and cholecystitis were identified by codes 574 and 575 in ICD8. In ICD9 code 576 includes part of code 575 in ICD8, and code 575 is formed from part of 575 and part of 576 in ICD9.

Changes in the crude death rate for each 'avoidable' condition for the whole EC between 1974–78 and 1980–84 are shown in Table 2.2. These differences were greater than the changes attributable to discrepancies in coding between ICD8 and ICD9 for every condition. Apart from asthma, for which mortality increased by 27 per cent, the

Table 2.1. Comparison of the number of deaths coded according to ICD8 and ICD9 in a 25 per cent sample of all deaths in England and Wales in 1978 Codes

	Age Group (years)	ICD codes		Number of deaths		Change (%)
		ICD8	ICD9	ICD8	ICD9	
Tuberculosis	1–64	010–019	010–018, 137	86	84	−2
Malignant neoplasm of cervix uteri	15–64	180	180	277	277	0
Malignant neoplasm of body of uterus	15–64	182	179,182	102	101	−1
Hodgkin's disease	1–64	201	201	124	124	0
Chronic rheumatic heart disease	1–44	393–398	393–398	59	36	−39
All respiratory diseases	1–14	460–519	460–519	64	62	−3
Asthma	1–44	493	493	74	81	+9
Appendicitis	1–64	540–543	540–543	15	16	+7
Abdominal hernia	1–64	550–553	550–553	36	34	−6
Cholelithiasis and cholecystitis	1–64	574–575	574–575.1, 576.1	24	25	+4
Hypertensive disease	45–64	400–404	401–405	292	298	+2
Cerebrovascular disease	45–64	430–438	430–438	1986	2056	+4

Table 2.2. Change in EC death rate per 100 000 between 1974–78 and 1980–84 for 'avoidable' causes of death

	Age Group	ICD Codes		Death rate		Change (%)
		ICD8	ICD9	ICD8	ICD9	
Tuberculosis	5–64	010–019	010–018, 137	2.05	1.08	−47
Malignant neoplasm of cervix uteri	15–64	180	180	4.89	3.83	−22
Malignant neoplasm of cervix and body of uterus	15–54	182	179,182	6.23	4.38	−30
Hodgkin's disease	5–64	201	201	1.25	0.95	−24
Chronic rheumatic heart disease	5–44	393–398	393–398	1.05	0.35	−66
All respiratory diseases	1–14	460–519	460–519	3.01	1.98	−34
Asthma	5–44	493	493	0.50	0.63	27
Appendicitis	5–64	540–543	540–543	0.35	0.14	−59
Abdominal hernia	5–64	550–553	550–553	0.35	0.20	−42
Cholelithiasis and cholecystitis	5–64	574–575	574–575.1, 561.1	0.83	0.35	−58
Hypertension and cerebrovascular disease	35–64	400–404, 430–438	401–405, 430–438	52.47	41.48	−21
Maternal deaths	All	630–678	630–676	20.49	11.74	−43
Perinatal deaths				18.49	12.17	−34
All causes	5–64			316.26	291.50	−8
All causes	1+			1067.19	1054.03	−1

decline in mortality from each 'avoidable' cause ranged from 21 to 67 per cent, while the decline in all-cause mortality was only 2 per cent. This is consistent with the finding of Charlton and Velez (1986) that between 1950 and 1980 mortality from 'avoidable' causes declined faster than all-cause mortality for countries as diverse as the United States, France, Japan, Italy, Sweden, and England and Wales.

The changes in 'avoidable' mortality in the EC attributable to the introduction of ICD9 appear negligible for 10 causes of death, and could not account for the whole of the decrease seen in cholecystitis and chronic rheumatic heart disease or the increase seen in asthma.It has been shown that, in England and Wales at least, there is a continuing increase in asthma deaths that cannot be accounted for by the change in ICD.

Data were also collected for indicators of social conditions and health services inputs. The choice of these was limited, since similar data needed to be available for all countries. The meaning of these will, nevertheless, not be the same between countries, and they should only be used for within-country comparisons.

Analysis and presentation

The atlas is divided into two sections. In the first section the geographical distribution of 'avoidable mortality' over the 451 administrative areas of the EC in 1980–84 is presented in maps and tables. In the second section, changes in 'avoidable' mortality between the time periods 1974–78 and 1980–84 are described. Since Spain and Portugal were not within the EC, they did not provide data for the 1974–78 atlas, and are therefore not included in the analysis of changes over time in the 1980–84 Atlas. The 1980–84 data for the Federal Republic of Germany and for the Netherlands has been aggregated to the 1974–78 boundaries for comparison over time. Thus, the analysis of changes over time is presented for the 360 areas described in the *EC Atlas of 'Avoidable Death'* 1974–78, rather than for the 451 areas described in the first section of this atlas.

Analysis and presentation of data for 1980–84

Since local age- and sex-specific mortality rates would be unreliable due to the small numbers of deaths involved, indirect age standardization (standardized mortality ratios — SMRs) was employed (see Armitage 1971). The two sexes were combined, since we did not consider that the avoidability of death would depend on gender. For malignant neoplasm of the cervix uterus and malignant neoplasm of the cervix and body uterus, the deaths are age-standardized to the female population.

For each disease group and each of the 451 areas included in the study, SMRs were calculated in two different ways:

(1) using the age-specific death rates for the EC as a whole for that disease;

(2) using the age-specific death rates pertaining to the area's own country.

The first method was used to show between-country variation with all data standardized to a common standard (whole EC = 100). The second method was used to show within–country variation (whole country = 100).

Age-standardization was not employed for maternal and perinatal mortality. The EC standard for maternal mortality was taken to be the crude death rate per 100 000 births for the whole EC. The EC standard for perinatal mortality was the crude perinatal death rate per 1000 births. For between-country comparisons the SMR for each administrative area was calculated as the ratio of the crude rate for that area to the crude rate for the whole EC, multiplied by 100. For within-country comparisons of maternal and perinatal mortality the standard used was the crude death rate for that country. The SMR for an administrative area of that country was then the crude rate for that area divided by the crude rate for the country, multiplied by 100.

The following statistical tests were carried out on the resulting SMRs to examine:

(1) whether SMRs validly describe the data;

(2) whether the degree of heterogeneity between different areas is greater than could be expected by chance;

(3) for each area, whether the SMR is significantly higher than 100 (the standard).

Tests (1) and (2) above are chi-squared tests as described by Gail (1978). Test (3) is as described in Armitage (1971): a one-sided test was chosen because we are only interested in highlighting excess mortality, since the ideal is to have no deaths, or very few. Test (1) examines whether the death ratios (local/EC and local/national) for the different age groups are similar, this being a necessary requirement for the SMR to validly describe the data. For no cause of 'avoidable' mortality was there evidence of SMRs being inappropriate. For perinatal and maternal mortality the appropriate rates were calculated (perinatal: rate per 1000 births; maternal: rate per 100 000 births). Test (2) was also carried out on these, and they were also tested for whether they were significantly greater than national and EC standard rates for the appropriate period.

The SMRs for 1980–84 are not directly comparable with those for 1974–78, in that an SMR of 100 in 1980–84 does not imply the same level of mortality as an SMR of 100 in 1974–78, because the age-specific mortality rates on which the SMRs are based differ for the two time periods. The age-specific mortality rates for the countries included in the 1974–78 atlas changed between the two time periods, decreasing for all diseases except asthma, where they increased. Further, the addition of two new countries, Spain and Portugal, to the 1980–84 atlas changes the EC standard reducing the age-specific death rates for diseases where mortality is low in Spain and Portugal, and increasing it for diseases where mortality is high.

Maps

A large map of Europe (Miller oblated stereographic projection) was divided into sections. This was distributed to participating centres, where administrative boundaries were drawn on to the maps, which were then returned to the co-ordinating centre. The boundaries were then digitized (converted into a series of latitude and longitude co-ordinates) in a form suitable for the INFOMAP computer mapping package (Claymore Services Ltd 1988).

Two sets of maps produced in this way were designed to show up different aspects of mortality variations. Six shading intervals were used for all maps. The two methods of allocating areas to intervals are described below. Histograms showing the distribution of SMRs are shown on each map.

Whole EC, sextile intervals

These maps are intended to show between-country variations. They show the rankings of areas when mortality is compared with a common EC standard. Mortality data for each area were age-standardized using the age-specific death rates of the EC as a whole (SMR for whole EC = 100), and these SMRs were then placed in rank order. One-sixth of the areas are placed in each shading interval.

The sextiles are indicated on the maps by the following colours:

Top sextile (highest mortality)	1	Red
	2	Dark-Orange
	3	Light-Orange
	4	Yellow
	5	Light-Green
Bottom sextile (lowest mortality)	6	Dark-Green

The maps of perinatal and maternal mortality show the distribution of the maternal and perinatal SMRs. In the *EC Atlas of 'Avoidable Death'* for 1974–78 the maps illustrate the crude death rates. The crude rate would produce the same shading on the map as the SMRs because the SMR for each small area is its crude death rate divided by a constant (the EC crude rate). Thus the 1974–78 and 1980–84 EC maps of maternal and perinatal mortality use comparable shading. However, using the SMR rather than the crude rate to describe the intervals employed in shading gives a measure which is consistent with the measures used in mapping the other diseases.

The 1974–78 atlas included both maps of the EC based on sextile shading and maps where shading was based on the magnitude of SMRs, rather than their ranks described as 'middle intervals equal'. Maps using 'middle intervals equal' shading have not been included in the 1980–84 atlas.

On each map of the EC a histogram of frequencies of the SMRs is included to illustrate the amount of variability in the SMRs across small areas of the EC for mortality from the cause of death mapped. The histograms are based on a grouping interval of 20. The same grouping interval is used for every histogram, to provide a common scale on which variability of SMRs for different disease groups can be compared. The histogram intervals are different from the SMR ranges used in shading the maps.

Individual countries, sextile intervals

These maps are intended to show within-country variations in mortality, and separate maps have been produced for each country. Between-country comparisons of mortality levels should not be made using these maps. Here the mortality data for each area have been standardized to the age-specific death rates of the country to which they belong (SMR for whole country = 100), so the SMR for a small area indicates the extent to which that area differs from the country as a whole. It was important that for each disease a common yardstick should be employed to show variation within the different countries, so the 451 small-area SMRs based on national standards were ranked and divided into sextiles to create the shading intervals. The shading based on standardization using national rates illustrates the extent to which mortality in a small area differs from the average mortality in its own country, compared with the extent to which other small areas in the EC differ from the average mortality in their countries.

The shading of the individual country maps in the 1980–84 atlas is based on sextile groupings, while the shading on the individual country maps in the 1974–78 atlas was based on the magnitude of the SMRs rather than their ranks. The maps of individual countries in the two atlases are therefore not comparable. A histogram of the frequencies of the SMRs based on a grouping interval of 20 is presented on each map. They show in grey the distribution of small-area SMRs based on national standards for the 451 areas of the whole EC, and in black the distribution of SMRs for the country in the map. The histogram intervals are different from the SMR ranges used in shading the maps.

Tables

Tables showing the mortality indicators (standardized both to the EC and to the individual country) and whether they significantly exceed 100 (the SMR for the standard population) are given for each area of each country in Chapter 7 p.153. Whether an SMR for an area differs significantly from the standard, depends not only on the size of the SMR but also on the population size of the area and the overall mortality rate for the particular disease (both of which contribute to the 'expected' number of deaths in an area). The same SMR value in two areas which differ greatly in population size, may be significantly different from the standard in the area with the larger population, but not in the area with the smaller population. Also shown in tabular form are the actual numbers of deaths from each cause and the populations of each area.

Tables are also given showing indicators of social conditions and health service inputs. Since these data are not strictly comparable between countries, between-country variations should be treated with great caution.

Changes in 'avoidable' mortality between 1974–78 and 1980–84

To make comparisons between levels of 'avoidable' mortality in 1974–78 and in 1980–84, the mortality and population data must relate to the same geographical areas. There were 451 administrative areas in the EC in 1980–84 for the purposes of this study, but only 360 in 1974–78. For comparisons over time the data for 1980–84 have therefore been aggregated to the countries and boundaries used in 1974–78. The area boundaries used for comparison of mortality between 1974–78 and 1980–84 are the 360 areas described in the 1974–1978 atlas.

Maps

The shading in the maps of change is based on the ranks of the SMRs in the two time periods. Overall mortality rates have fallen for every disease except asthma. The shading indicates change in mortality relative to other areas in the EC, rather than absolute change. The SMRs used to describe mortality for 1974–78 are based on the EC standard used in the 1974–78 atlas. The SMRs used to describe mortality in 1980–84 are based on the EC 1980–84 age-specific rates calculated, excluding Spain and Portugal (this differs from the EC standard including Spain and Portugal). In each time period, areas with SMRs in the top two sextiles were rated as high in that time period, those in the middle two sextiles were rated as medium, and those in the bottom two sextiles rated as low. The shading scales for the maps of change between 1974–78 and 1980–84 were defined as follows:

1. Improved: changed from high (in top third) in 1974–78 to medium (middle third) or low (bottom third) in 1980–84 or changed from medium in 1974–78 to low in 1980–84.
2. Low–Low: low in 1974–78, low in 1980–84.
3. Medium–medium: medium in 1974–78, medium in 1980–84.
4. High–high: high in 1974–78, high in 1980–84.
5. Deteriorated: changed from low in 1974–78 to medium or high in 1980–84 or changed from medium in 1974–78 to high in 1980–84.

Figure 2.1 illustrates the shading areas for Hodgkin's disease in graphical form. In the maps representing change over time between 1974–78 and 1980–84 areas which deteriorated are shaded black, those which improved shaded white.

Spain and Portugal are not included in the analysis. In the Federal Republic of Germany and in the Netherlands the 1980–84 administrative areas have been aggregated to the 1974–78 areas. Greece is omitted from the analysis and maps of maternal and perinatal mortality (because data were not available for 1974–78) and of asthma (because data were not available for 1980–84).

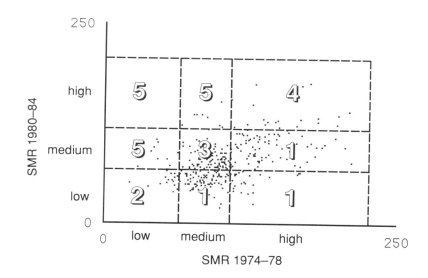

Figure 2.1. Shading method for maps of changes over time; Hodgkin's disease.

Tables

Changes in avoidable mortality at national level are shown in Tables 9.1.1 p.269 and 9.1.2 p.275.

The overall change in national 'avoidable' mortality is shown in Table 9.1.1. This gives the numbers of deaths, crude death rate and age-standardized death rate for each disease in each country for 1974–78 and for 1980–1984. The age-standardized death rate is taken to be the SMR (standardized to the EC rate) for the country, multiplied by the EC crude death rate for that time period. In the EC as a whole there has been a decrease in mortality from every cause of death studied, except for asthma where mortality has increased. National changes in mortality in different age-groups are shown in Table 9.1.2(b)–(l). The number of observed deaths and age-specific death rates and the change in age-specific death rates between the two time periods are given for each disease in each country. The pattern of change for most diseases is of a decrease in mortality in all age groups in all countries. The exceptions to this are asthma, where mortality has increased in most age-groups in most countries, and cervical cancer where there have been increases and decreases in different age-groups in different countries. Data on population changes in different age-groups are shown in Table 9.1.2(b).

Changes in avoidable mortality in the administrative areas of the EC are given in Table 9.1.3 (p.310). For each small area the age-standardized mortality rate for 1974–78 and for 1980–84 is shown, together with an indication of whether this is significantly high compared to the EC standard for that time period (the significance test is based on the SMR).

The age-standardized mortality rate is taken to be the SMR multiplied by the EC crude death rate. Mortality in the EC was lower in 1980–84 than in 1974–78 for each 'avoidable' cause of death except asthma. Since rates in 1980–84 are compared with a lower EC standard than rates in 1974–78, an area may have a significantly high rate in 1980–84 and a rate that is not significantly high in 1974–78, even if the actual rate is higher in 1974–78.

Graphs

The graphs plot the SMRs for 1980–84 against the SMRs for 1974–78. The SMRs are in both cases based on the EC standard for 1974–78. The graphs illustrate the extent to which areas changed relative to other areas in the EC in the two time periods.

2. METHODES

Selection des indicateurs d'évaluation des soins

Les indicateurs présentés dans cet atlas reposent sur la mortalité due à dix-sept groupes de causes. Ils ont été choisis dans le but de mesurer les résultats des services curatifs ou de prévention dans la population des zones géographiques considérées. Trois de ces causes de mortalité (cancer du poumon, cirrhose du foie, et accidents de la circulation) peuvent néanmoins être amendées au niveau national par la prévention primaire. En ce qui concerne les autres affections (tuberculose, cancers du col et du corps de l'utérus, maladie de Hodgkin, cardiopathies rhumatismales chroniques, affections respiratoires de l'enfance, asthme, appendicite, hernie, lithiase biliaire et cholécystite, hypertension et maladies vasculaires cérébrales, mortalité maternelle, mortalité périnatale, et un regroupement de maladies infectieuses telles que coqueluche etc ...) il est raisonnable de considérer qu'elles pourraient être soit prévenues (primitivement ou secondairement), soit traitées par les services de soins. Les indicateurs qui sont appelés 'indicateurs de morts évitables' sont censés donner l'alerte en cas d'insuffisances dans la délivrance des soins, même si d'autres explications sont possibles. Deux utilisations de ces indicateurs ont été envisagées dans l'atlas:

(1) examiner si géographiquement les résultats d'activité des services de santé sont égaux;
(2) fournir des signaux d'alarme qui encouragent les investigations dont l'objectif serait d'identifier les facteurs évitables et les autres problèmes au niveau local, de manière à ce que l'organisation des services de santé locaux soit améliorée.

La sélection des causes de décès, à inclure dans l'évaluation des services de soins, a commencé par la liste des quatorze groupements de maladies utilisés par Charlton *et al.* en 1983 dans leur étude des variations géographiques de l'Angleterre. Celle-ci était issue de la liste des 'événements sentinelles', compilée par un groupe de travail sur les maladies à prévenir et à traiter, aux Etats Unis (Rutstein *et al.* 1980).

A la première réunion du groupe de travail, une liste des causes fut examinée par tous les participants de la Communauté, bien que les membres des différents pays aient estimé diversement l'importance des différentes affections. Après examen, dix-sept groupes de maladies furent retenus comme indicateurs de la prévention primaire, de la prévention secondaire, et des soins curatifs. Le choix, des maladies qui a été fait, repose sur deux principes généraux: des interventions connues et efficaces sont applicables à chaque affection, et des soins appropriés peuvent être dispensés. Les tableaux de l'annexe A présentent, pour chacun des groupes d'affections sélectionnées, les codes de la Classification Internationale des Maladies, les groupes d'âge et les causes incluses ainsi que les raisons qui ont conduit le groupe d'étude à considérer ces décès comme 'évitables' (c'est-à-dire les facteurs qui contribuent éventuellement à la mortalité), et les services de soins et les autres interventions qui pourraient réduire la mortalité. Les dispensateurs principaux des soins ont été répertoriés et

les références les concernant sont indiquées. Des limites strictes d'âge furent arrêtées pour chaque catégorie d'affection en tant qu'indicateur de résultat des services médicaux. Ces groupes d'affections devaient couvrir la variété des différents services de santé. Ils n'incluent pas toutes les conditions où l'intervention médicale peut éviter le décès, pas plus que chaque décès dû à ces causes ne peut être considéré comme totalement évitable; toutefois, on escompte qu'une proportion substantielle pourrait être prévenue.

Des cartes et des tableaux furent réalisés afin de montrer les variations géographiques de la mortalité par les affections suivantes: tuberculose, cancer du col, maladie de Hodgkin, rhumatisme articulaire chronique, maladies hypertensive et cérébrovasculaire, maladies respiratoires de l'enfance, asthme, hernie abdominale, appendicite, cholélithiase et cholécystite, mortalité maternelle et périnatale. En outre, sont présentés des tableaux qui procurent le nombre de décès et les taux de mortalité par maladies infectieuses, dans chaque pays.

En raison des problèmes de déclaration et de codage, qui existent dans certains pays, les données sur les cancers du col et du corps de l'utérus furent réunies pour les groupes d'âge 15 à 54 ans. A l'intérieur de ce groupe d'âge, la plupart des décès ainsi classés sont probablement des cancers du col. Toutefois les cartes présentent soit les décès par cancer cervical, soit les décès par cancer cervical et cancer de l'utérus réunis.

Les trois indicateurs de prévention primaire (cancer du poumon, cirrhose du foie et accidents de la circulation routière) sont présentés par pays, seulement sous forme de tableaux, car les décès dûs à ces affections reflètent moins certainement que les autres maladies l'efficacité des services de soins locaux. La disparition de ces décès dépend probablement davantage des politiques nationales de santé et de facteurs exogènes aux services de santé locaux, (voir HATTON *et al.* 1981 sur les accidents de la route).

Données

L'Atlas Européen des Décès Evitables de 1974–78 incluait les données de mortalité de la Belgique, le Luxembourg, la République Fédérale d'Allemagne, le Danemark, la France, la Grèce, l'Italie, la République d'Irlande, les Pays-Bas, l'Angleterre, le Pays de Galles, l'Irlande du Nord, et l'Ecosse. Cet atlas ci, couvrant la période 1980–84, inclut en outre les données de l'Espagne et du Portugal.

Les données de mortalité furent fournies pour la période 1980–84 par chaque pays, exceptés la Grèce qui a fourni les données de 1980–82, l'Espagne et l'Italie celles de 1979–83. Les données sur l'asthme n'étaient pas disponibles par région administrative ni en Grèce ni au Portugal.

Les données de population furent fournies par chaque pays, pour les cinq années 1980–84 avec les exceptions suivantes: en Italie les données sont celles de 1979–83 ; dans quatre pays les données de la population sont disponibles par région seulement l'année de recensement. Les données de population de la France sont celles du recensement de 1982, et les données de population de la Grèce, l'Irlande, et l'Espagne sont celles du recensement de 1981. En France, Irlande, et Espagne, il a été considéré que ces données sont représentatives de la totalité de la période 1980, et en Grèce de la période 1980–82. Dans tous les pays les données proviennent des organismes officiels et la population est fondée sur les recensements, utilisant, le cas échéant, les estimations intercensitaires officielles. Les sources des données sont répertoriées dans l'annexe B.

Les participants de chaque pays sont responsables pour leur propre pays de la validité des données qui ont été fournies au centre coordonnateur, regroupées par sexe, âge, et région administrative (de résidence en France). L'objectif était de considérer des régions administratives comprenant environ 500 000 habitants mais comme il s'agissait d'utiliser les circonscriptions administratives existantes, la taille des régions varie néanmoins.

Dans le cadre de cette étude, la Communaué Européene compte 451 régions administratives en 1980–84, au lieu de 360 régions en 1974–78. L'inclusion de l'Espagne et du Portugal a ajouté 70 autres régions. En 1974-78, les données de la République Fédérale d'Allemagne étaient classées en onze régions géographiques. La population de ces zones était disproportionnée (en moyenne 5 594 000 habitants). Pour l'étude de 1980–84, la République Fédérale d'Allemagne a pu fournir les données selon 31 zones, comportant en moyenne 1 984 000 habitants, donc plus proches de la taille des populations des autres zones administratives des pays de la CEE. Enfin aux Pays-Bas, un district administratif de 1974–78 a été partagé en deux en 1980–84.

La 9ème révision de la Classification International des Maladies (CIM) fut introduite en 1979. Les causes de *l'Atlas Européen des Morts Evitables* de 1974–78 étaient classées avec la 8éme révision de la CIM. En 1980–84, elles le sont avec la 9ème révision. L'effet possible du changement de classification a été analysé à partir des résultats de la table de correspondance établie par L'Office of Population, Censuses and Surveys (OPCS). Un échantillon de 25 pour cent des décès, survenus en Angleterre-Galles en 1978, furent codés en fonction de la 8ème et en fonction de la 9ème (Tableau 2.1) La différence dans les décès assignés à telle ou telle rubrique était inférieure à 10 pour cent pour chacune des causes 'evitables', exception faite des cardiopathies rhumatismales chroniques.

En effet les hypothèses faites sur l'étiologie des cardiopathies rhumatismales chroniques ont changé entre les 8ème et 9ème révisions de la CIM. Dans la 8ème il était supposé que les maladies des valvules mitrales et aortiques (393–397) étaient d'origine rhumatismale, sauf si elles étaient spécifiées non-rhumatismales ou dues à l'artériosclérose ou à l'hypertension. Dans la 9ème révision les seules maladies des valvules mitrales aortiques considérées d'origine rhumatismale sont la sténose ou l'obstruction mitrale, les maladies et défaillances mitrales sans autre indication, les autres affections mitrales sans autre indication (394). Les autres affections mitrales et des valvules aortiques ne sont pas considérées d'origine rhumatismale si elles ne sont pas précisées spécifiquement d'origine rhumatismale. En revanche si les deux valvules mitrales et aortiques sont concernées, l'origine rhumatismale est considérée (396).

Les certificats de décès, qui comportent bronchite, bronchiolite, ou

Tableau 2.1. Comparaison du nombre des décès en fonction des codes de la CIM-8 et de la CIM-9, d'après un échantillon, au quart, de tous les décès de 1978 en Angleterre–Galles

	Group d'âge (ans)	Codes de la CIM		Nombre de décès		Changement en%
		CIM-8	CIM-9	CIM-8	CIM-9	
Tuberculose	1–64	010–019	010–018, 137	86	84	-2
Tumeur maligne du col de l'utérus	15–64	180	180	277	277	0
Tumeur maligne du corps de l'utérus	15–64	182	179, 182	102	101	−1
Maladie de Hodgkin	1–64	201	201	124	124	0
Cardiopathies rhumatismales chroniques	1–44	393–398	393–398	59	36	−39
Maladies de l'appareil respiratoire	1–14	460–519	460–519	64	62	−3
Asthme	1–44	493	493	74	81	+9
Appendicite	1–64	540–543	540–543	15	16	+7
Hernie abdominale	1–64	550–553	550–553	36	34	-6
Cholélithiase et cholécystite	1–64	574–575	574–575.1, 576.1	24	25	+4
Maladies hypertensives	45–64	400–404	401–405	292	298	+2
Maladies vasculaires cérébrales	45–64	430–438	430–438	2056	+4	1986

Tableau 2.2. Taux pour 100 000 et évolution de la mortalité européenne due à des causes 'évitables' entre 1974–78 et 1980–84

	Group d'âge (ans)	Codes de la CIM		Taux p. 100 000		Changement en %
		CIM-8	CIM-9	CIM-8	CIM-9	
Tuberculose	5–64	010–019	010–018, 137	2.05	1.08	–47
Tumeur maligne du col de l'utérus	15–64	180	180	4.89	3.83	–22
Tumeur maligne du corps de l'utérus	15–54	182	179, 182	6.23	4.38	–30
Maladie de Hodgkin	5–64	201	201	1.25	0.95	–24
Cardiopathies rhumatismales chroniques	5–44	393–398	393–398	1.05	0.35	–66
Maladies de l'appareil respiratoire	1–14	460–519	460–519	3.01	1.98	–34
Asthme	5–44	493	493	0.50	0.63	27
Appendicite	5–64	540–543	540–543	0.35	0.14	–59
Hernie abdominale	5–64	550–553	550–553	0.35	0.20	–42
Cholélithiase et cholécystite	5–64	574–575	574–575.1, 576.1	0.83	0.35	–58
Maladies hypertensives et maladies vasculaires cérébrales	35–64	400–404, 430–438	401–405, 430–438	52.47	41.48	–21
Mortalité maternelle	Toutes	630–678	630–676	20.49	11.74	–43
Mortalité périnatale				18.49	12.17	–34
Toutes causes	5–64			316.26	291.50	–8
Toutes causes	1+			1067.19	1054.03	–1

emphysème en cause initiale du décès, tout en mentionnant l'asthme, sont classés à l'asthme avec la 9ème mais pas avec la 8ème. Ceci a augmenté le nombre total des décès dus à l'asthme d'environ 28 pour cent dans tous les groupes d'âge, avec 313 décès dans la 8ème révision et 401 dans la 9ème révision. La différence entre les deux classifications était plus grande dans les groupes d'âge élevés. Dans le groupe 1–44 ans, qui contient les décès par asthme considérés comme 'évitables', le pourcentage de changement était de 9 pour cent. L'analyse des indices de mortalité relative par asthme en Angleterre–Galles, pour chaque année entre 1974 et 1984 montrait un accroissement constant, de la mortalité années, au courses des après qu'il ait été tenu compte du changement en 1979, de la CIM-8 à la CIM-9 (Burney-Lancet).

La cholélithiase et la cholécystite étaient classées sous les rubriques 574 et 575 dans la 8ème révision. Dans la 9ème révision, la rubrique 575 correspond à une partie de la rubrique 575 et une partie de la rubrique 576 de la 8ème révision; la rubrique 576 de la 9ème est formée de l'autre partie de la rubrique 575 de la 8ème.

Les changements des taux bruts de mortalité, pour chaque affection 'évitable', dans l'ensemble de la Communauté Européenne, entre 1974–78 et 1980–84, sont présentés sur le Tableau 2.2. Ces différences sont supérieures aux changements attribuables aux modifications intervenues dans le classement des causes entre la 8ème et la 9ème

révision de la CIM. Exception faite de l'asthme, où la mortalité a augmenté de 27 pour cent, le déclin de la mortalité due aux causes 'évitables' varie de 21 à 67 pour cent, tandis que la diminution de la mortalité totale a été de 2 pour cent seulement. Ceci corrobore les résultats de Charlton et Velez (1986) qui montrent qu'entre 1950 et 1980 la mortalité due aux causes 'évitables' a diminué plus vite que la totalité des causes, dans des pays aussi variés que les Etats-Unis, la France, le Japon, l'Italie, la Suède, et l'Angleterre–Galles.

Les changements intervenus dans la mortalité 'évitable' de la Communauté Européenne, et attribuables à l'introduction de la 9ème révision de la CIM, paraissent négligeables pour 10 causes de décès, et pourraient ne pas rendre compte en totalité de la décroissance observée dans les cholécystites et les cardiopathies rhumatismales chroniques, ni de l'augmentation observée pour l'asthme.

En Angleterre–Galles au moins, il a été démontré qu'une augmentation constante des décès par asthme ne peut être attribuée au changement de classification.

Les statistiques régionales de condition sociale et du système de santé furent également collectées. Le choix en a été limité car il manque des données comparables d'un pays à l'autre. En outre, la signification de ces données ne sera pas exactement la même et celles-ci doivent être utilisées surtout dans les comparaisons internes aux pays.

Analyse et présentation

L'atlas comporte deux sections. Dans la première, la distribution géographique de la mortalité 'évitable' parmi les 451 zones administratives de la Communauté Européenne, en 1980–84, est présentée sous forme de cartes et tableaux. Dans la seconde, sont décrites les évolutions entre 1974–78 et 1980–84 de la mortalité 'évitable'. Comme l'Espagne et le Portugal n'appartenaient pas à la Communauté Européenne, ces pays n'avaient pas fourni les données pour l'atlas de 1974–78, et ne sont donc pas inclus dans l'analyse des évolutions temporelles du second atlas. Pour ces comparaisons dans le temps, les données de 1980–84 de la République Fédérale d'Allemagne et des Pays-Bas ont été regroupées en fonction des limites régionales de 1974–78. Ainsi les évolutions temporelles sont présentées pour les 360 zones décrites dans l'Atlas Européen de 1974–78 et non, pour les 451 zones décrites dans le présent atlas.

Analyse et présentation des données de 1980–84

En raison du petit nombre de décès inclus, les taux spécifiques de mortalité par sexe et âge, au niveau local auraient été peu fiables. Une standardisation indirecte par âge a donc été employée (indice de mortalité relative, SMR, voir Armitage 1971 et Rumeau-Rouquette 1984). Les deux sexes ont été combinés puisqu'on considère que le caractère évitable des décès ne dépend pas du sexe. Dans les cancers du col de l'utérus et les cancers de l'utérus en général, les nombres de décès sont ajustés en fonction de la seule population féminine.

Pour chaque groupe de maladies des 451 régions incluses dans l'étude, les indices de mortalité relative ont été calculés de deux manières différentes:

(1) en utilisant les taux spécifiques par âge et par cause de la Communauté Européenne considérée comme un tout;
(2) en utilisant pour ses régions les taux spécifiques propres à chaque pays.

La première méthode fut employée pour montrer les variations entre pays par rapport à une référence commune (la CEE dans son ensemble = 100). La deuxième méthode était utilisée pour montrer les variations régionales internes à chaque pays (par rapport à sa norme nationale).

Il n'y a pas de standardisation par âge pour les mortalités maternelles et périnatales. La mortalité maternelle utilisée comme référence (mortalité type) est le taux brut de décès pour 100 000 naissances dans l'Europe Communautaire tout entière. La mortalité périnatale utilisée comme référence est le taux brut de mortalité périnatale pour 1000 naissances de la CEE. Pour comparer les pays entre eux, des indices comparatifs de mortalité ont été calculés : rapport du taux de la zone au taux de la Communauté Européenne × 100. Pour comparer les mortalités maternelles et périnatales dans les régions, à l'interieur d'un même pays, la référence utilisée a été le taux national de chaque pays, ainsi l'indice comparatif de mortalité d'une région de ce pays est le taux de cette région divisé par le taux national, multiplié par 100.

Des tests statistiques furent réalisés sur les indices de mortalité relative pour vérifier:

(1) si les indices décrivaient valablement les données;
(2) si le degré d'hétérogénéité entre les différentes régions était plus grand que celui dû au hasard;
(3) si l'indice était significativement plus élevé que 100 (la référence) dans chaque région.

Les tests (1) et (2), ci-dessus, sont des tests de chi deux décrits par Gail (1978). Le test (3) est décrit par Armitage (1971): un test unilatéral a été retenu en raison de la volonté de souligner l'excès de mortalité seulement puisque l'idéal serait de n'avoir aucun décès ou très peu. Le test (1) examine si les rapports de mortalité (local/Communauté Européenne et local/national) dans les différents groupes d'âge sont identiques, ceci étant une condition nécessaire pour que l'indice décrive valablement les données. Aucune cause de mort 'évitable' ne s'est montrée significativement inappropriée à l'utilisation de l'indice comparatif de mortalité. Des taux spécifiques furent calculés pour la motalité périnatale (taux pour 1000 naissances) et la mortalité maternelle (taux pour 100 000 naissances). Le test (2) a été appliqué également à ces taux et de même on a vérifié s'ils étaient significativement supérieurs aux taux standardisés de la Communauté durant la période considérée.

Les indices de mortalité relative (SMR) de 1980–84 ne sont pas directement comparables avec ceux de 1974–78 : un SMR de 100 en 1980–84 n'implique pas le même niveau de mortalité qu'un SMR de 100 en 1974–78, car les taux spécifiques de mortalité par âge, sur lesquels sont fondés les SMR, diffèrent d'une période à l'autre. Les taux spécifiques de mortalité par âge, des pays inclus dans l'atlas de 1974–78 ont changé entre les deux époques, diminuant pour toutes les affections, excepté l'asthme. En outre l'addition de deux pays, Espagne et Portugal, pour l'atlas de 1980–84 a modifié les références européennes, en réduisant les taux spécifiques de mortalité par âge, des affections où la mortalité est faible en Espagne et Portugal, et en les accroissant pour les affections où la mortalité y est élevée.

Cartes

Une grande carte d'Europe (projection Miller) fut divisée en sections, distribuée aux centres participants qui y portèrent les limites administratives avant de les réexpédier au centre coordinateur. Les limites furent alors converties (transformées) en coordonnées longitudinales et de latitude adaptées au système de cartographie automatique INFOMAP (Claymore Services Ltd 1988).

Deux ensembles de cartes ont été réalisés qui montrent différents aspects des variations de la mortalité. Six classes furent utilisées pour toutes les cartes, et deux méthodes de distribution des zones par classe sont décrits ci-dessous. Des histogrammes, montrant la distribution des indices comparatifs de mortalité, figurent sur chaque carte.

Ensemble Communautaire: répartition par sextile
Ces cartes doivent illustrer les variations entre les pays. Elles montrent le classement des régions quand la mortalité est comparée à une référence européenne commune. Les données de mortalité de chaque région furent standardisées par âge, à partir des taux spécifiques par âge de la Communauté toute entière (indice de mortalité relative pour la CEE dans son ensemble = 100) et ces indices furent ordonnés. Un sixième des régions fut placé dans chaque classe.

Les classes, en sextiles, sont indiquées sur les cartes par les couleurs suivantes:

Sextile supérieur (mortalité la plus élevée)	1	Rouge
	2	Orange-Foncé
	3	Orange-Clair
	4	Jaune
	5	Vert-Clair
Sextile inférieur (mortalité la plus faible)	6	Vert-Foncé

Les cartes de mortalité maternelle et périnatale montrent la distribution des indices comparatifs des mortalités maternelle et périnatale. Dans *l'Atlas Européen de la Mortalité 'Evitable'* de 1974–78 les cartes illustraient les taux bruts. La cartographie des taux bruts produirait les mêmes zonages que ceux obtenus par la cartographie des indices, car dans chaque zone l'indice est son taux divisé par une constante, le taux européen. En outre, les cartes de 1974–78 et 1980–84 de mortalité maternelle et périnatale utilisent des légendes comparables. Toutefois, utiliser les indices plutôt que les taux pour décrire les différences de mortalité conduit à réaliser une cartographie qui devient cohérente avec la cartographie des autres affections.

L'atlas de 1974–78 incluait à la fois des cartes de la Communauté Européenne fondées sur les classes en sextile, et des cartes qui étaient établies sur la base des écarts des indices comparatifs de mortalité — ou classes d'amplitude égale — plutôt que sur leur range. Les cartes avec classes d'amplitude égale n'ont plus été incluses dans cet atlas.

Sur chaque carte de la Communauté Européenne, l'histogramme des fréquences des indices comparatifs de mortalité est reproduit pour illustrer l'importance des variations de la mortalité due à cette cause dans les régions de la Communauté Européenne. L'amplitude des classes, choisies pour constituer les histogrammes (de SMR) est de vingt. Le même mode de regroupement a été utilisé pour chaque histogramme, afin de procurer une échelle commune sur laquelle la variabilité des indices des différentes affections est comparable. Les intervalles utilisés dans les histogrammes sont différents des classes d'indices utilisés dans la cartographie.

Pays: répartition par sextile

Ces cartes sont prévues pour montrer les variations internes à chaque pays; elles ont été produites séparément. Il n'est pas possible de comparer les niveaux de mortalité entre les différents pays à l'aide de ces cartes.

Ici, les données de mortalité de chaque région ont été standardisées à l'aide des taux spécifiques par âge du pays considéré (l'indice pour le pays dans son ensemble est la référence = 100); ainsi l'indice d'une petite région indique l'amplitude avec laquelle cette région diffère de l'ensemble du pays. Il était important d'employer pour chaque affection une mesure commune afin de montrer les variations internes aux pays ainsi les 451 indices des régions, établis sur la base nationale, ont été classés et subdivisés en sextiles pour créer les intervalles de classes cartographiées. Les trames, défines à partir de la standardisation qui repose sur les taux nationaux, illustrent l'amplitude avec laquelle la mortalité des régions diffère de la mortalité moyenne nationale, en comparaison de l'amplitude avec laquelle les autres régions de la Communauté Européenne diffèrent de la mortalité moyenne de leur propre pays.

Dans l'atlas de 1980–84, la légende des cartes de chaque pays repose sur le groupement des indices en sextiles, alors que, dans l'atlas de 1974–78, les cartes nationales avaient pour base l'amplitude des indices plutôt que leur classe. En conséquence, les cartes des pays ne sont pas comparables d'un atlas à l'autre. Un histogramme de la fréquence des indices régionaux, défini par un classement dont les intervalles sont d'une amplitude égale à 20, est présenté sur chaque carte. En gris, figure la distribution des indices des 451 régions de la Communauté Européenne fondés sur les taux nationaux, et, en noir, figure la distribution des indices du pays considéré. Les intervalles pris en compte dans les histogrammes sont différents des intervalles de classe des indices utilisés dans la cartographie.

Tableaux

Les indicateurs de mortalité (standardisés de deux manières), le résultat des tests de signification (indice de mortalité relative supérieur à 100), et les scores récapitulatifs sont donnés pour chaque région dans le Chapitre 7, page 153.

Si l'indice de mortalité relative d'une région diffère significativement de la référence, cela dépend non seulement du niveau de l'indice mais aussi de la taille de la population de la région et du taux de mortalité totale pour la cause considérée (chacune des deux contribue au nombre 'attendu' de décès dans la région). Une même valeur de l'indice dans deux régions, dont la taille de population diffère grandement, peut s'avérer significativement différente dans la région avec une population nombreuse, mais non significative dans une région comptant moins d'habitants. Les nombres observés de décès et les effectifs de la population concernée sont donc également présentés dans des tableaux, pour chaque région.

Enfin, les données sociales et les statistiques d'équipement en service de soins sont également présentées en tableaux. Toutefois, les dernières données n'étant pas absolument comparables d'un pays à l'autre les comparaisons inter-pays doivent être menées avec prudence.

Evolution de la mortalité 'évitable' entre 1974–78 et 1980–84

Pour permettre la comparaison du niveau de la mortalité 'évitable' entre les périodes 1974–78 et 1980–84, les données de mortalité et de population doivent concerner des zones géographiques identiques pour les deux périodes. En 1980–84, l'étude a inclus au total 451 zones administratives alors qu'en 1974–78, le nombre de zones n'était que de 360. Pour l'étude des évolutions dans le temps, nous avons donc dû agréger les données de la période 1980–84 en fonction du découpage des zones géographiques utilisé en 1974–78. Les zones prises en compte lors des comparaisons entre les deux périodes correspondent ainsi aux 360 zones définies dans l'atlas de 1974–78.

Cartes

Les trames utilisées pour les cartes relatives aux évolutions dans le temps, sont basées sur le classement des SMR observé sur les deux périodes. Les taux bruts de mortalité ont baissé pour l'ensemble des causes de décès à l'exception de l'asthme. Les trames indiquent l'évolution de la mortalité relativement aux autres zones et non les changements absolus survenus au sein d'une même zone. Les SMR calculés pour analyser la mortalité en 1974–78 sont basés sur la mortalité de référence de la Communauté entière utilisée dans l'atlas de 1974–78. Les SMR calculés pour analyser la mortalité en 1980–84, sont basés sur les taux spécifiques de décès de la Communauté en 1980–84 (Espagne et Portugal exclus). Pour chacune des deux périodes, les zones situées dans les deux sextiles supérieurs sont définies en tant que zones à mortalité élevée, celles situées dans les deux sextiles intermédiaires sont définies en tant que zones à mortalité moyenne, et celles correspondantes aux deux sextiles inférieurs sont définies en tant que zones à faible mortalité. Les trames utilisées pour les cartes indiquant l'évolution de la mortalité entre 1974–78 et 1980–84 sont définies ainsi:

1. Amélioration: évolution de mortalité élevée en 1974–78 à mortalité moyenne ou faible en 1980–84 *ou* évolution de mortalité moyenne en 1974–78 à mortalité faible en 1980–84.
2. Faible–faible: mortalité faible en 1974–78; mortalité faible en 1980–84.
3. Moyenne–moyenne : mortalité moyenne en 1974–78; mortalité moyenne en 1980–84.
4. Élevée–élevée : mortalité élevée en 1974–78; mortalité élevée en 1980–84.
5. Détérioration: évolution de faible mortalité en 1974–78 à mortalité moyenne ou élevée en 1980–84 *ou* évolution de mortalité moyenne en 1974–78 à mortalité élevée en 1980–84.

La Figure 2.1 illustre les trames utilisées pour les différentes zones dans le cas de la maladie de Hodgkin. Sur les cartes relatives à l'évolution entre 1974–78 et 1980–84, les zones pour lesquelles a été observée une détérioration sont représentées en noir et les zones pour lesquelles a été observée une amélioration sont représentées en blanc.

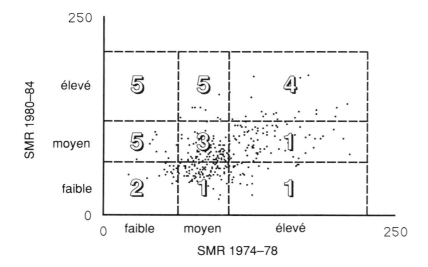

Figure 2.1. Evolution temporelle-constitution des classes cartographiques maladie du Hodgkin.

L'Espagne et le Portugal ne sont pas inclus dans cette analyse. En Allemagne Fédérale et aux Pays-Bas, les zones administratives de 1980–84 ont été agrégées selon celles de 1974–78. La Grèce est exclue de l'analyse pour la mortalité maternelle et périnatale (données non disponibles en 1974–78) et pour la mortalité par asthme (données non disponibles en 1980–84).

Tableaux

L'évolution générale de la mortalité 'évitable' par pays est indiquée au Tableau 9.1.1 (p.269). Ce tableau présente l'effectif des décès, le taux brut de décès, et le taux comparatif de décès selon l'âge pour chaque maladie, chaque pays, et pour les deux périodes 1974–78 et 1980–84. En multipliant le SMR du pays considéré (fondé sur les taux de mortalité de la Communauté) par le taux brut de décès de la Communauté, un taux comparatif de décès a été obtenu. La mortalité a diminué dans l'ensemble de la Communauté pour toutes les causes de décès étudiées, à l'exception de l'asthme dont le taux a progressé. L'évolution de la mortalité par pays pour différentes classes d'âge est indiquée au Tableau 9.1.2 (b)–(l) (p.275). Ce tableau présente l'effectif de décès, les taux spécifiques de décès par âge ainsi que l'évolution de ces taux entre les deux périodes pour chaque maladie et chaque pays. Pour l'ensemble des classes d'âge, on constate en général, une baisse de la mortalité quels que soient la maladie et le pays considérés. Les seules exceptions concernent l'asthme (progression de la mortalité pour la plupart des pays et des groupes d'âge) et les cancers du col de l'utérus (augmentation ou diminution selon les pays ou l'âge). Les données relatives aux changements de structure de population par groupe d'âge sont indiquées au Tableau 9.1.2(b).

L'évolution de la mortalité 'évitable' par zone est présentée au Tableau 9.1.3 (p.310). Pour chacune des zones, le taux de mortalité standardisé par âge est indiqué pour les deux périodes 1974–78 et 1980–84. Le résultat d'un test permettant de déterminer si ce taux est significativement plus élevé que la moyenne européenne est également fourni (ce test repose sur la valeur du SMR). Un taux comparatif de décès est obtenu en multipliant le SMR par le taux brut de décès européen. La mortalité dans la Communauté Européenne est moins élevée dans la période 1980–84 que dans la période 1974–78 pour l'ensemble des causes de mortalité 'évitable' à l'exception de l'asthme. Ceci implique que les taux en 1980–84 sont comparés à une mortalité de référence européenne moins élevée que pour les comparaisons de 1974–78. En conséquence, une zone peut avoir une mortalité significativement supérieure à la moyenne en 1980–84 et non significativement supérieure en 1974–78 alors que les taux de décès de cette zone étaient plus élevées en 1974–78.

Graphiques

Les graphiques indiquent la relation entre la valeur des SMR en 1980–84 et en 1974–78. Le calcul des SMR est, pour les deux périodes, basé sur les taux de décès spécifiques européens de la période 1974–78. Les graphiques illustrent dans quelle mesure la mortalité d'une zone a évolué comparativement à celles des autres zones d'une période à l'autre.

2. METHODEN

Auswahl von Indikatoren für die Bewertung von Gesundheitsleistungen

In diesem Atlas werden Indikatoren vorgestellt, die auf der Mortalität an 17 Krankheitsgruppen basieren. Diese Indikatoren wurden ausgewählt, um primär- und sekundärpräventive Aspekte von Gesundheitsleistungen von Bewohnern definierter geographischer Gebiete zu bewerten. Drei dieser ausgewählten Todesursachen (Lungenkrebs, Leberzirrhose und Kraftfahrzeugunfälle) wären überwiegend von primärpräventiven Massnahmen auf nationaler Ebene abhängig; für die übrigen (Tuberkulose, Cervix- und Korpus Krebs des Uterus, Morbus Hodgkin's, chronisch-rheumatische Herzkrankheit, Krankheiten der Atmungsorgane im Kindesalter, Asthma, Appendizitis, Hernie des Abdomen, Gallenblasenoperation, Hypertonie und Schlaganfall, Mütter- und Perinatal Sterblichkeit sowie eine Gruppe infektiöser Krankheiten (wie Keuchhusten) ist es mehr als wahrscheinlich, dass eine wirksame Behandlung order eine Primäroder Sekundärprävention durch die Gesundheitsdienste gegeben werden kann. Die Indikatoren die 'Indikatoren vermeidbarer Mortalität' genannt werden, sollen Warnsignale für mögliche Defizite der Gesundheitsversorgung darstellen, obwohl auch andere Erklärungen möglich sein können. Der Nutzen der Indikatoren in diesem Atlas wird vor allem darin gesehen:

(1) zu prüfen, ob die Resultate von Gesundheitsdiensten in Bezug auf spezielle geographische Regionen gleich sind;
(2) als Warnsignale zu dienen, die durch lokale Untersuchungen ergänzt werden sollen. Bei solchen Untersuchungen können vermeidbare Faktoren und andere Probleme erkannt werden, so dass die Handhabung der Lokalgesundheitsdienste verbessert werden kann.

Die Auswahl der Todesursachen, welche als Gesundheitsindikatoren benutzt werden sollten, begann mit einer modifizierten Liste von 14 Krankheiten, welche von Charlton und Mitarbeiter im Jahre 1983 in einer Studie geographischer Differenzen in England und Wales benutzt wurde. Diese, wiederum, stammte aus der Liste von 'einzigartigen Gesundheitsereignissen', welche von einer Arbeitsgruppe für präventive und behandelbare Krankheiten in den Vereinigten Staaten, wie oben erwähnt, erstellt wurde (Rutstein u.Mitarbeiter 1980).

Beim ersten 'Workshop' der Arbeitsgruppe wurde eine Liste von Krankheiten von den Teilnehmern aller beteiligten EG-Länder diskutiert, um die unterschiedliche Beurteilung in Bezug auf die Bedeutung bestimmter Krankheiten einzubeziehen. Auf Grund dieser Diskussion, wurden 17 Krankheiten als Indikatoren für Primär- und Sekundärprävention und kurative Dienste ausgewählt. Grundprinzip für die Auswahl dieser Krankheiten war, dass in Bezug auf jede Krankheit eine wirksame Intervention durch das medizinische Versorgungssystem gegeben sein sollte. Die Tabellen im Anhang A belegen für jede der ausgewählten Krankheitsgruppen die ICD-Ziffern, den Altersbereich, die einbezogenen Krankheiten und Gründe, die für das Projekt-Team

massgeblich waren, diese Sterbefälle als 'vermeidbar' zu betrachten (z.B. Faktoren, die zur Mortalität beitragen können) sowie die gesundheitlichen und andere Massnahmen, die die Sterblichkeit verringern könnten. Ausschlaggebende Gesundheitsversorger (Dienste) wurden identifiziert; ausgewählte sachdienliche Referenzen sind angeführt. Feste Altersgruppen wurden ausgewählt, um die Richtigkeit von Mortalitätsdaten als Indikator für die Bewertung der Gesundheitsdienste zu erhöhen. Mit den Krankheiten sollte der Bereich verschiedener Gesundheitsdienste abgedeckt werden. Die Liste enthält jedoch weder alle Krankheiten, für die der Tod durch medizinische Intervention 'vermeidbar' ist, noch ist jeder Todesfall an diesen Ursachen 'vermeidbar', dennoch wird angenommen, dass ein hoher Prozentsatz dieser Sterbefälle verhindert werden kann.

Es wurden Karten und Tabellen angefertigt, die die lokalen geographischen Unterschiede in Bezug auf diese 'vermeidbaren' Todesursachen (Tuberkulose, Cervix-Krebs, Morbus Hodgkin's, chronisch-rheumatische Herzkrankheit, Hypertonie and Schlaganfall, respiratorische Krankheit im Kindesalter, Asthma, Hernie des Abdomens, Appendizitis, Gallenblasenentzündung und Gallengangentzündung, Müttersterblichkeit und perinatale Mortalität) darstellen. Ausserdem werden Tabellen wiedergegeben, die die Anzahl und Häufigkeit von Todesfällen an Infektionskrankheiten in jedem der Länder aufzeigen.

Wegen Kodierproblemen in einigen Ländern wurden die Daten für Cervix- und Korpus-Krebs des Uterus zusammengefasst, und zwar für die Altersgruppe 15–54 Jahre. Innerhalb dieser Altersgruppe sind wahrscheinlich alle Todesfälle auf Cervix-Karzinom zurückzuführen. Es werden Karten gezeigt, die sowohl die Sterbefälle an Cervix-Krebs als auch die an Cervix- und Corpus-Krebs des Uterus wiedergeben.

Für die drei Indikatoren, die sich auf Primärprävention beziehen (Lungenkrebs, Leberzirrhose und Kraftfahrzeugunfälle), werden Tabellen nur für das gesamte Land vorgestellt, da die Todesfälle an diesen Krankheiten weniger stark auf lokale Gesundheitsdienste und ihre Möglichkeiten zurückzuführen sind. Die 'Vermeidbarkeit' dieser Todesfälle hängt wahrscheinlich mehr von einer nationalen Gesundheitspolitik ab, sowie von Faktoren, die ausserhalb der direkten Kontrolle durch lokale Gesundheitsdienste liegen.

Die Daten

Der *EG-Atlas über 'Vermeidbare' Mortalität* für die Jahre 1974–78 beinhaltete Mortalitätsdaten von Belgien, Luxemburg, Bundesrepublik Deutschland, Dänemark, Frankreich, Griechenland, Irland, Niederlande, England und Wales, Nordirland und Schottland. Dieser Atlas, der sich auf die Jahre 1980–84 erstreckt, umfässt nun auch Spanien und Portugal.

Von jedem Land wurden Mortalitätsdaten für den Zeitraum 1980–84 bereitgestellt, mit Ausnahme von Griechenland, das Daten für 1980–82 lieferte, sowie Spanien und Italien, deren Daten sich auf 1970–83 beziehen. Angaben über Asthma standen für Griechenland und Portugal nicht in administrativer Untergliederung zur Verfügung.

Bevölkerungsdaten wurden von den Ländern für den 5-Jahreszeitraum zur Verfügung gestellt; Ausnahmen bildeten: Italien mit Daten für 1979–83 und vier weitere Länder, die nur über regionalisierte Zensusdaten von einem der 5 Jahre verfügten. Die Bevölkerungsdaten von Frankreich beziehen sich auf 1982; für Griechenland, Irland und Spanien jeweils auf 1981. Es wurde deshalb unterstellt, dass die Daten für Frankreich, Irland und Spanien im gesamten Zeitraum, und von Griechenland für 1980–82 repräsentativ waren.

Die Daten stammen von offiziellen Ämtern; Bevölkerungsdaten z.B. beruhen auf Zensusergebnissen, wobei amtliche Fortschreibungen über Änderungen zwischen den Zensen, falls vorhanden, benutzt wurden. Die Datenquellen sind in Anhang B angegeben. Die Vertreter eines jeden Landes zeichnen verantwortlich, dass die dem Koordinationszentrum übermittelten Daten nach Alter, Geschlecht und administrativen Gebietseinheiten gegliedert, korrekt sind. Es war das Ziel, administrative Einheiten mit rund 500 000 Einwohnern abzugrenzen; da aber existierende Verwaltungseinheiten benutzt werden mussten, variieren die Gebietseinheiten in der Bevölkerungsgrösse. Es gab für Zwecke dieser Studie 451 administrative Einheiten in der EG für 1980–84, dagegen waren es für 1974–78 360 Regionen. Die Aufnahme von Spanien und Portugal vergrösserte die Anzahl der Regionen um 70. Daten für die Bundesrepublik Deutschland für 1974–78 waren in 11 geographische Einheiten untergliedert. Die Bevölkerung dieser administrativen Einheiten war überproportional gross (im Durchschnitt 5.594.000 Einwohner). Für die Studie über den Zeitraum 1980–84, konnte die Bundesrepublik Deutschland Daten für 31 Gebietseinheiten mit einer durchschnittlichen Bevölkerung von 1.984.000 Einwohnern liefern, und damit den Bevölkerungsgrössen der Gebietseinheiten der übrigen EG-Länder näherkommen. In den Niederlanden wurde ein Distrikt, Zeitspanne 1974–78, in 1980–84 in zwei Einheiten unterteilt.

Die neunte Revision der Internationalen Klassifikation von Krankheiten wurde in 1979 eingeführt. ICD 8-Codes wurden für die Klassifikation der Todesursachen im *EG-Atlas über 'vermeidbare' Sterbefälle* für 1974–78 benutzt; dagegen ICD 9-Codes für den Atlas für 1980–84. Ein möglicher Einfluss der Änderung der ICD auf die Sterblichkeit wurde durch Anwendung eines OPCS 'Umsteigeschlüssels' überprüft, wobei eine Stichprobe von 25 Prozent aller in England und Wales aufgetretenen Sterbefälle sowohl nach der ICD 8 als auch der ICD 9 signiert wurden (Tabelle 2.1). Der Unterschied, der den einzelnen Krankheiten zugeordneten Sterbefälle, war geringer als 10 Prozent in Bezug auf die 'vermeidbaren' Ursachen, mit Ausnahme der chronisch-rheumatischen Herzkrankheiten.

Die Annahmen über die Ätiologie der chronisch-rheumatischen Herzkrankheiten haben sich zwischen der IDC8 und ICD9 gewandelt. Bei der ICD8 wurde unterstellt, dass Mitral- oder Aortenfehler (393–396) rheumatisch bedingt waren; es sei denn, sie waren als nicht-rheumatisch bezeichnet oder als Folge einer Arteriosklerose oder eines Bluthochdrucks angegeben. Nach der ICD9 werden Mitral- oder Aortenfehler nur dann mit rheumatischer Genese angenommen, wenn eine Mitralstenose oder Verengung, Mitralkrankheit und Mitralversagen, ohne zusätzliche spezifische Indikation angegeben ist. Bei anderen Aortenklappenerkrankungen wird nicht von rheumatischer Ursache ausgegangen. Gleichwohl wird eine rheumatische Erkrankung unterstellt, wenn sowohl Mitral- als auch Aortenklappenfehler beteiligt sind.

Todesbescheinigungen   die   Bronchitis,   Bronchielitis   oder

Tabelle 2.1. Gegenüberstellung von Sterbefällen aus einer 25 prozentigen Stichprobe aller in England und Wales in 1978 Gestorben, signiert nach der ICD8 und ICD9

Krankheit	Alters-gruppe (Jahre)	ICD Codes		Anzahl der Sterbefälle		Änderung in%
		ICD8	ICD9	ICD8	ICD9	
Tuberkulose	1–64	010–019	010–018, 137	86	84	−2
Bösartige Neubilding des Cervix Uteri	15–64	180	180	277	277	0
Bösartige Neubilding des Corpus Uteri	15–64	182	179,182	102	101	−1
Morbus Hodgkin's	1–64	201	201	124	124	0
Chronisch-rheumatische Herzkrankheiten	1–44	393–398	393–398	59	36	−39
Alle Krankheiten der Atmungsorgane	1–14	460–519	460–519	64	62	−3
Asthma	1–44	493	493	74	81	+9
Appendizitis	1–64	540–543	540–543	15	16	+7
Hernie des Abdomens (Eingeweidebrüche)	1–64	550–553	550–553	36	34	−6
Gallenblasen- und Gallengangsentzündung	1–64	574–575	574–575.1, 576.1	24	25	+4
Bluthochdruckskrankheiten	45–64	400–404	401–405	292	298	+2
Hirngefässkrankheiten	45–64	430–438	430–438	1986	2056	+4

Tabelle 2.2. Änderung der Mortalitätsrate je 100.000 Einwohner zwischen 1974–78 und 1980–84 für 'vermeidbare' Todesursachen

Krankheit	Altersgruppe (Jahre)	ICD Codes		Mortalitäts rate		Änderung in %
		ICD8	ICD9	ICD8	ICD9	
Tuberkulose	5–64	010–019	010–018, 137	2.05	1.08	−47
Bösartige Neubildung des Cervix Uteri	15–64	180	180	4.89	3.83	−22
Bösartige Neubildung des Corpus Uteri	15–54	182	179,182	6.23	4.38	−30
Morbus Hodgkin's	5–64	201	201	1.25	0.95	−24
Chronisch-rheumatische Herzkrankheiten	5–44	393–398	393–398	1.05	0.35	−66
Alle Krankheiten der Atmungswege	1–14	460–519	460–519	3.01	1.98	−34
Asthma	5–44	493	493	0.50	0.63	27
Appendizitis	5–64	540–543	540–543	0.35	0.14	−59
Hernie des Abdomen (Eingeweidebrüche)	5–64	550–553	550–553	0.35	0.20	−42
Gallenblasen- und Gallengangsentzündung	5–64	574–575	574–575.1, 576.1	0.83	0.35	−58
Bluthochdruck und Hirngefässkrankheiten	35–64	400–404, 430–438	401–405, 430–438	52.47	41.48	−21
Müttersterbefälle	All	630–678	630–676	20.49	11.74	−43
Perinatalsterbefälle				18.49	12.17	−34
Alle Todesursachen	5–64			316.26	291.50	−8
Alle Todesursachen	1+			1067.19	1054.03	−1

Emphysem als ursachliches Leiden aufwiesen und bei denen auch Asthma erwähnt wurde, wurden nach der ICD9 im Gegensatz zur ICD8 als Asthma verschlüsselt. Dies führte zu einem Anstieg von 28 Prozent der als Asthma signierten Sterbfälle über alle Altersgruppen, dabei standen 313 als Asthma signierten Sterbefällen nach der ICD8, 401 Fällen bei Verschlüsselung nach der ICD9 gegenüber. Der Unterschied zwischen beiden Klassifikationen war in höheren Altersgruppen stärker ausgeprägt. Im Altersbereich 1–44 Jahre, auf den die als 'vermeidbar' betrachteten Sterbefälle entfallen, betrug der prozentale Unterschied 9 Prozent. Eine Analyse der SMR für Asthma zwischen 1974 und 1984 in England und Wales, zeigte einen konzentrierten Anstieg der Mortalität über Zeit, sogar dann wenn der Wechsel von der ICD8 zur ICD9 im Jahre 1979 berücksichtigt wurde (Burney, Lancet 1986).

Gallenblasen- und Gallengangsentzündung wurden nach der ICD8 mit den Ziffern 574 und 575 signiert. Nach der ICD9 enthält die Signiernummer 576 Teile von 575 der ICD8, und die Ziffer 575 setzt sich aus Teilen von 575 und 576 in der ICD9 zusammen.

Änderungen der rohen Mortalitätsrate wurden für jede 'vermeidbare' Krankheit für die EG insgesamt, zwischen 1974–78 und 1980–84 in Tabelle 2.2 wiedergegeben. Die Unterschiede waren bei jeder Krankheit grösser als die Veränderungen, die sich aus dem Wechsel von der ICD8 zur ICD9 erklären lassen. Mit Ausnahme von Asthma, für das ein Mortalitätsanstieg von 27 Prozent registriert wurde,

bewegte sich der Rückgang der Mortalität für die einzelnen 'vermeidbaren' Ursachen von 21 bis 67 Prozent, wohingegen die Gesamtmortalität nur um 2 Prozent sank. Dies stimmt mit der Untersuchung von Charlton und Velez (1986) überein, nach der im Zeitraum 1950–1980 die 'vermeidbaren' Ursachen rascher als die Gesamtmortalität zurückgingen, und zwar in so ganz unterschiedlichen Ländern wie die Vereinigten Staaten, Frankreich, Japan, Italien und England und Wales.

Die Veränderungen der 'vermeidbaren' Mortalität in der EG aufgrund der Einführung der ICD9, scheinen bei 10 Todesursachen unwesentlich zu sein, und können den Rückgang bei den Gallenerkrankungen und chronisch-rheumatischen Herzkrankheiten, oder den Anstieg bei Asthma nicht erklären. Für England und Wales zumindest, konnte gezeigt werden, dass es einen kontinuierlichen Anstieg von Asthma-Sterbefällen gibt, der durch den Wechsel in der ICD nicht erklärt werden kann.

Es wurden auch Daten für Sozialindikatoren und Gesundheitsdienstleistungen eingeholt. Die Auswahl dieser Angaben war begrenzt, weil vergleichbare Daten für alle Länder vorhanden sein mussten. Die Bedeutung dieser Indikatoren bezieht sich jedoch keineswegs auf die zwischen den Ländern bestehenden Unterschiede, und sollten daher nur für den Vergleich innerhalb eines Landes genutzt werden.

Analyse und Präsentation

Der Atlas ist in zwei Teile untergliedert. Im ersten Teil wird die geographische Verteilung der 'vermeidbaren' Mortalität auf die 451 Gebietseinheiten der EG für 1980–84, in Karten und Tabellen dargestellt. Im zweiten Teil werden die Veränderungen der 'vermeidbaren' Mortalität zwischen den Zeitabschnitten 1974–78 und 1980–84 beschrieben. Da Spanien und Portugal nicht zur EG gehörten, lieferten sie zum Atlas für 1974–78 keine Daten und sind infolgedessen, in die Analyse der zeitlichen Veränderung im Atlas für 1980–84 nicht eingeschlossen. Die Daten für 1980–84 mussten für einen Zeitvergleich für die Bundersrepublik Deutschland und für die Niederlande, auf die Gebietsgrenzen für 1974–78 zusammengefasst werden. Aus diesem Grunde wurde die Analyse zeitlicher Veränerungen, für die im EG-Atlas für 'vermeidbare' Sterbefälle 1974–78 beschriebenen 360 Regionen durchgeführt, und nicht für die 451 Regionen die im ersten Teil dieses Atlas beschrieben sind.

Analyse und Präsentation der Daten für 1980–84

Da lokale alters- und geschlechtsspezifische Mortalitätsraten wegen der geringen Zahl von Todesfällen ungenau werden, wurde die indirekte Altersstandardisierung ('standardisierte Mortalitätsquotienten' — SMR) gewählt (siehe Armitage 1971). Die Daten für beide Geschlechtsgruppen wurden zusammengefasst, da wir nicht annehmen dass die 'Vermeidbarkeit' von Todesfällen vom Geschlecht abhänge. Die Sterbefälle an Cervix- und Korpus-Krebs des Uterus wurden altersstandardisiert auf die Anteile der weiblichen Bevölkerung bezogen.

Für jede Krankheitsgruppe und jede der 451 in der Studie untersuchten Regionen, wurden 'Standardisierte Mortalitätsquotienten' (SMR) auf zwei verschiedene Arten berechnet:

(1) indem die altersspezifischen Raten der EG insgesamt als Standard zugrunde gelegt, und
(2) indem die altersspezifischen Raten des jeweiligen Landes zugrunde gelegt wurden.

Die erste Methode wurde angewandt, um Unterschiede zwischen den Ländern herauszuarbeiten, dadurch dass alle Daten auf einem gemeinsamen Standard (gesamte EG = 100) bezogen wurden. Die zweite Methode wurde benutzt, um Differenzen innerhalb des Landes aufzuzeigen (das gesamte Land = 100).

Eine Altersstandardisierung wurde nicht bei der Mütter-und Perinatalsterblichkeit angewandt. Als EG-Standard wurde die rohe Sterberate für 100.000 Geburten angenommen. EG-Standard für die perinatale Mortalität war die rohe perinatale Sterberate je 1000 Geburten. Zum Vergleich zwischen den Ländern wurde der 'Standardiesierte Mortalitäts-Quotient (SMR)' für jede Gebietseinheit als Quotient aus roher Sterberate für diese Region, und der rohen Sterberate für die gesamte EG ermittelt und mit 100 multipliziert. Bei Vergleichen der Mütter- und Perinatalsterblichkeit innerhalb der Länder, wurde als Standard die rohe Sterberate für das betreffende Land gewählt. Die SMR für eine bestimmte regionale Gebietseinheit dieses Landes wurde dann als Quotient aus roher Rate für dieses Gebiet, und roher Rate für das Land ermittelt, und mit 100 multipliziert.

Die folgenden statistischen Tests wurden auf der Basis der standardisierten Mortalitätsquotienten durchgeführt, um zu prüfen:

(1) ob die standardisierten Mortalitätsquotienten die Daten triftig beschreiben;
(2) ob die Unterschiede in Bezug auf verschiedene Regionen grösser sind als nach der Wahrscheinlichkeit zu erwarten wäre;
(3) ob für jede Region der standardisierte Mortaliätsindex ausschlaggebend grösser als 100 ist.

Die Tests (1)und (2) sind CHI-QUADRAT Tests wie sie von Gail (1978) beschrieben wurden, der Test (3) wurde von Armitage (1971) dargestellt. Von uns wurde der einseitige Test ausgewählt, weil wir nur erhöhte Mortalität zeigen wollten, zumal im Idealfall nur wenige oder keine Sterbefälle auftreten. Der Test (1) untersucht, ob die Verhältnisse (lokal/EG und lokal/national) für die verschiedenen Altersgruppen gleich sind. Dies ist eine Voraussetzung dafür, dass mit den standardisierten Mortalitätsindizes die Daten triftig beschrieben werden können. Für keine 'vermeidbare' Todesursache gab es ausschlaggebende Beweise, dass die standardisierten Mortalitätsquotienten nicht anwendbar wären. Für die Perinatal- und Müttersterblichkeit wurden die Raten folgendermassen berechnet (Perinatalfälle je 1000 Geburten: Müttersterblichkeit: Fälle je 100 000 Geburten. Der Test (2) wurde auch in Bezug auf diese Raten angewendet, um zu prüfen, ob sie für den betreffenden Zeitabschnitt signifikant grösser als der nationale oder der EG-Durchschnitt waren.

Die SMR für 1980-1984 sind nicht unmittelbar mit denen für 1974-1978 vergleichbar, weil eine SMR von 100 für 1980-1984 nicht das gleiche Mortalitätsniveau angibt wie eine SMR gleich 100 für 1974-1978; dies ist in den unterschiedlichen altersspezifischen Mortalitäsraten begründet, auf denen die SMRn für die zwei Zeitspannen basieren. Die altersspezifischen Mortalitätraten der Länder, die im Atlas 1974-1978 enthalten sind, haben sich während dieser beiden Zeitspannen verändert, und zwar mit rückläufiger Tendenz für alle Krankheiten, mit Ausnahme von Asthma für das sie zunahmen. Darüberhinaus hat sich der EG Standard durch die Erweiterung um Spanien und Portugal im Atlas für 1980-1984 verändert, so dass sich die altersspezifischen Raten für Krankheiten, bei denen die Sterblichkeit in Spanien und Portugal niedrig war, veringerten, und für Krankheiten wo die Mortalität hoch ist, zunahmen.

Karten

Eine grosse Europakarte (Miller's stereographische Projektion) wurde in Abschnitte eingeteilt. Diese Karte wurde an die teilnehmenden Zentren zur Eintragung ihrer Grenzen verteilt und an das Koordinierungszentrum zurückgeschickt. Die Grenzen wurden dann digitalisiert in eine Serie von Längs- und Querkoordinaten übertragen, und zwar in einer für das INFOMAP Computer-Karten-Programm (Claymore Services Ltd 1988) passenden Form.

Zwei Gruppen von Karten wurden erstellt, um die verschiedenen Aspekte der Mortalitätsunterschiede aufzuzeigen. Sechs Schattierabstufungen liegen allen Karten zugrunde: die zwei Methoden, die benutzt wurden, die Regionen einzuteilen, werden im folgenden beschrieben:-Histogramme, die die Verteilung der standardisierten Mortalitätsindizes aufzeigen, sind auf jeder Karte zu sehen.

Gesamt-EG, Sechstil-Intervalle

Diese Karten haben den Zweck, Unterschiede zwischen den Ländern aufzuzeigen. Sie zeigen die Rangordnung der Regionen, wenn die Mortalität mit einem gemeinsamen EG-Standard verglichen wird. Die Mortalitätsdaten für jede Region wurden altersstandardisiert, indem die altersspezifischen Mortalitätsraten der EG insgesamt (SMR für die EG insgesamt = 100) benutzt wurden: diese SMRn wurden dann der Grösse nach geordnet. Ein Sechstel der Regionen wurde jeweils einem Schattierintervall zugeordnet.

Die Sechstile werden in den Karten durch folgende Farben gekennzeichnet:

Oberstes Sechstil (höchste Mortalität)	1	Rot
	2	Dunkel-Orange
	3	Hell-Orange
	4	Gelb
	5	Hell-Grün
Unterstes Sechstil (geringste Mortalität)	6	Dunkel-Grün

Die Karten für Perinatal- und Mütterserblichkeit zeigen die Verteilung der entsprechenden SMR. Im *EG-Atlas über 'vermeidbare Sterbefälle' 1974–1978* sind die rohen Sterberaten in den Karten wiedergegeben. Diese rohen Raten würden die gleichen farblichen Abstufungen wie SMR ergeben, weil die SMR für jede Regionaleinheit nichts anderes ist als die rohe Sterberate dividiert durch eine Konstante (rohe Rate der EG). So gesehen, weisen die EG-Karten über die Mütter- und Perinatalsterblichkeit von 1974–78 und 1980–84 vergleichbare Farbgebung auf. Benutzt man jedoch die SMR statt der rohen Rate zur Beschreibung der Schattierung im Zeitintervall, so gibt man damit ein Mass vor das mit der Kartendarstellung für die anderen Krankheiten übereinstimmt.

Der Atlas für 1974–78 enthält sowohl Karten der EG die auf Schattierung von Sechstilen beruhen, als auch Karten die mehr auf die Grösse der SMR als auf ihre Rangfolge, beschrieben als 'gleiche mittlere Intervalle', abgestellt sind. Karten, denen 'gleiche mittlere Intervalle' zugrunde liegen, sind im Atlas 1980–84 nicht enthalten.

Auf jeder Karte der EG ist ein Histogramm der Frequenzen der SMR enthalten, um die Schwankungen in SMR für Mortalität der kartographisch dargestellten Todesursachen über kleine Regionen der EG zu zeigen. Histogramme, die auf einer Gruppierung von zwanzig beruhen, geben die Häufigkeitsverteilung der SMR wieder. Diese Gruppierungen der Histogramme wurden so gewählt, dass sie für alle Krankheitsgruppen gleich sind, um eine gemeinsame Vergleichsskala zu bilden.

Einzelne Länder, Sechstil-Intervalle

Diese Karten sollen die Unterschiede der Mortalität innerhalb eines Landes zeigen; für jedes Land wurden dafür eigene Karten angefertigt. Mit diesen Karten sollten keine Vergleiche zwischen den Ländern angestellt werden. Es wurden die Mortalitätsdaten jeder Region auf die altersspezifische Mortalitätsrate des jeweiligen Landes standardisiert (SMR für das gesamte Land = 100), also ist die SMR ein Mass für eine kleine Gebietseinheit, insoweit dieses Gebiet vom Landesdurchschnitt abweicht. Es war wichtig an jede Krankheit einen gleichen Massstab anzulegen, um die Abweichung innerhalb der verschiedenen Länder aufzuzeigen; auf diese Weise werden 451 Regionen, bezogen auf nationalen Standard, in ein Rangfolge gebracht und in Sechstile untergeteilt, um daraus die Schattierungen zu gewinnen. Die Schattierungen, die auf einem Standard nationaler Raten beruhen, zeigen wie stark die Mortalität einer kleinen Gebietseinheit von der durchschnittlichen Mortalität des eigenen Landes abweicht, verglichen mit dem Abweichungsausmass anderer kleiner Gebietseinheiten der EG und der Durchschnittsmortalität ihres Landes.

Die Schattierung der Karten der einzelnen Länder im Atlas für 1980–84 beruht auf Sechstil Gruppen, wohingegen die Schattierung der Länderkarten im Atlas 1974–78 mehr auf der Grösse der SMR als auf ihrer Reihenfolge beruhte. Die Karten der einzelnen Länder in den beiden Atlanten sind deshalb nicht vergleichbar. Ein Häufigkeitshistogramm der SMRn stützt sich auf ein Intervall von 20 und wird in jeder Karte dargestellt. Sie zeigen in grau die Verteilung der SMRn kleiner Gebiete, auf einem für die 451 Gebiete der EG insgesamt beruhenden National-Standard, und in schwarz die Verteilung der SMRn für das jeweilige Land. Die Histogramm-Intervalle sind unterschiedlich zu dem SMR-Bereich, der bei der Schattierung der Karten benutzt wird.

Tabellen

Tabellen, die die Mortalitätsindizes (standardisiert sowohl auf die EG als auch auf das jeweilige Land) sowie Angaben enthalten, ob diese Indizes signifikant von 100 (=SMR der Standardbevölkerung) abweichen, befinden sich im Abschnitt 7, Seite 153 für jedes Gebiet in jedem Land. Ob eine SMR für eine Region signifikant vom Standard abweicht, hängt nicht nur von ihrer Grösse, sondern auch von der Bevölkerungsgrösse der Region, sowie von der Gesamtmortalitätsrate der betreffenden Krankheit ab (beide tragen zu der 'erwarteten' Zahl der Sterbefälle der Region bei). Ein gleicher SMR-Wert für zwei Regionen die sich stark in der Grösse der Bevölkerung unterscheiden, können für die Region mit der grösseren Bevölkerung signifikant abweichen, hingegen für die mit der kleineren Bevölkerung nicht.

In Tabellenform sind auch die Zahlen der Sterbefälle an jeder Krankheit und die Bevölkerung jeder Region dargestellt. Zusätzlich werden Tabellen mit den Indikatoren für soziale Bedingungen und Gesundheitsleistungen aufgeführt. Da diese Daten genaugenommen, zwischen Ländern nicht vergleichbar sind, sollten Unterschiede zwischen den Ländern mit grosser Vorsicht betrachtet werden.

Änderungen der 'vermeidbaren' Mortalität zwischen 1974–78 und 1980–84

Um Vergleiche zwischen Ausmass der 'vermeidbaren' Mortalität für 1974–78 gegenüber 1980–84 anstellen zu können, müssen sich die Mortalitäts- und Bevölkerungsdaten auf die gleichen Gebietseinheiten beziehen. Für 1980–84 gab es 451 administrative Gebietseinheiten, aber nur 360 für 1974–78. Aus Gründen eines zeitlichen Vergleichs mussten die Daten für 1974–78 auf die Länder und Grenzen, wie sie in 1974–78 benutzt wurden, aggregiert werden. Als Gebietsgrenzen für einen Mortalitätsvergleich zwischen 1974–78 und 1980–84, dienen die 360 Regionen wie sie im Atlas für 1970–74 beschrieben sind.

Karten

Die Schattierung in den Karten zur Darstellung der Veränderungen, beruht auf der Rangfolge der SMRn in den zwei Zeitspannen. Die Gesamtmortalitätsraten waren mit Ausnahme von Asthma rückläufig. Die Schattierung gibt eher die relative Änderung der Mortalität im Vergleich zu anderen Regionen der EG, als die absolute Änderung wieder. Die SMRn, die zur Beschreibung der Mortalität für 1974–78 herangezogen wurden, beruhten auf dem EG-Standard der im EG-Atlas1974–78 als Massstab galt. Die SMRn zur Darstellung der Mortalität von 1980–84, werden auf der Basis altersspezifischer Raten der EG für 1980–84 ohne Spanien und Portugal berechnet (dies unterscheidet sich vom EG-Standard einschliesslich Spanien und Portugal). In jedem Zeitraum wurden Gebiete mit SMR in den beiden höchsten Sechstilen, als hoch für die jeweilige Periode gewertet; Gebiete in den beiden mittleren Sechstilen, wurden als mittel- und schliesslich solche in den beiden unteren Sechstilen als gering eingestuft. Die Einteilung der Schattierung in den Karten zur Darstellung der Änderung zwischen 1974–78 und 1980–84, wurde wie folgt festgelegt:

1. Verbessert: Wechsel von Hoch (oberes Drittel) 1974–78 zu mittel oder niedrig (unterstes Drittel) 1980–84, oder Wechsel von mittel (mittleres Drittel) 1974–78 zu niedrig 1980–84.
2. Niedrig–niedrig: niedrig 1974–78, niedrig 1980–84.
3. Mittel–mittel: mittel 1974–78, mittel 1980–84.
4. Hoch–hoch: hoch 1974–1978, hoch 1980–1984.
5. Verschlechtert: Wechsel von niedrig in 1974–78 nach mittel, oder hoch in 1980–84, oder Wechsel von mittel zu hoch in 1980–84.

Abbildung 2.1 zeigt die schattierten Gebiete für Morbus Hodgkin's graphisch dargestellt. In den Karten die einen Zeitwechsel (der Mortalität) zwischen 1974–78 und 1980–84 wiedergeben, werden Gebiete die eine Verschlechterung zeigen schwarz schattiert, die die eine Verbesserung aufweisen, weiss dargestellt.

Spanien und Portugal sind in diese Analyse nicht mit einbezogen. Für die Bundesrepublik Deutschland und für die Niederlande, wurden

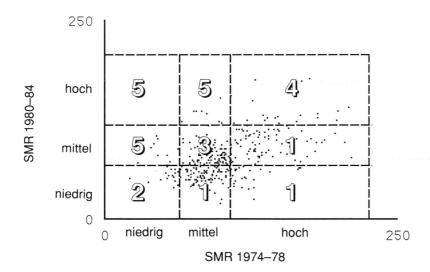

Abb. 2.1. Schattierungsmethode für Karten die Änderungen über Zeitspanne darstellen; Morbus Hodgkin.

die Verwaltungsgebietseinheiten von 1980–84 auf den Stand von 1974–78 gebracht. Griechenland ist von der Analyse der Mütter- und Säuglingssterblichkeit ausgeschlossen (weil die Daten für 1974–78 nicht verfügbar waren), und bei Asthma (weil die Daten für 1980–84 nicht zur Verfügung standen).

Tabellen

Änderungen der 'vermeidbaren' Mortalität auf nationaler Ebene werden in Tabelle 9.1.1 (S.269) und in Tabelle 9.1.2 (S.275) wiedergegeben.

Die gesamte Veränderung der 'vermeidbaren' Mortalität auf Landesebene wird auf Tabelle 9.1.1 gezeigt. Hier wird die Anzahl der Todesfälle, die rohe Mortalitätsrate und altersstandardisierte Mortalitätsrate für jede Krankheit in jedem Land, sowohl für 1974–78 als auch 1980–84 aufgeführt. Bei der altersstandardisierten Mortalitätsrate wird unterstellt, dass sie durch Multiplikation der SMR (Standardisiert auf die EG-Rate) des Landes, mit der rohen Mortalitätsrate der EG für diesen Zeitraum ermittelt wird. In der gesamten EG gab es einen Rückgang der Mortalität an jeder untersuchten Todesursache, mit Ausnahme von Asthma für das die Mortalität anstieg. Änderungen in Mortalität in den Ländern für verschiedene Altersgruppen, werden in Tabelle 9.1.2 (b)–(l) gezeigt. Die Zahl der beobachteten Sterbefälle und altersspezifischen Mortalitätsraten sowie die Veränderungen bei den altersspezifischen Mortalitätsraten zwischen den beiden Zeiträumen, werden für jede Krankheit in jedem Land dargestellt. Die Veränderungsraten in Mortalität der meisten Krankheiten, zeigen in allen Ländern über alle Altersgruppen eine fallende Tendenz. Ausnahmen davon bilden Asthma, für das die Mortalität in den meisten Altersgruppen und in der Mehrzahl der Länder anstieg, sowie das Cervix-Karzinom, für das sowohl eine Zunahme als auch ein Rückgang in verschiedenen Altersgruppen und unterschiedlichen Ländern festgestellt wurde. Angaben über Bevölkerungsänderungen werden für verschiedene Altersgruppen in Tabelle 9.1.2 (b) gezeigt.

Änderungen der 'vermeidbaren' Mortalität in verschiedenen administrativen Gebietseinheiten der EG werden in Tabelle 9.1.3 (S.310) wiedergegeben. Für jede kleinere Gebietseinheit wird sowohl die altersstandardisierte Mortalitätsrate für 1974–78 als auch für 1980–84 gezeigt,mit dem Zusatz, ob sie verglichen mit dem EG-Standard für den jeweiligen Zeitraum signifikant hoch ist (die Signifikanzprüfung basiert auf dem SMR). Die altersstandardisierte Rate ergibt sich durch Multiplikation der SMR mit der rohen Mortalitätsrate der EG. Die Mortalität war in der EG für die Zeitspanne 1980–84 bei jeder 'vermeidbaren' Todesursache, mit Ausnahme von Asthma, geringer als für die Zeitspanne 1974–78. Da die Raten für 1980–84 mit einem geringeren EG-Standard als für 1974–78, verglichen wurden kann ein Gebiet eine signifikant hohe Rate für 1980–84 und eine nicht–signifikant hohe Rate für 1974–78 aufweisen, selbst dann wenn die aktuelle Rate für 1974–78 höher ist.

Graphische Darstellungen

In den Kurven sind die SMRn für 1980–84 gegen die für 1974–78 eingezeichnet. Die SMR sind in beiden Fällen auf den EG-Standard von 1974–78 bezogen. Die graphischen Darstellungen verdeutlichen inwieweit sich Gebiete, im Vergleich mit anderen Regionen der EG, in den beiden Zeiträumen verändert haben.

3. DEFINITIONS

Age-specific death rate: the number of deaths in a specific age group per 100 000 population in that age group.

Age-standardized death rate: the SMR for an area multiplied by the crude death rate of the reference population (whole of EC or individual country).

Areas: administrative areas for local health services in particular countries. These were chosen on the basis of availability of data. The populations of these areas were intended to be approximately 500 000 but depend in practice on the organization of health services or the availability of information on mortality in individual countries.

'Avoidable' deaths: death from specific diseases (within selected age groups) for which mortality should be wholly or substantially avoidable when appropriate medical care is sought and provided in good time.

Expected deaths: expected deaths are the sum of the products of the age-specific death rates for the reference population (whole of EC or the individual country) and the age-specific populations for the area studied.

ICD number: code assigned to cause(s) of death by the International Classification of Diseases/8th or 9th revision.

Maternal death rate: the number of deaths associated with childbirth per 100 000 live and still births.

Maternal 'SMR': the percentage ratio of the crude maternal death rate in the area studied to the crude maternal death rate in the reference population (whole of EC or individual country).

Perinatal death rate: the number of still births and deaths in the first week of life per 1000 live and still births.

Perinatal 'SMR': the percentage ratio of the crude perinatal death rate in the area studied to the crude perinatal death rate in the reference population (whole of EC or individual country).

Standardized mortality ratio (SMR): the percentage ratio of the number of deaths observed in the area studied to the number expected from the standard age-specific death rates.

3. DEFINITIONS

Taux spécifiques de mortalité par âge: nombre de décès dans un groupe d'âge particulier pour 100 000 habitants du groupe d'âge considéré.

Taux comparatifs de mortalité: SMR de la zone, multiplié par le taux brut de décès de la population de référence (Communauté tout entière ou pays individuel selon le cas).

Régions: zones administratives correspondant dans certains pays aux secteurs sanitaires. Ces zones ont été choisies on fonction de l'échelon de diffusion des données statistiques. Le nombre d'habitants devait être d'environ 500 000, mais en pratique il dépend de l'organisation des services médicaux ou de la disponibilité des informations sur la mortalité propres à chaque Etat.

Décès 'évitables': affections particulières dont la mortalité devrait être complètement ou en grande partie évitée, à certains âges définis, si des soins médicaux appropriés étaient prodigués en temps utile.

Décès attendus: ils résultent de la somme des produits des taux spécifiques de la population de référence (Communauté toute entière, ou pays individuel)par la population correspondante de chaque zone étudiée.

Code de la CIM: code attribué aux affections responsables du décès par la Classification Internationale des Maladies, 8ème ou 9ème Révision.

Taux de mortalité maternelle: nombre de décès concernant les mères, associé à la naissance, rapporté au nombre de naissances totales (pour 100 000).

Indice comparatif de mortalité maternelle: rapport, en pourcentage, du taux de mortalité maternelle dans la région étudiée au taux de mortalité maternelle dans la population de référence (Communauté toute entière ou pays individuel selon le cas).

Taux de mortalité périnatale: nombre de mort-nés et de décès de la première semaine de vie, rapporté au nombre de naissances totales (pour 1000).

Indice comparatif de mortalité périnatale: rapport, en pourcentage, du taux de mortalité périnatale dans la région étudiée au taux de mortalité périnatale dans la population de référence (Communauté toute entière ou pays individuel selon le cas).

Indice de mortalité relative (SMR): rapport, en pourcentage, du nombre de décès observés dans la région étudiée au nombre de décès attendus (voir ci-dessus).

3. DEFINITIONEN

Alterspezifische Mortalitätsrate: die Zahl der Sterbefälle in einer spezifischen Altersgruppe, bezogen auf 100 000 der Bevölkerung dieser Altersgruppe.

Altersstandardisierte Mortalitätsrate: SMR für eine Gebietseinheit, multipliziert mit der rohen Mortalitätsrate der Referenzbevölkerung (EG insgesamt oder einzelnes Land.)

Regionen: Verwaltungseinheiten für die regionalen Gesundheitsdienste in einzelnen Ländern. Diese wurden nach dem Vorhandensein der Daten ausgewählt. Die Bevölkerung der Regionen sollte ungefähr 500 000 betragen; dies hängt jedoch von der Organisation der Gesundheitsdienste oder der Verfügbarkeit der Mortalitätsdaten in den einzelnen Ländern ab.

'Vermeidbare' Sterbefälle: Sterbefälle an spezifischen Krankheiten (innerhalb ausgewählter Altersgruppen) für die die Sterblichkeit ganz oder zum Grossteil vermeidbar sein sollte, wäre medizinische Behandlung in Anspruch genommen und rechtzeitig gewährt.

Erwartete Todesfälle: die erwartete Anzahl von Todesfällen ergibt sich aus der Summe der Produkte der altersspezifischen Mortalitätsraten der Standardbevölkerung (Gesamt-EG oder individuelles Land) und den altersspezifischen Bevölkerungsanteilen für die untersuchte Region.

ICD-Kategorie: Todesursache/n zugeteilte/n Ziffer/n des Kodex der Internationalen Klassifikation der Krankheiten 8.oder 9.Revision.

Müttersterblichkeit: die Zahl der im Zusammenhang mit Geburt verstorbenen Frauen, bezogen auf 100 000 Lebend- und Totgeburten.

Mütter 'SMR': Prozent-Quotient aus der rohen Mütter-Mortalitätsrate in der untersuchten Region, und der rohen Mütter-Mortalitätsrate der Referenzbevölkerung (EG insgesamt oder einzelnes Land.)

Perinatale Sterblichkeit: die Zahl von Totgeburten und Säuglingssterbefällen in der ersten Lebenswoche bezogen auf 1000 Lebend- und Totgeburten.

Perinatal 'SMR': Prozent-Quotient aus der rohen Perinatal-Mortalitätsrate der untersuchten Region, und der rohen Perinatal-Mortalitätsrate der Referenzbevölkerung (EG insgesamt oder einzelnes Land).

'Standardisierter Mortalitäts quotient' (SMR): Verhältniszahl in Prozenten, gebildet aus der Zahl der beobachteten Todesfälle in der untersuchten Region und der Zahl von Sterbefällen, wie sie nach den altersspezifischen Sterberaten des Standards zu erwarten wären.

4. INTERPRETATION OF THE MAPS/DATA AND SUGGESTIONS FOR FOLLOW–UP

The maps and tables in this atlas show mortality, socio-economic status and health service resources by area, both within a country framework and within an EC framework. There are limitations, however, in the use of this information to make both within-country and between-country comparisons. There may be differences between countries and, to a lesser extent, between areas in the same country, in the reliability and comparability of the data. Data on health service resources and social indicators, for example, are not always available for the same year(s) for all countries, and for some countries no data are available. The definitions used differ from country to country.

Observed variation in mortality between countries and areas may be an artefact due to variations in data collection, that is diagnosis, certification, and coding of deaths. Disease classification between countries was shown to vary by Kelson and Heller (1983), who found that for acute respiratory disease there were marked differences in the recording of diagnoses between eight EC countries. These differences were attributed to the way doctors complete death certificates and to coding. However, other authors have shown that misclassification of cause of death could not explain the whole difference between areas (Diehl and Gau 1982). The range of differences in levels of 'avoidable' mortality shown in this atlas are thus unlikely to be due to chance alone or to differences in the coding and certification of death.

Alternatively, the variation may be due to an uneven distribution of disease incidence or prevalence, or geographical variations in the provision, efficiency, and effectiveness of health services. For those diseases where morbidity is avoidable (e.g. childhood infections and tuberculosis) incidence and prevalence are influenced by the availability and appropriate use of services for the primary prevention of diseases (i.e. immunization) and health promotion. For those diseases where not all deaths are avoidable by timely and appropriate intervention (e.g. asthma) variation in disease incidence or prevalence between areas should be taken into account when examining variation in mortality. For those diseases where deaths are substantially avoidable by adequate and timely health service intervention irrespective of the incidence or prevalence (e.g. cervical cancer), variation in incidence or prevalence may explain but does not justify variation in mortality.

Case fatality may be influenced by the availability of services, the uptake of services and the efficiency and effectiveness of services. The uptake of services may be influenced by their acceptability, ease of access to them, perception of need by patients, social factors, and family and social support. A detailed review of the circumstances of 17 deaths from hypertension in one area in England (Singal *et al.* 1985) showed, for example, that the following potentially 'avoidable factors' may have contributed to the deaths:

Patient:

(a) failure to recognize the gravity of the symptoms;
(b) delay in seeking advice;

(c) failure to keep appointment;
(d) habits likely to cause ill health;
(e) failure to change habits;
(f) confusion over medication;
(g) omitting to take medicine.

Primary care doctor:

(a) missed opportunity for screening, case finding, or early diagnosis;
(b) failure to carry out investigations for diagnosis;
(c) inappropriate selection of drugs;
(d) inadequate dosage of drugs;
(e) failure to monitor blood pressure.

First hospital contact:

(a) delay in providing treatment;
(b) inappropriate treatment;
(c) patient not seen by sufficiently senior doctor.

Subsequent hospital contact:

(a) too long a time between appointments;
(b) patient not seen by sufficiently senior doctor;
(c) drugs not changed when necessary;
(d) dosage not changed when necessary;
(e) inappropriate initial treatment.

Hospital in-patient episode:

(a) inappropriate treatment;
(b) inappropriate early discharge;
(c) inadequate follow-up.

A description of variation in potentially 'avoidable' mortality between areas is only the first step in a series of investigations (Charlton *et al.* 1984). Any explanation of this variation may require further investigation, and some examples of ways in which this might be done are outlined:

Trends in the indicators

This may require the updating of indicators for a further 5-year period and the development of methods to show both the changes in mortality between the two periods and year on year trends over the 10-year period for the whole group of diseases and for those diseases and areas where the number of deaths permits such analyses. A description of differences between areas and countries, in changes and trends in mortality may lead to hypotheses for further investigation (Charlton and Velez 1986; Charlton *et al.* 1986).

Macro-studies

An attempt may be made in these studies to explain variation in mortality, between areas and countries, using aggregate data (routinely available or specially collected) on disease incidence, or prevalence, case fatality, treatment patterns, diagnosis, certification and coding patterns, socio-economic factors, health service provision, and expenditure on health (Charlton *et al.* 1984*a,b*; Charlton and Lakhani 1985; Bauer and Charlton 1986). There are a number of problems in the reliability of aggregate data and comparability of data between areas and countries. There may also be interactions between the variables, which make the interpretation of such analyses difficult. For example, socio-economic factors may affect the uptake of services and their timely and appropriate use, and thus influence mortality. The availability of health services may directly influence mortality. However, socio-economic factors may also be associated with the availability of services, in that socially deprived areas may have a lower availability and quality of service.

Despite these problems with interpretation, such studies provide a useful and relatively inexpensive first-line investigation of variation in mortality, particularly between areas at the two extremes of the distribution (i.e. comparing areas with high and low mortality).

Mackenbach *et al.* (1990) have reviewed 11 aggregate data studies on 'avoidable' mortality and health services published since 1983. They concluded that:

—the low levels of mortaltity from amenable causes which presently prevail in industrialized countries do probably reflect, at least in part, the increased effectiveness of health services.

—geographical variation in mortality from amenable causes has not yet been shown to reflect differences of health services.

—if geographical variation in mortality does reflect such differences, the latter arise from circumstances other than the level of supply, for example from more specific aspects of health care delivery, and are probably closely related to socio-economic circumstances.

It is improbable that more aggregate data studies will contribute to a further understanding of the determinants of 'avoidable' mortality. In-depth studies at the individual level are much more likely to produce new knowledge of factors limiting the effectiveness of health services.

Micro-studies

These studies may involve the investigation of individual deaths in an attempt to identify factors that either explain variation in mortality or identify 'avoidable factors' (i.e. aspects of service availability, uptake, appropriate use, efficiency, and effectiveness that may have contributed to the mortality). There are several stages in such investigations. The first stage is an examination of death certificates and health records to check the diagnoses, certification, and coding of causes of death for each case. This will establish how many deaths may still be classified as 'avoidable', in keeping with the study definition. The next stage may be to map all such deaths within small areas, to investigate clustering, and hence develop hypotheses for future investigation. The third stage is a detailed, confidential enquiry into each death, to identify potentially 'avoidable factors', for example, as previously described for hypertension. The problem with these studies is that the evidence on 'avoidable factors' tends to be subjective and circumstantial and some of these factors may also apply to cases who have survived. In order to help assess the importance of different 'avoidable factors', it may be necessary to study controls as well (i.e. cases matched for age, sex, diagnosis, and area of residence, but who survived). Before undertaking any confidential enquiry, criteria of what constitutes 'avoidable factors' should be established.

Standardized questionnaires, lists of potentially 'avoidable factors' and guidelines for the classification of factors for each disease would have to be prepared. The confidential enquiry may be carried out by sending questionnaires to doctors involved in the management of each case and also by extracting information from medical care records, if these are available. The questionnaires may then be examined by independent assessors, who would use the lists and guidelines to determine the part each 'avoidable factor' plays in each case. Differences between cases and controls in 'avoidable factors', or common factors observed in a large number of cases and also for a number of diseases, may identify shortcomings in service provision and uptake that are amenable to intervention.

Confidential enquiries on maternal, perinatal, asthma, hypertension, cervical cancer, and perioperative deaths have shown such shortcomings and have led to service improvements in the UK (Singal *et al.* 1985; Buck *et al.* 1987). In the United Kingdom further investigations into the relationship between incidence, treatment and outcome are being carried out on stroke, cancer of the cervix, and cancer of the bladder. United Kingdom regional health authorities are introducing routine investigations into 'avoidable' mortality. The COMAC-EPI has set up an EC working party to study incidence, treatment, and outcome in asthma.

4. INTERPRETATION DES RESULTATS ET PERSPECTIVES D'AVENIR

Les cartes et les tableaux de cet atlas montrent la mortalité et quelques aperçus de l'état économique, des ressources du système de santé par région, à la fois dans la cadre national et dans le cadre européen. Il y a toutefois des limites à l'utilisation de cette information dans les comparaisons intra- et inter-pays. La validité et la comparabilité des données peuvent différer entre les pays et, dans une moindre mesure, entre les régions d'un même pays. Par exemple, les données sur les ressources de santé et les indicateurs sociaux ne sont pas toujours disponibles les mêmes années dans tous les pays, et dans certains cas, aucune donnée n'est disponible. Les définitions utilisés different d'un pays à l'autre.

Les variations de la mortalité observées entre les pays et les régions peuvent être artificielles et dépendre de variantes dans la collecte des données, c'est-à-dire du diagnostic, de la certification, et du codage des décès. Kelson et Heller (1983) ont montré que le classement des maladies varie d'un pays à l'autre : ils trouvèrent de nettes différences entre huit pays de la CEE, dans la déclaration des maladies respiratoires aiguës au niveau du diagnostic. Ces divergences furent attribuées à la manière dont les médecins rédigent le certificat de décès, et subsidiairement au codage. Néanmoins, d'autres auteurs (Diehl et Gau 1982) soutiennent que les nuances de classement ne peuvent expliquer la totalité des différences entre régions. Les différences importantes des niveaux de la mortalité 'évitable', qui sont montrées dans cet atlas, sont vraisemblablement très peu dues au seul hasard ou à des différences de certification et de codage des causes de décès.

Inversement, les différences de mortalité peuvent découler des variations de l'incidence ou de la prévalence des maladies ou encore des disparités dans la déliverance des soins, l'efficacité, et le rendement des services. Par exemple, la morbidité due aux maladies infectieuses de l'enfance, ou à la tuberculose, peut être évitée, et la fréquence de la maladie dépend de la disponibilité et de l'utilisation appropriée des services de prévention primaire, c'est-à-dire la vaccination et la promotion de la santé. Pour d'autres maladies, par exemple l'asthme, tous les décès ne sont pas évitables mais l'intervention appropriée en temps utile, et les différences d'intensité de la maladie selon les régions, devraient être prises en compte dans l'analyse des variations de la mortalité. Dans d'autres affections enfin, le cancer du col par exemple, les décès sont en grande partie évitables par une intervention adéquate et à temps des services de santé, indépendamment de l'incidence et de la prévalence, dont les variations peuvent expliquer mais non justifier la variation de la mortalité.

La fatalité peut être influencée par la disponibilité des services, leur rapidité d'intervention, leur rendement, et leur efficacité. La rapidité d'intervention des services peut dépendre de leur implantation, leur accessibilité, mais aussi de la perception qu'en ont les patients, et enfin, de facteurs sociaux et familiaux. Une revue détaillée des circonstances dans lesquelles dix-sept décès dûs à l'hypertension se produisirent dans une région d'Angleterre (Singal et al. 1985) a mis en évidence vingt-trois facteurs potentiellement évitables, qui avaient contribué au décès, et qui sont les suivants:

Du coté du patient:

(a) non-reconnaissance de la gravité des symptômes;
(b) délai dans la prise de conseil;
(c) manquement au rendez-vous;
(d) habitudes néfastes à la santé;
(e) difficulté à changer d'habitudes;
(f) confusion sur le traitement;
(g) oubli de prendre les médicaments.

Soins primaires, médicin:

(a) absence d'examen ou de diagnostic précoce;
(b) défaillance à entreprendre les investigations nécessaires au diagnostic;
(c) choix des médicaments inadapté;
(d) dosage des médicaments inadéquat;
(e) contrôle insuffisant de la pression sanguine.

Premier recours hospitalier:

(a) délai dans la mise en oeuvre d'un traitement;
(b) traitement inapproprié;
(c) patient non examiné par un médecin expérimenté.

Recours hospitalier ultérieur:

(a) délai trop long entre rendez-vous;
(b) patient non examiné par un médecin expérimenté;
(c) médicaments non changés quand nécessaire;
(d) dosage des médicaments non modifié quand nécessaire;
(e) traitement initial inadapté.

Episode d'hospitalisation:

(a) traitement inadapté;
(b) sortie prématurée;
(c) surveillance inadéquate.

La description des variations par région de la 'mortalité potentiellement évitable' n'est que la première étape d'une série d'investigations sur les services de santé (Charlton et al. 1984a). Toute explication de ces variations suppose des recherches supplémentaires: quelques exemples d'orientations possibles sont suggérés ci-dessous.

Tendances des indicateurs

Ceci requiert la mise à jour des indicateurs pour une période ultérieure de cinq années ainsi que le développement de méthodes permettant de montrer à la fois les changements de la mortalité entre les deux périodes, et la tendance année par année sur les dix années pour l'ensemble des affections et les maladies dans les régions où le nombre de décès permettrait une telle analyse. La description des différences dans les changements et les tendances de la mortalité selon les régions et les pays, pourrait conduire aux hypothèses des investigations supplémentaires (Charlton et Velez 1986; Charlton *et al.* 1986).

Etudes macroscopiques

Dans ces études on peut tenter d'expliquer les variations de la mortalité, selon les régions et les pays en utilisant des données agrégées ordinairement disponibles, ou spécialement collectées, sur l'incidence ou la prévalence des affections, la létalité, les catégories de traitement, les diagnostics, les modèles de certification et de codage, les facteurs socio-économiques, l'equipement sanitaire, et les dépenses (Charlton *et al.* 1984 *a,b*; Charlton et Lakhani 1985; Bauer et Charlton 1986). Les données agrégées posent des problèms de validité et de comparaison entre régions et pays. Il peut également y avoir interaction entre les variables, ce qui complique l'interprétation de ces analyses. Par exemple, les facteurs socio-economiques peuvent agir sur la qualité des services, leur utilisation adaptée en temps utile, et de là, influer sur la mortalité. La disponibilité des services de santé peut influencer directement la mortalité. Néanmoins, les facteurs socio-économiques sont également associés avec la disponibilité des services, en ce que les régions socialement défavorisées disposent d'une moindre qualité et disponibilité des services.

En dépit de ces problèmes d'interprétation, de telles études produisent une première investigation utile et peu onéreuse, des variations de la mortalité, en particulier entre les zones situées aux extrémités de la distribution, c'est-à-dire comparant les régions à haute et basse mortalité.

Mackenbach *et al.* (1990) ont passé en revue 11 études de données agrégées, publiées depuis 1983, sur la relation entre mortalité 'évitable' et services de santé. Ils en ont conclu que :

— Les faibles niveaux de la mortalité due à des causes 'evitables', qui actuellement prévalent dans les pays industrialisés, reflètent en partie au moins une efficacité accrue des services de santé.

— Il n'a pas été possible de mettre en évidence une relation directe entre les variations géographiques de la mortalité de causes 'évitable' et les différences dans les services de santé.

— Si des variations géographiques de la mortalité reflètent des différences de services, d'autres circonstances que le niveau de l'offre, par exemple des aspects plus spécifiques de la délivrance des soins, interviennent qui sont probablement davantage liés aux conditions socio-économiques.

Il est peu probable que le développement des études sur les données agrégées contribue à une meilleure compréhension des déterminants de la mortalité 'évitable'. En revanche, des études approfondies, menées au niveau individuel, renouveleraient vraisemblablement la connaissance des facteurs qui limitent la portée des services de soins.

Etudes microscopiques

Il s'agit de mettre en oeuvre des études de cas afin d'identifier les facteurs qui, soit expliquent les changements de la mortalité, soit font apparaitre les facteurs évitables, c'est-à-dire certains aspects de la disponibilité (qualité, utilisation, rendement et efficacité) des services, ayant pu contribuer à la mortalité. Plusieurs étapes sont nécessaires dans de telles recherches. La première peut être un examen approfondi des certificats de décès et des dossiers hospitaliers pour vérifier les diagnostics, la certification, et le codage des causes de décès dans chaque cas. Ceci permettrait d'établir combien de décès peuvent être classés comme 'évitables' compte tenu de la définition de l'étude.

L'étape suivante pourrait être la cartographie de tous ces décès, à l'intérieur de petites zones, pour inventorier les regroupements et de là développer les hypothèses d'une recherche ultérieure. La troisième étape pourrait être une enquête confidentielle mais détaillée, de chaque décès, de manière à identifier les éventuels 'facteurs évitables' tels ceux décrits par exemple pour l'hypertension ou les anesthésies (Tiret *et al.* 1986). Le problème, dans de telles enquêtes, est que la mise en évidence des 'facteurs évitables' tend à être subjective et circonstancielle, en outre certains de ces mêmes facteurs pourraient être appliqués aux cas qui ont survécu. De manière à établir l'importance des différents 'facteurs évitables', il pourrait être nécessaire d'étudier les témoins, c'est-à-dire des cas appariés par sexe, âge, diagnostic et zone de résidence, mais ayant survécu. Avant d'entreprendre une enquête confidentielle, les critères de ce qui constitue les 'facteurs évitables' doivent être établis.

Des questionnaires homogènes, des listes de facteurs potentiellement évitables, et des directives pour le classement des facteurs de chaque affection devraient être préparés. L'enquête confidentielle pourrait être entreprise en envoyant des questionnaires aux médecins impliqués dans chaque cas et aussi en extrayant l'information des dossiers médicaux, s'ils sont disponibles. Les questionnaires pourraient ensuite être examinés (revus) par des experts indépendants, qui utiliseraient les listes et les recommandations, et détermineraient dans quelle mesure chaque 'facteur évitable' s'applique à chaque cas. Les différences entre les cas et les témoins dans les 'facteurs évitables', ou les facteurs communs observés dans un grand nombre de cas et aussi pour certaines affections, permettraient peut être d'identifier les insuffisances dans la prestation des services et ce qui est susceptible de être amélioré par une intervention. Des enquêtes confidentielles sur les mortalités maternelle et périnatale, sur l'asthme, l'hypertension, les décès du cancer, et les décès péri-opératoires ont contribué à mettre en évidence certaines imperfections, et à conduire à l'amélioration des services (Singal *et al.* 1985; Buck *et al.* 1987 au Royaume-Uni; Hatton et Tiret 1983 en France). Au Royaume-Uni des investigations ultérieures sur la relation entre incidence, traitement et issue, sont actuellement entreprises sur l'accident vasculaire cérébral, le cancer du col de l'utérus, et le cancer de la vessie. Les autorités sanitaires régionales du Royaume-Uni introduisent des investigations de 'routine' sur la mortalité 'évitable'. En France, une recherche sur l'incidence de la morbidité maternelle grave et les facteurs d'évitement de la mortalité maternelle a été entreprise. Le COMAC-EPI a établi un groupe de travail européen pour étudier l'incidence, le traitement, et l'issue de l'asthme.

4. INTERPRETATION DER KARTEN UND DATEN UND VORSCHLÄGE FÜR WEITERE UNTERSUCHUNGEN

Die Karten und Tabellen in diesem Atlas zeigen die Mortalität, den sozio-ökonomischen Status und Gesundheitsdienstleistungen in Bezug auf Regionen, sowohl im Rahmen eines jeden Landes als auch im Rahmen der EG insgesamt. Es gibt jedoch Grenzen des Nutzens dieser Information, sowohl in Bezug auf jedes Land als auch in Bezug auf Vergleiche zwischen den Ländern. Es können Unterschiede zwischen den Ländern und in geringerem Masse, zwischen den Regionen eines nämlichen Landes, in Bezug auf die Gültigkeit und Vergleichbarkeit der Daten auftreten. Daten über Gesundheitsdienstleistungen und soziale Indikatoren sind z.B. nicht immer für die gleichen Jahre und für alle Länder verfügbar; für einige Länder fehlen diese Angaben überhaupt. Die benutzten Definitionen unterscheiden sich von Land zu Land.

Die ermittelten Abweichungen der Mortalität zwischen Ländern und Regionen können auch ein Artefakt sein, der auf Unterschieden in der Datensammlung, Diagnose, Auswahl und Signierung der Todesursache beruht. Die Klassifikation von Krankheiten ist unterschiedlich, wie von Kelson und Heller (1983) gezeigt wurde. Sie fanden, dass sich bei akuten respiratorischen Erkrankungen grosse Unterschiede in der Benennung von Diagnosen zwischen acht EG-Ländern zeigten. Diese Unterschiede wurden darauf zurückgeführt, wie Ärzte die Todesbescheinigung ausgefüllt hatten und wie kodiert wurde. Andere Autoren haben jedoch gezeigt, dass diese Differenzen bei der Klassifizierung nicht den gesamten Unterschied zwischen Regionen erklären könnte (Diehl und Gau (1982). Der Unterschiedsbereich der 'vermeidbaren' Mortalitätsgrade der in diesem Atlas gezeigt wird, lässt sich wohl kaum als Zufallsprodukt, oder mit Unterschieden beim Kodieren und Ausstellen der Todesbescheinigungen erklären.

Andererseits können Abweichungen auch auf Unterschieden in der Inzidenz und Prävalenz der Krankheiten, oder auf geographischen Unterschieden in der Versorgungsdichte und Effektivität von Gesundheitsdiensten beruhen. Für einige Krankheiten, z.B. den Infektionskrankheiten bei Kindern und der Tuberkulose, sind Todesfälle vermeidbar: die Inzidenz und Prävalenz der Krankheit wird stark durch die Bereitstellung und angemessene Anwendung von primärpräventiven Massnahmen durch die Gesundheitsdienste, z.B. Impfung, und die Gesundheitserziehung beeinflusst. Bei einigen Krankheiten, z.B. Asthma, lassen sich nicht alle Todesfälle durch zeitgerechte und richtige medizinische Intervention vermeiden. Die unterschiedliche Inzidenz und Prävalenz zwischen Regionen sollte in Betracht gezogen werden, wenn Unterschiede in der Mortalität zu beurteilen sind. Für andere Krankheiten, z.B. Cervix-Krebs, lassen sich Sterbefälle in grösserem Umfang durch adäquate und zeitgerechte medizinische Intervention vermeiden, unabhängig von der Grösse der Inzidenz oder Prävalenz; durch Unterschiede in der Inzidenz oder Prävalenz lassen sich zwar Abweichungen in der Mortalität erklären, aber nicht rechtfertigen.

Die Letalität kann durch die Bereitstellung von Gesundheitsdiensten, der Inanspruchnahme und Wirksamkeit von Gesundheitsdienstleistungen beeinflusst werden. Die Inanspruchnahme von Gesundheitsdienstleistungen lässt sich durch ihre Annehmbarkeit, leichte Erreichbarkeit, Wahrnehmung der Notwendigkeit einer medizinischen Intervention durch die Patienten, soziale Faktoren, familiäre und soziale Unterstützung beeinflussen. Eine ausführliche Untersuchung der Umstände von siebzehn Todesfällen an Hypertonie in einer Region Englands (Singal u. Mitarbeiter 1985), zeigte 23 möglicherweise 'vermeidbare Faktoren' die zu diesen Todesfällen beigetragen haben:

Patient:

(a) Nichterkennen der schwerwiegenden Symptome;
(b) Zeitliche Verzögerung bei der Konsultation;
(c) Nichteinhaltung von Terminen;
(d) gesundheitsschädigende Gewohnheiten;
(e) mangelnde Veränderung von Verhaltensweisen;
(f) Verwirrung hinsichtlich der Medikation;
(g) Nichteinnahme von Medikamenten.

Primärversorgung, Arzt:

(a) verpasste Gelegenheit für eine Gesamtuntersuchung. Klärung der Krankheit;
(b) Nichtausführen diagnostischer Massnahmen;
(c) falsche Auswahl von Medikamenten;
(d) inadäquate Dosierung der Medikamente;
(e) keine Blutdrucküberwachung.

Erster Krankenhauskontakt:

(a) Verzögerung im Beginn der Behandlung;
(b) falsche Behandlung;
(c) Patient wurde nicht durch einen erfahreneren Kollegen gesehen.

Nachfolgender Krankenhauskontakt:

(a) zu grosser Zeitraum zwischen den Terminen;
(b) Patient wurde nicht durch einen erfahreneren Kollegen gesehen;
(c) die Medikamente wurden nicht bei Bedarf gewechselt;
(d) die Dosierung wurde nicht bei Bedarf gewechselt;
(e) falsche primäre Behandlung.

Krankenhausaufenthalt (stationäre Behandlung):

(a) falsche Behandlung;
(b) zu frühe Entlassung;
(c) inadäquates Verfolgen der Krankengeschichte (follow-up).

Eine Beschreibung der Schwankungen möglicherweise 'vermeidbarer' Mortalität zwischen den Regionen, ist nur der erste Schritt in einer Reihe von Untersuchungen der Gesundheitsdienste (Charlton u. Mitarbeiter 1984a). Jede Erklärung für die Abweichungen muss auf zusätzliche Untersuchungen zurückgreifen: hier werden dafür einige Beispiele aufgezeigt.

Tendenzen der Indikatoren

Eine Untersuchung von Tendenzen erfordert die Aktualisierung der Indikatoren für weitere 5 Jahre und die Entwicklung von Methoden, die sowohl die Veränderungen der Mortalität zwischen zwei Perioden, als auch die Veränderung in einzelnen Jahren über einen 10 Jahreszeitraum für die Gruppe von Krankheiten insgesamt und für solche Krankheiten und Regionen aufzeigt, bei denen die Anzahl der Todesfälle eine solche Analyse erlaubt. Eine Beschreibung der Unterschiede zwischen Regionen und Ländern in Bezug auf Änderungen und Tendenzen der Mortalität, könnte zu Hypothesen und weiteren Untersuchungen führen (Charlton u.Velez 1986; Charlton u.Mitarbeiter 1986).

Makrostudien

Bei diesen Studien könnte versucht werden, Unterschiede der Mortalität zwischen Regionen und Ländern durch Aggregatsdaten zu erklären (Routinedaten oder speziell zu diesem Zweck gesammelte Daten über Krankheitshäufigkeit oder Prävalenz, Letalität, Behandlungsweisen, Diagnosen, Zertifikation und Kodierungspraktiken, sozioökonomische Faktoren, sowie Gesundheitsdienstleistungen und finanziellen Ausgaben für die Gesundheit: (Bauer u. Charlton 1986; Charlton u. Mitarbeiter 1984a,b; Charlton u. Lakhani 1985).

Es gibt eine Reihe von Problemen hinsichtlich der Triftigkeit von aggregierten Daten und der Vergleichbarkeit von Daten zwischen Regionen und Ländern. Es bestehen darüber hinaus Abhängigkeiten zwischen den 'Variablen', die eine solche Interpretation und Analyse schwierig machen. Sozio-ökonomische Faktoren z.B. können die Inanspruchnahme von Gesundheitsdiensten, deren zeitgerechte und richtige Nutzung und dadurch die Mortalität beeinflussen. Das Vorhandensein von Gesundheitsdiensten kann dadurch die Mortalität beeinflussen, sozio-ökonomische Faktoren können aber auch mit der Bereitstellung von Dienstleistungen in der Weise verknüpft sein, so dass in sozial rückständigen Regionen schlechtere und weniger gut zugängliche Dienste vorhanden sind.

Trotz dieser Probleme bei der Auswertung, stellen solche Studien eine nützliche und relativ kostengünstige Methode zur Untersuchung der Mortalität zwischen Regionen im Extrembereich der Verteilung dar, d.h. für den Vergleich von Regionen mit hoher und niedriger Mortalität.

Mackenbach u. Mitarbeiter (1990) haben 11 Studien mit aggregierten Daten über 'vermeidbare' Sterbefälle untersucht, die seit 1983 veröffentlicht wurden. Sie kamen zu dem Schluss dass:

—die geringe Mortalität an behandelbaren Krankheiten, die gegenwärtig in den industrialisierten Ländern vorherrscht, zumindest teilweise die gestiegene Wirksamkeit medizinischer Dienste reflektiert;

—geographische Schwankungen in Mortalität behandelbarer Krankheiten bis jetzt noch nicht gezeigt haben, dass sie Unterschiede der Gesundheitsdienste wiedergeben;

—wenn geographische Schwankungen in Mortalität tatsächlich solche Unterschiede wiedergeben, dann sind diese auf andere Umstände zurückzuführen als auf den Grad der Versorgung, nämlich auf mehr spezifische Aspekte der gesundheitlichen Versorgung, und wahrscheinlich eng mit den sozio-ökonomischen Verhältnissen verbunden.

Es ist unwahrscheinlich, dass weitere Studien anhand von aggregierten Daten zu einem vertieften Verständnis bestimmter Faktoren der 'vermeidbaren' Mortalität beitragen können. Tiefgehende Studien auf der Basis von Einzelfällen sind besser geeignet neue Erkenntnisse über Faktoren zu vermitteln, die die Wirksamkeit von Gesundheitsdiensten begrenzen.

Mikrostudien

Diese Studien können auch die Untersuchung einzelner Todesfälle einschliessen, mit dem Versuch die Faktoren herauszufinden, die die Unterschiede der Mortalität erklären oder die 'vermeidbaren' Faktoren identifizieren, d.h. Aspekte der Gesundheitsdienste in Bezug auf Verfügbarkeit, Inanspruchnahme, angemessenem Gebrauch, Nutzleistung und Wirksamkeit im Hinblick auf die Sterblichkeit zu untersuchen; die erste Stufe kann eine Untersuchung von Todesbescheinigungen und Unterlagen von Gesundheitsdiensten sein, um die Diagnose, die Dokumentation und Kodierung jedes Sterbefalles zu überprüfen. Dabei kann geklärt werden, wieviele Todesfälle als 'vermeidbar' im Sinne der Definition dieser Studie eingeordnet werden können.

Die nächste Stufe könnte die Eintragung solcher Todesfälle in einer Karte für kleine Regionen sein, um herauszufinden ob sich diese auf bestimmte Bereiche konzentrieren, um daraus Hypothesen für weitere Untersuchungen ableiten zu können.

Die dritte Stufe könnte eine ausführliche, vertrauliche Untersuchung jedes einzelnen Todefalles sein, um mögliche 'vermeidbare' Faktoren zu finden, z.B. in der Weise wie es zuvor für Hypertonie beschrieben wurde. Die Schwierigkeit solcher Studien liegt darin, dass der Beweis 'vermeidbare' Faktoren subjektiv ausgelegt und auch auf solche Fälle übertragen wird, die überlebt haben. Um die Bedeutung einzelner 'vermeidbarer' Faktoren zu untersuchen, wird es notwendig sein, diese bestimmten Kontrollen zu unterwerfen, d.h. auch Fälle zu untersuchen, die im Bezug auf Alter, Geschlecht, Diagnose und Wohnort vergleichbar sind, die aber überlebt haben.

Bevor man aber mit einer vertraulichen Untersuchung beginnt, sollte man Kriterien für die Beschaffenheit 'vermeidbarer' Faktoren festlegen. Standardisierte Fragebogen, Listen von möglicherweise 'vermeidbaren' Faktoren und Richtlinien für die Klassifikation von Faktoren für jede Krankheit müssten vorbereitet werden. Die vertauliche Untersuchung kann mit Hilfe von Fragebogen an die behandelnden Ärzte und durch Einbeziehen von Informationen aus Krankenhausunterlagen und Aufzeichnungen aus Patienten-Karteien, falls diese vorhanden sind, vorgenommen werden. Die Fragebogen können dann durch unabhängige Untersucher überprüft werden, die auf der Basis von Listen und Richtlinien feststellen, welche Rolle der jeweilige 'vermeidbare' Faktor in jedem Einzelfalle spielt.

Unterschiede zwischen Fällen und Kontrollen in 'vermeidbaren' Faktoren oder allgemeinen Faktoren, die bei einer grossen Zahl von Fällen beobachtet werden können und die auch auf eine Anzahl von Krankheiten zutreffen, können Defizite in Vorsorge, in Gesundheitsdiensten und deren Nutzung identification und die darüberhinaus Eingriffen zugänglich sind.

Vertrauliche Untersuchungen über Mütter-und Perinatalsterbefälle, Sterbefälle an Asthma, Hypertonie, Cervix-Krebs und Sterbefälle vor,-während und nach Operationen haben solche Defizite gezeigt, und dann zu Verbesserungen bei den Gesundheitsdiensten in Gross-Britannien geführt (Singal u.Mitarbeiter 1985; Buck u.Mitarbeiter 1987).

In Gross-Britannien wurden weitere Untersuchungen über den Zusammenhang von Inzidenz, Behandlung und Erfolg bei Schlaganfall, Cervix-und Blasenkrebs durchgeführt.

Gesundheitsbehörden in den Regionen sind dabei Routine-Untersuchungen im Bezug auf 'vermeidbare' Sterblichkeit einzuführen.

Die COMAC-EPI hat eine EG-Arbeitsgruppe zur Untersuchung von Inzidenz, Behandlung und Erfolg bei Asthma, eingesetzt.

5. REFERENCES

1 Armitage, P. (1971). *Statistical methods in medical research.* Blackwell Scientific, Oxford.

2 Bauer, R.L. and Charlton, J.R.H. (1986). Area variation in mortality from diseases amenable to medical intervention: the contribution of differences in morbidity. *International Journal of Epidemiology,* **15**,408–12.

3 Buck N., Devlin, H.B., and Lunn, J.N.(1987). *Report of the confidential enquiry into perioperative deaths.* Nuffield Provincial Hospitals Trust and the King's Fund for Hospitals, London.

4 Burney, P. (1986). Asthma mortality in England and Wales: evidence for a further increase. 1974–78. *Lancet,* **ii**, 323.

5 Charlton, J.R.H. and Lakhani, A. (1985). Is the Jarman underprivileged area score valid? *British Medical Journal,* **290**, 1714–16.

6 Charlton, J.R.H. and Velez, R. (1986). Some international comparisons of mortality amenable to medical intervention. *British Medical Journal,* **292**, 295–301.

7 Charlton, J.R.H., Hartley, R.M., Silver, R., and Holland, W.W. (1983). Geographical variation in mortality from conditions amenable to medical intervention in England and Wales. *Lancet, i,* 691–6.

8 Charlton, J.R.H., Bauer, R., and Lakhani, A. (1984*a*). Outcome measures for district and regional health care planners. *Community Medicine,* **6**, 306–15.

9 Charlton, J.R.H., Prochazka, A., and Lakhani, A. (1984*b*). Death from appendicitis outside hospital? *Lancet,* **ii**, 399.

10 Charlton, J.R.H., Lakhani, A., and Aristidou, M. (1986). How have 'avoidable death' indices for England and Wales changed? 1974–78 compared with 1979–83. *Community Medicine,* **8**, 304–14.

11 Claymore Services Ltd (1988). INFO-MAP computer mapping package. Claymore Services Ltd, Station House, Wimple, Exeter.

12 Diehl, A.K. and Gau, D.W. (1982). Death certification by British doctors: a demographic analysis. *Journal of Epidemiology and Community Health,* **36**, 146–9.

13 Gail, M. (1978). The analysis of heterogeneity for indirect standardized mortality ratios. *Journal of the Royal Statistical Society,* **A141** (2), 224–34.

14 Kelson, M.C. and Heller, R.F. (1983). The effect of death certification and coding practices on observed differences in respiratory disease mortality in eight EC countries. *Revue d'Epidémiologie et de Santé Publique,* **31**, 423–32.

15 Rumeau-Rouquette, C., Breart, G., and Padieu, R. (1985). Méthodes en épidémiologie. Flammarion Médecine Sciences, Paris.

16 Rutstein, D.D., Berenberg, W., Chalmers, T.C., Child, C.G., *et al.* (1976). Measuring the quality of medical care. *New England Journal of Medicine,* **294**, 582–8.

17 Rutstein, D.D., Berenberg, W., Chalmers, T.C., Fishman, A.P., *et al.* (1980). Measuring the quality of medical care: second revision of tables and of indexes. *New England Journal of Medicine,* **302**, 1146.

18 Singal, G.M., Stillwell, P.J., Chambers, J., and Clews, B. (1985). *A confidential enquiry into premature preventable deaths.* Pilot study. Report to Walsall Health Authority, Walsall, England.

19 Tiret, L., Desmonts, J.M., Hatton, F., and Vourc'h, G. (1986). Complications associated with anaesthesia: a prospective survey in France. *Canadian Anaesthetists' Society Journal,* **33**, 336–44.

6. MAPS AND HISTOGRAMS FOR THE PERIOD 1980–84

Whole EC maps (pp.41–55)

1. These maps show SMRs (based on the EC standard) by disease and small area and are intended to show between-country variations.
2. Sextile intervals were used, the SMRs for each small area were ranked and one-sixth of the areas placed in each shading interval.
3. The histograms presented with the maps show the frequency distributions of the SMRs and are based on a grouping interval of 20. The same grouping interval is used for every histogram to provide a common scale on which variability of SMRs in different disease groups can be compared.

Individual country maps (pp.57–152)

1. These maps show SMRs (based on each country's own standard) by disease and small area and are intended to show within-country variation in an EC context.
2. SMRs were ranked and one-sixth of the areas placed in each shading interval.
3. The histograms presented with the maps show the frequency distributions of the SMRs and are based on a grouping interval of 20. The same grouping interval is used for every histogram to provide a common scale on which variability of SMRs in different disease groups can be compared. The histograms show in grey the distribution of small area SMRs based on national standards for the 451 areas of the whole EC, and in black the distribution of SMRs for the country in the map.

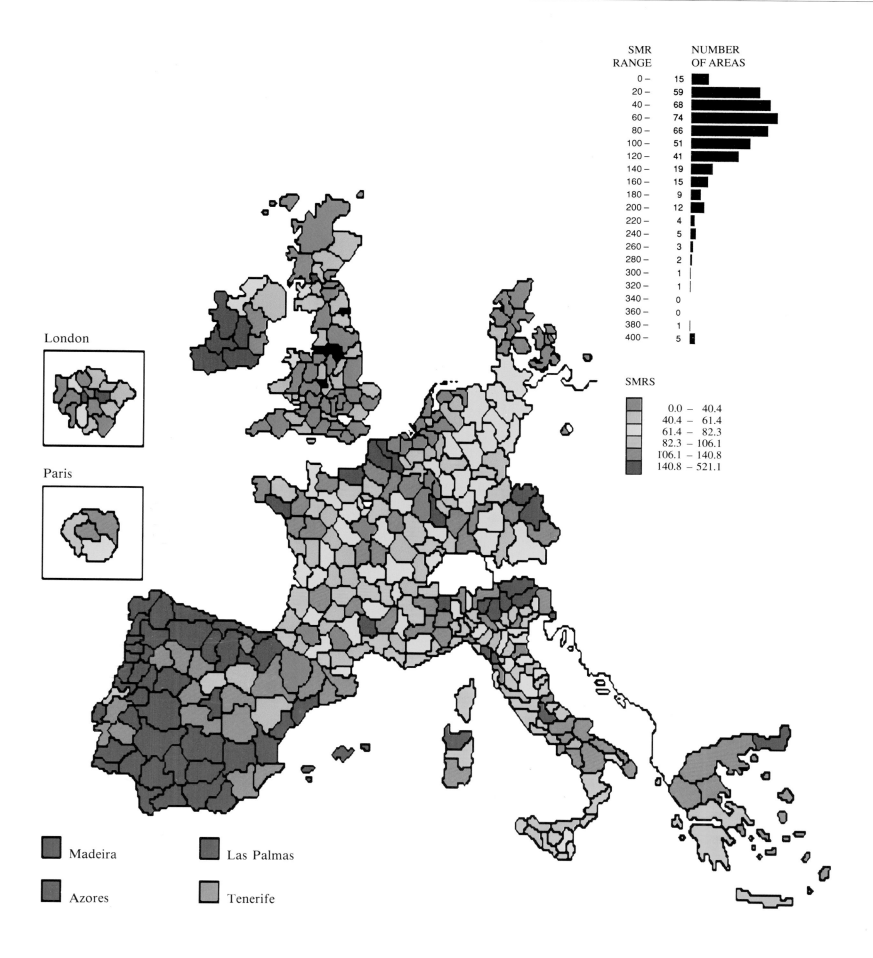

SMR RANGE	NUMBER OF AREAS
0 –	15
20 –	59
40 –	68
60 –	74
80 –	66
100 –	51
120 –	41
140 –	19
160 –	15
180 –	9
200 –	12
220 –	4
240 –	5
260 –	3
280 –	2
300 –	1
320 –	1
340 –	0
360 –	0
380 –	1
400 –	5

SMRS

0.0 – 40.4
40.4 – 61.4
61.4 – 82.3
82.3 – 106.1
106.1 – 140.8
140.8 – 521.1

London

Paris

Madeira

Las Palmas

Azores

Tenerife

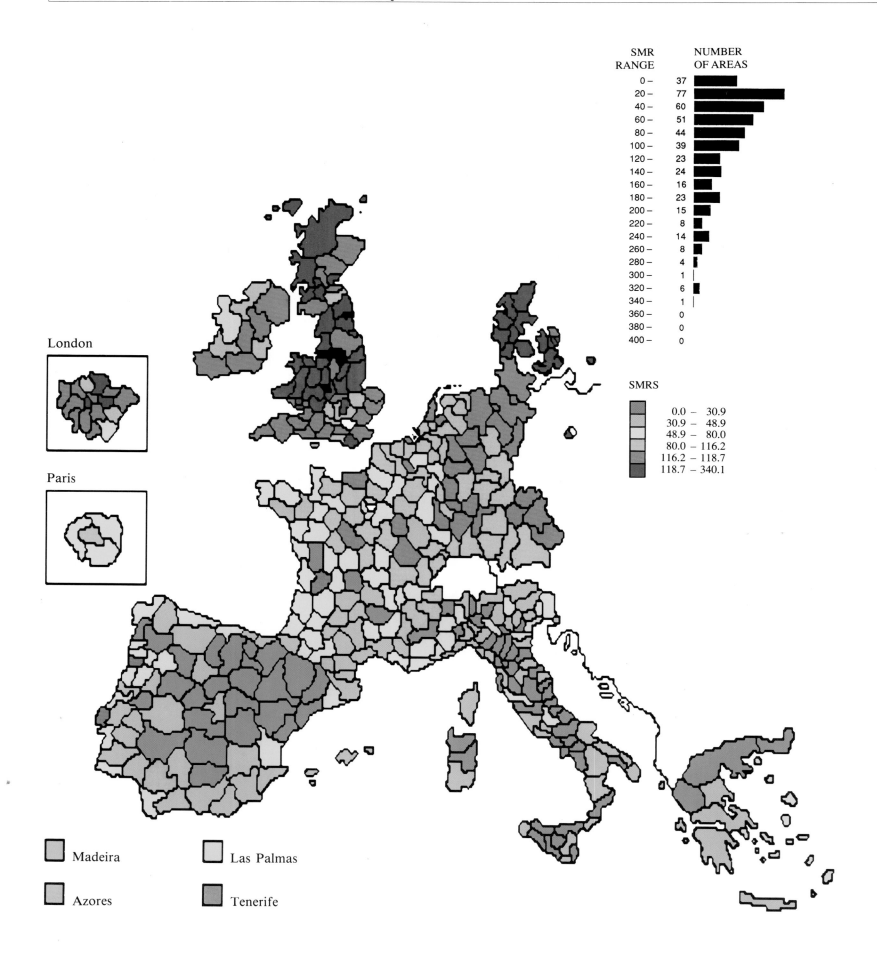

London

Paris

SMR
RANGE

NUMBER
OF AREAS

SMR RANGE	NUMBER OF AREAS
0 –	37
20 –	77
40 –	60
60 –	51
80 –	44
100 –	39
120 –	23
140 –	24
160 –	16
180 –	23
200 –	15
220 –	8
240 –	14
260 –	8
280 –	4
300 –	1
320 –	6
340 –	1
360 –	0
380 –	0
400 –	0

SMRS

	0.0 – 30.9
	30.9 – 48.9
	48.9 – 80.0
	80.0 – 116.2
	116.2 – 118.7
	118.7 – 340.1

Madeira

Las Palmas

Azores

Tenerife

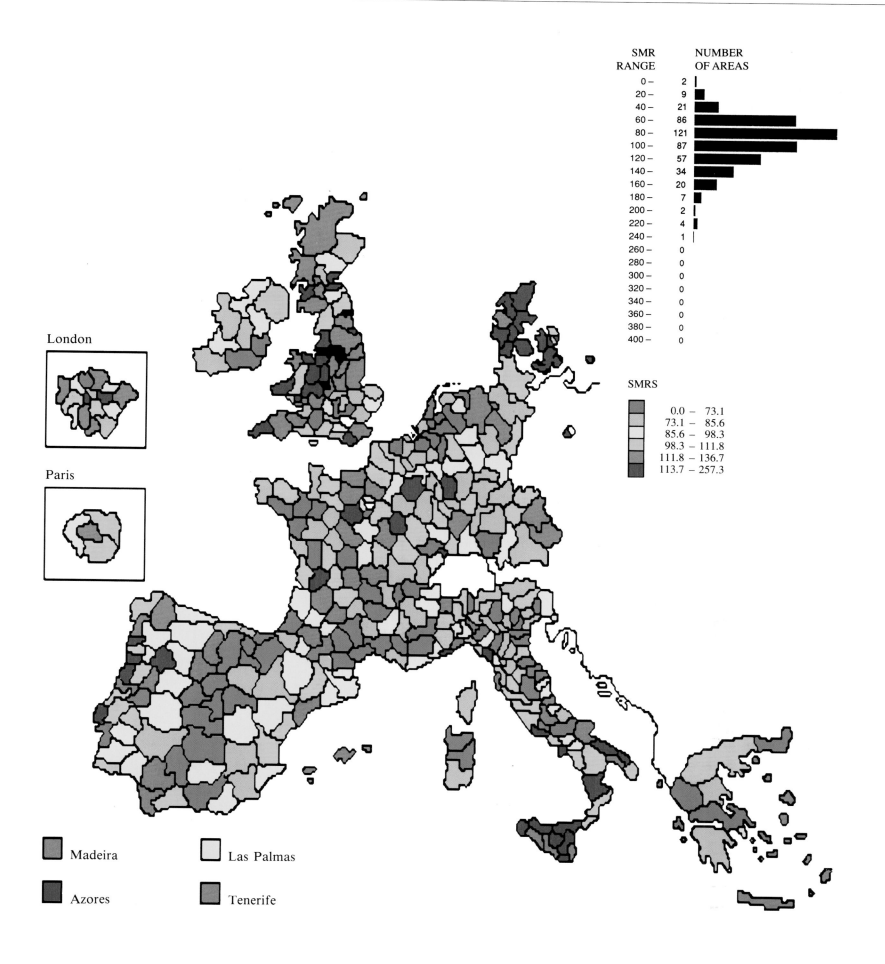

SMR RANGE	NUMBER OF AREAS
0 –	2
20 –	9
40 –	21
60 –	86
80 –	121
100 –	87
120 –	57
140 –	34
160 –	20
180 –	7
200 –	2
220 –	4
240 –	1
260 –	0
280 –	0
300 –	0
320 –	0
340 –	0
360 –	0
380 –	0
400 –	0

SMRS

0.0 –	73.1
73.1 –	85.6
85.6 –	98.3
98.3 –	111.8
111.8 –	136.7
113.7 –	257.3

London

Paris

Madeira   Las Palmas

Azores   Tenerife

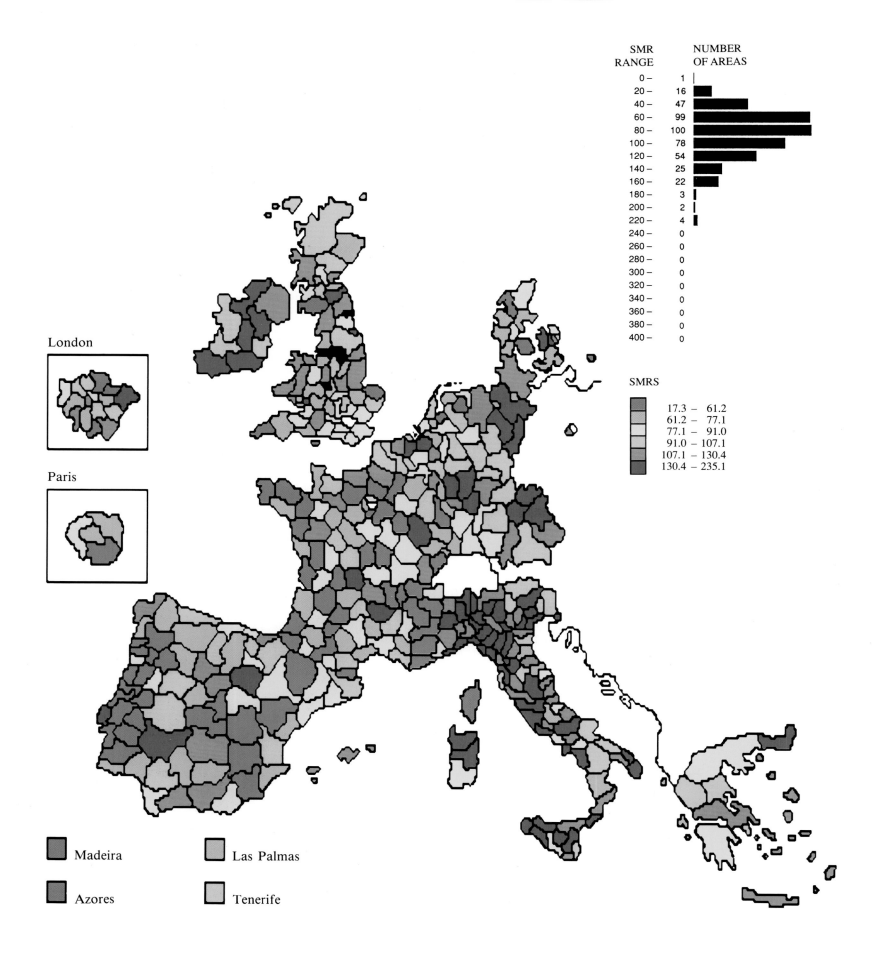

SMR RANGE	NUMBER OF AREAS
0 –	1
20 –	16
40 –	47
60 –	99
80 –	100
100 –	78
120 –	54
140 –	25
160 –	22
180 –	3
200 –	2
220 –	4
240 –	0
260 –	0
280 –	0
300 –	0
320 –	0
340 –	0
360 –	0
380 –	0
400 –	0

SMRS

17.3 – 61.2
61.2 – 77.1
77.1 – 91.0
91.0 – 107.1
107.1 – 130.4
130.4 – 235.1

London

Paris

Madeira

Azores

Las Palmas

Tenerife

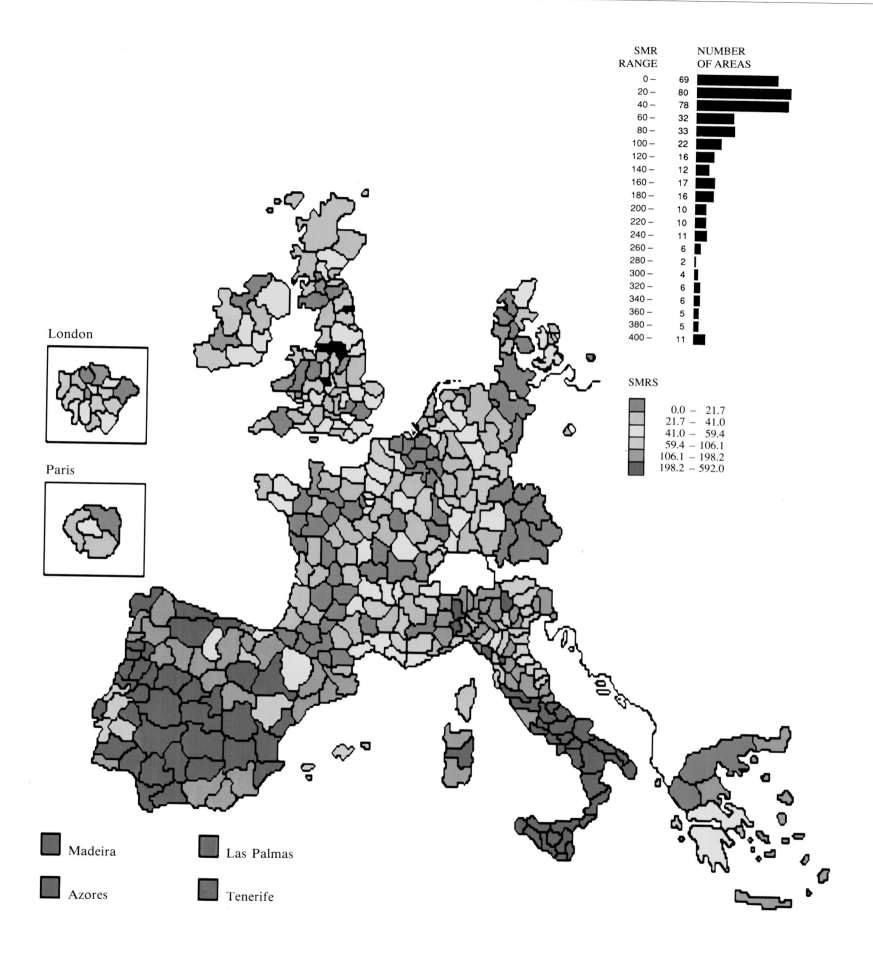

SMR RANGE	NUMBER OF AREAS
0 –	69
20 –	80
40 –	78
60 –	32
80 –	33
100 –	22
120 –	16
140 –	12
160 –	17
180 –	16
200 –	10
220 –	10
240 –	11
260 –	6
280 –	2
300 –	4
320 –	6
340 –	6
360 –	5
380 –	5
400 –	11

SMRS

0.0 – 21.7
21.7 – 41.0
41.0 – 59.4
59.4 – 106.1
106.1 – 198.2
198.2 – 592.0

London

Paris

Madeira

Azores

Las Palmas

Tenerife

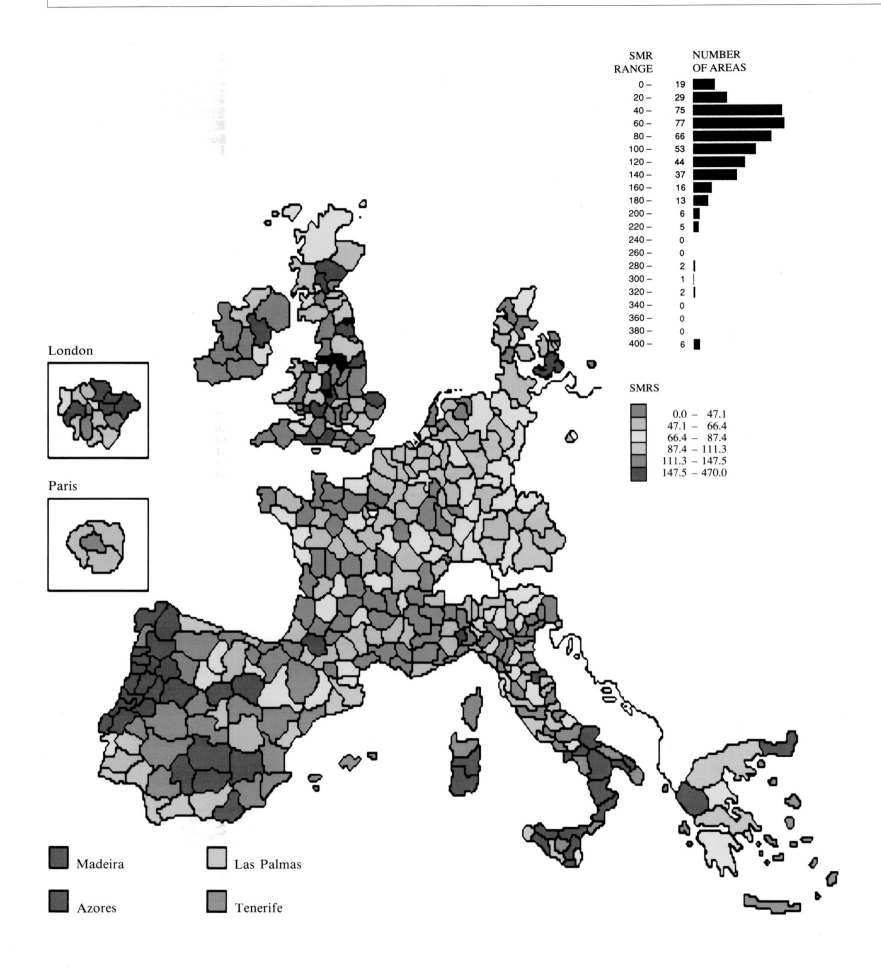

SMR RANGE | NUMBER OF AREAS
0 –	19
20 –	29
40 –	75
60 –	77
80 –	66
100 –	53
120 –	44
140 –	37
160 –	16
180 –	13
200 –	6
220 –	5
240 –	0
260 –	0
280 –	2
300 –	1
320 –	2
340 –	0
360 –	0
380 –	0
400 –	6

SMRS

0.0 – 47.1
47.1 – 66.4
66.4 – 87.4
87.4 – 111.3
111.3 – 147.5
147.5 – 470.0

London

Paris

Madeira

Azores

Las Palmas

Tenerife

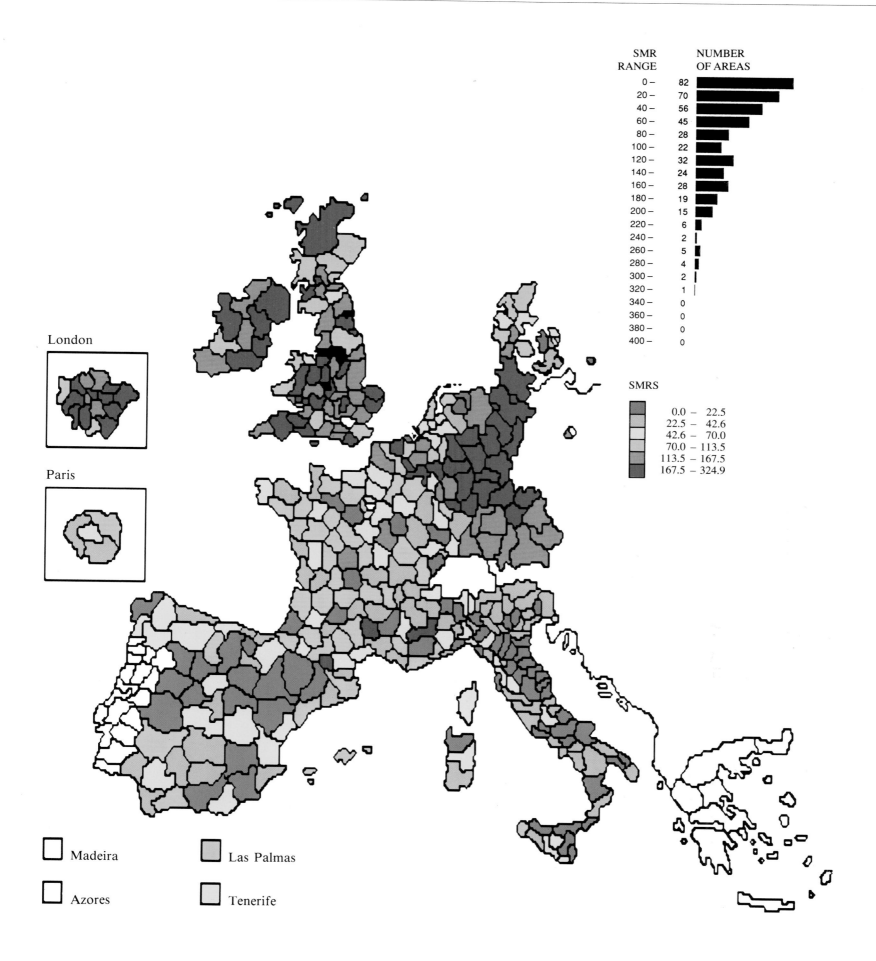

SMR
RANGE

NUMBER
OF AREAS

SMR RANGE	NUMBER OF AREAS
0 –	82
20 –	70
40 –	56
60 –	45
80 –	28
100 –	22
120 –	32
140 –	24
160 –	28
180 –	19
200 –	15
220 –	6
240 –	2
260 –	5
280 –	4
300 –	2
320 –	1
340 –	0
360 –	0
380 –	0
400 –	0

SMRS

0.0 – 22.5
22.5 – 42.6
42.6 – 70.0
70.0 – 113.5
113.5 – 167.5
167.5 – 324.9

London

Paris

Madeira

Azores

Las Palmas

Tenerife

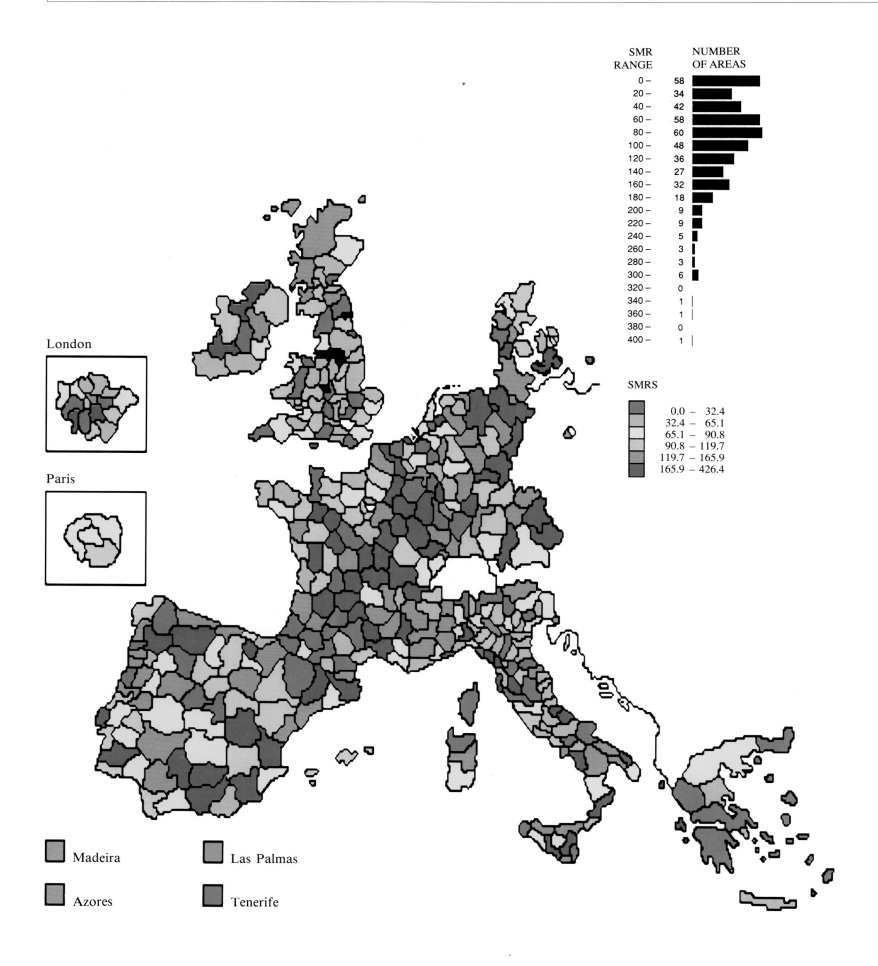

SMR RANGE	NUMBER OF AREAS
0 –	58
20 –	34
40 –	42
60 –	58
80 –	60
100 –	48
120 –	36
140 –	27
160 –	32
180 –	18
200 –	9
220 –	9
240 –	5
260 –	3
280 –	3
300 –	6
320 –	0
340 –	1
360 –	1
380 –	0
400 –	1

SMRS

0.0 – 32.4
32.4 – 65.1
65.1 – 90.8
90.8 – 119.7
119.7 – 165.9
165.9 – 426.4

London

Paris

Madeira

Azores

Las Palmas

Tenerife

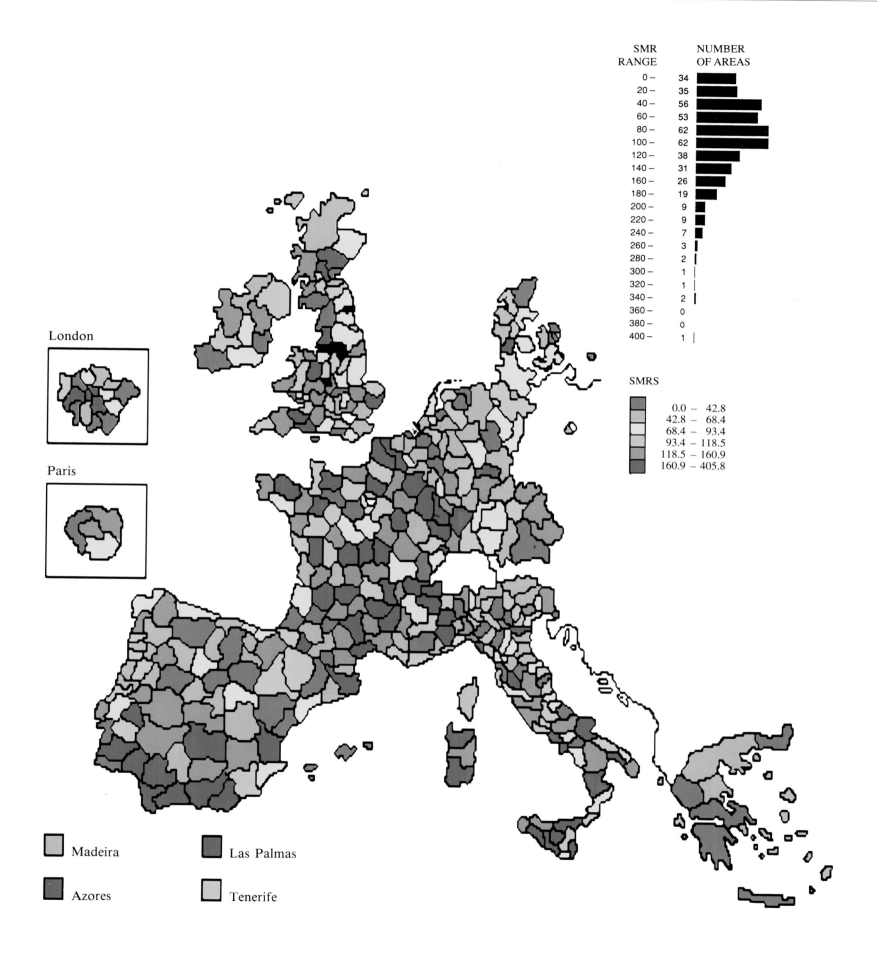

SMR
RANGE | NUMBER
OF AREAS
0 – | 34
20 – | 35
40 – | 56
60 – | 53
80 – | 62
100 – | 62
120 – | 38
140 – | 31
160 – | 26
180 – | 19
200 – | 9
220 – | 9
240 – | 7
260 – | 3
280 – | 2
300 – | 1
320 – | 1
340 – | 2
360 – | 0
380 – | 0
400 – | 1

SMRS

0.0 – 42.8
42.8 – 68.4
68.4 – 93.4
93.4 – 118.5
118.5 – 160.9
160.9 – 405.8

London

Paris

Madeira   Las Palmas

Azores   Tenerife

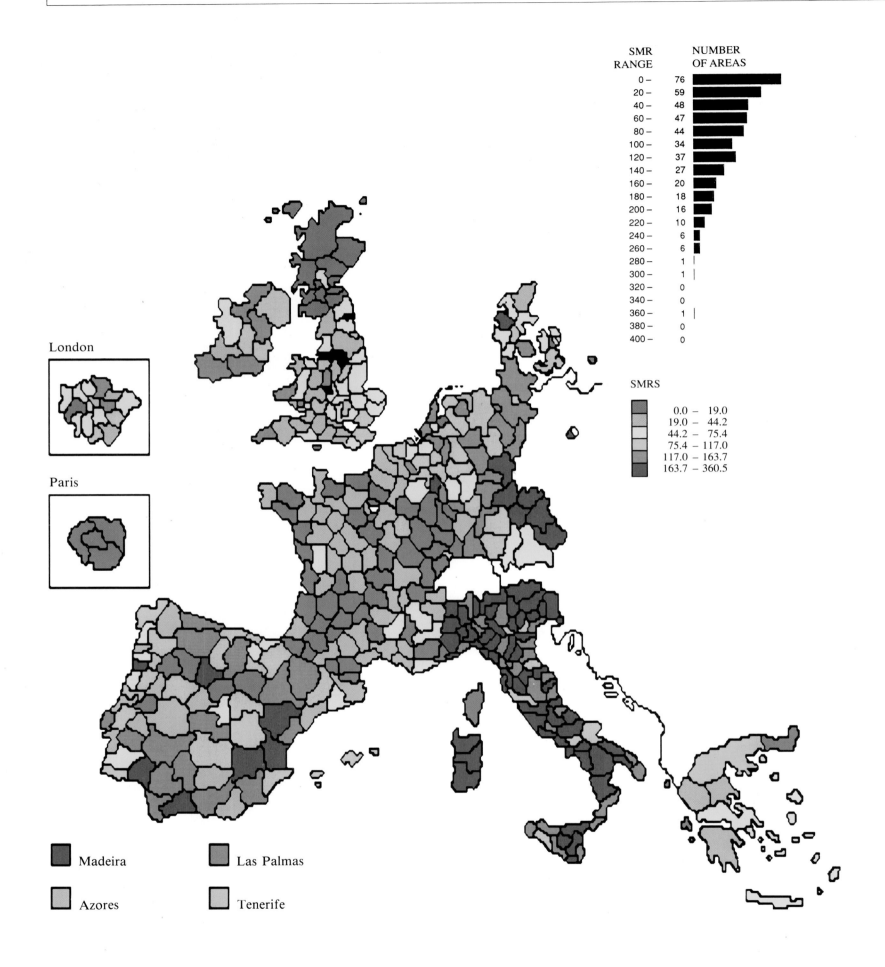

SMR RANGE	NUMBER OF AREAS
0 –	76
20 –	59
40 –	48
60 –	47
80 –	44
100 –	34
120 –	37
140 –	27
160 –	20
180 –	18
200 –	16
220 –	10
240 –	6
260 –	6
280 –	1
300 –	1
320 –	0
340 –	0
360 –	1
380 –	0
400 –	0

SMRS

	0.0 – 19.0
	19.0 – 44.2
	44.2 – 75.4
	75.4 – 117.0
	117.0 – 163.7
	163.7 – 360.5

London

Paris

Madeira   Las Palmas

Azores   Tenerife

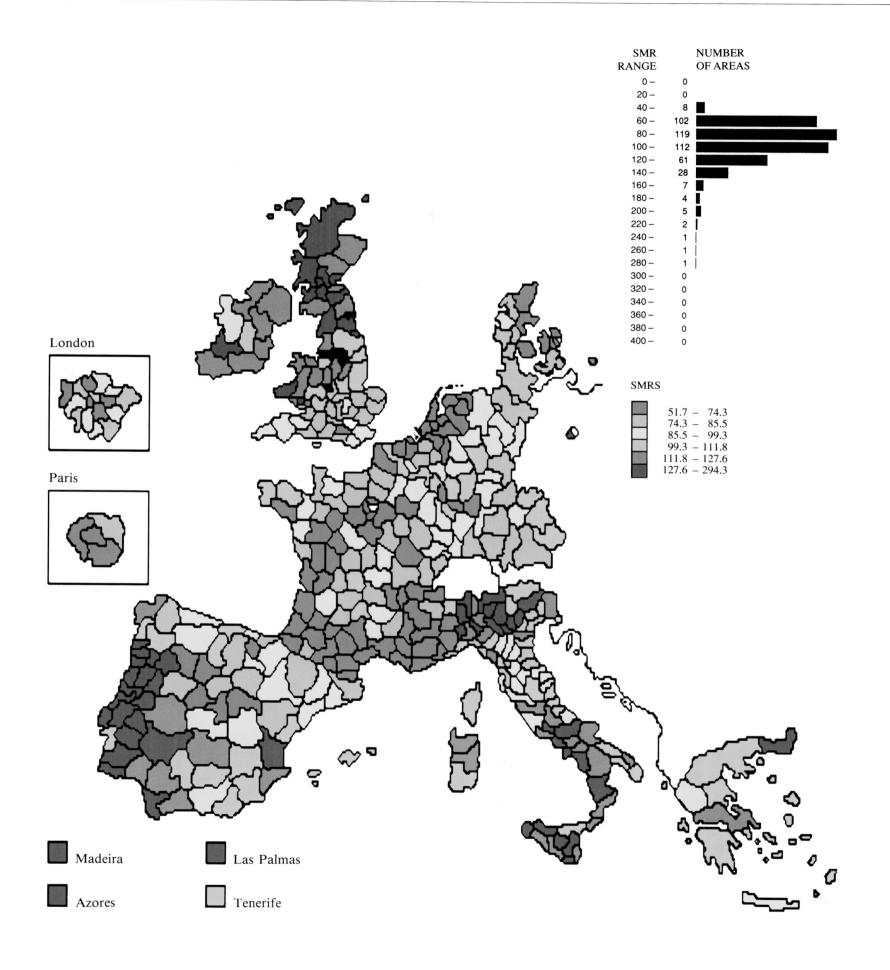

London

Paris

SMR RANGE	NUMBER OF AREAS
0 –	0
20 –	0
40 –	8
60 –	102
80 –	119
100 –	112
120 –	61
140 –	28
160 –	7
180 –	4
200 –	5
220 –	2
240 –	1
260 –	1
280 –	1
300 –	0
320 –	0
340 –	0
360 –	0
380 –	0
400 –	0

SMRS

51.7 – 74.3
74.3 – 85.5
85.5 – 99.3
99.3 – 111.8
111.8 – 127.6
127.6 – 294.3

Madeira   Las Palmas

Azores   Tenerife

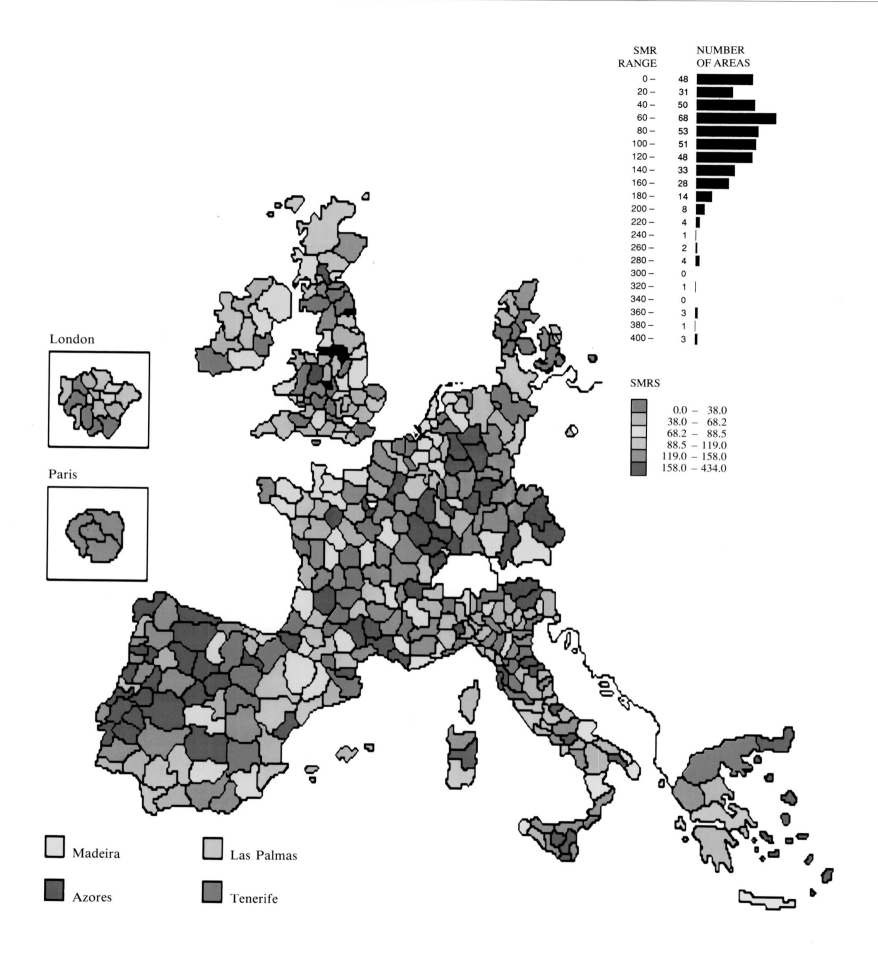

London

Paris

SMR
RANGE

NUMBER
OF AREAS

0 –	48
20 –	31
40 –	50
60 –	68
80 –	53
100 –	51
120 –	48
140 –	33
160 –	28
180 –	14
200 –	8
220 –	4
240 –	1
260 –	2
280 –	4
300 –	0
320 –	1
340 –	0
360 –	3
380 –	1
400 –	3

SMRS

0.0 – 38.0
38.0 – 68.2
68.2 – 88.5
88.5 – 119.0
119.0 – 158.0
158.0 – 434.0

Madeira

Las Palmas

Azores

Tenerife

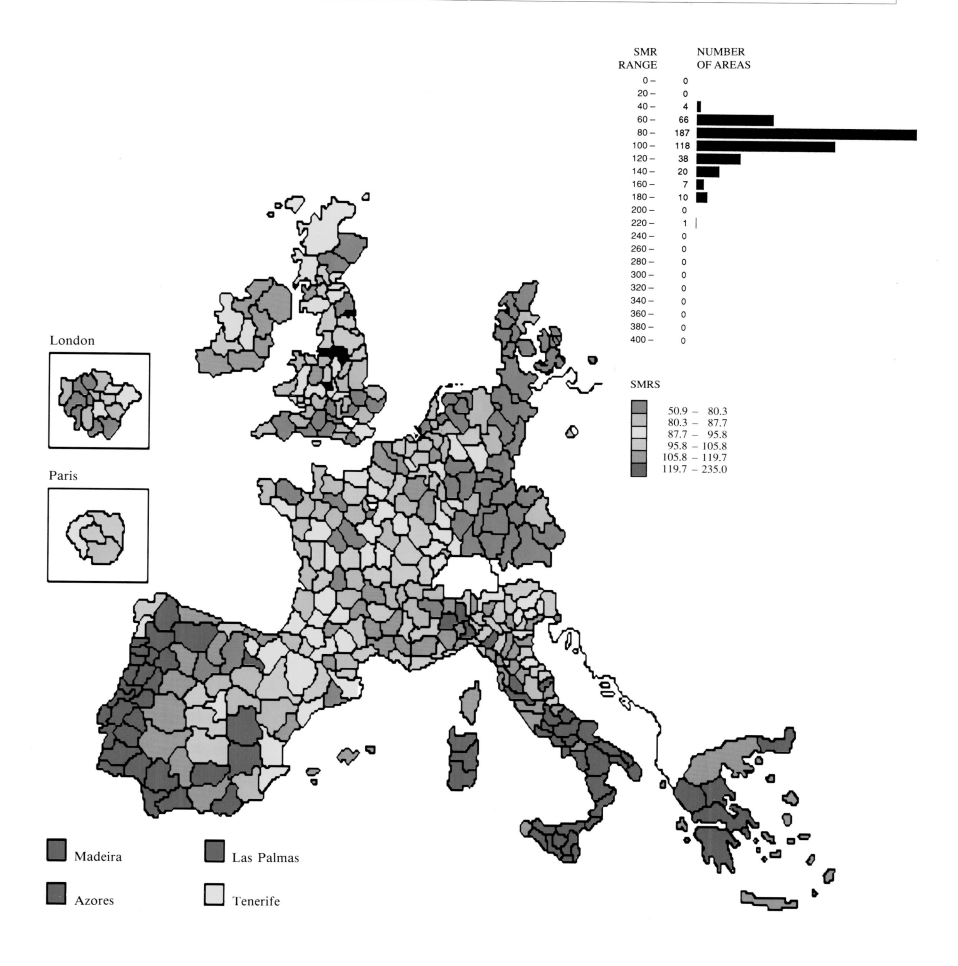

SMR RANGE | NUMBER OF AREAS
0 – 0
20 – 0
40 – 4
60 – 66
80 – 187
100 – 118
120 – 38
140 – 20
160 – 7
180 – 10
200 – 0
220 – 1
240 – 0
260 – 0
280 – 0
300 – 0
320 – 0
340 – 0
360 – 0
380 – 0
400 – 0

SMRS

50.9 – 80.3
80.3 – 87.7
87.7 – 95.8
95.8 – 105.8
105.8 – 119.7
119.7 – 235.0

London

Paris

Madeira

Azores

Las Palmas

Tenerife

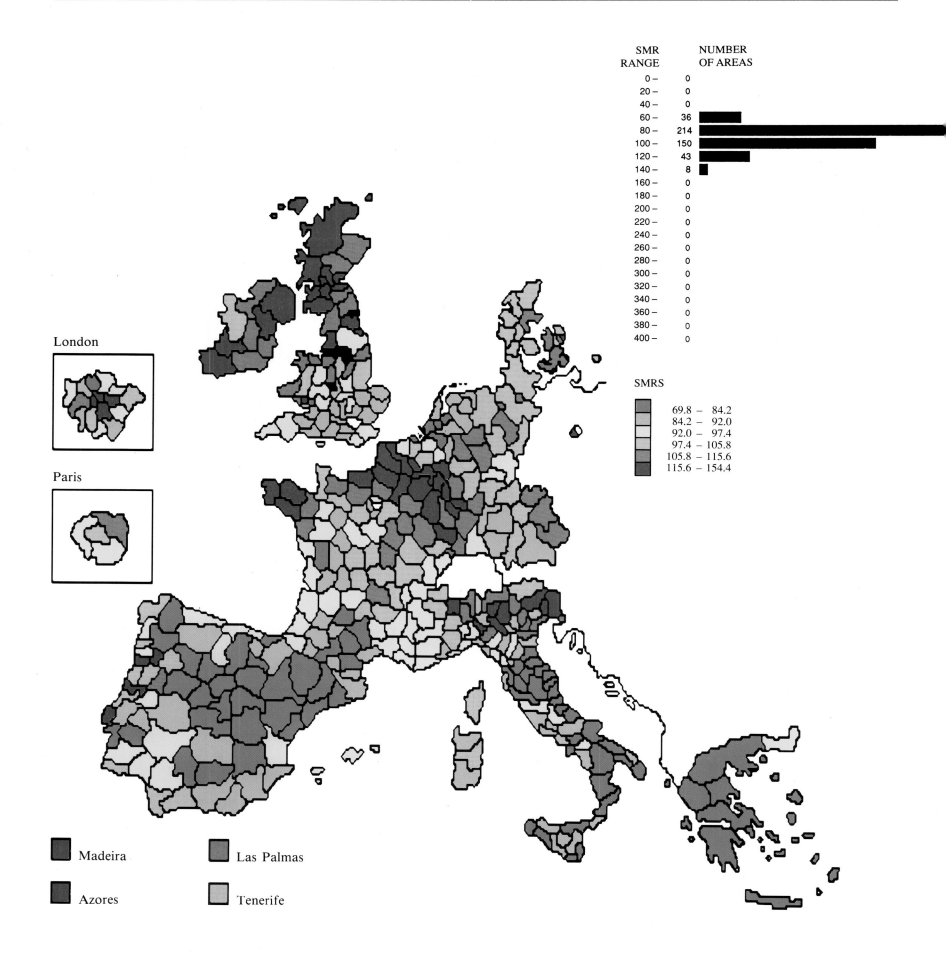

London

Paris

SMR RANGE	NUMBER OF AREAS
0 –	0
20 –	0
40 –	0
60 –	36
80 –	214
100 –	150
120 –	43
140 –	8
160 –	0
180 –	0
200 –	0
220 –	0
240 –	0
260 –	0
280 –	0
300 –	0
320 –	0
340 –	0
360 –	0
380 –	0
400 –	0

SMRS

69.8 – 84.2
84.2 – 92.0
92.0 – 97.4
97.4 – 105.8
105.8 – 115.6
115.6 – 154.4

Madeira

Azores

Las Palmas

Tenerife

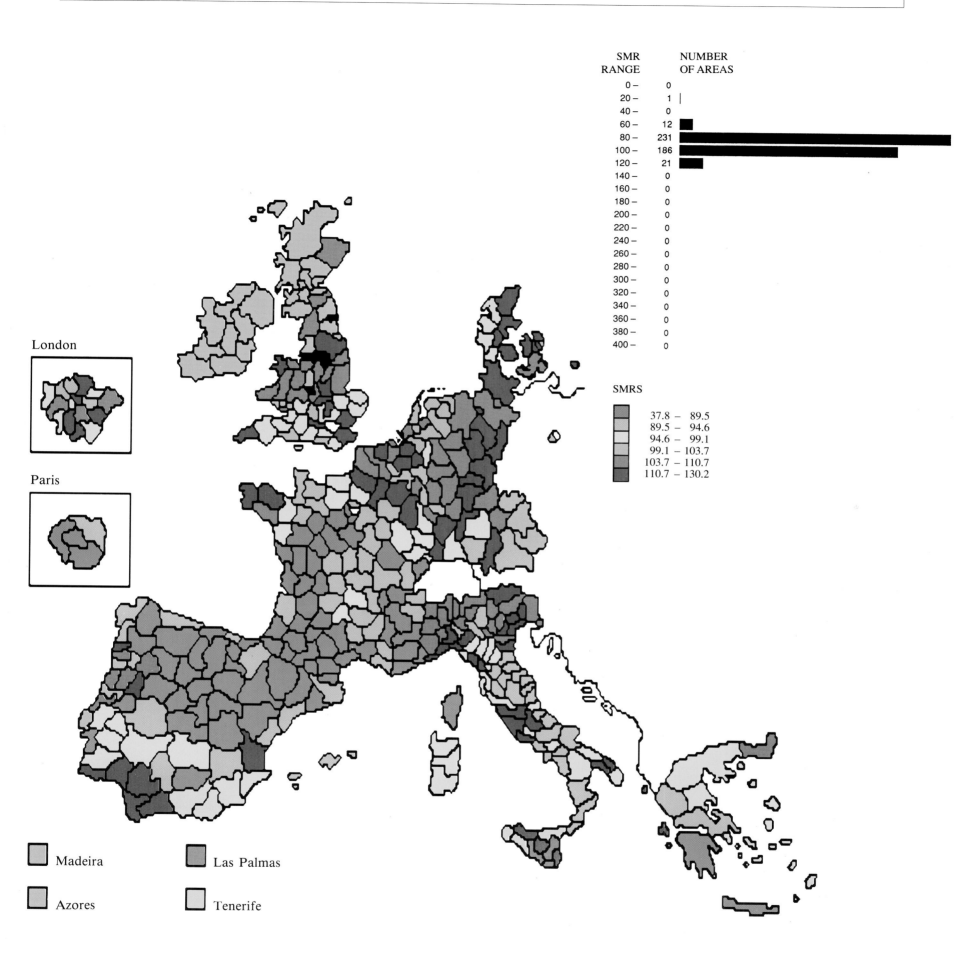

SMR RANGE	NUMBER OF AREAS
0 –	0
20 –	1
40 –	0
60 –	12
80 –	231
100 –	186
120 –	21
140 –	0
160 –	0
180 –	0
200 –	0
220 –	0
240 –	0
260 –	0
280 –	0
300 –	0
320 –	0
340 –	0
360 –	0
380 –	0
400 –	0

SMRS

37.8 – 89.5
89.5 – 94.6
94.6 – 99.1
99.1 – 103.7
103.7 – 110.7
110.7 – 130.2

London

Paris

Madeira

Azores

Las Palmas

Tenerife

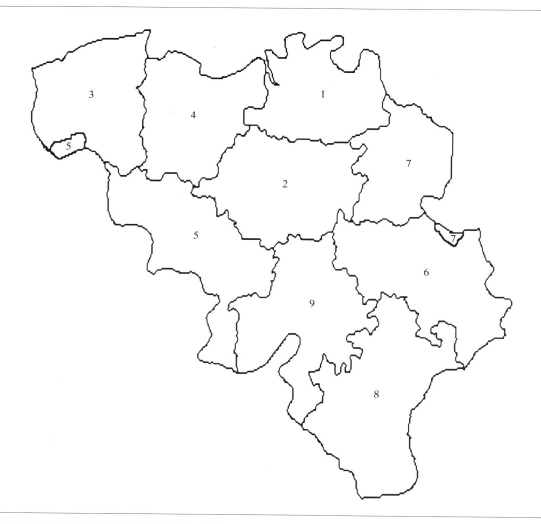

BELGIUM: TUBERCULOSIS MORTALITY AGES 5–64

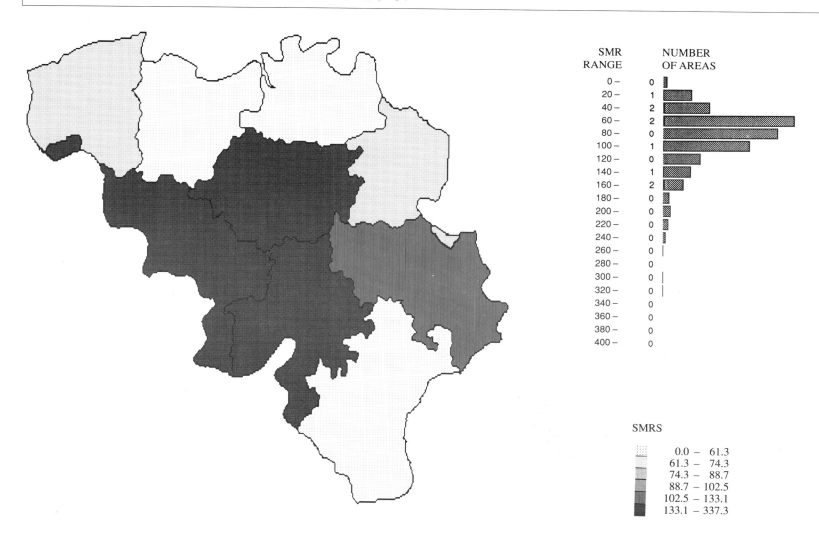

SMR RANGE	NUMBER OF AREAS
0 –	0
20 –	1
40 –	2
60 –	2
80 –	0
100 –	1
120 –	0
140 –	1
160 –	2
180 –	0
200 –	0
220 –	0
240 –	0
260 –	0
280 –	0
300 –	0
320 –	0
340 –	0
360 –	0
380 –	0
400 –	0

SMRS

0.0 – 61.3
61.3 – 74.3
74.3 – 88.7
88.7 – 102.5
102.5 – 133.1
133.1 – 337.3

BELGIUM: MALIGNANT NEOPLASM OF CERVIX UTERI MORTALITY AGES 15–64

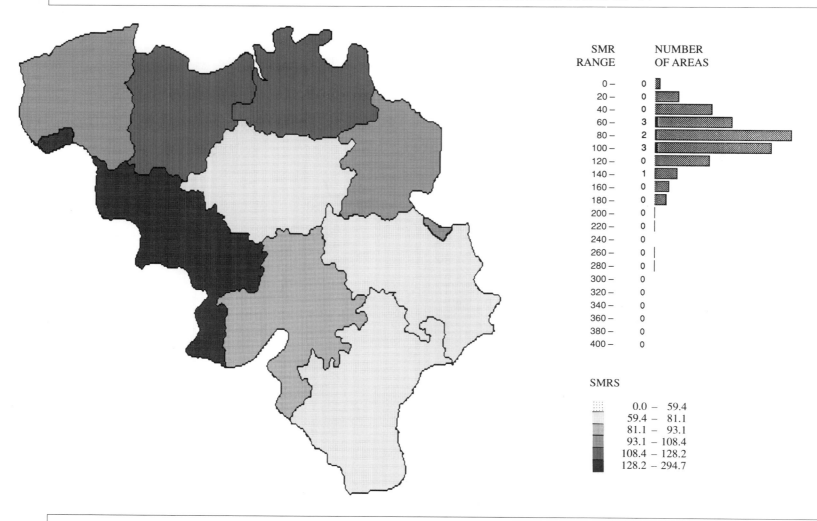

SMR RANGE	NUMBER OF AREAS
0 –	0
20 –	0
40 –	0
60 –	3
80 –	2
100 –	3
120 –	0
140 –	1
160 –	0
180 –	0
200 –	0
220 –	0
240 –	0
260 –	0
280 –	0
300 –	0
320 –	0
340 –	0
360 –	0
380 –	0
400 –	0

SMRS

	0.0 – 59.4
	59.4 – 81.1
	81.1 – 93.1
	93.1 – 108.4
	108.4 – 128.2
	128.2 – 294.7

BELGIUM: MALIGNANT NEOPLASM OF CERVIX AND BODY OF UTERUS MORTALITY AGES 15–54

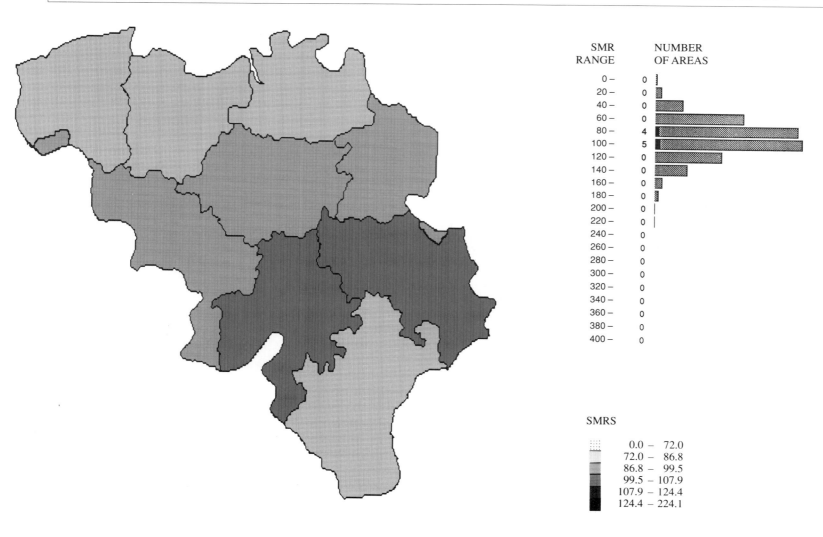

SMR RANGE	NUMBER OF AREAS
0 –	0
20 –	0
40 –	0
60 –	0
80 –	4
100 –	5
120 –	0
140 –	0
160 –	0
180 –	0
200 –	0
220 –	0
240 –	0
260 –	0
280 –	0
300 –	0
320 –	0
340 –	0
360 –	0
380 –	0
400 –	0

SMRS

	0.0 – 72.0
	72.0 – 86.8
	86.8 – 99.5
	99.5 – 107.9
	107.9 – 124.4
	124.4 – 224.1

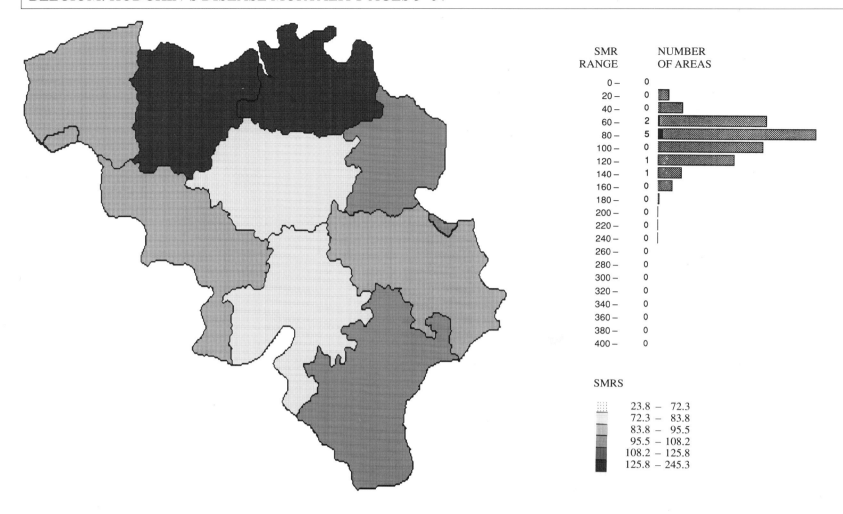

SMR RANGE	NUMBER OF AREAS
0 –	0
20 –	0
40 –	0
60 –	2
80 –	5
100 –	0
120 –	1
140 –	1
160 –	0
180 –	0
200 –	0
220 –	0
240 –	0
260 –	0
280 –	0
300 –	0
320 –	0
340 –	0
360 –	0
380 –	0
400 –	0

SMRS

23.8 – 72.3
72.3 – 83.8
83.8 – 95.5
95.5 – 108.2
108.2 – 125.8
125.8 – 245.3

BELGIUM: CHRONIC RHEUMATIC HEART DISEASE MORTALITY AGES 5–44

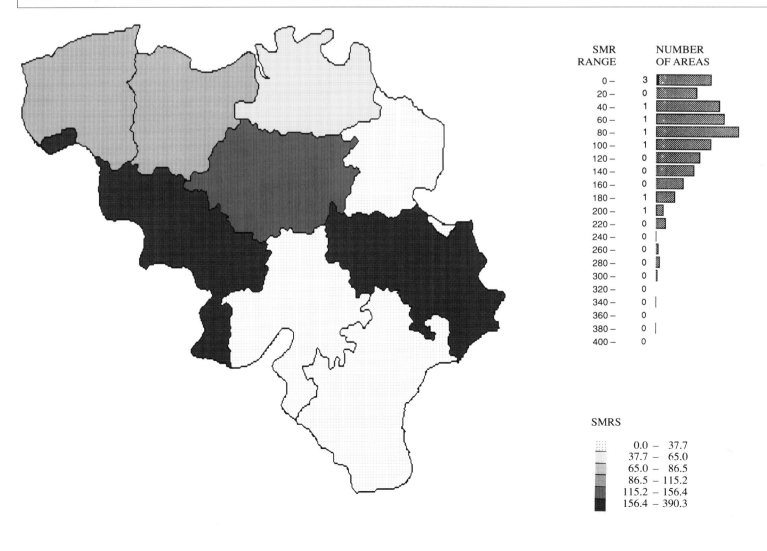

SMR RANGE	NUMBER OF AREAS
0 –	3
20 –	0
40 –	1
60 –	1
80 –	1
100 –	1
120 –	0
140 –	0
160 –	0
180 –	1
200 –	1
220 –	0
240 –	0
260 –	0
280 –	0
300 –	0
320 –	0
340 –	0
360 –	0
380 –	0
400 –	0

SMRS

0.0 – 37.7
37.7 – 65.0
65.0 – 86.5
86.5 – 115.2
115.2 – 156.4
156.4 – 390.3

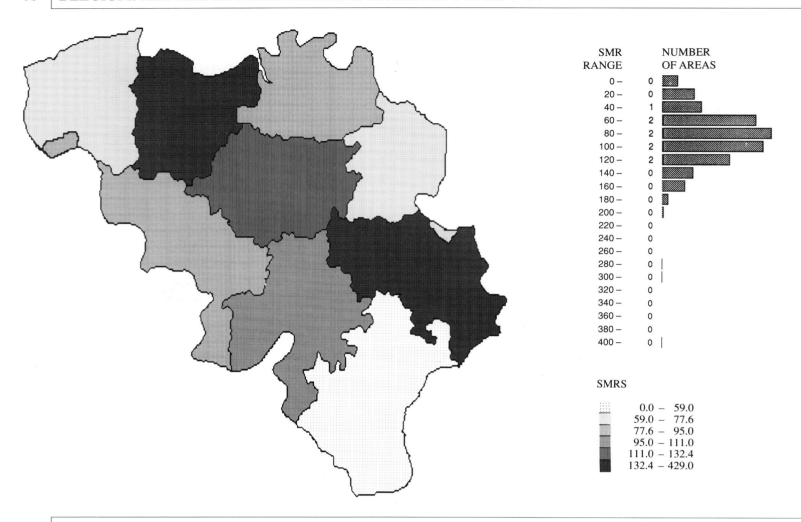

SMR RANGE | NUMBER OF AREAS

0 –	0
20 –	0
40 –	1
60 –	2
80 –	2
100 –	2
120 –	2
140 –	0
160 –	0
180 –	0
200 –	0
220 –	0
240 –	0
260 –	0
280 –	0
300 –	0
320 –	0
340 –	0
360 –	0
380 –	0
400 –	0

SMRS

	0.0 – 59.0
	59.0 – 77.6
	77.6 – 95.0
	95.0 – 111.0
	111.0 – 132.4
	132.4 – 429.0

BELGIUM: ASTHMA MORTALITY AGES 5–44

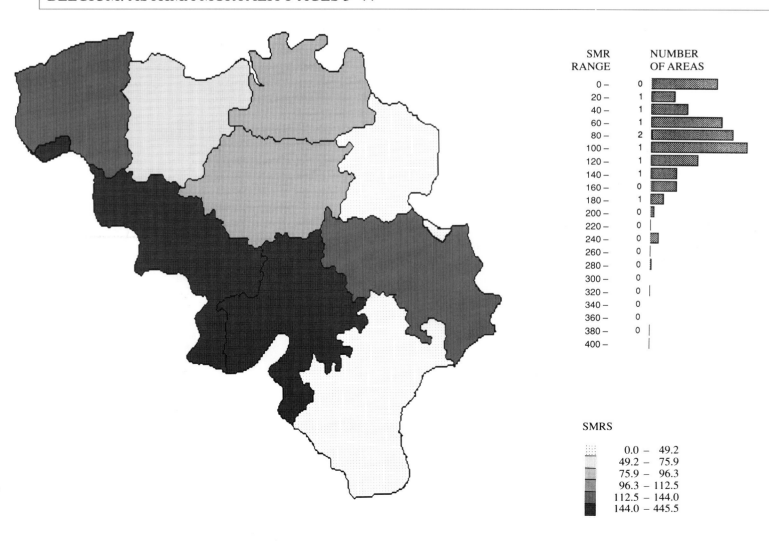

SMR RANGE | NUMBER OF AREAS

0 –	0
20 –	1
40 –	1
60 –	1
80 –	2
100 –	1
120 –	1
140 –	1
160 –	0
180 –	1
200 –	0
220 –	0
240 –	0
260 –	0
280 –	0
300 –	0
320 –	0
340 –	0
360 –	0
380 –	0
400 –	

SMRS

	0.0 – 49.2
	49.2 – 75.9
	75.9 – 96.3
	96.3 – 112.5
	112.5 – 144.0
	144.0 – 445.5

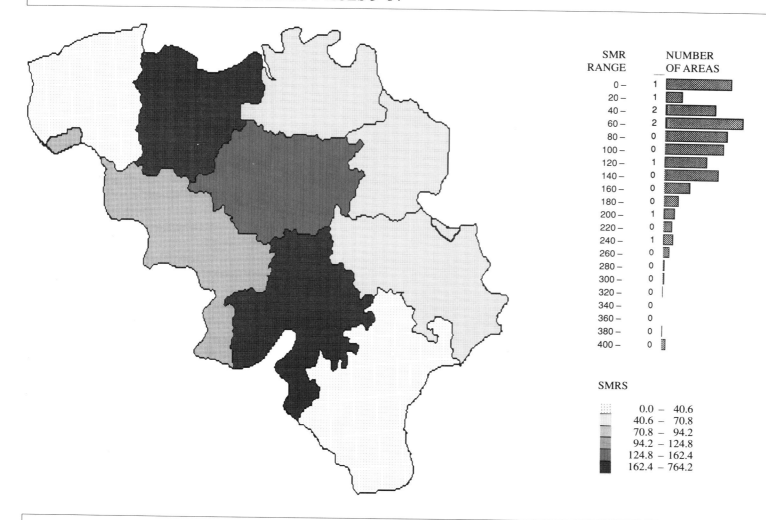

BELGIUM: APPENDICITIS MORTALITY AGES 5–64

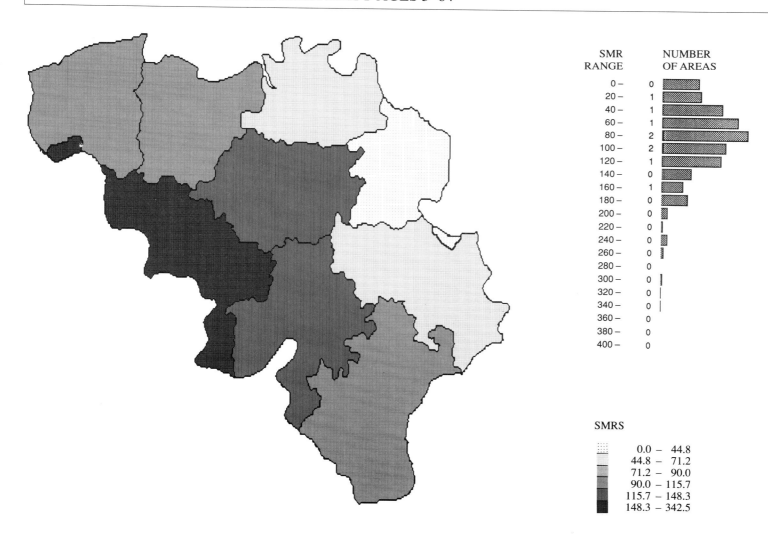

BELGIUM: ABDOMINAL HERNIA MORTALITY AGES 5–64

61

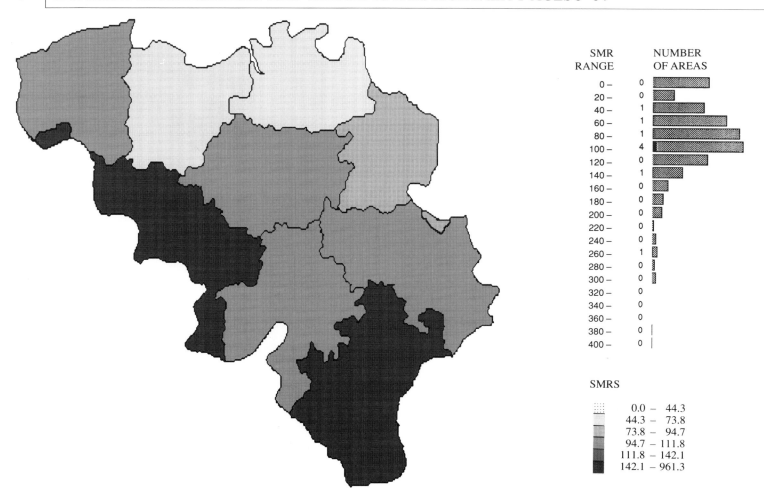

SMR RANGE   NUMBER OF AREAS

SMR RANGE	NUMBER OF AREAS
0 –	0
20 –	0
40 –	1
60 –	1
80 –	1
100 –	4
120 –	0
140 –	1
160 –	0
180 –	0
200 –	0
220 –	0
240 –	0
260 –	1
280 –	0
300 –	0
320 –	0
340 –	0
360 –	0
380 –	0
400 –	0

SMRS

	0.0 – 44.3
	44.3 – 73.8
	73.8 – 94.7
	94.7 – 111.8
	111.8 – 142.1
	142.1 – 961.3

BELGIUM: HYPERTENSIVE AND CEREBROVASCULAR DISEASES MORTALITY AGES 35–64

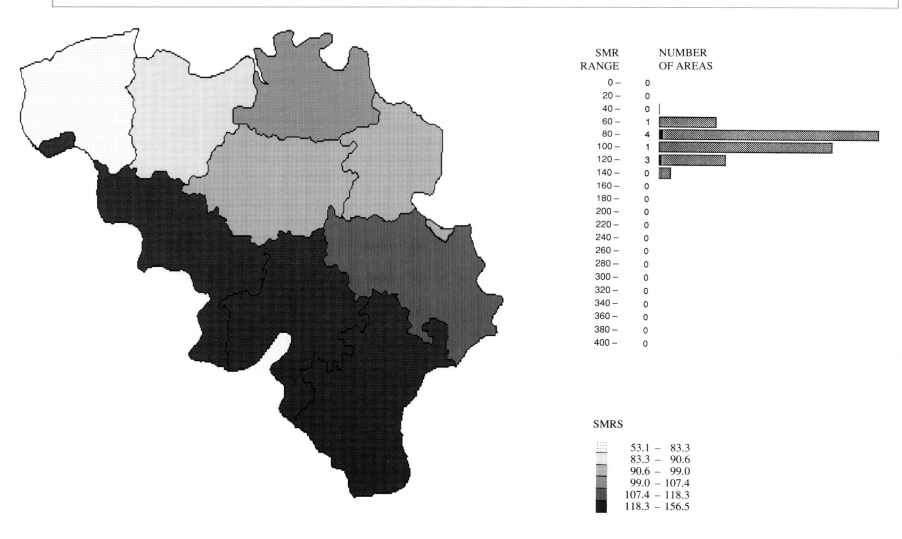

SMR RANGE   NUMBER OF AREAS

SMR RANGE	NUMBER OF AREAS
0 –	0
20 –	0
40 –	0
60 –	1
80 –	4
100 –	1
120 –	3
140 –	0
160 –	0
180 –	0
200 –	0
220 –	0
240 –	0
260 –	0
280 –	0
300 –	0
320 –	0
340 –	0
360 –	0
380 –	0
400 –	0

SMRS

	53.1 – 83.3
	83.3 – 90.6
	90.6 – 99.0
	99.0 – 107.4
	107.4 – 118.3
	118.3 – 156.5

BELGIUM: MATERNAL MORTALITY ALL AGES

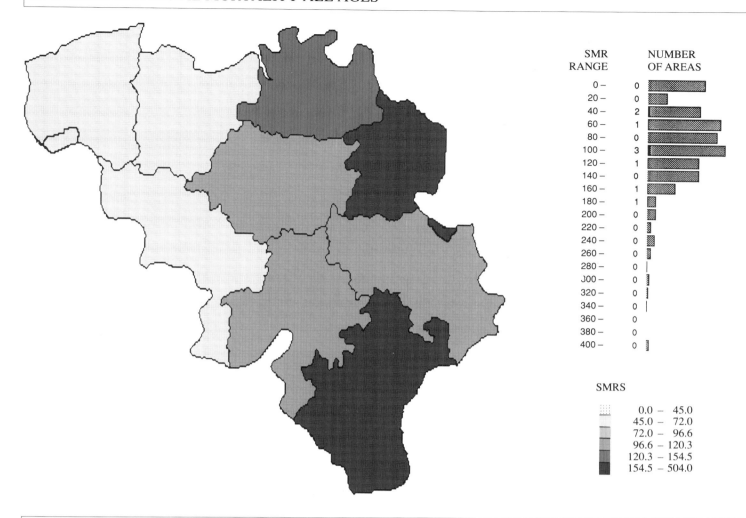

SMR RANGE	NUMBER OF AREAS
0 –	0
20 –	0
40 –	2
60 –	1
80 –	0
100 –	3
120 –	1
140 –	0
160 –	1
180 –	1
200 –	0
220 –	0
240 –	0
260 –	0
280 –	0
300 –	0
320 –	0
340 –	0
360 –	0
380 –	0
400 –	0

SMRS

	0.0 – 45.0
	45.0 – 72.0
	72.0 – 96.6
	96.6 – 120.3
	120.3 – 154.5
	154.5 – 504.0

BELGIUM: PERINATAL MORTALITY

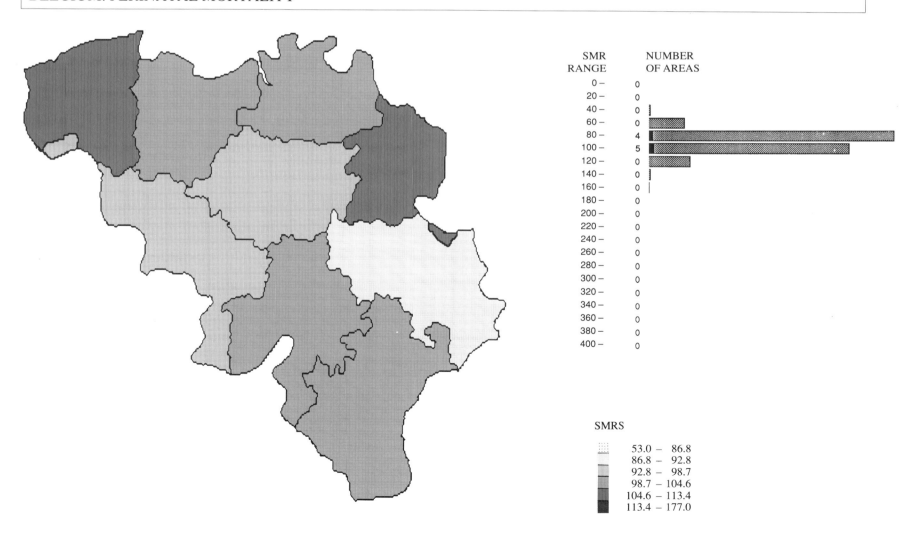

SMR RANGE	NUMBER OF AREAS
0 –	0
20 –	0
40 –	0
60 –	0
80 –	4
100 –	5
120 –	0
140 –	0
160 –	0
180 –	0
200 –	0
220 –	0
240 –	0
260 –	0
280 –	0
300 –	0
320 –	0
340 –	0
360 –	0
380 –	0
400 –	0

SMRS

	53.0 – 86.8
	86.8 – 92.8
	92.8 – 98.7
	98.7 – 104.6
	104.6 – 113.4
	113.4 – 177.0

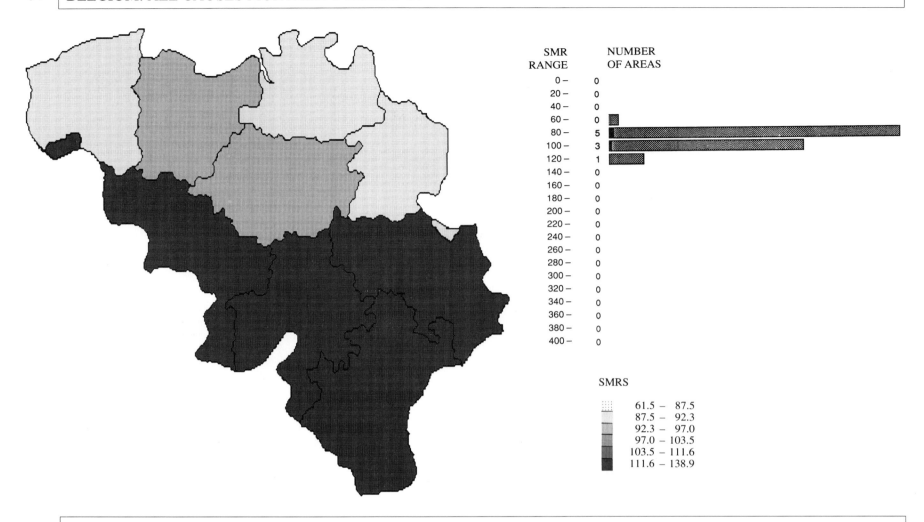

SMR RANGE	NUMBER OF AREAS
0 –	0
20 –	0
40 –	0
60 –	0
80 –	5
100 –	3
120 –	1
140 –	0
160 –	0
180 –	0
200 –	0
220 –	0
240 –	0
260 –	0
280 –	0
300 –	0
320 –	0
340 –	0
360 –	0
380 –	0
400 –	0

SMRS

    61.5 –   87.5
    87.5 –   92.3
    92.3 –   97.0
    97.0 – 103.5
  103.5 – 111.6
  111.6 – 138.9

BELGIUM: ALL CAUSES MORTALITY ALL AGES

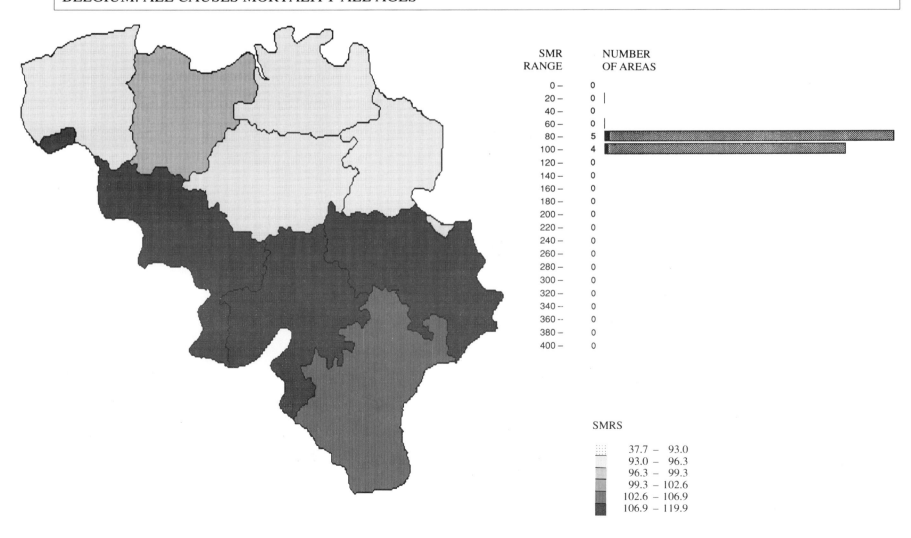

SMR RANGE	NUMBER OF AREAS
0 –	0
20 –	0
40 –	0
60 –	0
80 –	5
100 –	4
120 –	0
140 –	0
160 –	0
180 –	0
200 –	0
220 –	0
240 –	0
260 –	0
280 –	0
300 –	0
320 –	0
340 –	0
360 –	0
380 –	0
400 –	0

SMRS

    37.7 –   93.0
    93.0 –   96.3
    96.3 –   99.3
    99.3 – 102.6
  102.6 – 106.9
  106.9 – 119.9

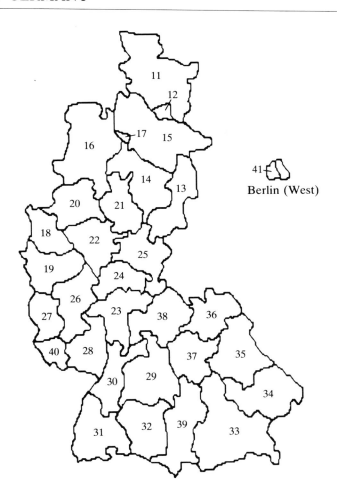

FEDERAL REPUBLIC OF GERMANY: TUBERCULOSIS MORTALITY AGES 5–64

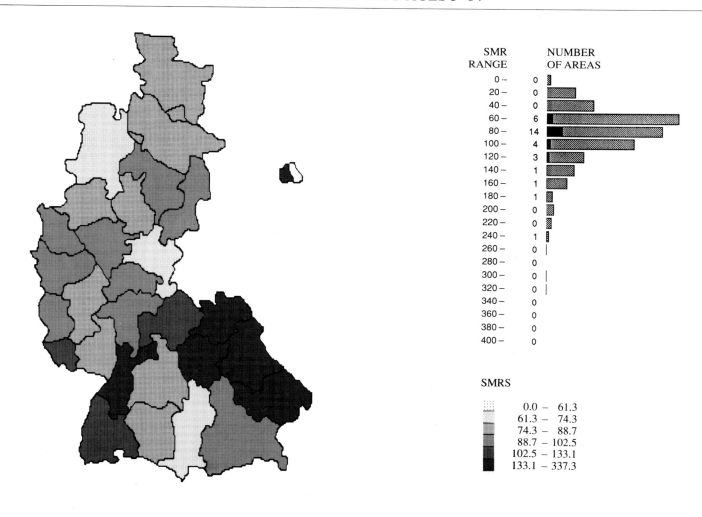

SMR RANGE	NUMBER OF AREAS
0 –	0
20 –	0
40 –	0
60 –	6
80 –	14
100 –	4
120 –	3
140 –	1
160 –	1
180 –	1
200 –	0
220 –	0
240 –	1
260 –	0
280 –	0
300 –	0
320 –	0
340 –	0
360 –	0
380 –	0
400 –	0

SMRS

0.0 – 61.3
61.3 – 74.3
74.3 – 88.7
88.7 – 102.5
102.5 – 133.1
133.1 – 337.3

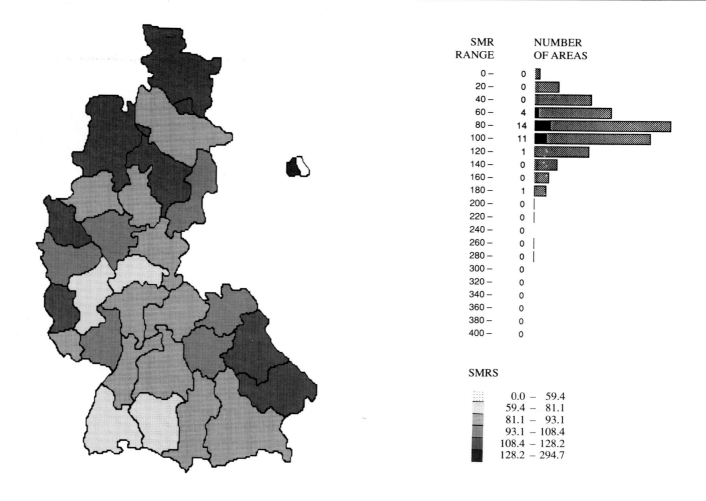

FEDERAL REPUBLIC OF GERMANY: MALIGNANT NEOPLASM OF CERVIX AND BODY OF UTERUS MORTALITY AGES 15–54

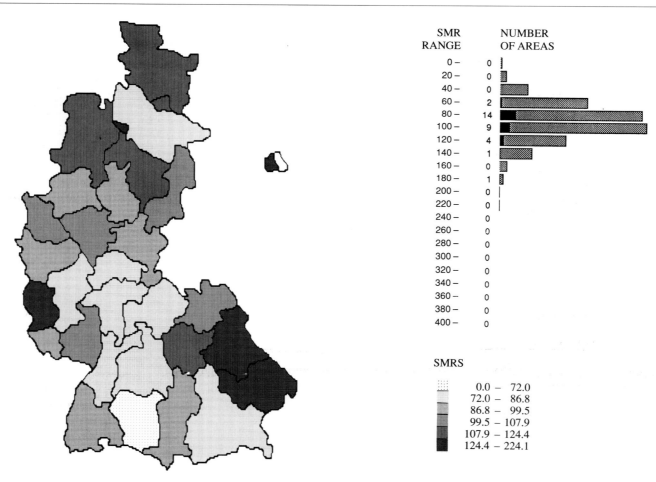

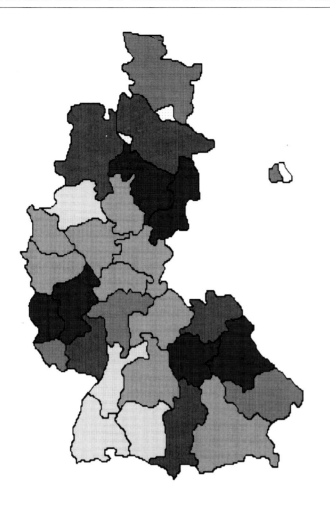

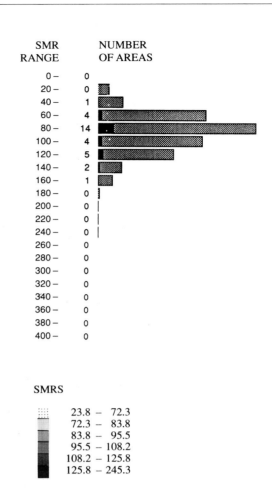

SMR RANGE	NUMBER OF AREAS
0 –	0
20 –	0
40 –	1
60 –	4
80 –	14
100 –	4
120 –	5
140 –	2
160 –	1
180 –	0
200 –	0
220 –	0
240 –	0
260 –	0
280 –	0
300 –	0
320 –	0
340 –	0
360 –	0
380 –	0
400 –	0

SMRS

	23.8 – 72.3
	72.3 – 83.8
	83.8 – 95.5
	95.5 – 108.2
	108.2 – 125.8
	125.8 – 245.3

FEDERAL REPUBLIC OF GERMANY: CHRONIC RHEUMATIC HEART DISEASE MORTALITY AGES 5–44

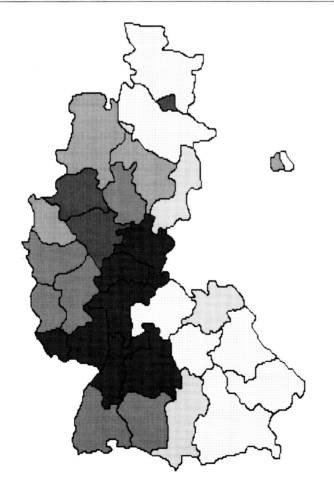

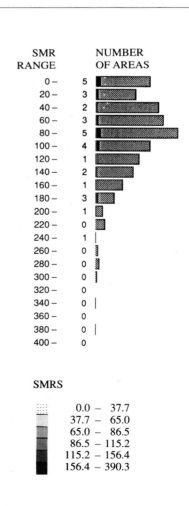

SMR RANGE	NUMBER OF AREAS
0 –	5
20 –	3
40 –	2
60 –	3
80 –	5
100 –	4
120 –	1
140 –	2
160 –	1
180 –	3
200 –	1
220 –	0
240 –	1
260 –	0
280 –	0
300 –	0
320 –	0
340 –	0
360 –	0
380 –	0
400 –	0

SMRS

	0.0 – 37.7
	37.7 – 65.0
	65.0 – 86.5
	86.5 – 115.2
	115.2 – 156.4
	156.4 – 390.3

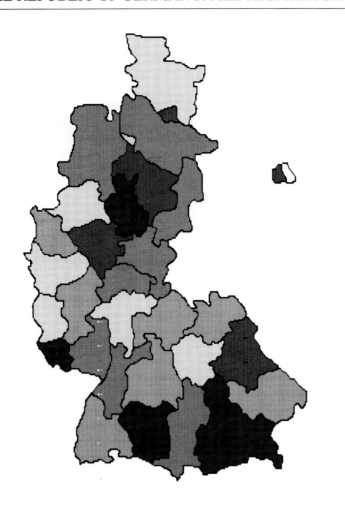

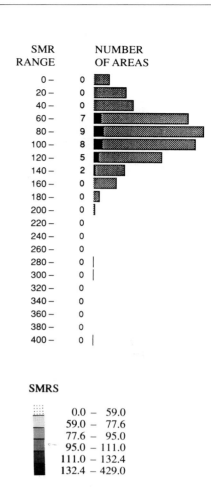

SMR RANGE	NUMBER OF AREAS
0 –	0
20 –	0
40 –	0
60 –	7
80 –	9
100 –	8
120 –	5
140 –	2
160 –	0
180 –	0
200 –	0
220 –	0
240 –	0
260 –	0
280 –	0
300 –	0
320 –	0
340 –	0
360 –	0
380 –	0
400 –	0

SMRS

	0.0 – 59.0
	59.0 – 77.6
	77.6 – 95.0
	95.0 – 111.0
	111.0 – 132.4
	132.4 – 429.0

FEDERAL REPUBLIC OF GERMANY: ASTHMA MORTALITY AGES 5–44

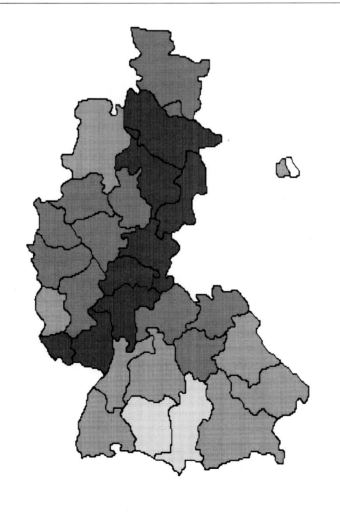

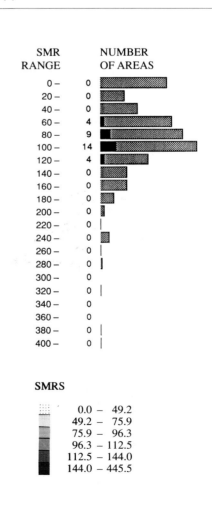

SMR RANGE	NUMBER OF AREAS
0 –	0
20 –	0
40 –	0
60 –	4
80 –	9
100 –	14
120 –	4
140 –	0
160 –	0
180 –	0
200 –	0
220 –	0
240 –	0
260 –	0
280 –	0
300 –	0
320 –	0
340 –	0
360 –	0
380 –	0
400 –	0

SMRS

	0.0 – 49.2
	49.2 – 75.9
	75.9 – 96.3
	96.3 – 112.5
	112.5 – 144.0
	144.0 – 445.5

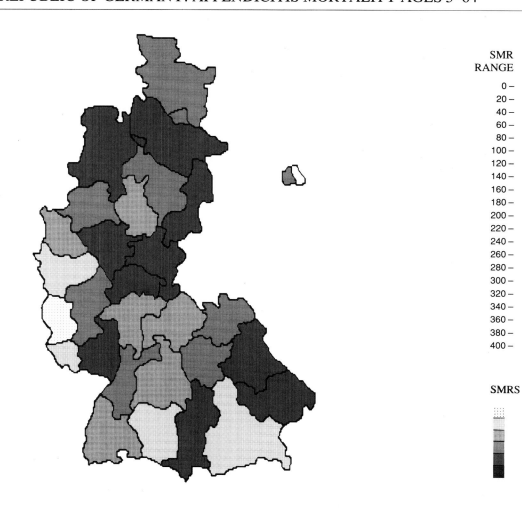

SMR RANGE	NUMBER OF AREAS
0 –	0
20 –	1
40 –	1
60 –	7
80 –	3
100 –	6
120 –	8
140 –	5
160 –	0
180 –	0
200 –	0
220 –	0
240 –	0
260 –	0
280 –	0
300 –	0
320 –	0
340 –	0
360 –	0
380 –	0
400 –	0

SMRS

	0.0 – 40.6
	40.6 – 70.8
	70.8 – 94.2
	94.2 – 124.8
	124.8 – 162.4
	162.4 – 764.2

FEDERAL REPUBLIC OF GERMANY: ABDOMINAL HERNIA MORTALITY AGES 5–64

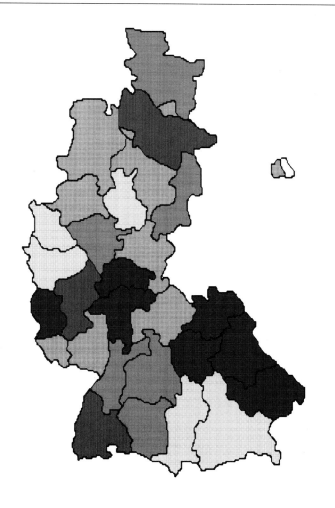

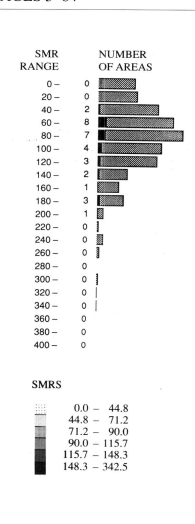

SMR RANGE	NUMBER OF AREAS
0 –	0
20 –	0
40 –	2
60 –	8
80 –	7
100 –	4
120 –	3
140 –	2
160 –	1
180 –	3
200 –	1
220 –	0
240 –	0
260 –	0
280 –	0
300 –	0
320 –	0
340 –	0
360 –	0
380 –	0
400 –	0

SMRS

	0.0 – 44.8
	44.8 – 71.2
	71.2 – 90.0
	90.0 – 115.7
	115.7 – 148.3
	148.3 – 342.5

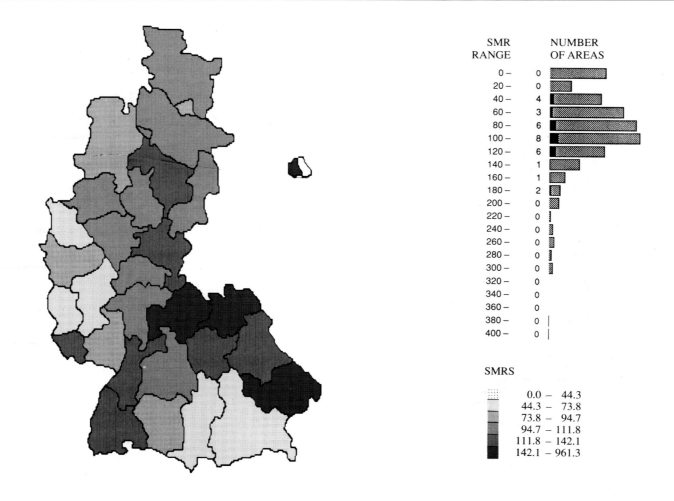

SMR RANGE	NUMBER OF AREAS
0 –	0
20 –	0
40 –	4
60 –	3
80 –	6
100 –	8
120 –	6
140 –	1
160 –	1
180 –	2
200 –	0
220 –	0
240 –	0
260 –	0
280 –	0
300 –	0
320 –	0
340 –	0
360 –	0
380 –	0
400 –	0

SMRS

	0.0 – 44.3
	44.3 – 73.8
	73.8 – 94.7
	94.7 – 111.8
	111.8 – 142.1
	142.1 – 961.3

FEDERAL REPUBLIC OF GERMANY: HYPERTENSIVE AND CEREBROVASCULAR DISEASES MORTALITY AGES 35–64

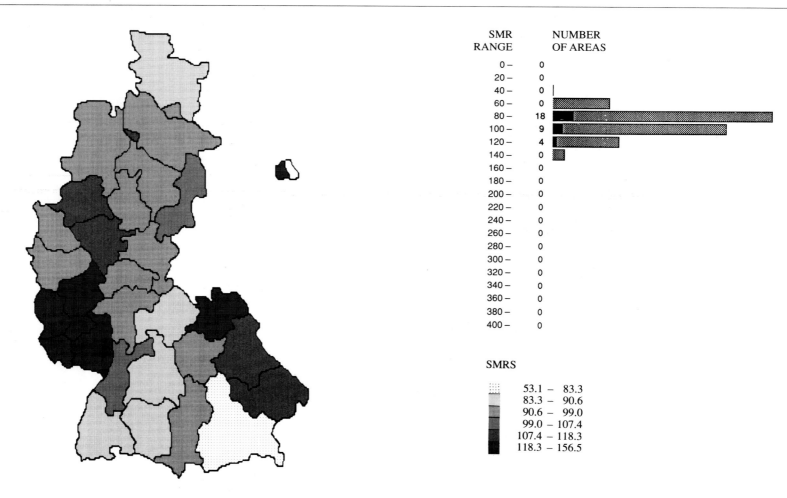

SMR RANGE	NUMBER OF AREAS
0 –	0
20 –	0
40 –	0
60 –	0
80 –	18
100 –	9
120 –	4
140 –	0
160 –	0
180 –	0
200 –	0
220 –	0
240 –	0
260 –	0
280 –	0
300 –	0
320 –	0
340 –	0
360 –	0
380 –	0
400 –	0

SMRS

	53.1 – 83.3
	83.3 – 90.6
	90.6 – 99.0
	99.0 – 107.4
	107.4 – 118.3
	118.3 – 156.5

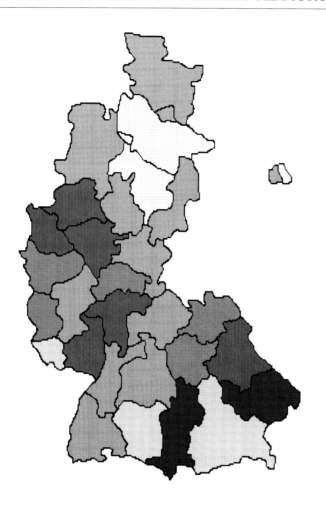

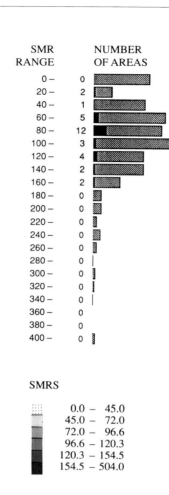

SMR RANGE	NUMBER OF AREAS
0 –	0
20 –	2
40 –	1
60 –	5
80 –	12
100 –	3
120 –	4
140 –	2
160 –	2
180 –	0
200 –	0
220 –	0
240 –	0
260 –	0
280 –	0
300 –	0
320 –	0
340 –	0
360 –	0
380 –	0
400 –	0

SMRS

	0.0 – 45.0
	45.0 – 72.0
	72.0 – 96.6
	96.6 – 120.3
	120.3 – 154.5
	154.5 – 504.0

FEDERAL REPUBLIC OF GERMANY: PERINATAL MORTALITY

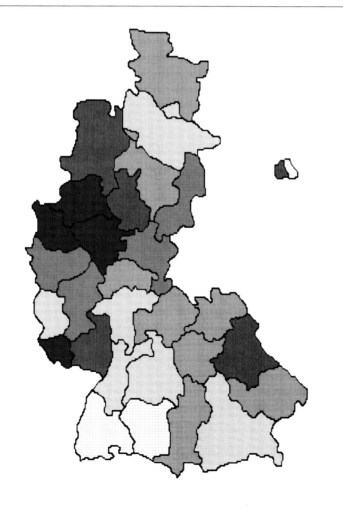

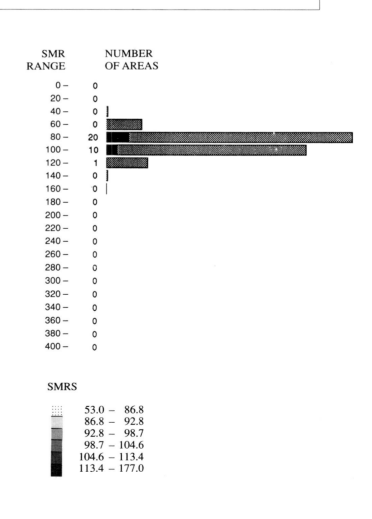

SMR RANGE	NUMBER OF AREAS
0 –	0
20 –	0
40 –	0
60 –	0
80 –	20
100 –	10
120 –	1
140 –	0
160 –	0
180 –	0
200 –	0
220 –	0
240 –	0
260 –	0
280 –	0
300 –	0
320 –	0
340 –	0
360 –	0
380 –	0
400 –	0

SMRS

	53.0 – 86.8
	86.8 – 92.8
	92.8 – 98.7
	98.7 – 104.6
	104.6 – 113.4
	113.4 – 177.0

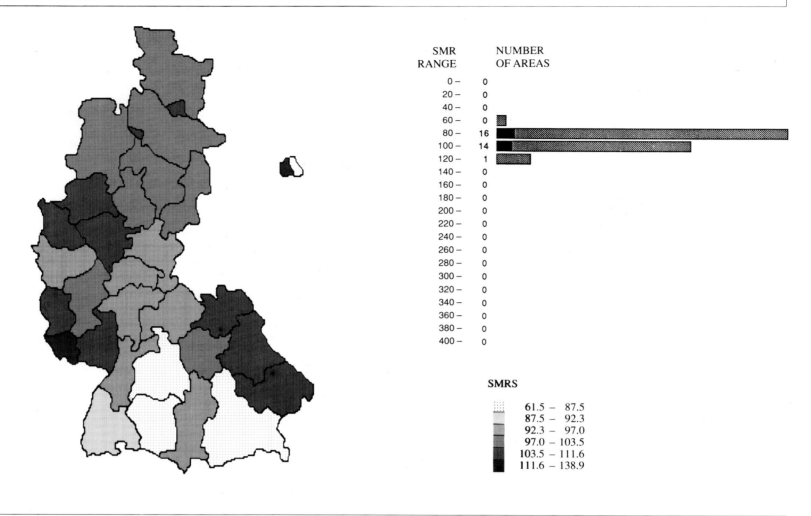

SMR RANGE	NUMBER OF AREAS
0 –	0
20 –	0
40 –	0
60 –	0
80 –	16
100 –	14
120 –	1
140 –	0
160 –	0
180 –	0
200 –	0
220 –	0
240 –	0
260 –	0
280 –	0
300 –	0
320 –	0
340 –	0
360 –	0
380 –	0
400 –	0

SMRS

61.5 – 87.5
87.5 – 92.3
92.3 – 97.0
97.0 – 103.5
103.5 – 111.6
111.6 – 138.9

FEDERAL REPUBLIC OF GERMANY: ALL CAUSES MORTALITY ALL AGES

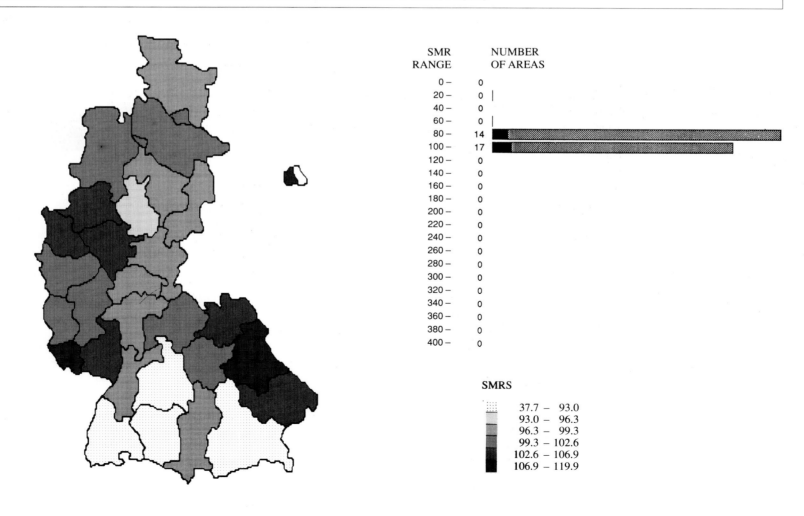

SMR RANGE	NUMBER OF AREAS
0 –	0
20 –	0
40 –	0
60 –	0
80 –	14
100 –	17
120 –	0
140 –	0
160 –	0
180 –	0
200 –	0
220 –	0
240 –	0
260 –	0
280 –	0
300 –	0
320 –	0
340 –	0
360 –	0
380 –	0
400 –	0

SMRS

37.7 – 93.0
93.0 – 96.3
96.3 – 99.3
99.3 – 102.6
102.6 – 106.9
106.9 – 119.9

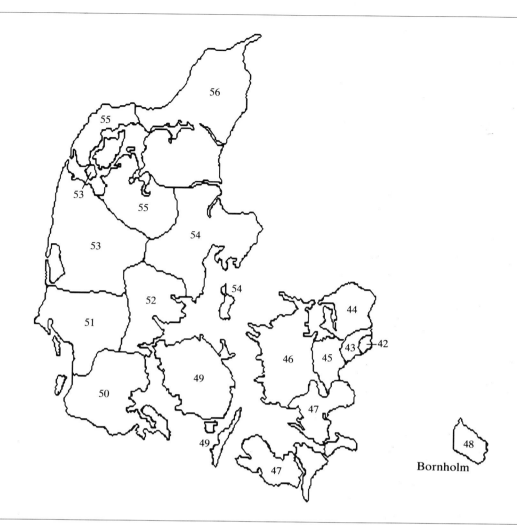

DENMARK: TUBERCULOSIS MORTALITY AGES 5–64

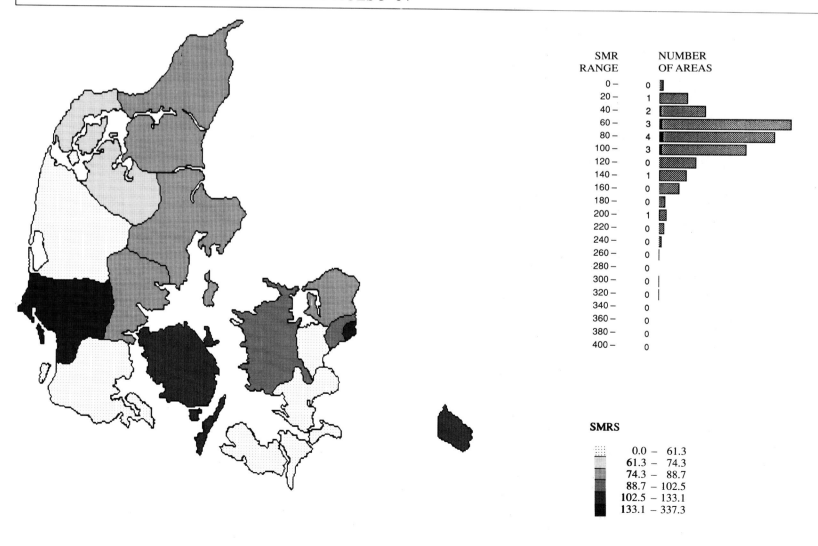

SMR RANGE	NUMBER OF AREAS
0 –	0
20 –	1
40 –	2
60 –	3
80 –	4
100 –	3
120 –	0
140 –	1
160 –	0
180 –	0
200 –	1
220 –	0
240 –	0
260 –	0
280 –	0
300 –	0
320 –	0
340 –	0
360 –	0
380 –	0
400 –	0

SMRS

0.0 – 61.3
61.3 – 74.3
74.3 – 88.7
88.7 – 102.5
102.5 – 133.1
133.1 – 337.3

DENMARK: MALIGNANT NEOPLASM OF CERVIX UTERI MORTALITY AGES 15–64

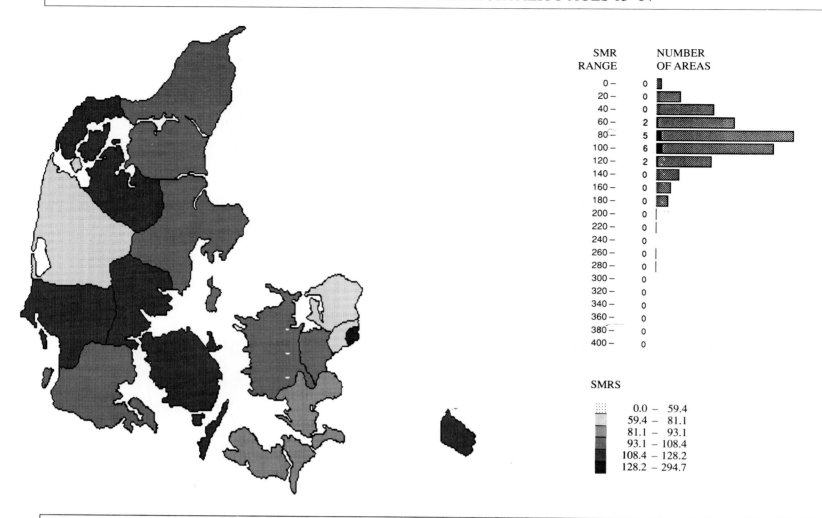

SMR RANGE	NUMBER OF AREAS	
0 –	0	
20 –	0	
40 –	0	
60 –	2	
80 –	5	
100 –	6	
120 –	2	
140 –	0	
160 –	0	
180 –	0	
200 –	0	
220 –	0	
240 –	0	
260 –	0	
280 –	0	
300 –	0	
320 –	0	
340 –	0	
360 –	0	
380 –	0	
400 –	0	

SMRS

	0.0 – 59.4
	59.4 – 81.1
	81.1 – 93.1
	93.1 – 108.4
	108.4 – 128.2
	128.2 – 294.7

DENMARK: MALIGNANT NEOPLASM OF CERVIX AND BODY OF UTERUS MORTALITY AGES 15–54

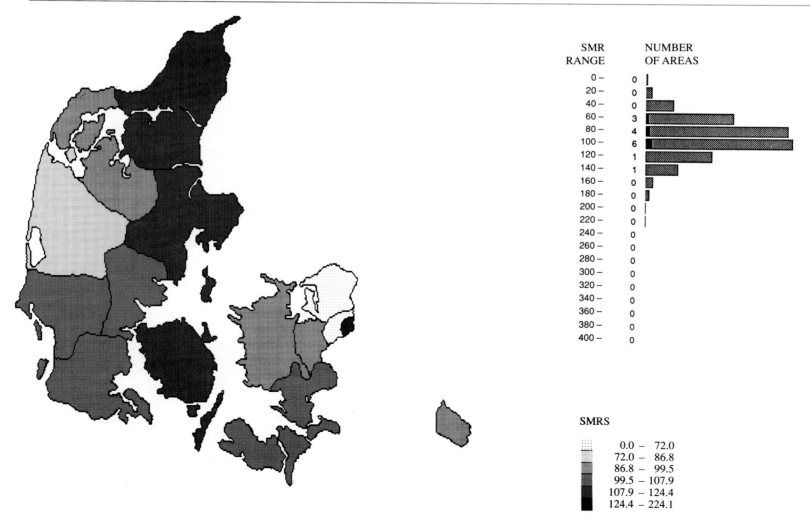

SMR RANGE	NUMBER OF AREAS	
0 –	0	
20 –	0	
40 –	0	
60 –	3	
80 –	4	
100 –	6	
120 –	1	
140 –	1	
160 –	0	
180 –	0	
200 –	0	
220 –	0	
240 –	0	
260 –	0	
280 –	0	
300 –	0	
320 –	0	
340 –	0	
360 –	0	
380 –	0	
400 –	0	

SMRS

	0.0 – 72.0
	72.0 – 86.8
	86.8 – 99.5
	99.5 – 107.9
	107.9 – 124.4
	124.4 – 224.1

DENMARK: HODGKIN'S DISEASE MORTALITY AGES 5–64

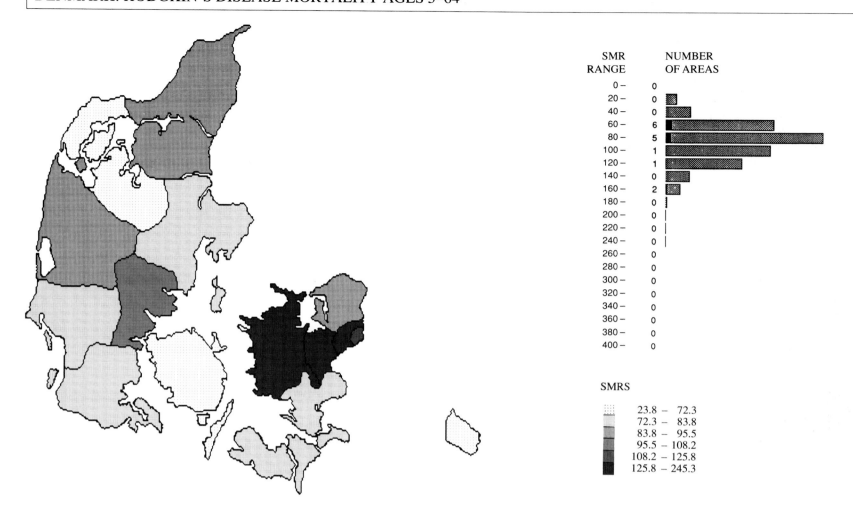

SMR RANGE	NUMBER OF AREAS
0 –	0
20 –	0
40 –	0
60 –	6
80 –	5
100 –	1
120 –	1
140 –	0
160 –	2
180 –	0
200 –	0
220 –	0
240 –	0
260 –	0
280 –	0
300 –	0
320 –	0
340 –	0
360 –	0
380 –	0
400 –	0

SMRS

	23.8 – 72.3
	72.3 – 83.8
	83.8 – 95.5
	95.5 – 108.2
	108.2 – 125.8
	125.8 – 245.3

DENMARK: CHRONIC RHEUMATIC HEART DISEASE MORTALITY AGES 5–44

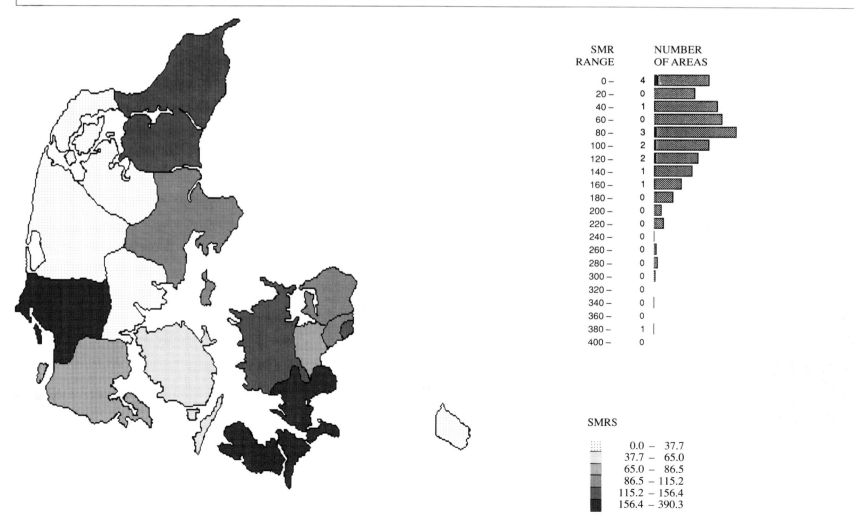

SMR RANGE	NUMBER OF AREAS
0 –	4
20 –	0
40 –	1
60 –	0
80 –	3
100 –	2
120 –	2
140 –	1
160 –	1
180 –	0
200 –	0
220 –	0
240 –	0
260 –	0
280 –	0
300 –	0
320 –	0
340 –	0
360 –	0
380 –	1
400 –	0

SMRS

	0.0 – 37.7
	37.7 – 65.0
	65.0 – 86.5
	86.5 – 115.2
	115.2 – 156.4
	156.4 – 390.3

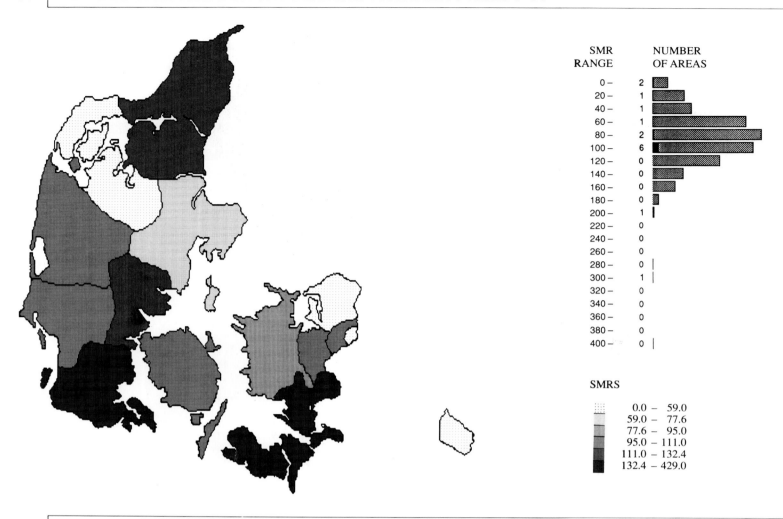

SMR RANGE	NUMBER OF AREAS
0 –	2
20 –	1
40 –	1
60 –	1
80 –	2
100 –	6
120 –	0
140 –	0
160 –	0
180 –	0
200 –	1
220 –	0
240 –	0
260 –	0
280 –	0
300 –	1
320 –	0
340 –	0
360 –	0
380 –	0
400 –	0

SMRS

	0.0 – 59.0
	59.0 – 77.6
	77.6 – 95.0
	95.0 – 111.0
	111.0 – 132.4
	132.4 – 429.0

DENMARK: ASTHMA MORTALITY AGES 5–44

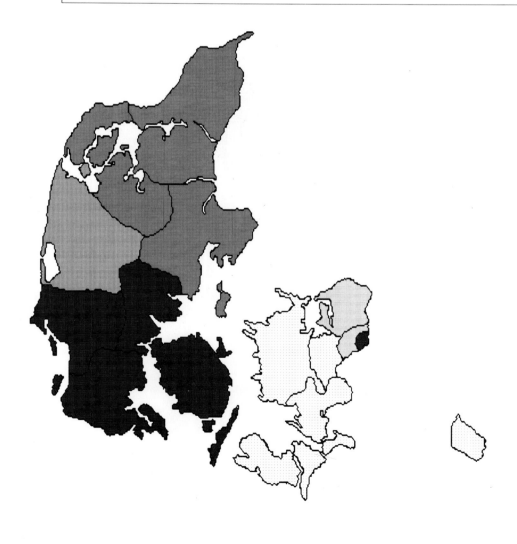

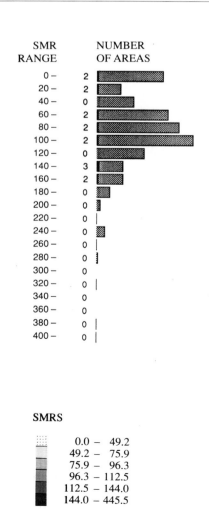

SMR RANGE	NUMBER OF AREAS
0 –	2
20 –	2
40 –	0
60 –	2
80 –	2
100 –	2
120 –	0
140 –	3
160 –	2
180 –	0
200 –	0
220 –	0
240 –	0
260 –	0
280 –	0
300 –	0
320 –	0
340 –	0
360 –	0
380 –	0
400 –	0

SMRS

	0.0 – 49.2
	49.2 – 75.9
	75.9 – 96.3
	96.3 – 112.5
	112.5 – 144.0
	144.0 – 445.5

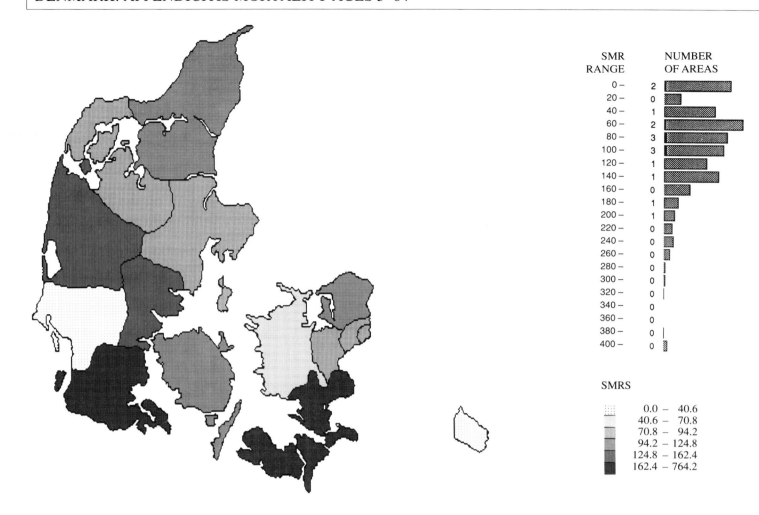

SMR RANGE | NUMBER OF AREAS
0 – | 2
20 – | 0
40 – | 1
60 – | 2
80 – | 3
100 – | 3
120 – | 1
140 – | 1
160 – | 0
180 – | 1
200 – | 1
220 – | 0
240 – | 0
260 – | 0
280 – | 0
300 – | 0
320 – | 0
340 – | 0
360 – | 0
380 – | 0
400 – | 0

SMRS

0.0 – 40.6
40.6 – 70.8
70.8 – 94.2
94.2 – 124.8
124.8 – 162.4
162.4 – 764.2

DENMARK: ABDOMINAL HERNIA MORTALITY AGES 5–64

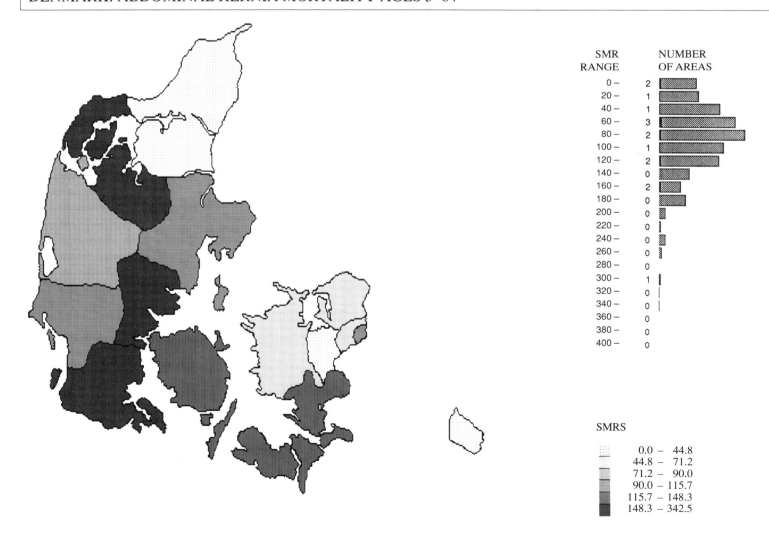

SMR RANGE | NUMBER OF AREAS
0 – | 2
20 – | 1
40 – | 1
60 – | 3
80 – | 2
100 – | 1
120 – | 2
140 – | 0
160 – | 2
180 – | 0
200 – | 0
220 – | 0
240 – | 0
260 – | 0
280 – | 0
300 – | 1
320 – | 0
340 – | 0
360 – | 0
380 – | 0
400 – | 0

SMRS

0.0 – 44.8
44.8 – 71.2
71.2 – 90.0
90.0 – 115.7
115.7 – 148.3
148.3 – 342.5

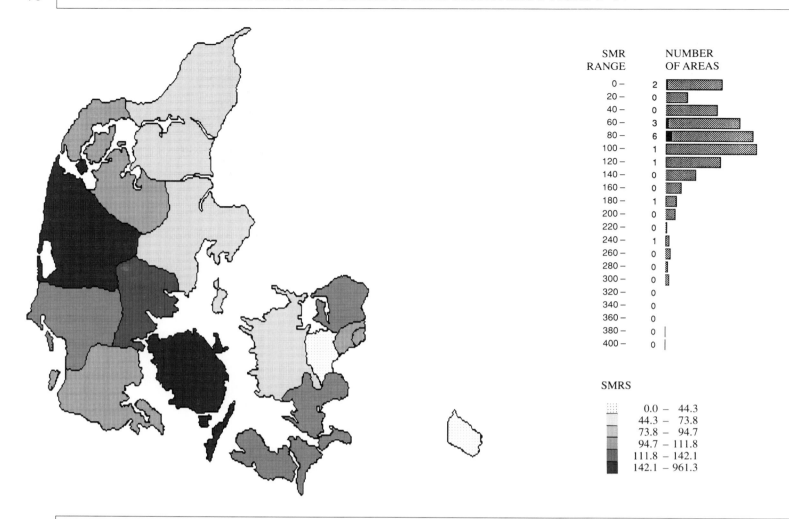

SMR RANGE	NUMBER OF AREAS
0 –	2
20 –	0
40 –	0
60 –	3
80 –	6
100 –	1
120 –	1
140 –	0
160 –	0
180 –	1
200 –	0
220 –	0
240 –	1
260 –	0
280 –	0
300 –	0
320 –	0
340 –	0
360 –	0
380 –	0
400 –	0

SMRS

	0.0 – 44.3
	44.3 – 73.8
	73.8 – 94.7
	94.7 – 111.8
	111.8 – 142.1
	142.1 – 961.3

DENMARK: HYPERTENSIVE AND CEREBROVASCULAR DISEASES MORTALITY AGES 35–64

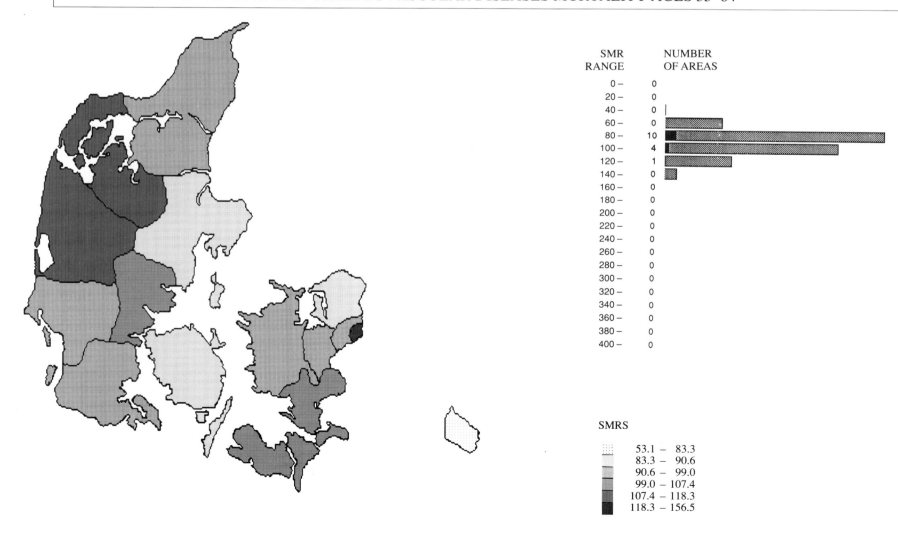

SMR RANGE	NUMBER OF AREAS
0 –	0
20 –	0
40 –	0
60 –	0
80 –	10
100 –	4
120 –	1
140 –	0
160 –	0
180 –	0
200 –	0
220 –	0
240 –	0
260 –	0
280 –	0
300 –	0
320 –	0
340 –	0
360 –	0
380 –	0
400 –	0

SMRS

	53.1 – 83.3
	83.3 – 90.6
	90.6 – 99.0
	99.0 – 107.4
	107.4 – 118.3
	118.3 – 156.5

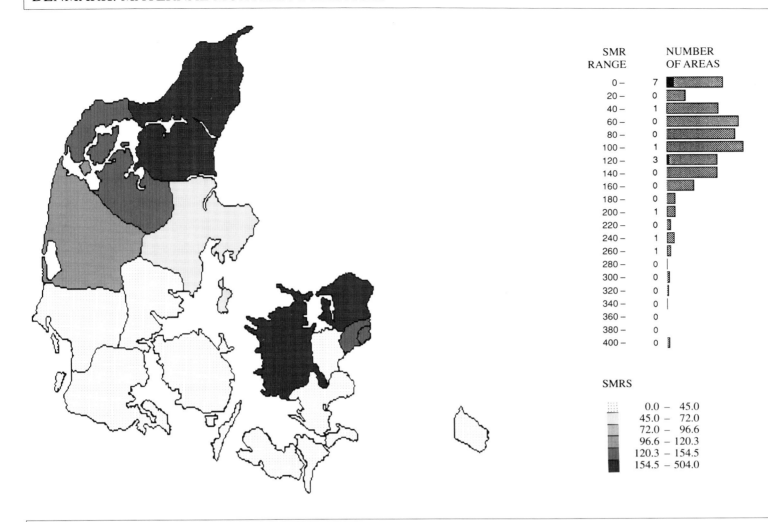

SMR RANGE	NUMBER OF AREAS
0 –	7
20 –	0
40 –	1
60 –	0
80 –	0
100 –	1
120 –	3
140 –	0
160 –	0
180 –	0
200 –	1
220 –	0
240 –	1
260 –	1
280 –	0
300 –	0
320 –	0
340 –	0
360 –	0
380 –	0
400 –	0

SMRS

	0.0 – 45.0
	45.0 – 72.0
	72.0 – 96.6
	96.6 – 120.3
	120.3 – 154.5
	154.5 – 504.0

DENMARK: PERINATAL MORTALITY

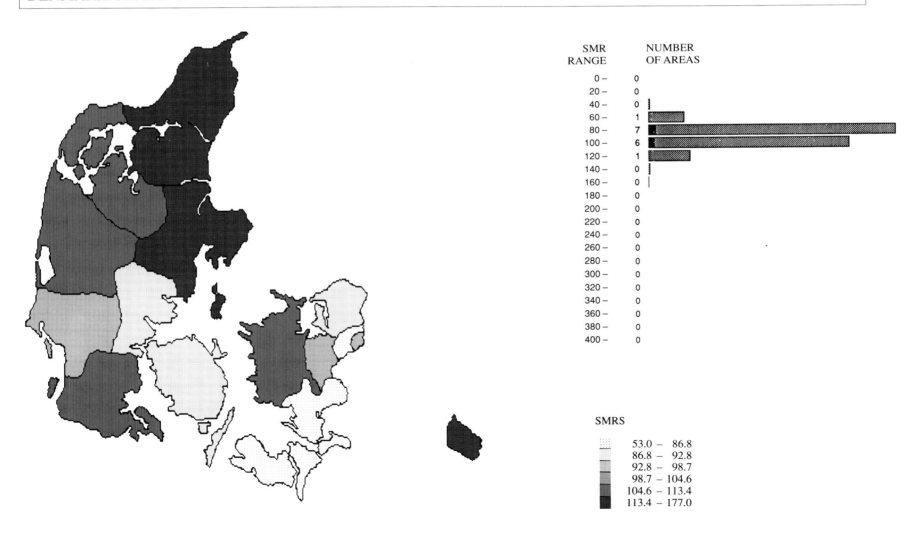

SMR RANGE	NUMBER OF AREAS
0 –	0
20 –	0
40 –	0
60 –	1
80 –	7
100 –	6
120 –	1
140 –	0
160 –	0
180 –	0
200 –	0
220 –	0
240 –	0
260 –	0
280 –	0
300 –	0
320 –	0
340 –	0
360 –	0
380 –	0
400 –	0

SMRS

	53.0 – 86.8
	86.8 – 92.8
	92.8 – 98.7
	98.7 – 104.6
	104.6 – 113.4
	113.4 – 177.0

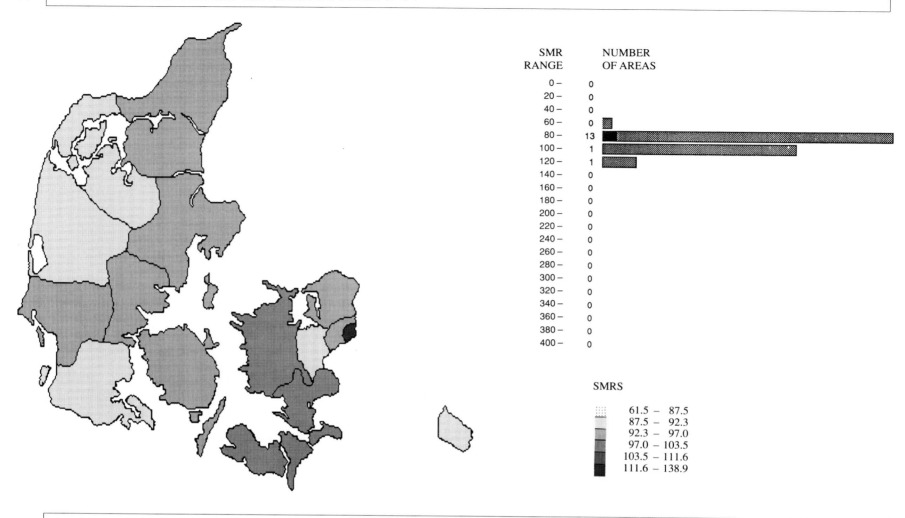

SMR
RANGE

NUMBER
OF AREAS

0 –	0
20 –	0
40 –	0
60 –	0
80 –	13
100 –	1
120 –	1
140 –	0
160 –	0
180 –	0
200 –	0
220 –	0
240 –	0
260 –	0
280 –	0
300 –	0
320 –	0
340 –	0
360 –	0
380 –	0
400 –	0

SMRS

61.5 –	87.5
87.5 –	92.3
92.3 –	97.0
97.0 –	103.5
103.5 –	111.6
111.6 –	138.9

DENMARK: ALL CAUSES MORTALITY ALL AGES

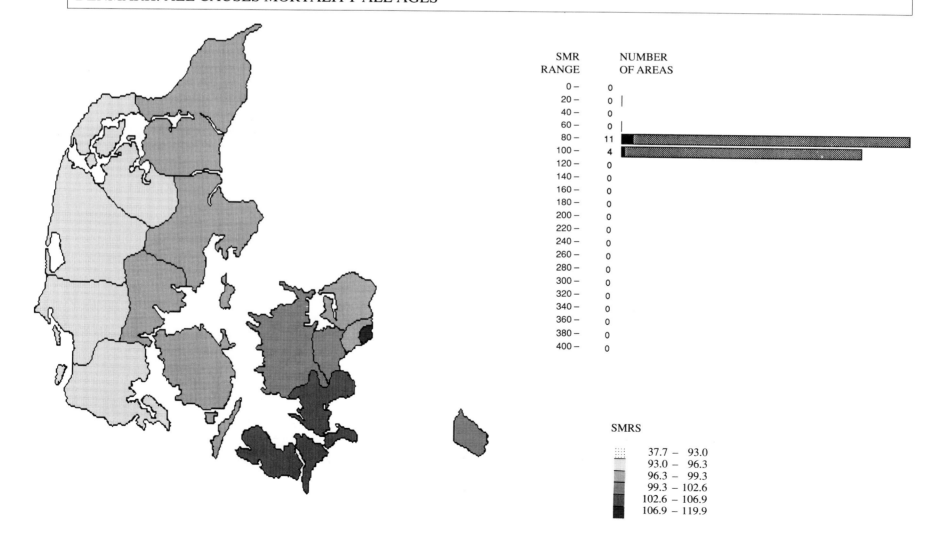

SMR
RANGE

NUMBER
OF AREAS

0 –	0
20 –	0
40 –	0
60 –	0
80 –	11
100 –	4
120 –	0
140 –	0
160 –	0
180 –	0
200 –	0
220 –	0
240 –	0
260 –	0
280 –	0
300 –	0
320 –	0
340 –	0
360 –	0
380 –	0
400 –	0

SMRS

37.7 –	93.0
93.0 –	96.3
96.3 –	99.3
99.3 –	102.6
102.6 –	106.9
106.9 –	119.9

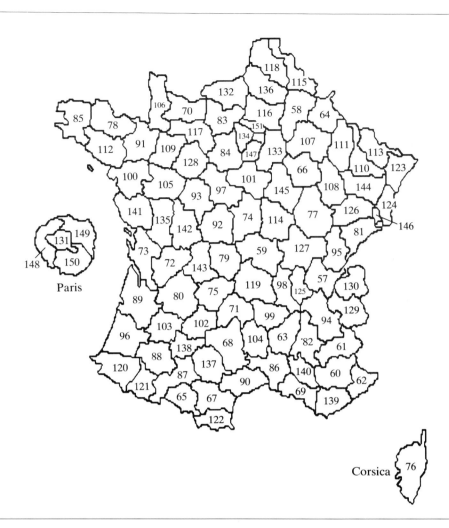

FRANCE: TUBERCULOSIS MORTALITY AGES 5–64

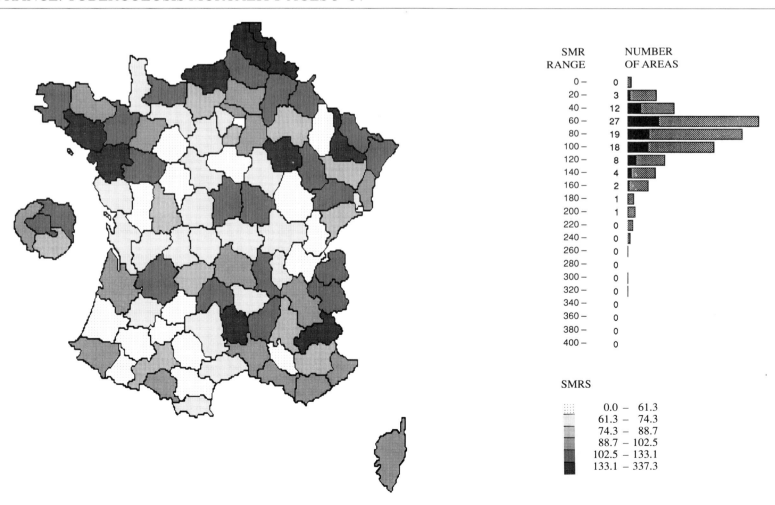

SMR RANGE	NUMBER OF AREAS
0 –	0
20 –	3
40 –	12
60 –	27
80 –	19
100 –	18
120 –	8
140 –	4
160 –	2
180 –	1
200 –	1
220 –	0
240 –	0
260 –	0
280 –	0
300 –	0
320 –	0
340 –	0
360 –	0
380 –	0
400 –	0

SMRS

	0.0 – 61.3
	61.3 – 74.3
	74.3 – 88.7
	88.7 – 102.5
	102.5 – 133.1
	133.1 – 337.3

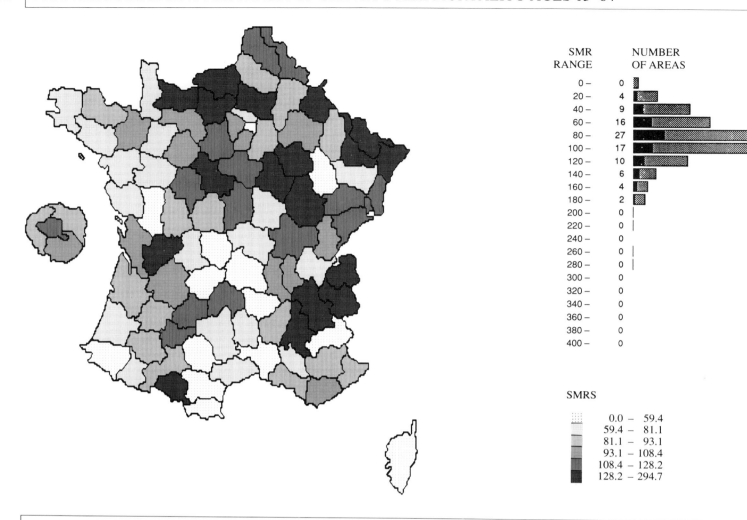

SMR RANGE	NUMBER OF AREAS
0 –	0
20 –	4
40 –	9
60 –	16
80 –	27
100 –	17
120 –	10
140 –	6
160 –	4
180 –	2
200 –	0
220 –	0
240 –	0
260 –	0
280 –	0
300 –	0
320 –	0
340 –	0
360 –	0
380 –	0
400 –	0

SMRS

	0.0 – 59.4
	59.4 – 81.1
	81.1 – 93.1
	93.1 – 108.4
	108.4 – 128.2
	128.2 – 294.7

FRANCE: MALIGNANT NEOPLASM OF CERVIX AND BODY OF UTERUS MORTALITY AGES 15–54

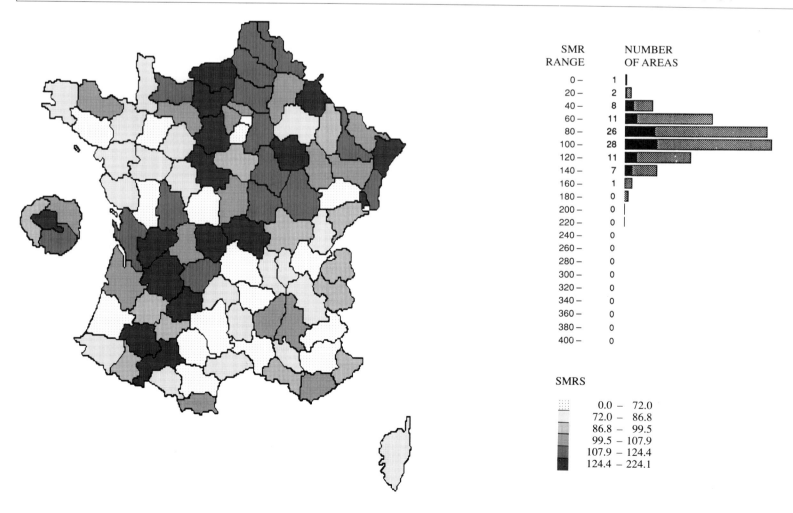

SMR RANGE	NUMBER OF AREAS
0 –	1
20 –	2
40 –	8
60 –	11
80 –	26
100 –	28
120 –	11
140 –	7
160 –	1
180 –	0
200 –	0
220 –	0
240 –	0
260 –	0
280 –	0
300 –	0
320 –	0
340 –	0
360 –	0
380 –	0
400 –	0

SMRS

	0.0 – 72.0
	72.0 – 86.8
	86.8 – 99.5
	99.5 – 107.9
	107.9 – 124.4
	124.4 – 224.1

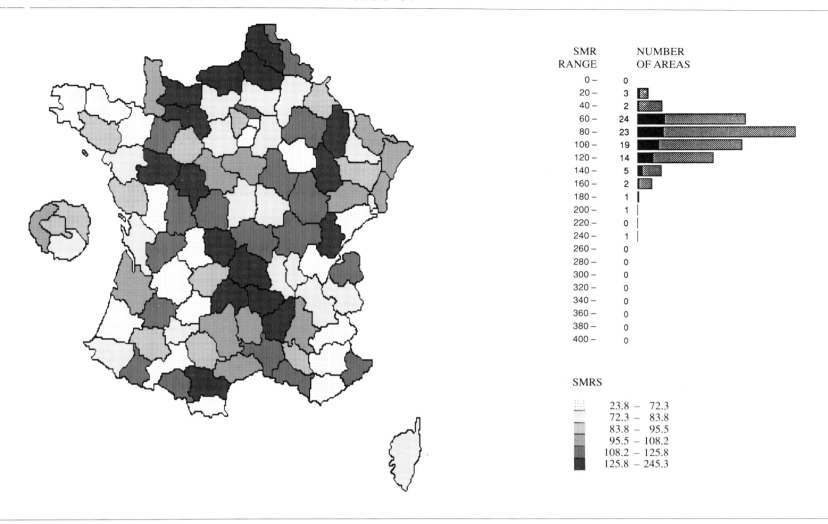

SMR RANGE	NUMBER OF AREAS
0 –	0
20 –	3
40 –	2
60 –	24
80 –	23
100 –	19
120 –	14
140 –	5
160 –	2
180 –	1
200 –	1
220 –	0
240 –	1
260 –	0
280 –	0
300 –	0
320 –	0
340 –	0
360 –	0
380 –	0
400 –	0

SMRS

23.8 – 72.3
72.3 – 83.8
83.8 – 95.5
95.5 – 108.2
108.2 – 125.8
125.8 – 245.3

FRANCE: CHRONIC RHEUMATIC HEART DISEASE MORTALITY AGES 5–44

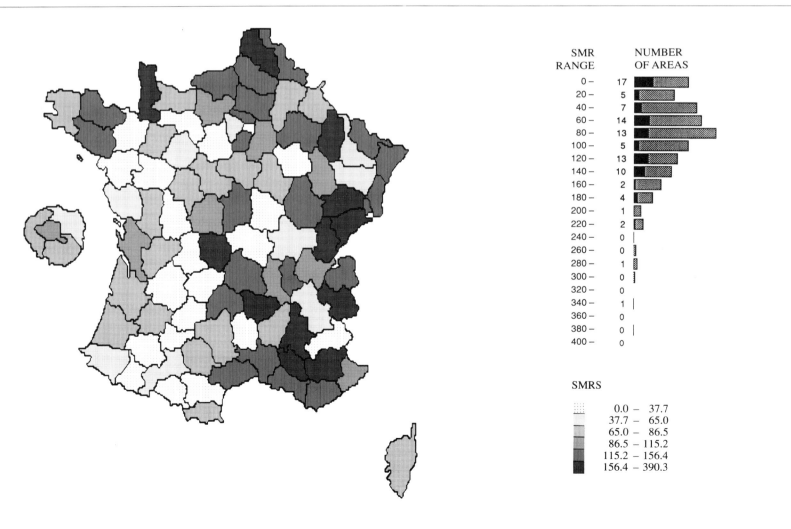

SMR RANGE	NUMBER OF AREAS
0 –	17
20 –	5
40 –	7
60 –	14
80 –	13
100 –	5
120 –	13
140 –	10
160 –	2
180 –	4
200 –	1
220 –	2
240 –	0
260 –	0
280 –	1
300 –	0
320 –	0
340 –	1
360 –	0
380 –	0
400 –	0

SMRS

0.0 – 37.7
37.7 – 65.0
65.0 – 86.5
86.5 – 115.2
115.2 – 156.4
156.4 – 390.3

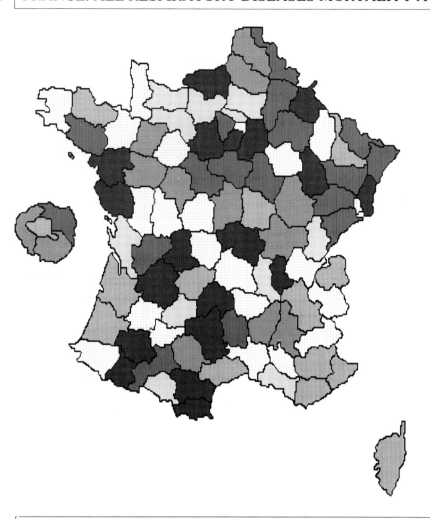

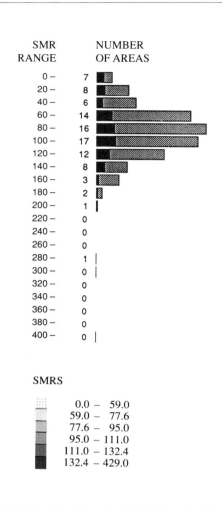

SMR RANGE	NUMBER OF AREAS	
0 –	7	
20 –	8	
40 –	6	
60 –	14	
80 –	16	
100 –	17	
120 –	12	
140 –	8	
160 –	3	
180 –	2	
200 –	1	
220 –	0	
240 –	0	
260 –	0	
280 –	1	
300 –	0	
320 –	0	
340 –	0	
360 –	0	
380 –	0	
400 –	0	

SMRS

	0.0 – 59.0
	59.0 – 77.6
	77.6 – 95.0
	95.0 – 111.0
	111.0 – 132.4
	132.4 – 429.0

FRANCE: ASTHMA MORTALITY AGES 5–44

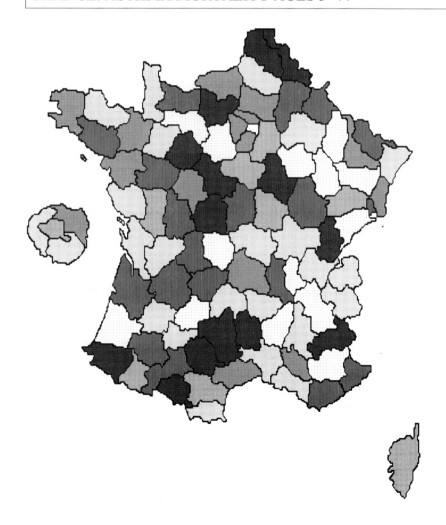

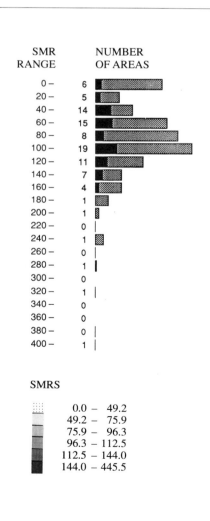

SMR RANGE	NUMBER OF AREAS	
0 –	6	
20 –	5	
40 –	14	
60 –	15	
80 –	8	
100 –	19	
120 –	11	
140 –	7	
160 –	4	
180 –	1	
200 –	1	
220 –	0	
240 –	1	
260 –	0	
280 –	1	
300 –	0	
320 –	1	
340 –	0	
360 –	0	
380 –	0	
400 –	1	

SMRS

	0.0 – 49.2
	49.2 – 75.9
	75.9 – 96.3
	96.3 – 112.5
	112.5 – 144.0
	144.0 – 445.5

FRANCE: APPENDICITIS MORTALITY AGES 5–64

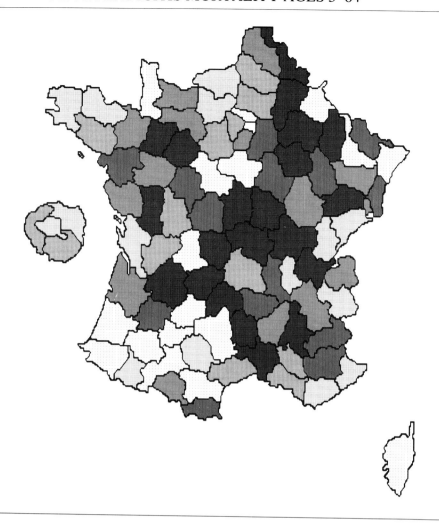

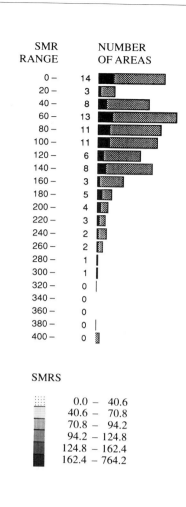

SMR RANGE	NUMBER OF AREAS
0 –	14
20 –	3
40 –	8
60 –	13
80 –	11
100 –	11
120 –	6
140 –	8
160 –	3
180 –	5
200 –	4
220 –	3
240 –	2
260 –	2
280 –	1
300 –	1
320 –	0
340 –	0
360 –	0
380 –	0
400 –	0

SMRS

	0.0 – 40.6
	40.6 – 70.8
	70.8 – 94.2
	94.2 – 124.8
	124.8 – 162.4
	162.4 – 764.2

FRANCE: ABDOMINAL HERNIA MORTALITY AGES 5–64

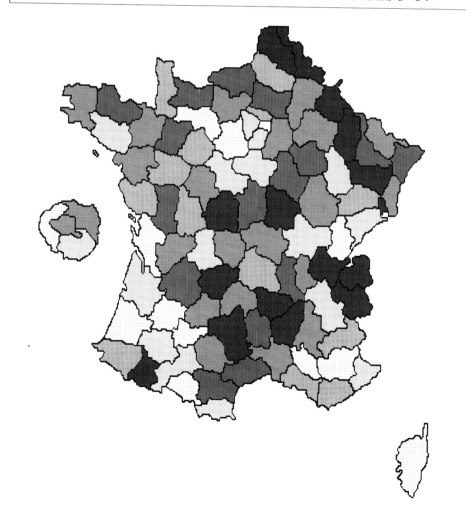

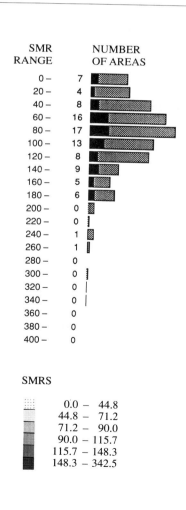

SMR RANGE	NUMBER OF AREAS
0 –	7
20 –	4
40 –	8
60 –	16
80 –	17
100 –	13
120 –	8
140 –	9
160 –	5
180 –	6
200 –	0
220 –	0
240 –	1
260 –	1
280 –	0
300 –	0
320 –	0
340 –	0
360 –	0
380 –	0
400 –	0

SMRS

	0.0 – 44.8
	44.8 – 71.2
	71.2 – 90.0
	90.0 – 115.7
	115.7 – 148.3
	148.3 – 342.5

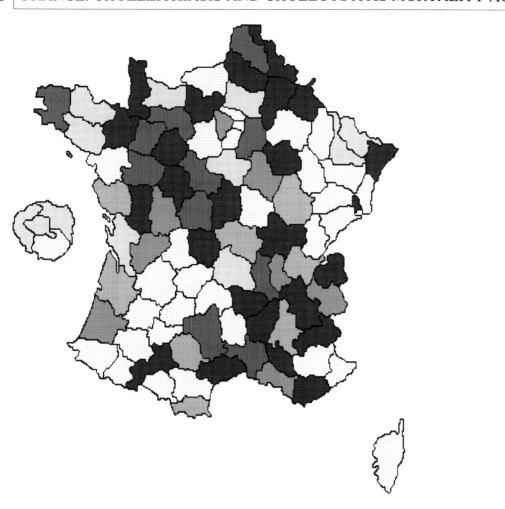
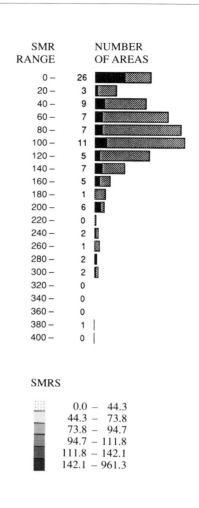

SMR RANGE	NUMBER OF AREAS
0 –	26
20 –	3
40 –	9
60 –	7
80 –	7
100 –	11
120 –	5
140 –	7
160 –	5
180 –	1
200 –	6
220 –	0
240 –	2
260 –	1
280 –	2
300 –	2
320 –	0
340 –	0
360 –	0
380 –	1
400 –	0

SMRS

	0.0 – 44.3
	44.3 – 73.8
	73.8 – 94.7
	94.7 – 111.8
	111.8 – 142.1
	142.1 – 961.3

FRANCE: HYPERTENSIVE AND CEREBROVASCULAR DISEASES MORTALITY AGES 35–64

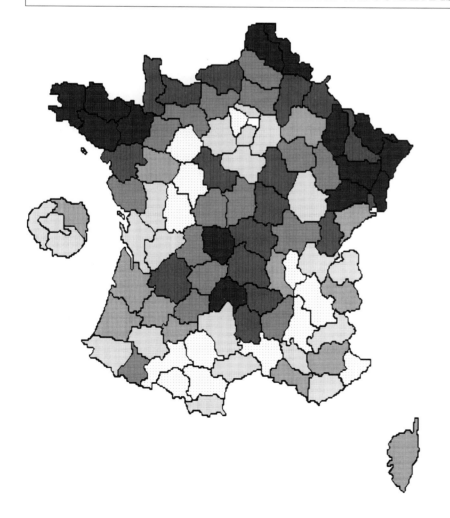
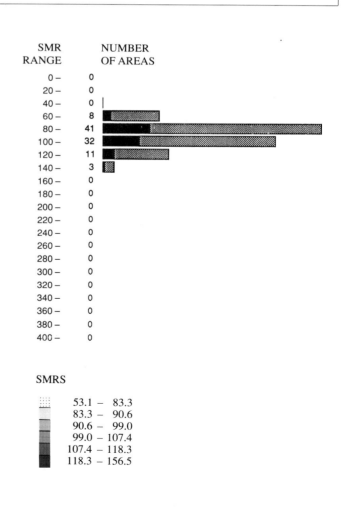

SMR RANGE	NUMBER OF AREAS
0 –	0
20 –	0
40 –	0
60 –	8
80 –	41
100 –	32
120 –	11
140 –	3
160 –	0
180 –	0
200 –	0
220 –	0
240 –	0
260 –	0
280 –	0
300 –	0
320 –	0
340 –	0
360 –	0
380 –	0
400 –	0

SMRS

	53.1 – 83.3
	83.3 – 90.6
	90.6 – 99.0
	99.0 – 107.4
	107.4 – 118.3
	118.3 – 156.5

FRANCE: MATERNAL MORTALITY ALL AGES

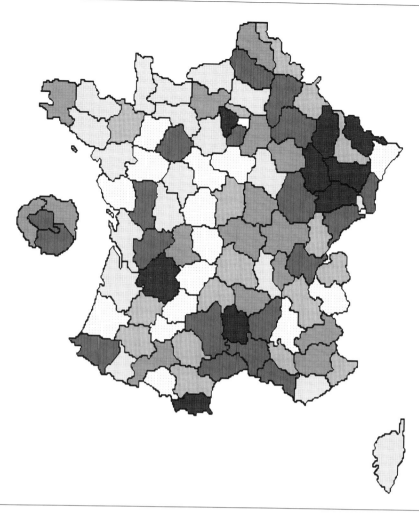

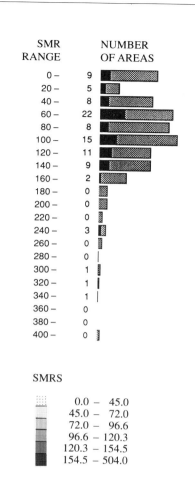

SMR RANGE	NUMBER OF AREAS
0 –	9
20 –	5
40 –	8
60 –	22
80 –	8
100 –	15
120 –	11
140 –	9
160 –	2
180 –	0
200 –	0
220 –	0
240 –	3
260 –	0
280 –	0
300 –	1
320 –	1
340 –	1
360 –	0
380 –	0
400 –	0

SMRS

	0.0 – 45.0
	45.0 – 72.0
	72.0 – 96.6
	96.6 – 120.3
	120.3 – 154.5
	154.5 – 504.0

FRANCE: PERINATAL MORTALITY

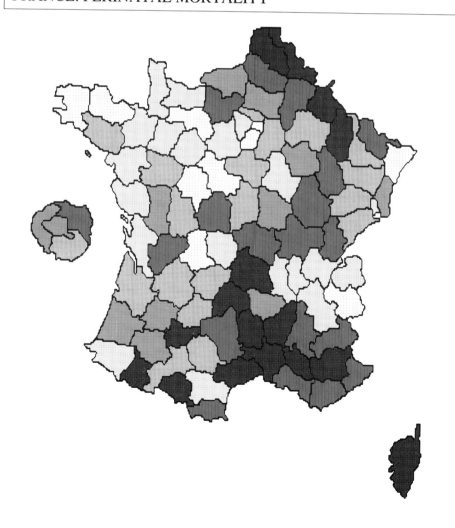

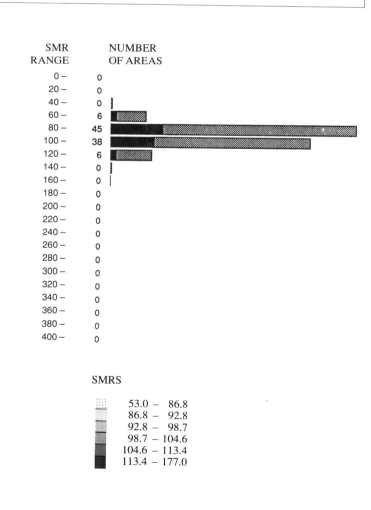

SMR RANGE	NUMBER OF AREAS
0 –	0
20 –	0
40 –	0
60 –	6
80 –	45
100 –	38
120 –	6
140 –	0
160 –	0
180 –	0
200 –	0
220 –	0
240 –	0
260 –	0
280 –	0
300 –	0
320 –	0
340 –	0
360 –	0
380 –	0
400 –	0

SMRS

	53.0 – 86.8
	86.8 – 92.8
	92.8 – 98.7
	98.7 – 104.6
	104.6 – 113.4
	113.4 – 177.0

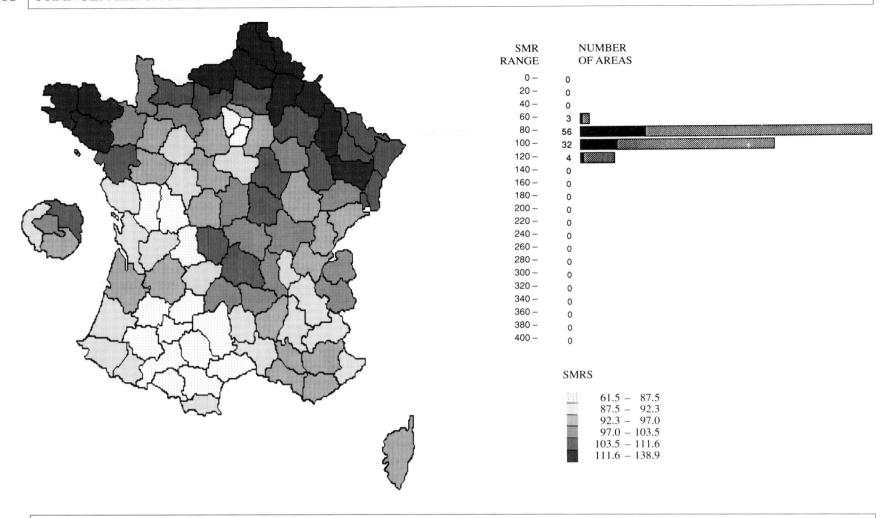

SMR RANGE	NUMBER OF AREAS
0 –	0
20 –	0
40 –	0
60 –	3
80 –	56
100 –	32
120 –	4
140 –	0
160 –	0
180 –	0
200 –	0
220 –	0
240 –	0
260 –	0
280 –	0
300 –	0
320 –	0
340 –	0
360 –	0
380 –	0
400 –	0

SMRS

61.5 – 87.5
87.5 – 92.3
92.3 – 97.0
97.0 – 103.5
103.5 – 111.6
111.6 – 138.9

FRANCE: ALL CAUSES MORTALITY ALL AGES

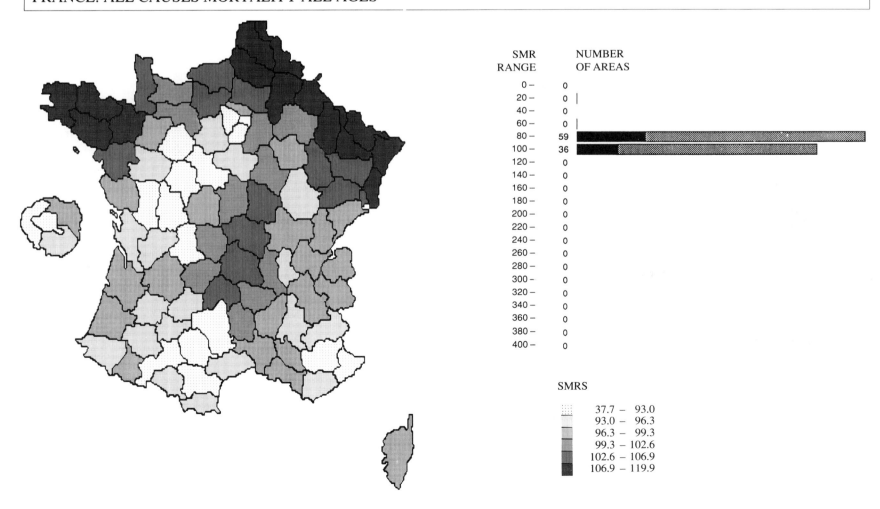

SMR RANGE	NUMBER OF AREAS
0 –	0
20 –	0
40 –	0
60 –	0
80 –	59
100 –	36
120 –	0
140 –	0
160 –	0
180 –	0
200 –	0
220 –	0
240 –	0
260 –	0
280 –	0
300 –	0
320 –	0
340 –	0
360 –	0
380 –	0
400 –	0

SMRS

37.7 – 93.0
93.0 – 96.3
96.3 – 99.3
99.3 – 102.6
102.6 – 106.9
106.9 – 119.9

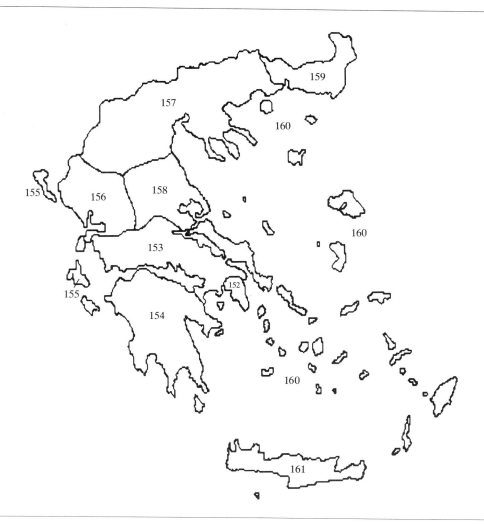

GREECE: TUBERCULOSIS MORTALITY AGES 5–64

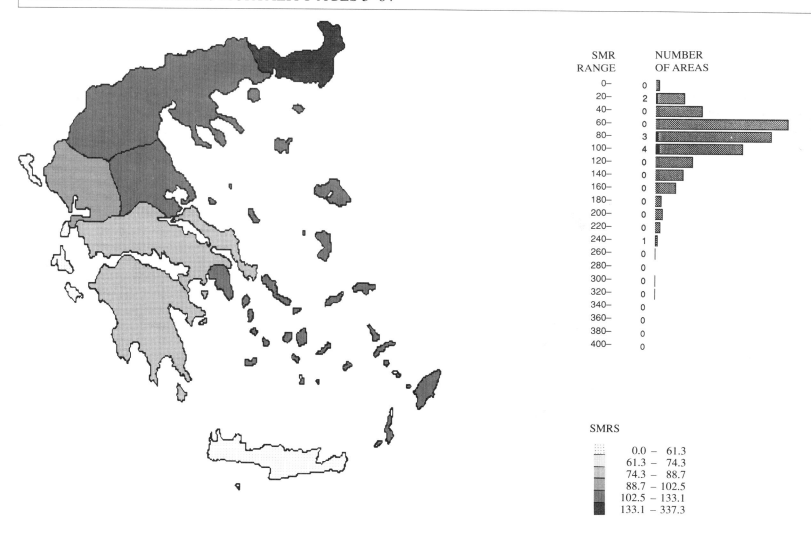

SMR RANGE	NUMBER OF AREAS
0–	0
20–	2
40–	0
60–	0
80–	3
100–	4
120–	0
140–	0
160–	0
180–	0
200–	0
220–	0
240–	1
260–	0
280–	0
300–	0
320–	0
340–	0
360–	0
380–	0
400–	0

SMRS

0.0 – 61.3
61.3 – 74.3
74.3 – 88.7
88.7 – 102.5
102.5 – 133.1
133.1 – 337.3

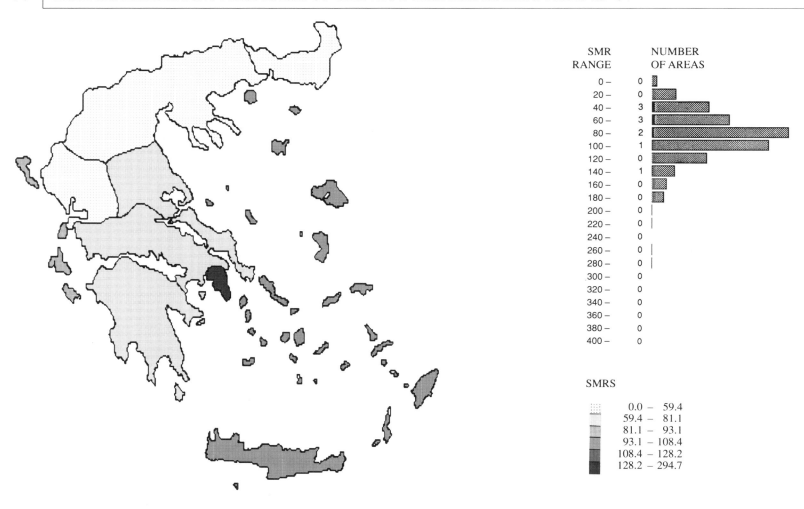

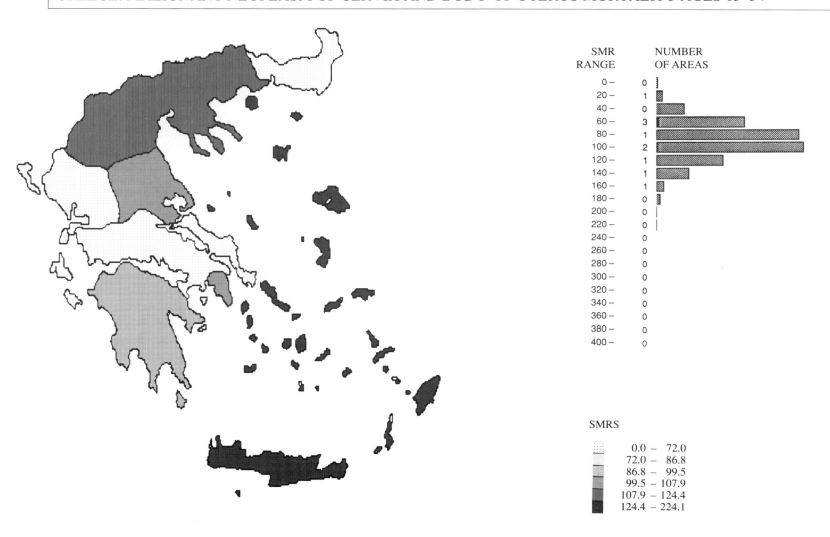

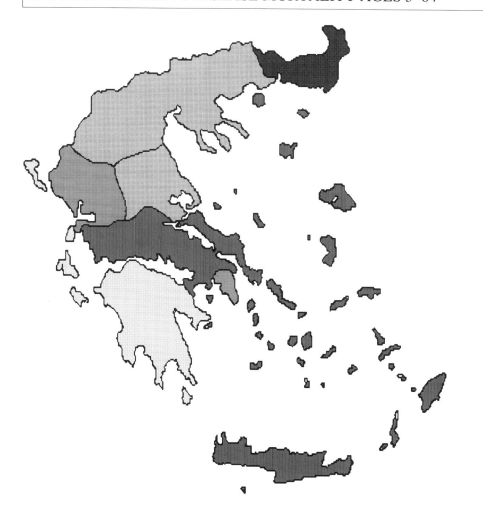

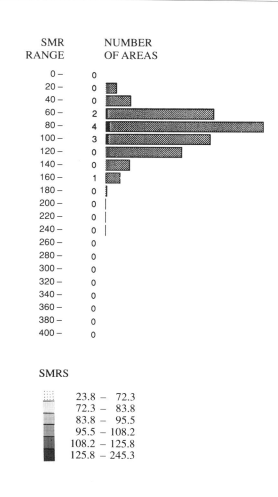

SMR RANGE	NUMBER OF AREAS
0 –	0
20 –	0
40 –	0
60 –	2
80 –	4
100 –	3
120 –	0
140 –	0
160 –	1
180 –	0
200 –	0
220 –	0
240 –	0
260 –	0
280 –	0
300 –	0
320 –	0
340 –	0
360 –	0
380 –	0
400 –	0

SMRS

	23.8 – 72.3
	72.3 – 83.8
	83.8 – 95.5
	95.5 – 108.2
	108.2 – 125.8
	125.8 – 245.3

GREECE: CHRONIC RHEUMATIC HEART DISEASE MORTALITY AGES 5–44

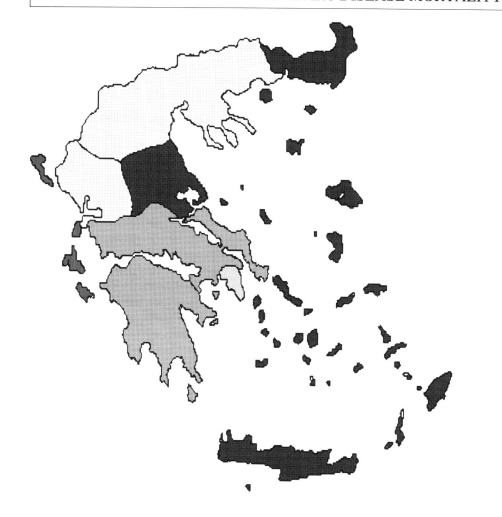

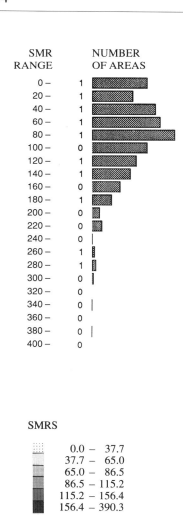

SMR RANGE	NUMBER OF AREAS
0 –	1
20 –	1
40 –	1
60 –	1
80 –	1
100 –	0
120 –	1
140 –	1
160 –	0
180 –	1
200 –	0
220 –	0
240 –	0
260 –	1
280 –	1
300 –	0
320 –	0
340 –	0
360 –	0
380 –	0
400 –	0

SMRS

	0.0 – 37.7
	37.7 – 65.0
	65.0 – 86.5
	86.5 – 115.2
	115.2 – 156.4
	156.4 – 390.3

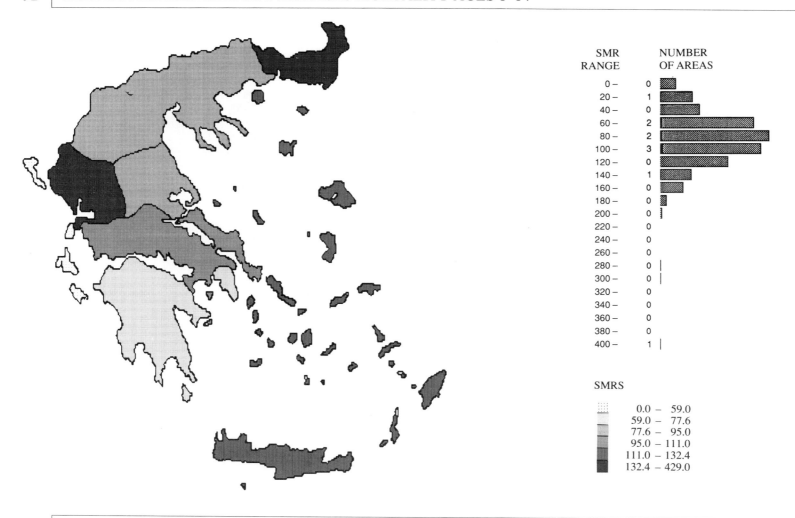

SMR RANGE	NUMBER OF AREAS	
0 –	0	
20 –	1	
40 –	0	
60 –	2	
80 –	2	
100 –	3	
120 –	0	
140 –	1	
160 –	0	
180 –	0	
200 –	0	
220 –	0	
240 –	0	
260 –	0	
280 –	0	
300 –	0	
320 –	0	
340 –	0	
360 –	0	
380 –	0	
400 –	1	

SMRS

	0.0 – 59.0
	59.0 – 77.6
	77.6 – 95.0
	95.0 – 111.0
	111.0 – 132.4
	132.4 – 429.0

GREECE: ASTHMA MORTALITY AGES 5–44

DATA FOR THIS MAP ARE NOT AVAILABLE FOR GREECE

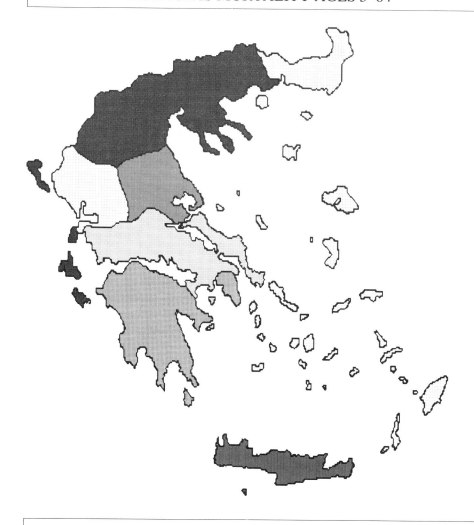

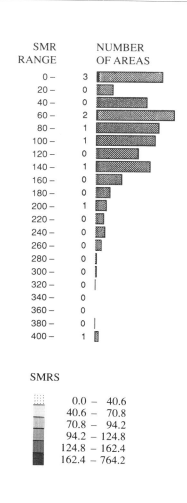

SMRS

	0.0 – 40.6
	40.6 – 70.8
	70.8 – 94.2
	94.2 – 124.8
	124.8 – 162.4
	162.4 – 764.2

GREECE: ABDOMINAL HERNIA MORTALITY AGES 5–64

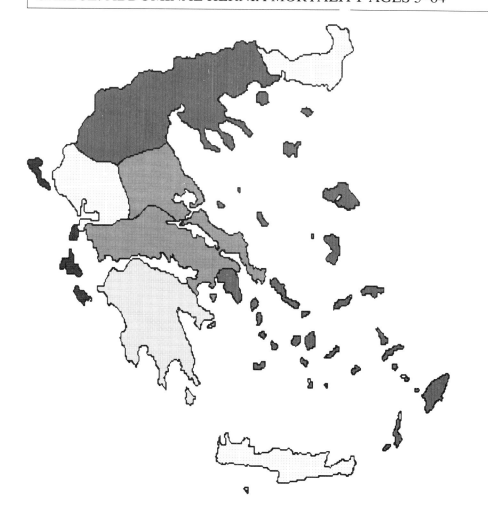

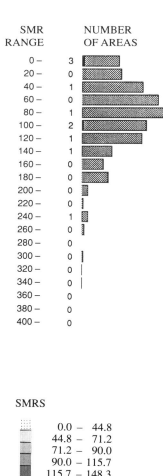

SMRS

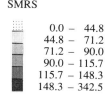

	0.0 – 44.8
	44.8 – 71.2
	71.2 – 90.0
	90.0 – 115.7
	115.7 – 148.3
	148.3 – 342.5

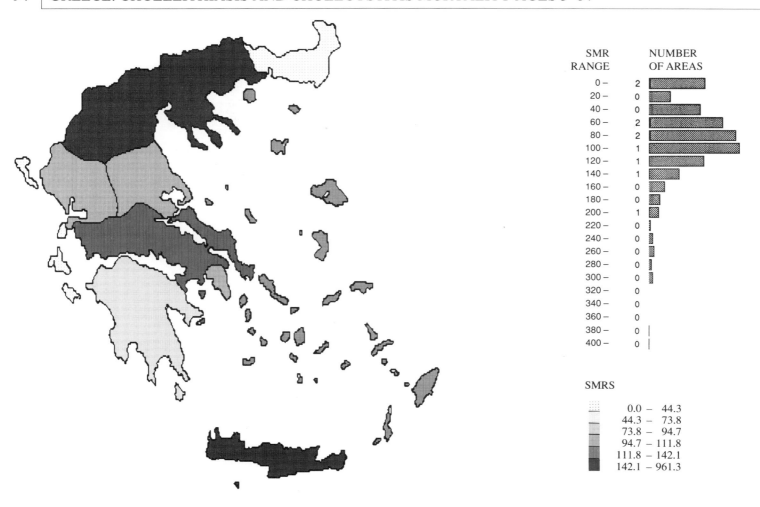

SMR RANGE	NUMBER OF AREAS
0 –	2
20 –	0
40 –	0
60 –	2
80 –	2
100 –	1
120 –	1
140 –	1
160 –	0
180 –	0
200 –	1
220 –	0
240 –	0
260 –	0
280 –	0
300 –	0
320 –	0
340 –	0
360 –	0
380 –	0
400 –	0

SMRS

	0.0 – 44.3
	44.3 – 73.8
	73.8 – 94.7
	94.7 – 111.8
	111.8 – 142.1
	142.1 – 961.3

GREECE: HYPERTENSIVE AND CEREBROVASCULAR DISEASES MORTALITY AGES 35–64

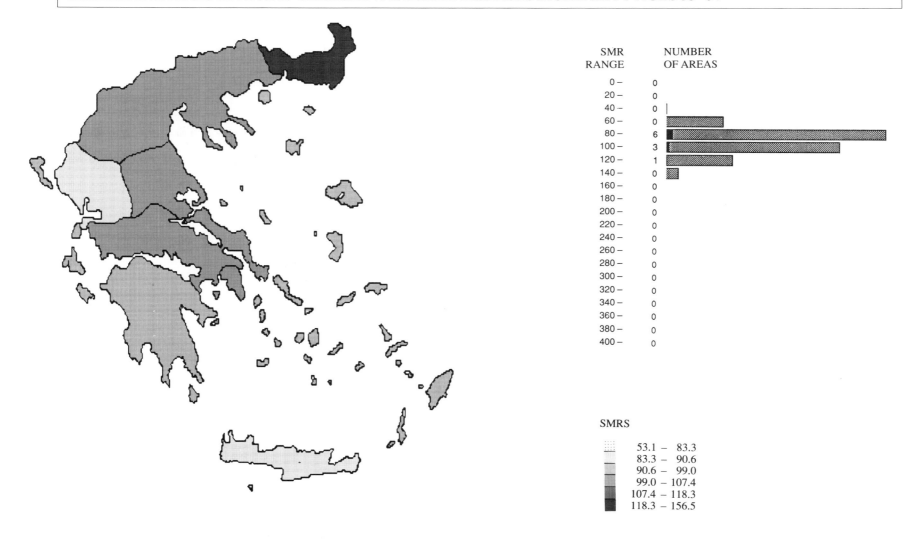

SMR RANGE	NUMBER OF AREAS
0 –	0
20 –	0
40 –	0
60 –	0
80 –	6
100 –	3
120 –	1
140 –	0
160 –	0
180 –	0
200 –	0
220 –	0
240 –	0
260 –	0
280 –	0
300 –	0
320 –	0
340 –	0
360 –	0
380 –	0
400 –	0

SMRS

	53.1 – 83.3
	83.3 – 90.6
	90.6 – 99.0
	99.0 – 107.4
	107.4 – 118.3
	118.3 – 156.5

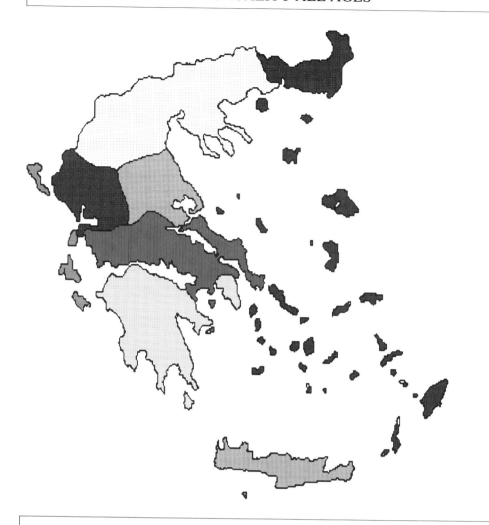

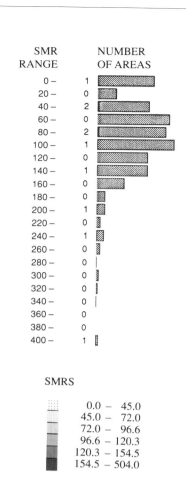

SMR RANGE	NUMBER OF AREAS
0 –	1
20 –	0
40 –	2
60 –	0
80 –	2
100 –	1
120 –	0
140 –	1
160 –	0
180 –	0
200 –	1
220 –	0
240 –	1
260 –	0
280 –	0
300 –	0
320 –	0
340 –	0
360 –	0
380 –	0
400 –	1

SMRS

	0.0 – 45.0
	45.0 – 72.0
	72.0 – 96.6
	96.6 – 120.3
	120.3 – 154.5
	154.5 – 504.0

GREECE: PERINATAL MORTALITY

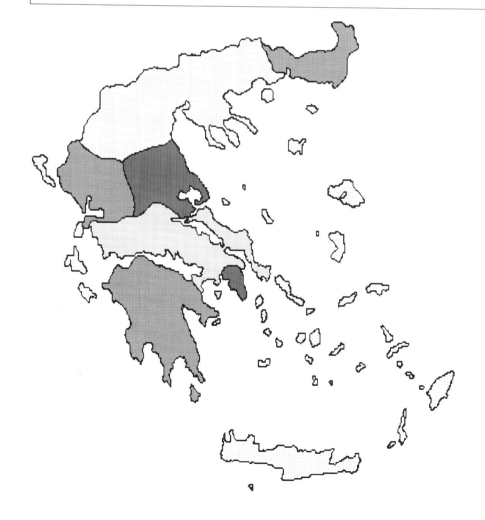

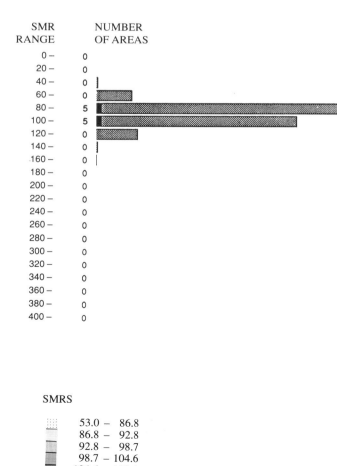

SMR RANGE	NUMBER OF AREAS
0 –	0
20 –	0
40 –	0
60 –	0
80 –	5
100 –	5
120 –	0
140 –	0
160 –	0
180 –	0
200 –	0
220 –	0
240 –	0
260 –	0
280 –	0
300 –	0
320 –	0
340 –	0
360 –	0
380 –	0
400 –	0

SMRS

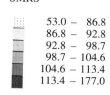

	53.0 – 86.8
	86.8 – 92.8
	92.8 – 98.7
	98.7 – 104.6
	104.6 – 113.4
	113.4 – 177.0

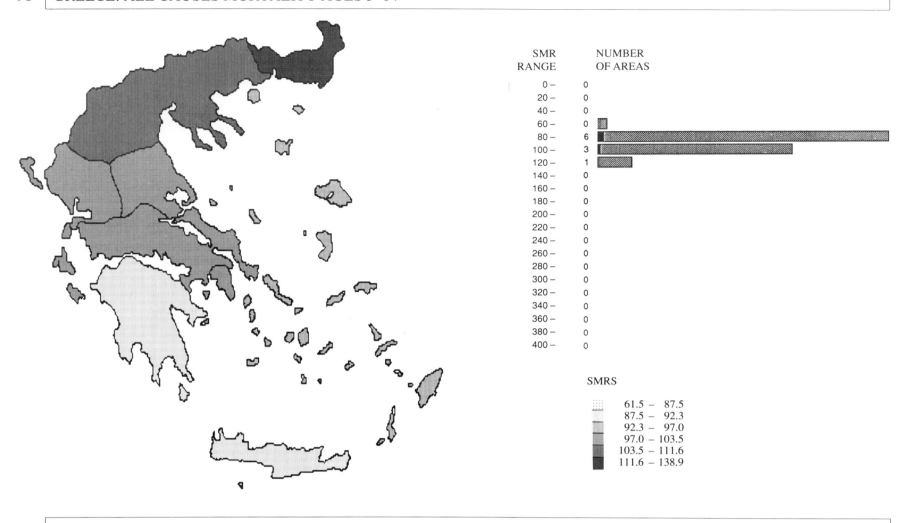

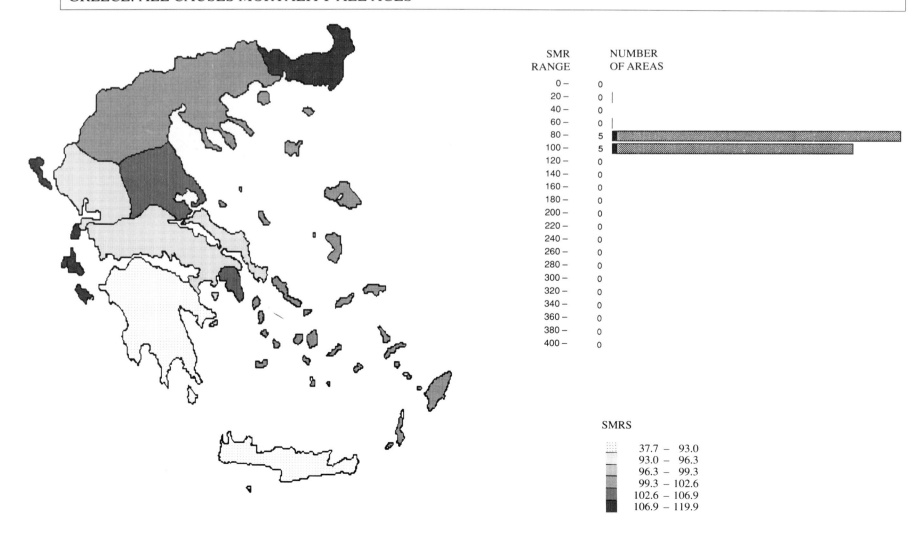

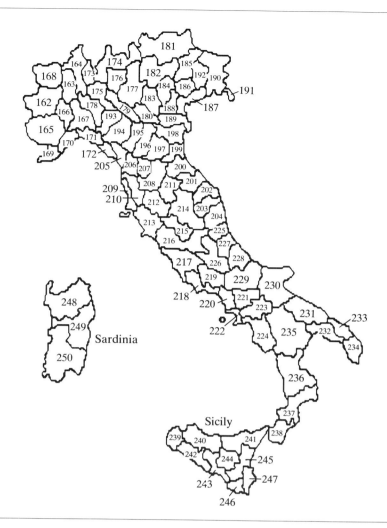

ITALY: TUBERCULOSIS MORTALITY AGES 5–64

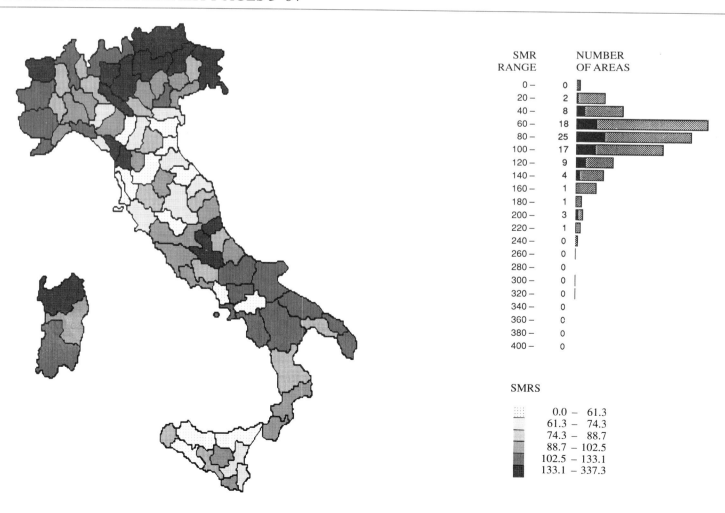

SMR RANGE	NUMBER OF AREAS
0 –	0
20 –	2
40 –	8
60 –	18
80 –	25
100 –	17
120 –	9
140 –	4
160 –	1
180 –	1
200 –	3
220 –	1
240 –	0
260 –	0
280 –	0
300 –	0
320 –	0
340 –	0
360 –	0
380 –	0
400 –	0

SMRS

	0.0 – 61.3
	61.3 – 74.3
	74.3 – 88.7
	88.7 – 102.5
	102.5 – 133.1
	133.1 – 337.3

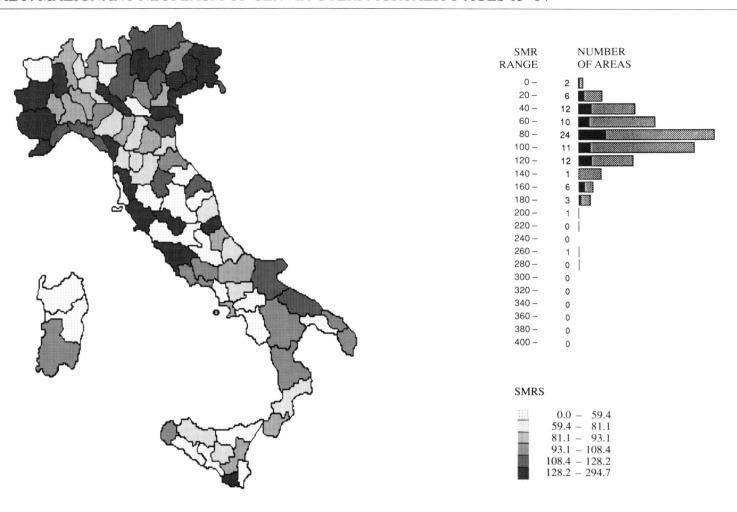

SMR RANGE	NUMBER OF AREAS
0 –	2
20 –	6
40 –	12
60 –	10
80 –	24
100 –	11
120 –	12
140 –	1
160 –	6
180 –	3
200 –	1
220 –	0
240 –	0
260 –	1
280 –	0
300 –	0
320 –	0
340 –	0
360 –	0
380 –	0
400 –	0

SMRS

	0.0 – 59.4
	59.4 – 81.1
	81.1 – 93.1
	93.1 – 108.4
	108.4 – 128.2
	128.2 – 294.7

ITALY: MALIGNANT NEOPLASM OF CERVIX AND BODY OF UTERUS MORTALITY AGES 15–54

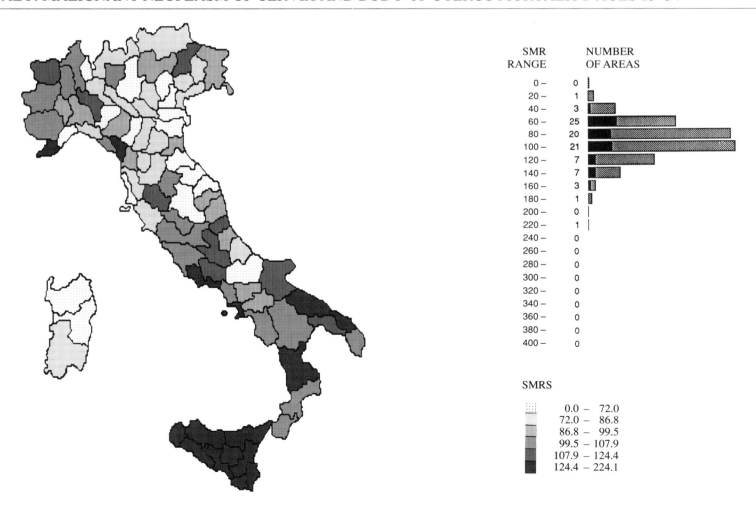

SMR RANGE	NUMBER OF AREAS
0 –	0
20 –	1
40 –	3
60 –	25
80 –	20
100 –	21
120 –	7
140 –	7
160 –	3
180 –	1
200 –	0
220 –	1
240 –	0
260 –	0
280 –	0
300 –	0
320 –	0
340 –	0
360 –	0
380 –	0
400 –	0

SMRS

	0.0 – 72.0
	72.0 – 86.8
	86.8 – 99.5
	99.5 – 107.9
	107.9 – 124.4
	124.4 – 224.1

ITALY: HODGKIN'S DISEASE MORTALITY AGES 5–64

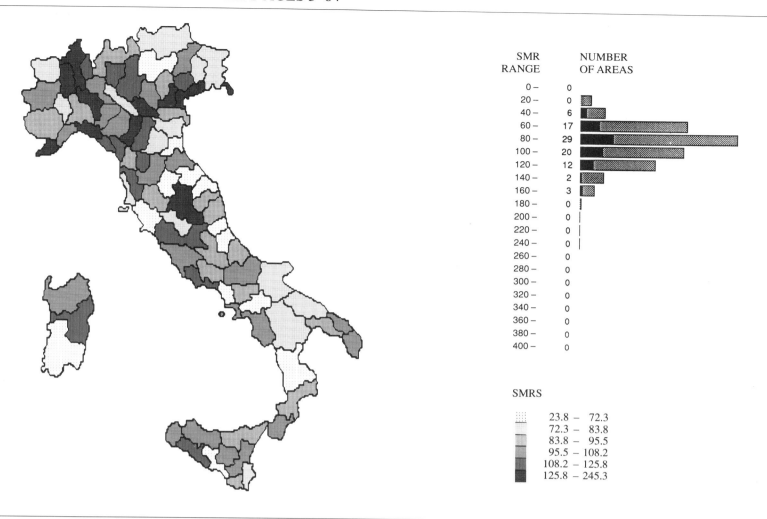

SMR RANGE	NUMBER OF AREAS
0 –	0
20 –	0
40 –	6
60 –	17
80 –	29
100 –	20
120 –	12
140 –	2
160 –	3
180 –	0
200 –	0
220 –	0
240 –	0
260 –	0
280 –	0
300 –	0
320 –	0
340 –	0
360 –	0
380 –	0
400 –	0

SMRS

	23.8 – 72.3
	72.3 – 83.8
	83.8 – 95.5
	95.5 – 108.2
	108.2 – 125.8
	125.8 – 245.3

ITALY: CHRONIC RHEUMATIC HEART DISEASE MORTALITY AGES 5–44

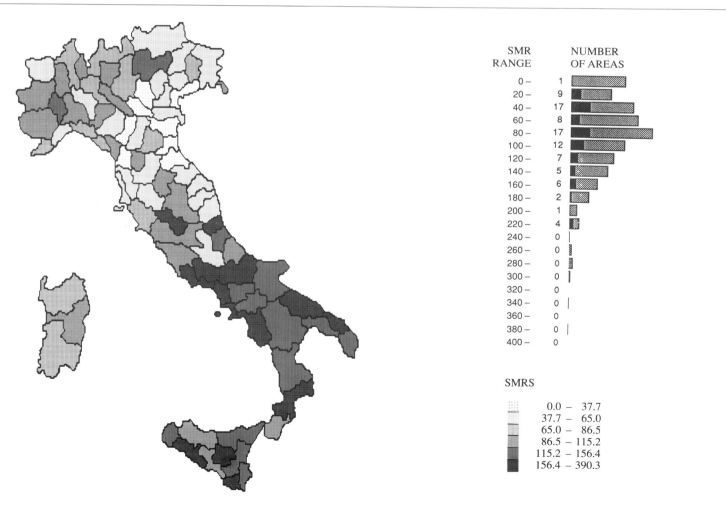

SMR RANGE	NUMBER OF AREAS
0 –	1
20 –	9
40 –	17
60 –	8
80 –	17
100 –	12
120 –	7
140 –	5
160 –	6
180 –	2
200 –	1
220 –	4
240 –	0
260 –	0
280 –	0
300 –	0
320 –	0
340 –	0
360 –	0
380 –	0
400 –	0

SMRS

	0.0 – 37.7
	37.7 – 65.0
	65.0 – 86.5
	86.5 – 115.2
	115.2 – 156.4
	156.4 – 390.3

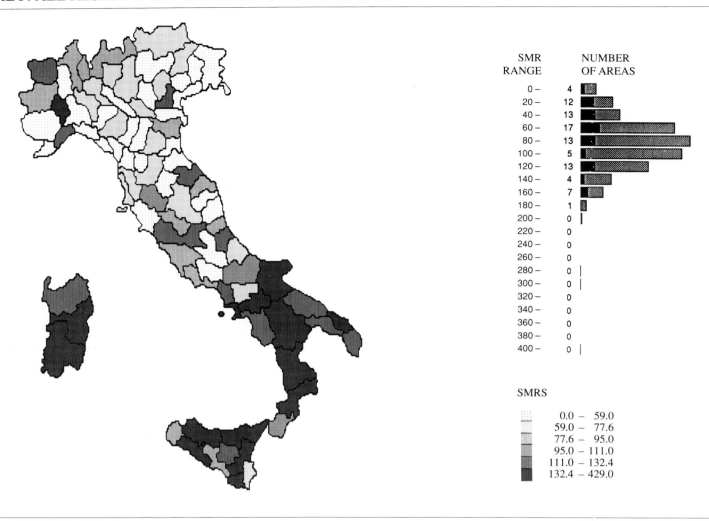

SMR RANGE	NUMBER OF AREAS	
0 –	4	
20 –	12	
40 –	13	
60 –	17	
80 –	13	
100 –	5	
120 –	13	
140 –	4	
160 –	7	
180 –	1	
200 –	0	
220 –	0	
240 –	0	
260 –	0	
280 –	0	
300 –	0	
320 –	0	
340 –	0	
360 –	0	
380 –	0	
400 –	0	

SMRS

	0.0 – 59.0
	59.0 – 77.6
	77.6 – 95.0
	95.0 – 111.0
	111.0 – 132.4
	132.4 – 429.0

ITALY: ASTHMA MORTALITY AGES 5–44

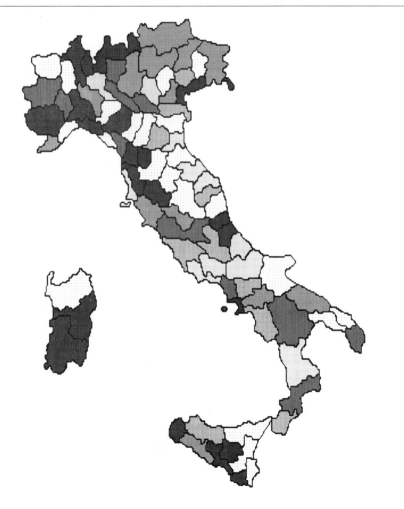

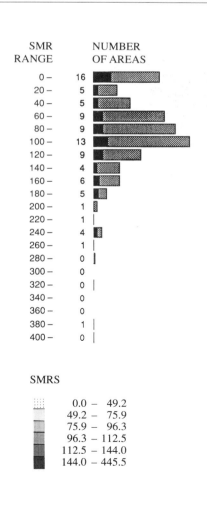

SMR RANGE	NUMBER OF AREAS	
0 –	16	
20 –	5	
40 –	5	
60 –	9	
80 –	9	
100 –	13	
120 –	9	
140 –	4	
160 –	6	
180 –	5	
200 –	1	
220 –	1	
240 –	4	
260 –	1	
280 –	0	
300 –	0	
320 –	0	
340 –	0	
360 –	0	
380 –	1	
400 –	0	

SMRS

	0.0 – 49.2
	49.2 – 75.9
	75.9 – 96.3
	96.3 – 112.5
	112.5 – 144.0
	144.0 – 445.5

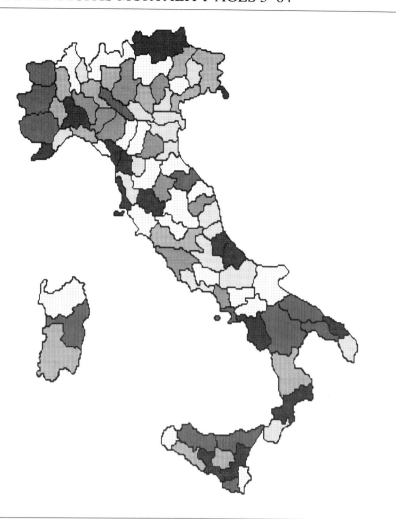

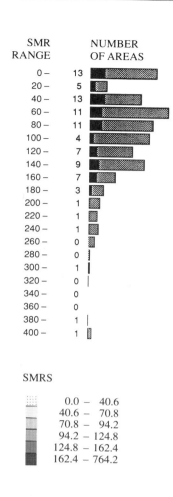

SMR RANGE	NUMBER OF AREAS
0 –	13
20 –	5
40 –	13
60 –	11
80 –	11
100 –	4
120 –	7
140 –	9
160 –	7
180 –	3
200 –	1
220 –	1
240 –	1
260 –	0
280 –	0
300 –	1
320 –	0
340 –	0
360 –	0
380 –	1
400 –	1

SMRS

	0.0 – 40.6
	40.6 – 70.8
	70.8 – 94.2
	94.2 – 124.8
	124.8 – 162.4
	162.4 – 764.2

ITALY: ABDOMINAL HERNIA MORTALITY AGES 5–64

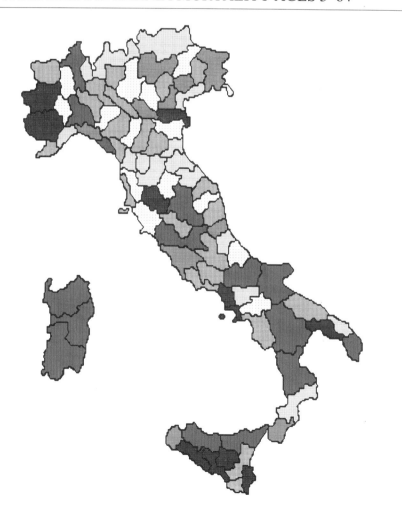

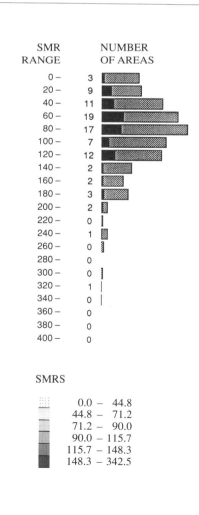

SMR RANGE	NUMBER OF AREAS
0 –	3
20 –	9
40 –	11
60 –	19
80 –	17
100 –	7
120 –	12
140 –	2
160 –	2
180 –	3
200 –	2
220 –	0
240 –	1
260 –	0
280 –	0
300 –	0
320 –	1
340 –	0
360 –	0
380 –	0
400 –	0

SMRS

	0.0 – 44.8
	44.8 – 71.2
	71.2 – 90.0
	90.0 – 115.7
	115.7 – 148.3
	148.3 – 342.5

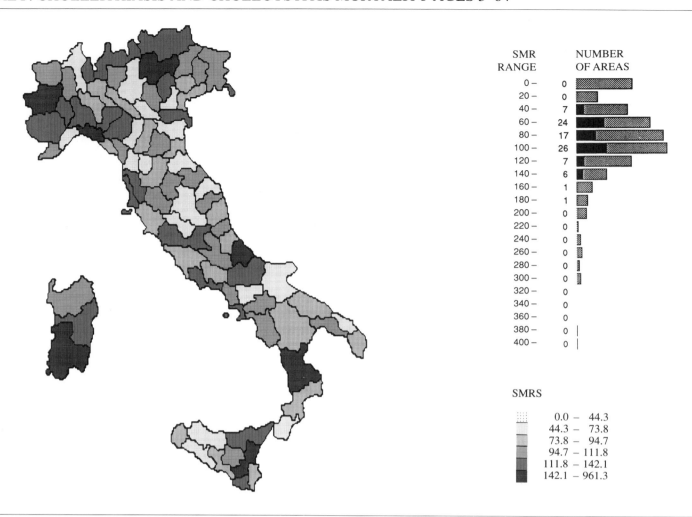

SMR RANGE	NUMBER OF AREAS
0 –	0
20 –	0
40 –	7
60 –	24
80 –	17
100 –	26
120 –	7
140 –	6
160 –	1
180 –	1
200 –	0
220 –	0
240 –	0
260 –	0
280 –	0
300 –	0
320 –	0
340 –	0
360 –	0
380 –	0
400 –	0

SMRS

	0.0 – 44.3
	44.3 – 73.8
	73.8 – 94.7
	94.7 – 111.8
	111.8 – 142.1
	142.1 – 961.3

ITALY: HYPERTENSIVE AND CEREBROVASCULAR DISEASES MORTALITY AGES 35–64

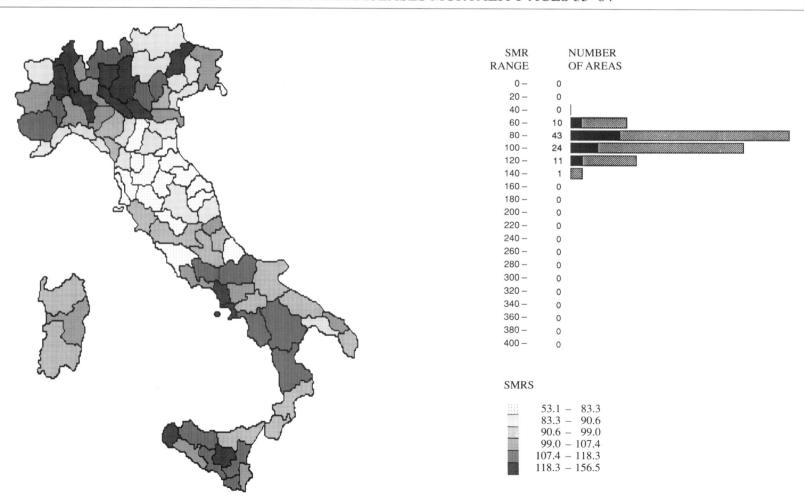

SMR RANGE	NUMBER OF AREAS
0 –	0
20 –	0
40 –	0
60 –	10
80 –	43
100 –	24
120 –	11
140 –	1
160 –	0
180 –	0
200 –	0
220 –	0
240 –	0
260 –	0
280 –	0
300 –	0
320 –	0
340 –	0
360 –	0
380 –	0
400 –	0

SMRS

	53.1 – 83.3
	83.3 – 90.6
	90.6 – 99.0
	99.0 – 107.4
	107.4 – 118.3
	118.3 – 156.5

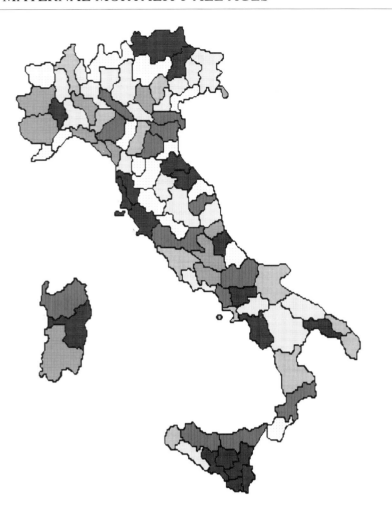

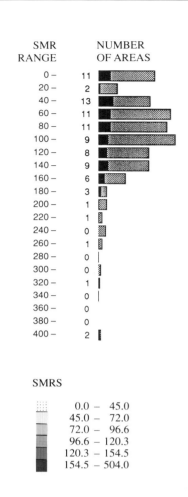

SMR RANGE	NUMBER OF AREAS
0 –	11
20 –	2
40 –	13
60 –	11
80 –	11
100 –	9
120 –	8
140 –	9
160 –	6
180 –	3
200 –	1
220 –	1
240 –	0
260 –	1
280 –	0
300 –	0
320 –	1
340 –	0
360 –	0
380 –	0
400 –	2

SMRS

	0.0 – 45.0
	45.0 – 72.0
	72.0 – 96.6
	96.6 – 120.3
	120.3 – 154.5
	154.5 – 504.0

ITALY: PERINATAL MORTALITY

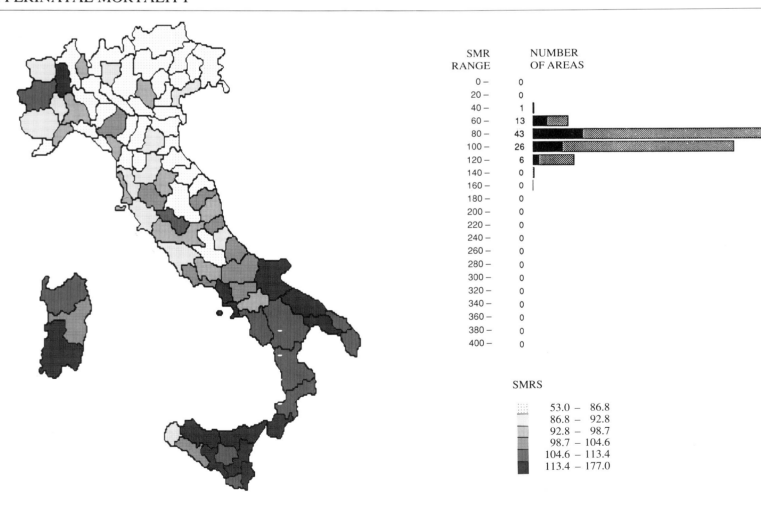

SMR RANGE	NUMBER OF AREAS
0 –	0
20 –	0
40 –	1
60 –	13
80 –	43
100 –	26
120 –	6
140 –	0
160 –	0
180 –	0
200 –	0
220 –	0
240 –	0
260 –	0
280 –	0
300 –	0
320 –	0
340 –	0
360 –	0
380 –	0
400 –	0

SMRS

	53.0 – 86.8
	86.8 – 92.8
	92.8 – 98.7
	98.7 – 104.6
	104.6 – 113.4
	113.4 – 177.0

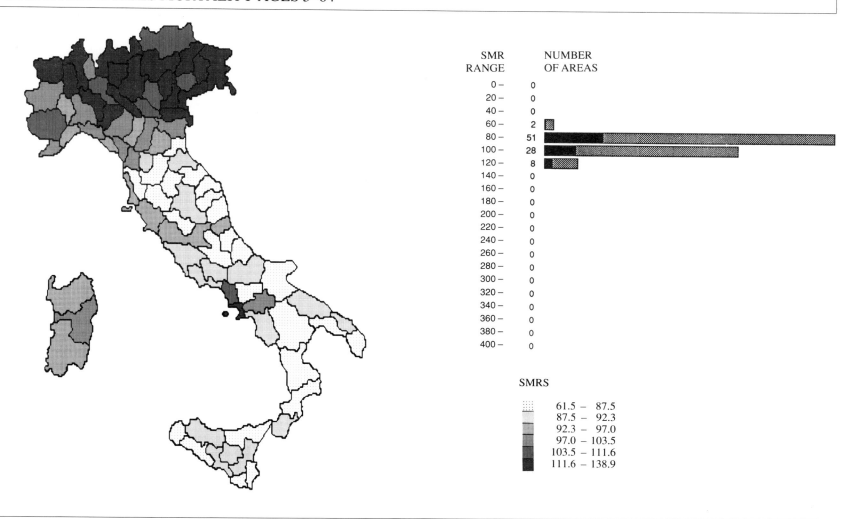

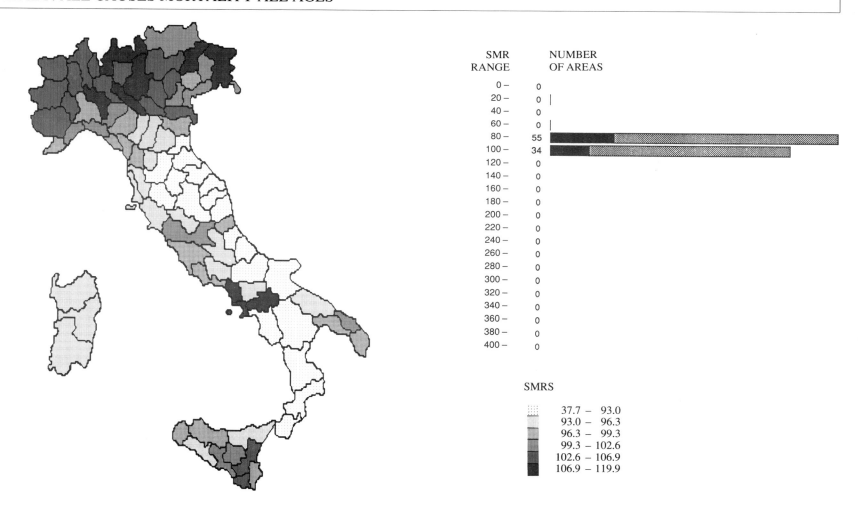

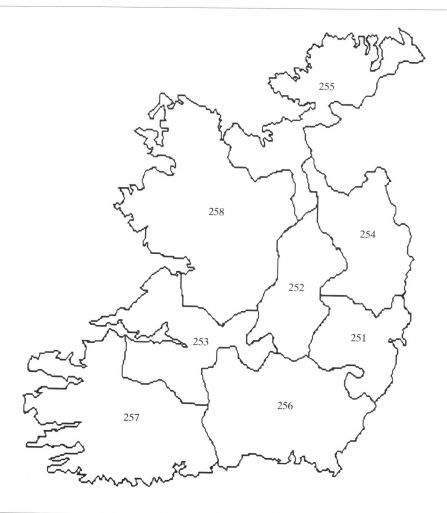

IRELAND: TUBERCULOSIS MORTALITY AGES 5–64

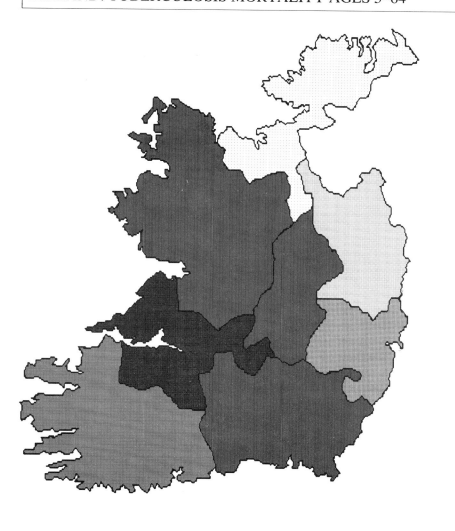

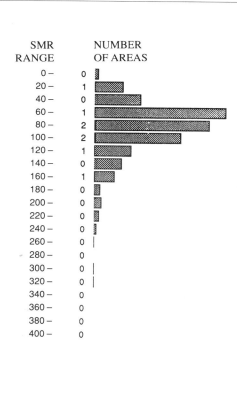

SMR RANGE	NUMBER OF AREAS
0 –	0
20 –	1
40 –	0
60 –	1
80 –	2
100 –	2
120 –	1
140 –	0
160 –	1
180 –	0
200 –	0
220 –	0
240 –	0
260 –	0
280 –	0
300 –	0
320 –	0
340 –	0
360 –	0
380 –	0
400 –	0

SMRS

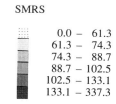

	0.0 – 61.3
	61.3 – 74.3
	74.3 – 88.7
	88.7 – 102.5
	102.5 – 133.1
	133.1 – 337.3

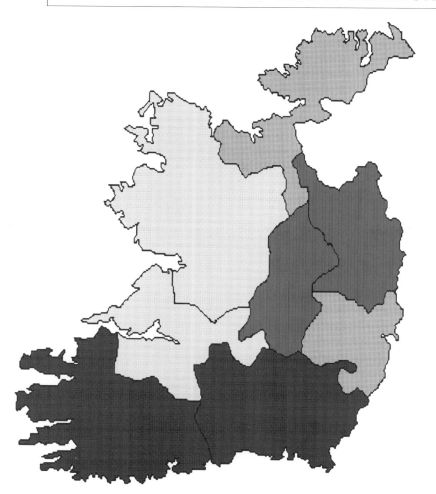

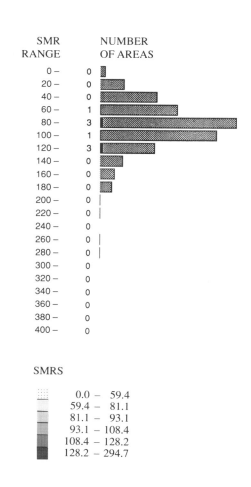

SMR RANGE	NUMBER OF AREAS
0 –	0
20 –	0
40 –	0
60 –	1
80 –	3
100 –	1
120 –	3
140 –	0
160 –	0
180 –	0
200 –	0
220 –	0
240 –	0
260 –	0
280 –	0
300 –	0
320 –	0
340 –	0
360 –	0
380 –	0
400 –	0

SMRS

0.0 – 59.4
59.4 – 81.1
81.1 – 93.1
93.1 – 108.4
108.4 – 128.2
128.2 – 294.7

IRELAND: MALIGNANT NEOPLASM OF CERVIX AND BODY OF UTERUS MORTALITY AGES 15–54

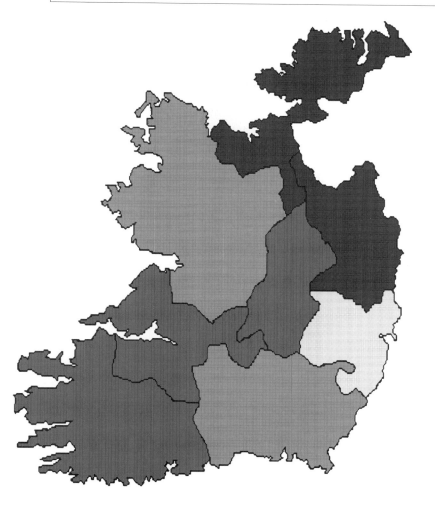

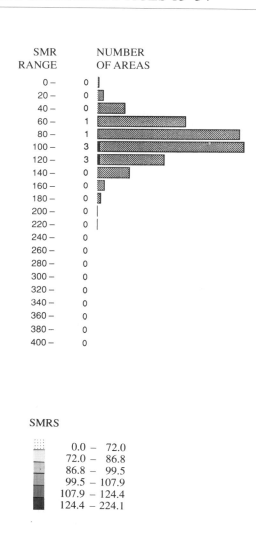

SMR RANGE	NUMBER OF AREAS
0 –	0
20 –	0
40 –	0
60 –	1
80 –	1
100 –	3
120 –	3
140 –	0
160 –	0
180 –	0
200 –	0
220 –	0
240 –	0
260 –	0
280 –	0
300 –	0
320 –	0
340 –	0
360 –	0
380 –	0
400 –	0

SMRS

0.0 – 72.0
72.0 – 86.8
86.8 – 99.5
99.5 – 107.9
107.9 – 124.4
124.4 – 224.1

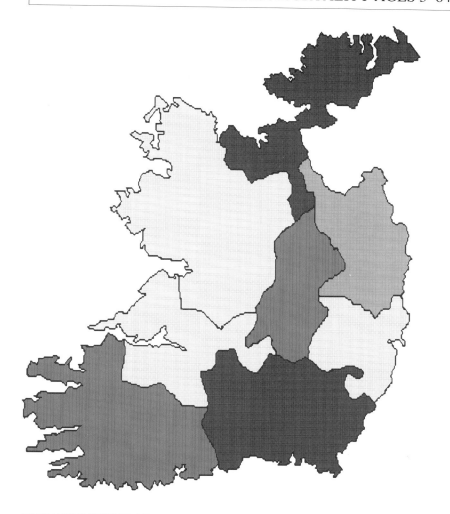

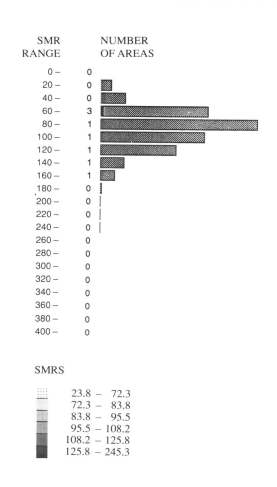

SMR RANGE	NUMBER OF AREAS
0 –	0
20 –	0
40 –	0
60 –	3
80 –	1
100 –	1
120 –	1
140 –	1
160 –	1
180 –	0
200 –	0
220 –	0
240 –	0
260 –	0
280 –	0
300 –	0
320 –	0
340 –	0
360 –	0
380 –	0
400 –	0

SMRS

23.8 – 72.3
72.3 – 83.8
83.8 – 95.5
95.5 – 108.2
108.2 – 125.8
125.8 – 245.3

IRELAND: CHRONIC RHEUMATIC HEART DISEASE MORTALITY AGES 5–44

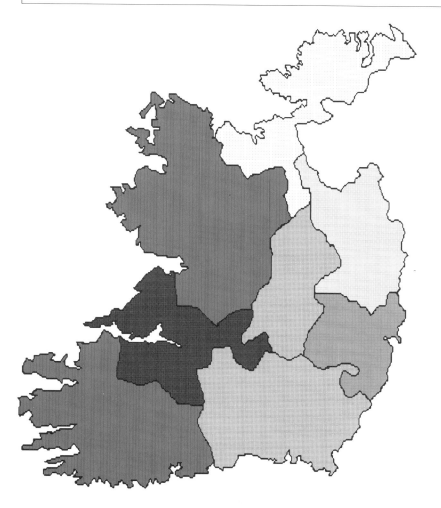

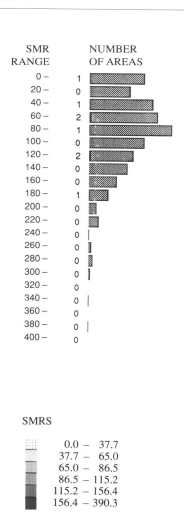

SMR RANGE	NUMBER OF AREAS
0 –	1
20 –	0
40 –	1
60 –	2
80 –	1
100 –	0
120 –	2
140 –	0
160 –	0
180 –	1
200 –	0
220 –	0
240 –	0
260 –	0
280 –	0
300 –	0
320 –	0
340 –	0
360 –	0
380 –	0
400 –	0

SMRS

0.0 – 37.7
37.7 – 65.0
65.0 – 86.5
86.5 – 115.2
115.2 – 156.4
156.4 – 390.3

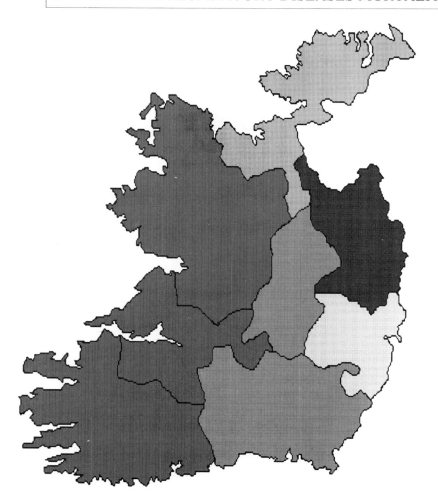

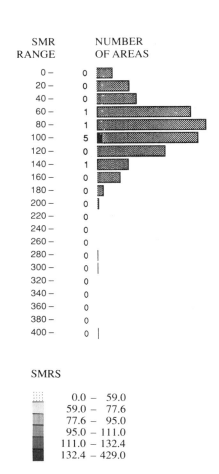

SMR RANGE | NUMBER OF AREAS

0 –	0
20 –	0
40 –	0
60 –	1
80 –	1
100 –	5
120 –	0
140 –	1
160 –	0
180 –	0
200 –	0
220 –	0
240 –	0
260 –	0
280 –	0
300 –	0
320 –	0
340 –	0
360 –	0
380 –	0
400 –	0

SMRS

| 0.0 – 59.0 |
| 59.0 – 77.6 |
| 77.6 – 95.0 |
| 95.0 – 111.0 |
| 111.0 – 132.4 |
| 132.4 – 429.0 |

IRELAND: ASTHMA MORTALITY AGES 5–44

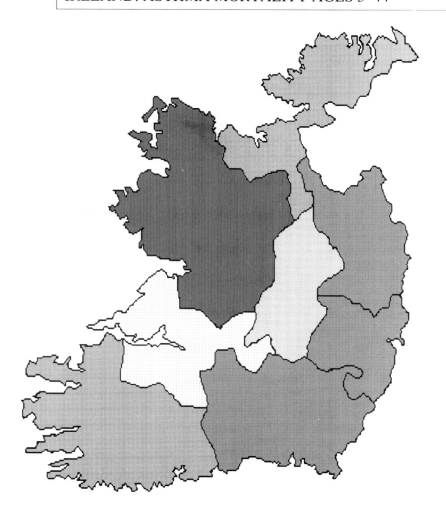

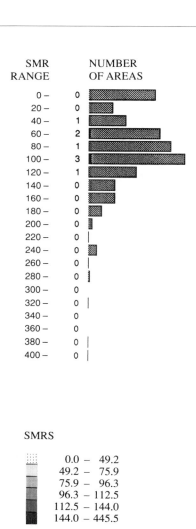

SMR RANGE | NUMBER OF AREAS

0 –	0
20 –	0
40 –	1
60 –	2
80 –	1
100 –	3
120 –	1
140 –	0
160 –	0
180 –	0
200 –	0
220 –	0
240 –	0
260 –	0
280 –	0
300 –	0
320 –	0
340 –	0
360 –	0
380 –	0
400 –	0

SMRS

| 0.0 – 49.2 |
| 49.2 – 75.9 |
| 75.9 – 96.3 |
| 96.3 – 112.5 |
| 112.5 – 144.0 |
| 144.0 – 445.5 |

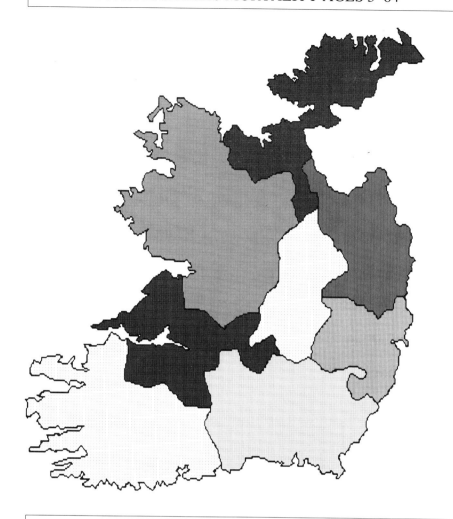

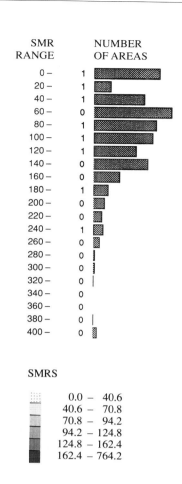

SMR RANGE	NUMBER OF AREAS
0 –	1
20 –	1
40 –	1
60 –	0
80 –	1
100 –	1
120 –	1
140 –	0
160 –	0
180 –	1
200 –	0
220 –	0
240 –	1
260 –	0
280 –	0
300 –	0
320 –	0
340 –	0
360 –	0
380 –	0
400 –	0

SMRS

	0.0 – 40.6
	40.6 – 70.8
	70.8 – 94.2
	94.2 – 124.8
	124.8 – 162.4
	162.4 – 764.2

IRELAND: ABDOMINAL HERNIA MORTALITY AGES 5–64

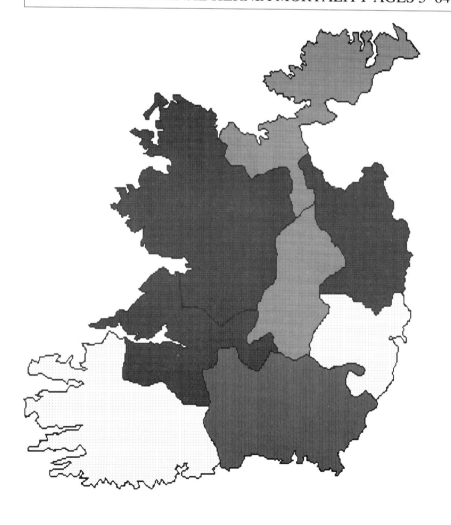

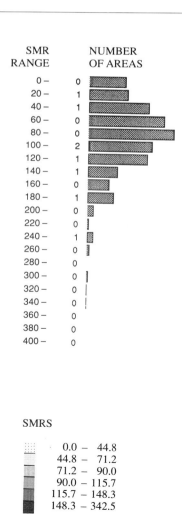

SMR RANGE	NUMBER OF AREAS
0 –	0
20 –	1
40 –	1
60 –	0
80 –	0
100 –	2
120 –	1
140 –	1
160 –	0
180 –	1
200 –	0
220 –	0
240 –	1
260 –	0
280 –	0
300 –	0
320 –	0
340 –	0
360 –	0
380 –	0
400 –	0

SMRS

	0.0 – 44.8
	44.8 – 71.2
	71.2 – 90.0
	90.0 – 115.7
	115.7 – 148.3
	148.3 – 342.5

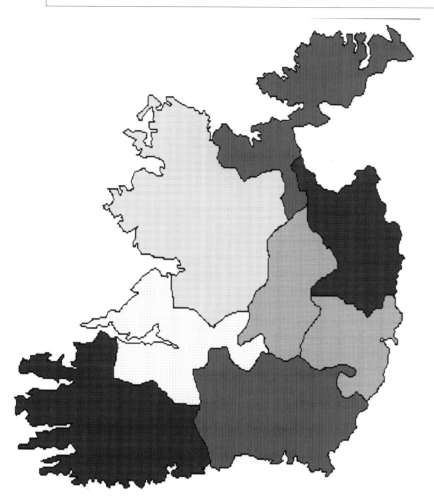

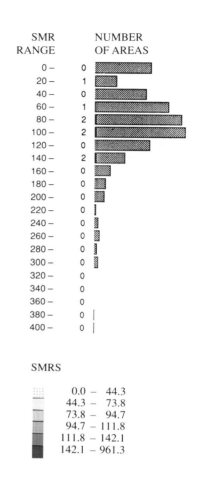

SMR RANGE	NUMBER OF AREAS
0 –	0
20 –	1
40 –	0
60 –	1
80 –	2
100 –	2
120 –	0
140 –	2
160 –	0
180 –	0
200 –	0
220 –	0
240 –	0
260 –	0
280 –	0
300 –	0
320 –	0
340 –	0
360 –	0
380 –	0
400 –	0

SMRS

0.0 – 44.3
44.3 – 73.8
73.8 – 94.7
94.7 – 111.8
111.8 – 142.1
142.1 – 961.3

IRELAND: HYPERTENSIVE AND CEREBROVASCULAR DISEASES MORTALITY AGES 35–64

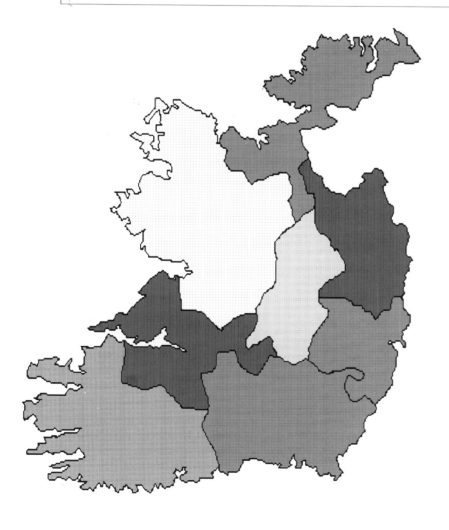

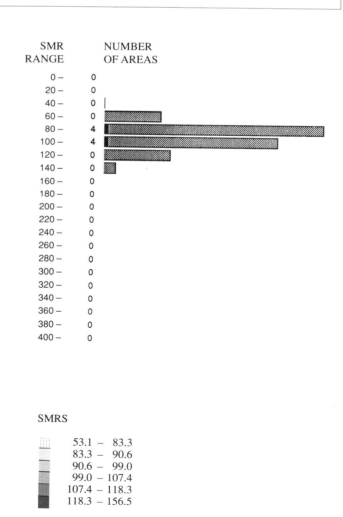

SMR RANGE	NUMBER OF AREAS
0 –	0
20 –	0
40 –	0
60 –	0
80 –	4
100 –	4
120 –	0
140 –	0
160 –	0
180 –	0
200 –	0
220 –	0
240 –	0
260 –	0
280 –	0
300 –	0
320 –	0
340 –	0
360 –	0
380 –	0
400 –	0

SMRS

53.1 – 83.3
83.3 – 90.6
90.6 – 99.0
99.0 – 107.4
107.4 – 118.3
118.3 – 156.5

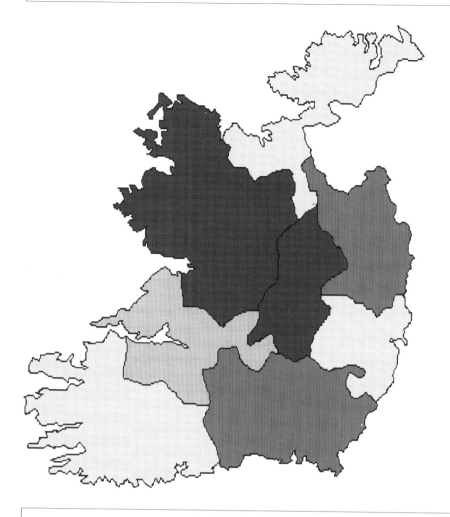

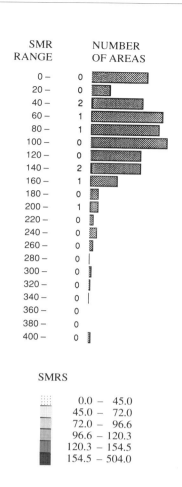

SMR RANGE	NUMBER OF AREAS
0 –	0
20 –	0
40 –	2
60 –	1
80 –	1
100 –	0
120 –	0
140 –	2
160 –	1
180 –	0
200 –	1
220 –	0
240 –	0
260 –	0
280 –	0
300 –	0
320 –	0
340 –	0
360 –	0
380 –	0
400 –	0

SMRS

	0.0 – 45.0
	45.0 – 72.0
	72.0 – 96.6
	96.6 – 120.3
	120.3 – 154.5
	154.5 – 504.0

IRELAND: PERINATAL MORTALITY

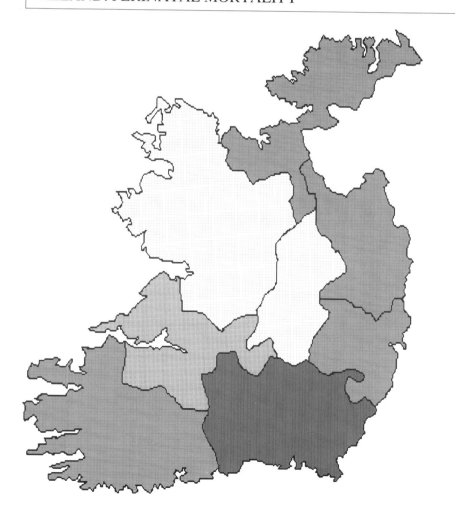

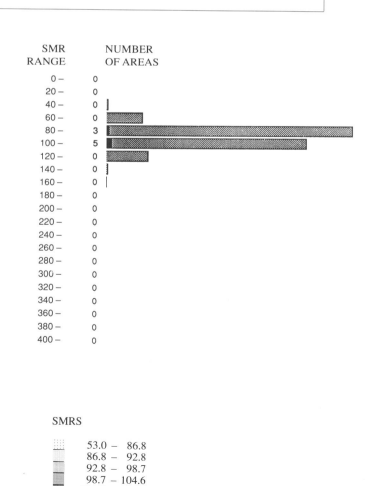

SMR RANGE	NUMBER OF AREAS
0 –	0
20 –	0
40 –	0
60 –	0
80 –	3
100 –	5
120 –	0
140 –	0
160 –	0
180 –	0
200 –	0
220 –	0
240 –	0
260 –	0
280 –	0
300 –	0
320 –	0
340 –	0
360 –	0
380 –	0
400 –	0

SMRS

	53.0 – 86.8
	86.8 – 92.8
	92.8 – 98.7
	98.7 – 104.6
	104.6 – 113.4
	113.4 – 177.0

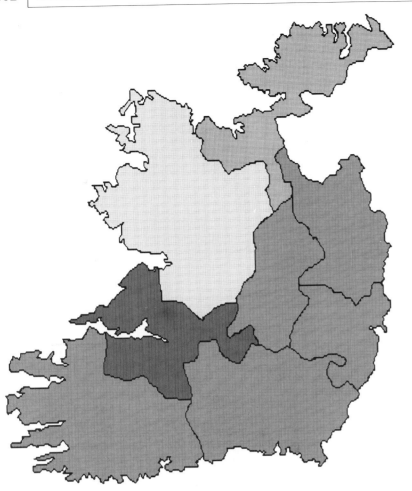

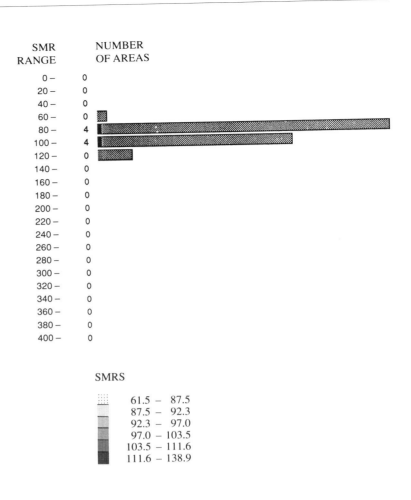

SMR RANGE   NUMBER OF AREAS

SMR RANGE	NUMBER OF AREAS
0 –	0
20 –	0
40 –	0
60 –	0
80 –	4
100 –	4
120 –	0
140 –	0
160 –	0
180 –	0
200 –	0
220 –	0
240 –	0
260 –	0
280 –	0
300 –	0
320 –	0
340 –	0
360 –	0
380 –	0
400 –	0

SMRS

	61.5 – 87.5
	87.5 – 92.3
	92.3 – 97.0
	97.0 – 103.5
	103.5 – 111.6
	111.6 – 138.9

IRELAND: ALL CAUSES MORTALITY ALL AGES

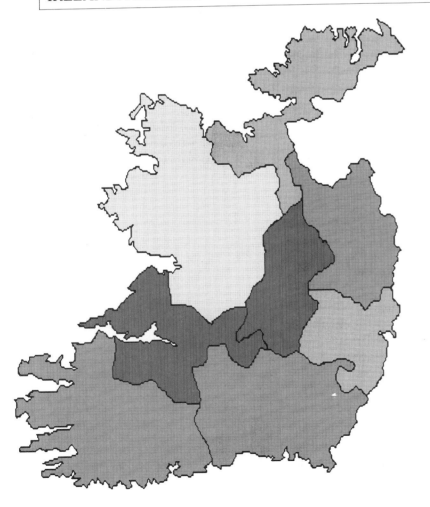

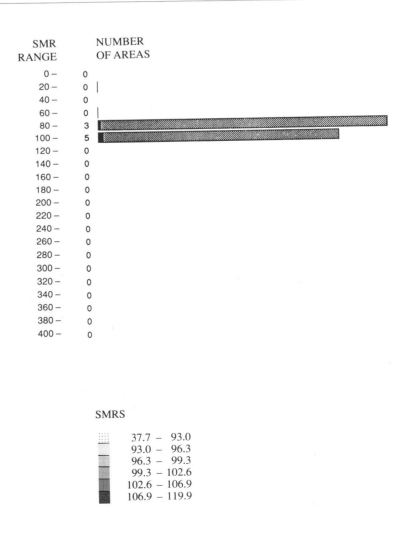

SMR RANGE	NUMBER OF AREAS
0 –	0
20 –	0
40 –	0
60 –	0
80 –	3
100 –	5
120 –	0
140 –	0
160 –	0
180 –	0
200 –	0
220 –	0
240 –	0
260 –	0
280 –	0
300 –	0
320 –	0
340 –	0
360 –	0
380 –	0
400 –	0

SMRS

	37.7 – 93.0
	93.0 – 96.3
	96.3 – 99.3
	99.3 – 102.6
	102.6 – 106.9
	106.9 – 119.9

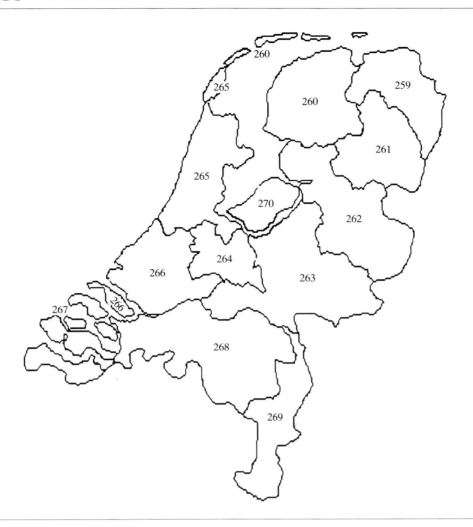

NETHERLANDS: TUBERCULOSIS MORTALITY AGES 5–64

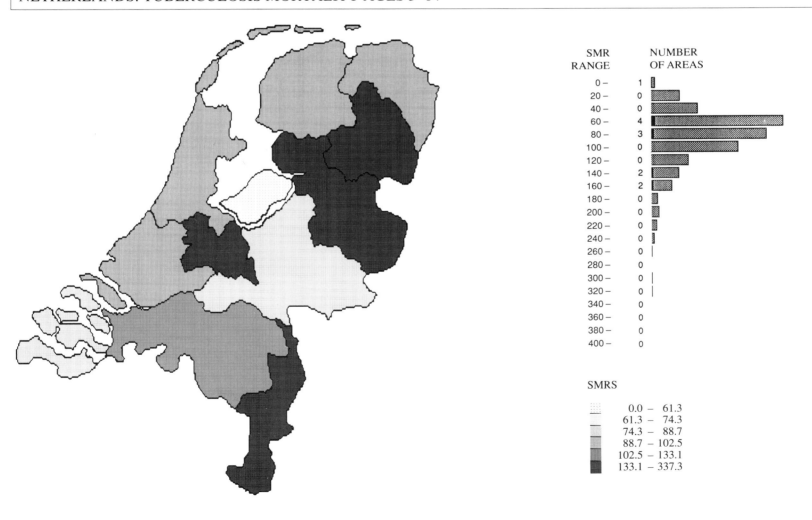

SMR RANGE	NUMBER OF AREAS
0 –	1
20 –	0
40 –	0
60 –	4
80 –	3
100 –	0
120 –	0
140 –	2
160 –	2
180 –	0
200 –	0
220 –	0
240 –	0
260 –	0
280 –	0
300 –	0
320 –	0
340 –	0
360 –	0
380 –	0
400 –	0

SMRS

0.0 – 61.3
61.3 – 74.3
74.3 – 88.7
88.7 – 102.5
102.5 – 133.1
133.1 – 337.3

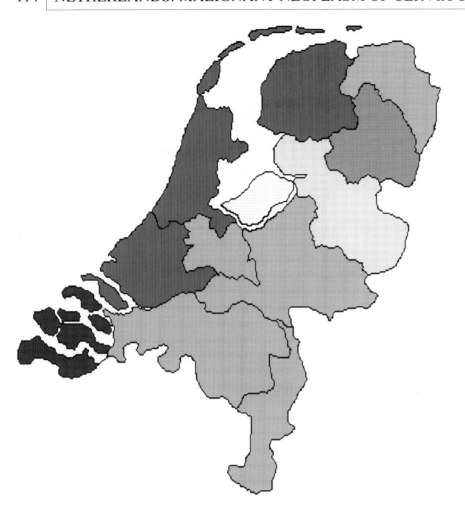

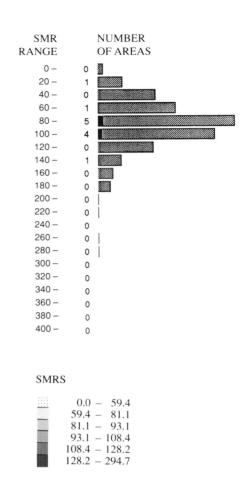

SMR RANGE	NUMBER OF AREAS
0 –	0
20 –	1
40 –	0
60 –	1
80 –	5
100 –	4
120 –	0
140 –	1
160 –	0
180 –	0
200 –	0
220 –	0
240 –	0
260 –	0
280 –	0
300 –	0
320 –	0
340 –	0
360 –	0
380 –	0
400 –	0

SMRS

	0.0 – 59.4
	59.4 – 81.1
	81.1 – 93.1
	93.1 – 108.4
	108.4 – 128.2
	128.2 – 294.7

NETHERLANDS: MALIGNANT NEOPLASM OF CERVIX AND BODY OF UTERUS MORTALITY AGES 15–54

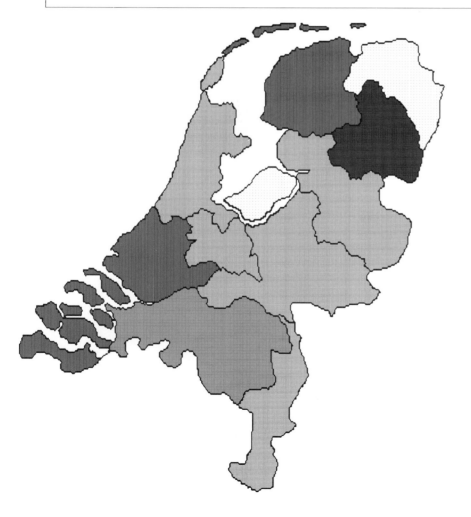

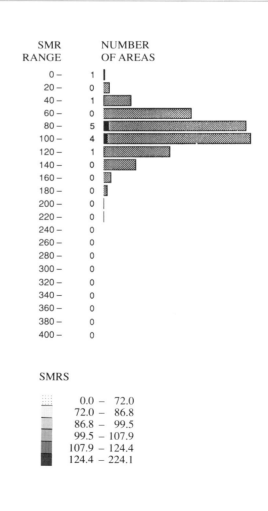

SMR RANGE	NUMBER OF AREAS
0 –	1
20 –	0
40 –	1
60 –	0
80 –	5
100 –	4
120 –	1
140 –	0
160 –	0
180 –	0
200 –	0
220 –	0
240 –	0
260 –	0
280 –	0
300 –	0
320 –	0
340 –	0
360 –	0
380 –	0
400 –	0

SMRS

	0.0 – 72.0
	72.0 – 86.8
	86.8 – 99.5
	99.5 – 107.9
	107.9 – 124.4
	124.4 – 224.1

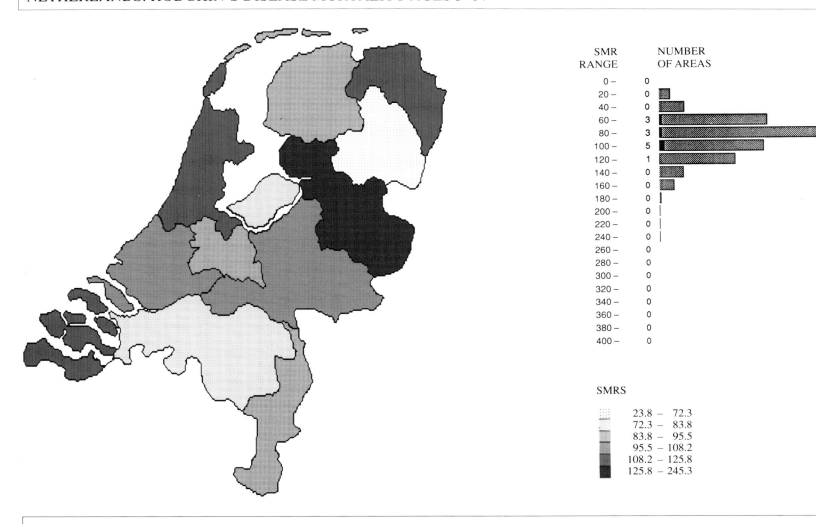

SMR RANGE	NUMBER OF AREAS
0 –	0
20 –	0
40 –	0
60 –	3
80 –	3
100 –	5
120 –	1
140 –	0
160 –	0
180 –	0
200 –	0
220 –	0
240 –	0
260 –	0
280 –	0
300 –	0
320 –	0
340 –	0
360 –	0
380 –	0
400 –	0

SMRS

	23.8 – 72.3
	72.3 – 83.8
	83.8 – 95.5
	95.5 – 108.2
	108.2 – 125.8
	125.8 – 245.3

NETHERLANDS: CHRONIC RHEUMATIC HEART DISEASE MORTALITY AGES 5–44

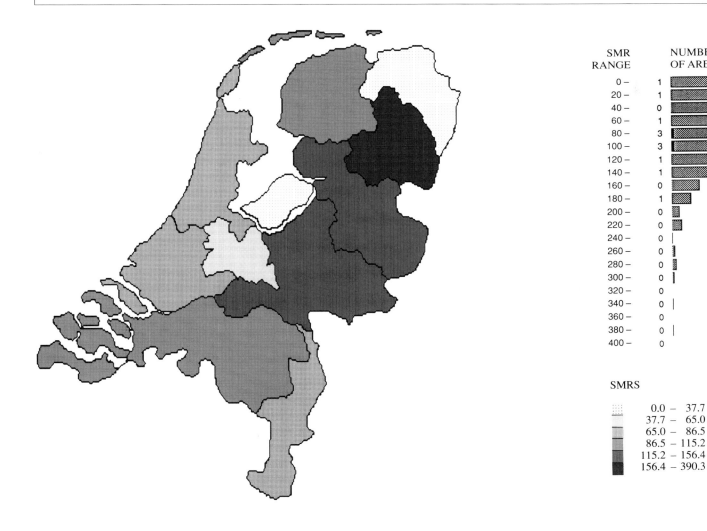

SMR RANGE	NUMBER OF AREAS
0 –	1
20 –	1
40 –	0
60 –	1
80 –	3
100 –	3
120 –	1
140 –	1
160 –	0
180 –	1
200 –	0
220 –	0
240 –	0
260 –	0
280 –	0
300 –	0
320 –	0
340 –	0
360 –	0
380 –	0
400 –	0

SMRS

	0.0 – 37.7
	37.7 – 65.0
	65.0 – 86.5
	86.5 – 115.2
	115.2 – 156.4
	156.4 – 390.3

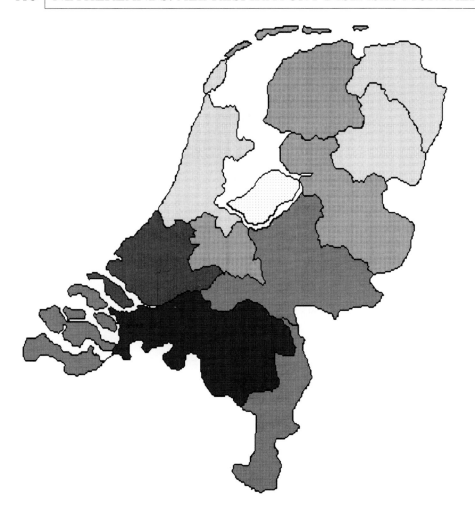

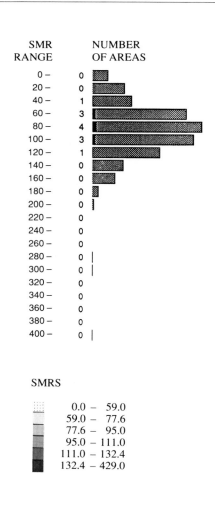

SMR RANGE	NUMBER OF AREAS
0 –	0
20 –	0
40 –	1
60 –	3
80 –	4
100 –	3
120 –	1
140 –	0
160 –	0
180 –	0
200 –	0
220 –	0
240 –	0
260 –	0
280 –	0
300 –	0
320 –	0
340 –	0
360 –	0
380 –	0
400 –	0

SMRS

	0.0 – 59.0
	59.0 – 77.6
	77.6 – 95.0
	95.0 – 111.0
	111.0 – 132.4
	132.4 – 429.0

NETHERLANDS: ASTHMA MORTALITY AGES 5–44

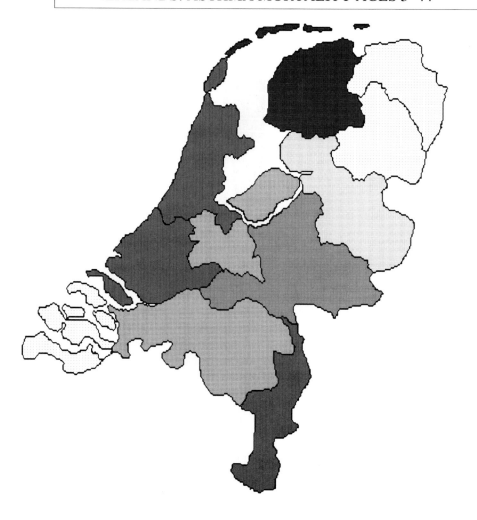

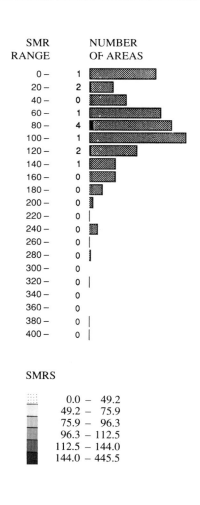

SMR RANGE	NUMBER OF AREAS
0 –	1
20 –	2
40 –	0
60 –	1
80 –	4
100 –	1
120 –	2
140 –	1
160 –	0
180 –	0
200 –	0
220 –	0
240 –	0
260 –	0
280 –	0
300 –	0
320 –	0
340 –	0
360 –	0
380 –	0
400 –	0

SMRS

	0.0 – 49.2
	49.2 – 75.9
	75.9 – 96.3
	96.3 – 112.5
	112.5 – 144.0
	144.0 – 445.5

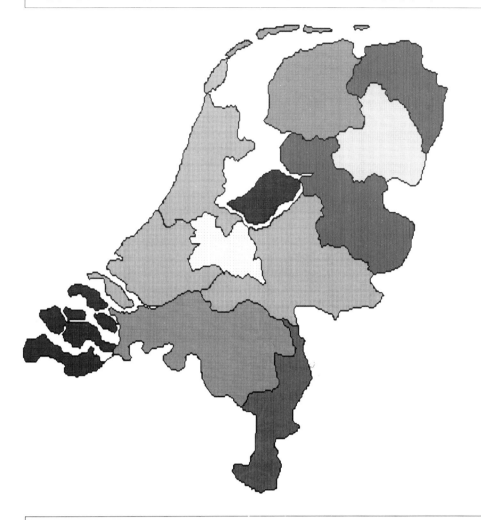

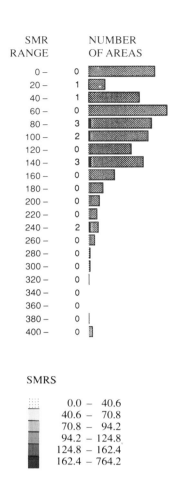

SMR RANGE	NUMBER OF AREAS
0 –	0
20 –	1
40 –	1
60 –	0
80 –	3
100 –	2
120 –	0
140 –	3
160 –	0
180 –	0
200 –	0
220 –	0
240 –	2
260 –	0
280 –	0
300 –	0
320 –	0
340 –	0
360 –	0
380 –	0
400 –	0

SMRS

	0.0 – 40.6
	40.6 – 70.8
	70.8 – 94.2
	94.2 – 124.8
	124.8 – 162.4
	162.4 – 764.2

NETHERLANDS: ABDOMINAL HERNIA MORTALITY AGES 5–64

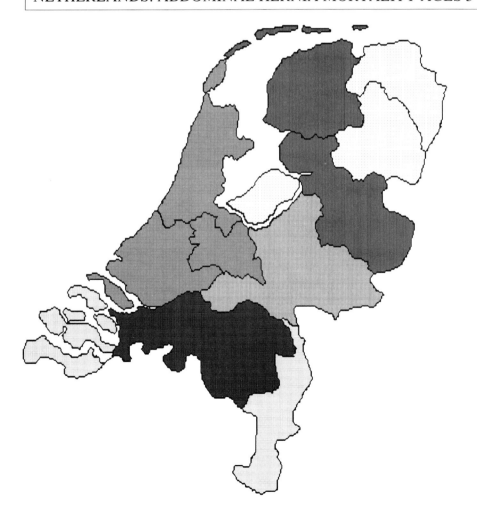

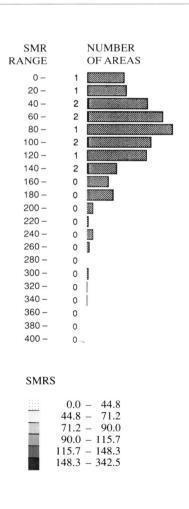

SMR RANGE	NUMBER OF AREAS
0 –	1
20 –	1
40 –	2
60 –	2
80 –	1
100 –	2
120 –	1
140 –	2
160 –	0
180 –	0
200 –	0
220 –	0
240 –	0
260 –	0
280 –	0
300 –	0
320 –	0
340 –	0
360 –	0
380 –	0
400 –	0

SMRS

	0.0 – 44.8
	44.8 – 71.2
	71.2 – 90.0
	90.0 – 115.7
	115.7 – 148.3
	148.3 – 342.5

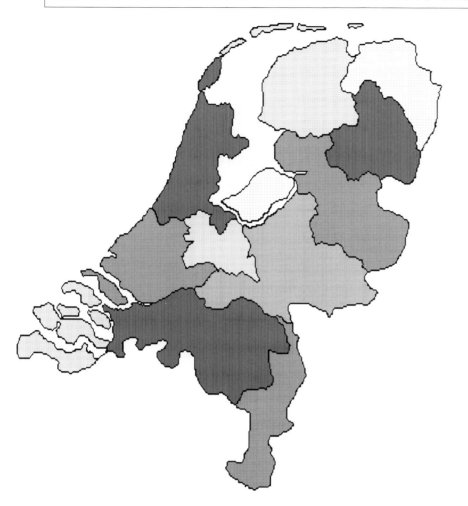

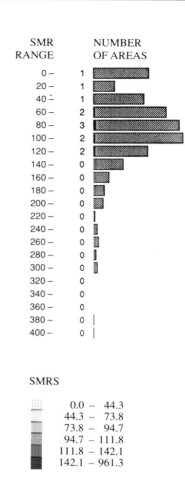

SMR RANGE	NUMBER OF AREAS	
0 –	1	
20 –	1	
40 –	1	
60 –	2	
80 –	3	
100 –	2	
120 –	2	
140 –	0	
160 –	0	
180 –	0	
200 –	0	
220 –	0	
240 –	0	
260 –	0	
280 –	0	
300 –	0	
320 –	0	
340 –	0	
360 –	0	
380 –	0	
400 –	0	

SMRS

	0.0 – 44.3
	44.3 – 73.8
	73.8 – 94.7
	94.7 – 111.8
	111.8 – 142.1
	142.1 – 961.3

NETHERLANDS: HYPERTENSIVE AND CEREBROVASCULAR DISEASES MORTALITY AGES 35–64

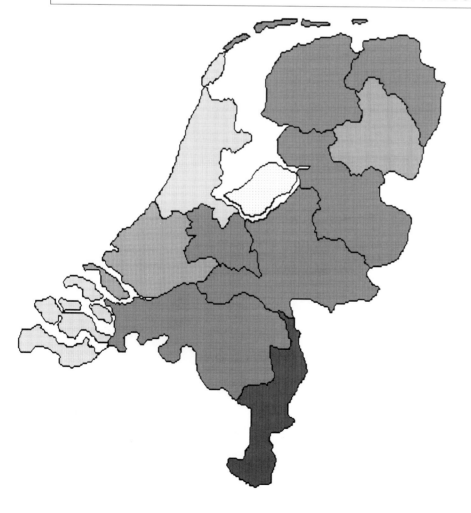

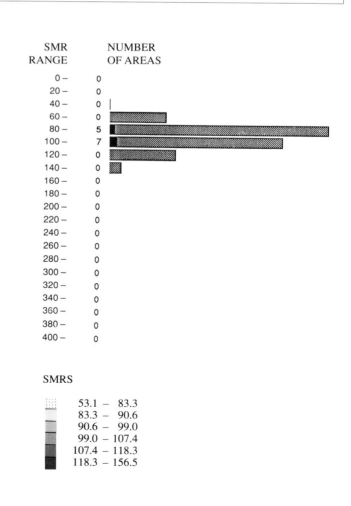

SMR RANGE	NUMBER OF AREAS	
0 –	0	
20 –	0	
40 –	0	
60 –	0	
80 –	5	
100 –	7	
120 –	0	
140 –	0	
160 –	0	
180 –	0	
200 –	0	
220 –	0	
240 –	0	
260 –	0	
280 –	0	
300 –	0	
320 –	0	
340 –	0	
360 –	0	
380 –	0	
400 –	0	

SMRS

	53.1 – 83.3
	83.3 – 90.6
	90.6 – 99.0
	99.0 – 107.4
	107.4 – 118.3
	118.3 – 156.5

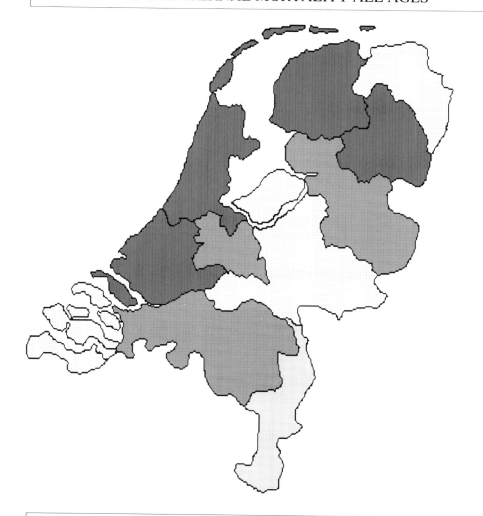

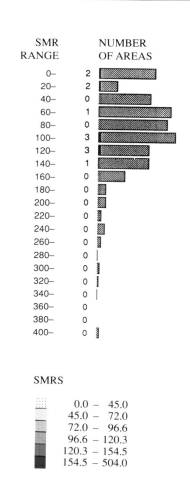

SMR RANGE	NUMBER OF AREAS
0–	2
20–	2
40–	0
60–	1
80–	0
100–	3
120–	3
140–	1
160–	0
180–	0
200–	0
220–	0
240–	0
260–	0
280–	0
300–	0
320–	0
340–	0
360–	0
380–	0
400–	0

SMRS

	0.0 – 45.0
	45.0 – 72.0
	72.0 – 96.6
	96.6 – 120.3
	120.3 – 154.5
	154.5 – 504.0

NETHERLANDS: PERINATAL MORTALITY

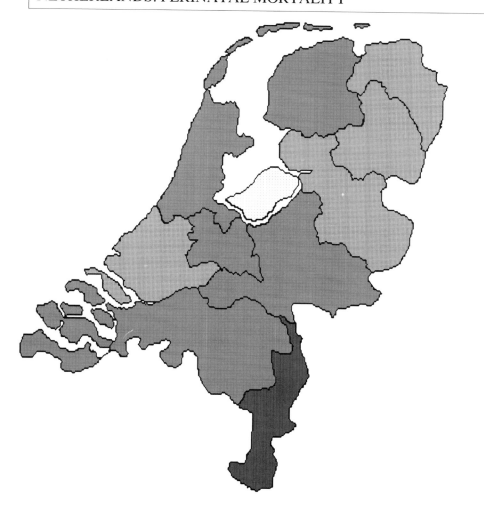

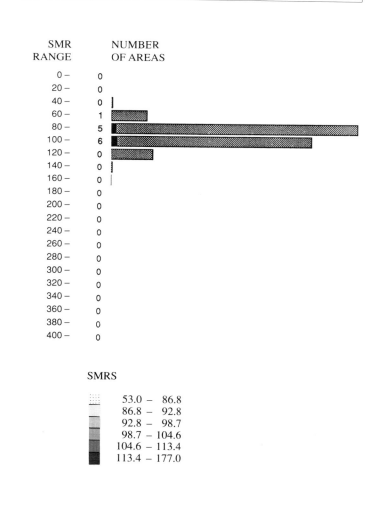

SMR RANGE	NUMBER OF AREAS
0 –	0
20 –	0
40 –	0
60 –	1
80 –	5
100 –	6
120 –	0
140 –	0
160 –	0
180 –	0
200 –	0
220 –	0
240 –	0
260 –	0
280 –	0
300 –	0
320 –	0
340 –	0
360 –	0
380 –	0
400 –	0

SMRS

	53.0 – 86.8
	86.8 – 92.8
	92.8 – 98.7
	98.7 – 104.6
	104.6 – 113.4
	113.4 – 177.0

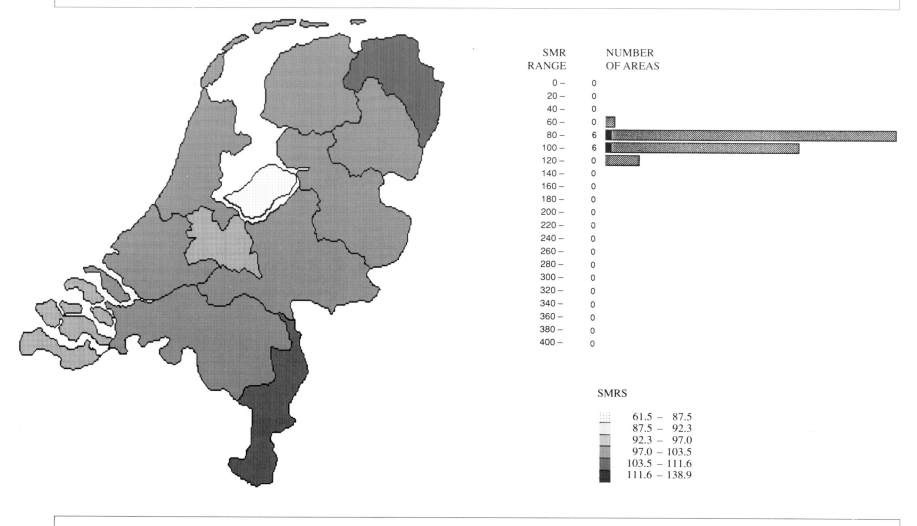

SMR RANGE | NUMBER OF AREAS

0 –	0
20 –	0
40 –	0
60 –	0
80 –	6
100 –	6
120 –	0
140 –	0
160 –	0
180 –	0
200 –	0
220 –	0
240 –	0
260 –	0
280 –	0
300 –	0
320 –	0
340 –	0
360 –	0
380 –	0
400 –	0

SMRS

61.5 – 87.5
87.5 – 92.3
92.3 – 97.0
97.0 – 103.5
103.5 – 111.6
111.6 – 138.9

NETHERLANDS: ALL CAUSES MORTALTY ALL AGES

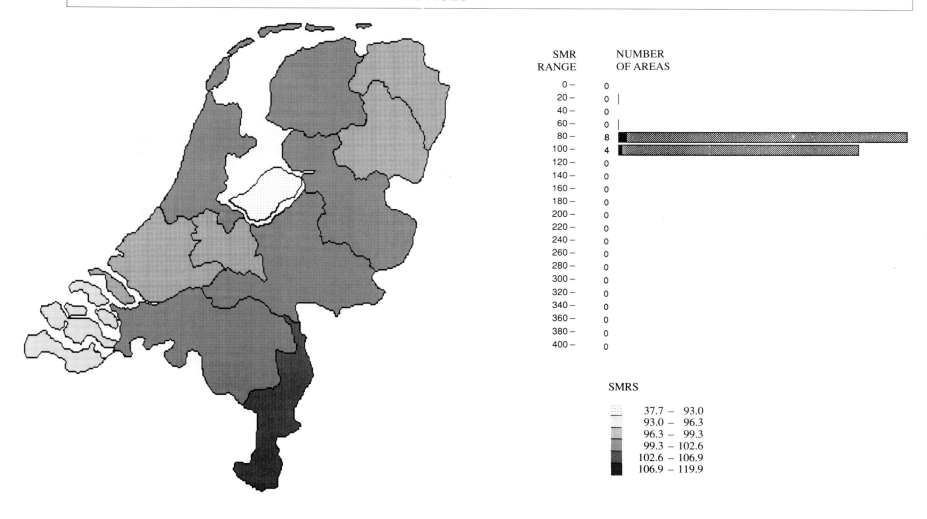

SMR RANGE | NUMBER OF AREAS

0 –	0
20 –	0
40 –	0
60 –	0
80 –	8
100 –	4
120 –	0
140 –	0
160 –	0
180 –	0
200 –	0
220 –	0
240 –	0
260 –	0
280 –	0
300 –	0
320 –	0
340 –	0
360 –	0
380 –	0
400 –	0

SMRS

37.7 – 93.0
93.0 – 96.3
96.3 – 99.3
99.3 – 102.6
102.6 – 106.9
106.9 – 119.9

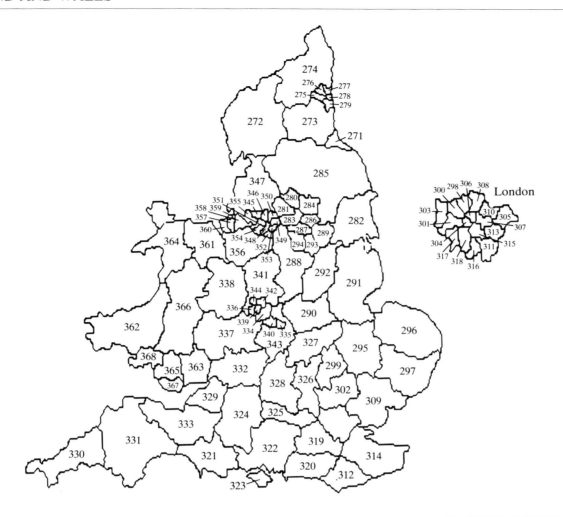

ENGLAND AND WALES: TUBERCULOSIS MORTALITY AGES 5–64

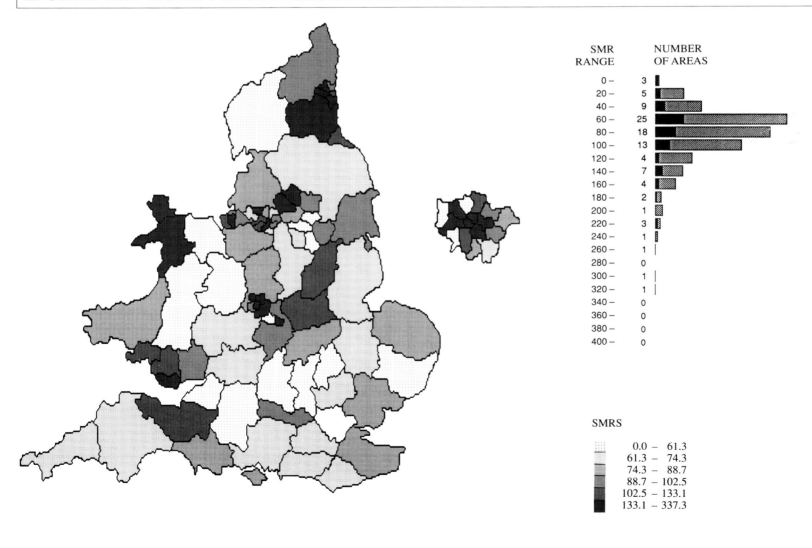

SMR RANGE	NUMBER OF AREAS
0 –	3
20 –	5
40 –	9
60 –	25
80 –	18
100 –	13
120 –	4
140 –	7
160 –	4
180 –	2
200 –	1
220 –	3
240 –	1
260 –	1
280 –	0
300 –	1
320 –	1
340 –	0
360 –	0
380 –	0
400 –	0

SMRS

	0.0 – 61.3
	61.3 – 74.3
	74.3 – 88.7
	88.7 – 102.5
	102.5 – 133.1
	133.1 – 337.3

ENGLAND AND WALES: MALIGNANT NEOPLASM OF CERVIX UTERI MORTALITY AGES 15–64

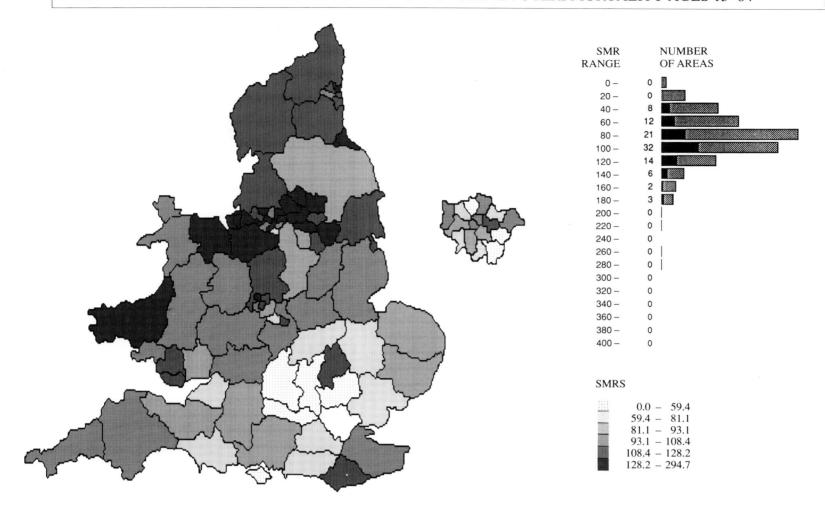

SMR RANGE	NUMBER OF AREAS
0 –	0
20 –	0
40 –	8
60 –	12
80 –	21
100 –	32
120 –	14
140 –	6
160 –	2
180 –	3
200 –	0
220 –	0
240 –	0
260 –	0
280 –	0
300 –	0
320 –	0
340 –	0
360 –	0
380 –	0
400 –	0

SMRS

	0.0 – 59.4
	59.4 – 81.1
	81.1 – 93.1
	93.1 – 108.4
	108.4 – 128.2
	128.2 – 294.7

ENGLAND AND WALES: MALIGNANT NEOPLASM OF CERVIX AND BODY OF UTERUS MORTALITY AGES 15–54

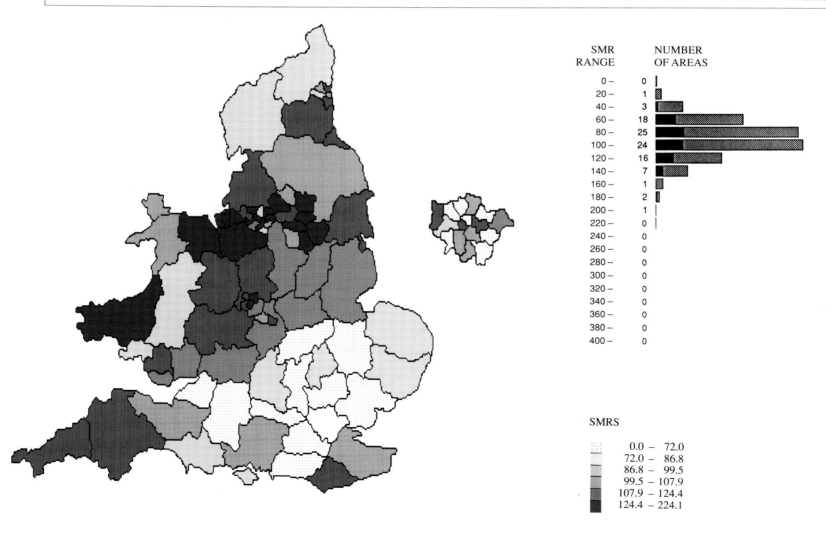

SMR RANGE	NUMBER OF AREAS
0 –	0
20 –	1
40 –	3
60 –	18
80 –	25
100 –	24
120 –	16
140 –	7
160 –	1
180 –	2
200 –	1
220 –	0
240 –	0
260 –	0
280 –	0
300 –	0
320 –	0
340 –	0
360 –	0
380 –	0
400 –	0

SMRS

	0.0 – 72.0
	72.0 – 86.8
	86.8 – 99.5
	99.5 – 107.9
	107.9 – 124.4
	124.4 – 224.1

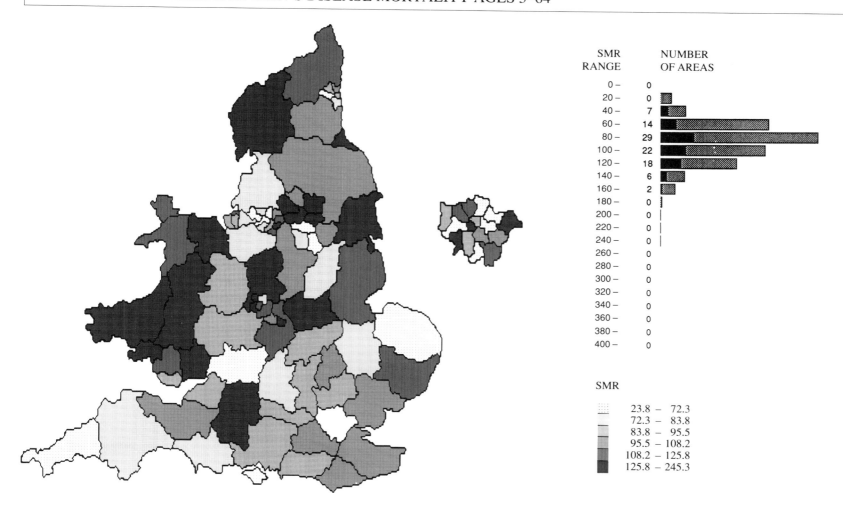

SMR RANGE	NUMBER OF AREAS
0 –	0
20 –	0
40 –	7
60 –	14
80 –	29
100 –	22
120 –	18
140 –	6
160 –	2
180 –	0
200 –	0
220 –	0
240 –	0
260 –	0
280 –	0
300 –	0
320 –	0
340 –	0
360 –	0
380 –	0
400 –	0

SMR

23.8 – 72.3
72.3 – 83.8
83.8 – 95.5
95.5 – 108.2
108.2 – 125.8
125.8 – 245.3

ENGLAND AND WALES: CHRONIC RHEUMATIC HEART DISEASE MORTALITY AGES 5–44

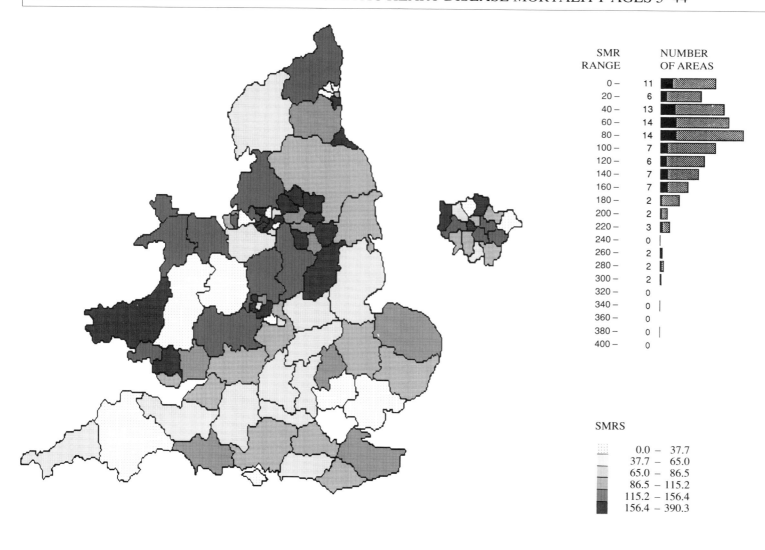

SMR RANGE	NUMBER OF AREAS
0 –	11
20 –	6
40 –	13
60 –	14
80 –	14
100 –	7
120 –	6
140 –	7
160 –	7
180 –	2
200 –	2
220 –	3
240 –	0
260 –	2
280 –	2
300 –	2
320 –	0
340 –	0
360 –	0
380 –	0
400 –	0

SMRS

0.0 – 37.7
37.7 – 65.0
65.0 – 86.5
86.5 – 115.2
115.2 – 156.4
156.4 – 390.3

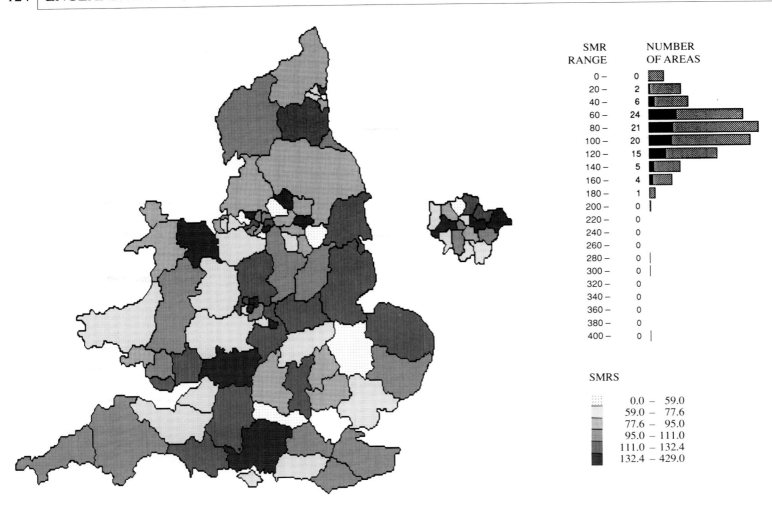

SMR RANGE	NUMBER OF AREAS
0 –	0
20 –	2
40 –	6
60 –	24
80 –	21
100 –	20
120 –	15
140 –	5
160 –	4
180 –	1
200 –	0
220 –	0
240 –	0
260 –	0
280 –	0
300 –	0
320 –	0
340 –	0
360 –	0
380 –	0
400 –	0

SMRS

	0.0 – 59.0
	59.0 – 77.6
	77.6 – 95.0
	95.0 – 111.0
	111.0 – 132.4
	132.4 – 429.0

ENGLAND AND WALES: ASTHMA MORTALITY AGES 5–44

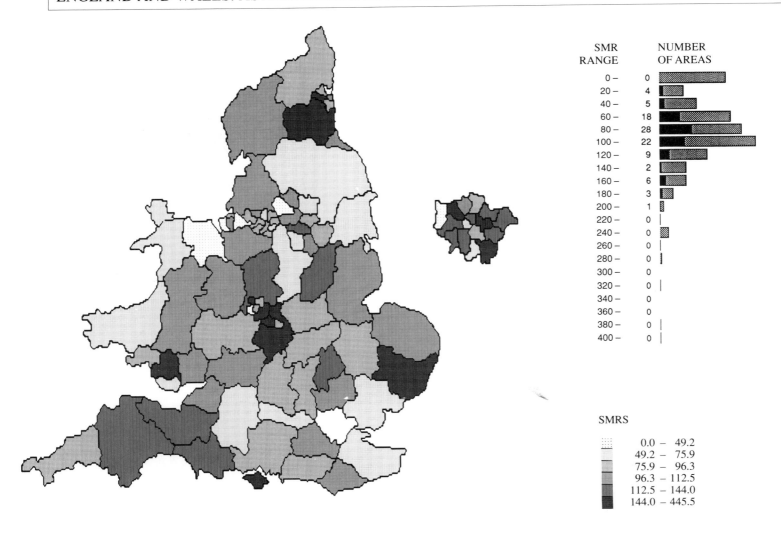

SMR RANGE	NUMBER OF AREAS
0 –	0
20 –	4
40 –	5
60 –	18
80 –	28
100 –	22
120 –	9
140 –	2
160 –	6
180 –	3
200 –	1
220 –	0
240 –	0
260 –	0
280 –	0
300 –	0
320 –	0
340 –	0
360 –	0
380 –	0
400 –	0

SMRS

	0.0 – 49.2
	49.2 – 75.9
	75.9 – 96.3
	96.3 – 112.5
	112.5 – 144.0
	144.0 – 445.5

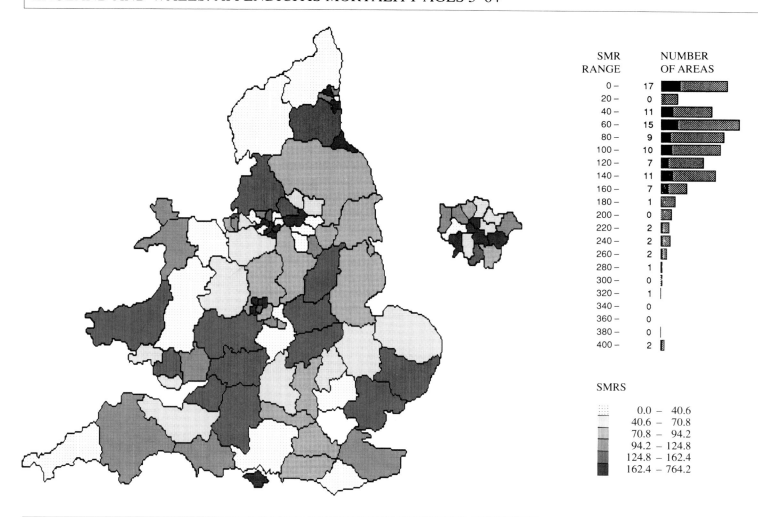

SMR RANGE	NUMBER OF AREAS
0 –	17
20 –	0
40 –	11
60 –	15
80 –	9
100 –	10
120 –	7
140 –	11
160 –	7
180 –	1
200 –	0
220 –	2
240 –	2
260 –	2
280 –	1
300 –	0
320 –	1
340 –	0
360 –	0
380 –	0
400 –	2

SMRS

	0.0 – 40.6
	40.6 – 70.8
	70.8 – 94.2
	94.2 – 124.8
	124.8 – 162.4
	162.4 – 764.2

ENGLAND AND WALES: ABDOMINAL HERNIA MORTALITY AGES 5–64

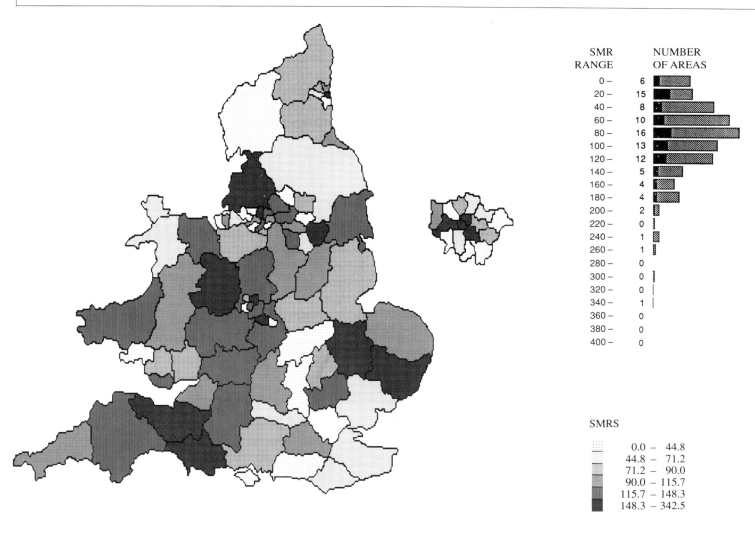

SMR RANGE	NUMBER OF AREAS
0 –	6
20 –	15
40 –	8
60 –	10
80 –	16
100 –	13
120 –	12
140 –	5
160 –	4
180 –	4
200 –	2
220 –	0
240 –	1
260 –	1
280 –	0
300 –	0
320 –	0
340 –	1
360 –	0
380 –	0
400 –	0

SMRS

	0.0 – 44.8
	44.8 – 71.2
	71.2 – 90.0
	90.0 – 115.7
	115.7 – 148.3
	148.3 – 342.5

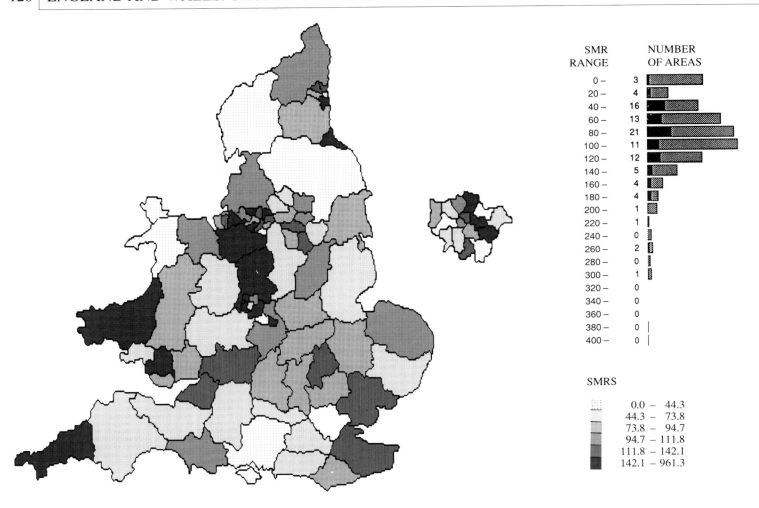

SMR RANGE	NUMBER OF AREAS
0 –	3
20 –	4
40 –	16
60 –	13
80 –	21
100 –	11
120 –	12
140 –	5
160 –	4
180 –	4
200 –	1
220 –	1
240 –	0
260 –	2
280 –	0
300 –	1
320 –	0
340 –	0
360 –	0
380 –	0
400 –	0

SMRS

	0.0 – 44.3
	44.3 – 73.8
	73.8 – 94.7
	94.7 – 111.8
	111.8 – 142.1
	142.1 – 961.3

ENGLAND AND WALES: HYPERTENSIVE AND CEREBROVASCULAR DISEASES MORTALITY AGES 35–64

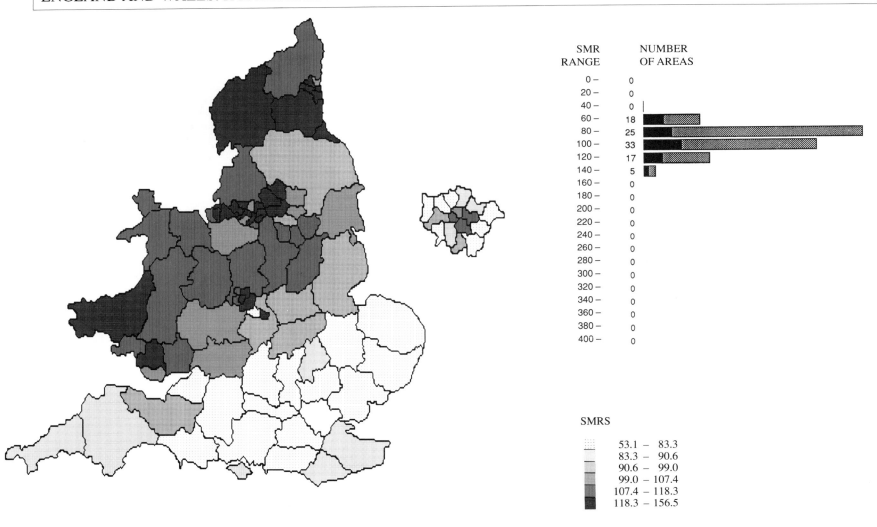

SMR RANGE	NUMBER OF AREAS
0 –	0
20 –	0
40 –	0
60 –	18
80 –	25
100 –	33
120 –	17
140 –	5
160 –	0
180 –	0
200 –	0
220 –	0
240 –	0
260 –	0
280 –	0
300 –	0
320 –	0
340 –	0
360 –	0
380 –	0
400 –	0

SMRS

	53.1 – 83.3
	83.3 – 90.6
	90.6 – 99.0
	99.0 – 107.4
	107.4 – 118.3
	118.3 – 156.5

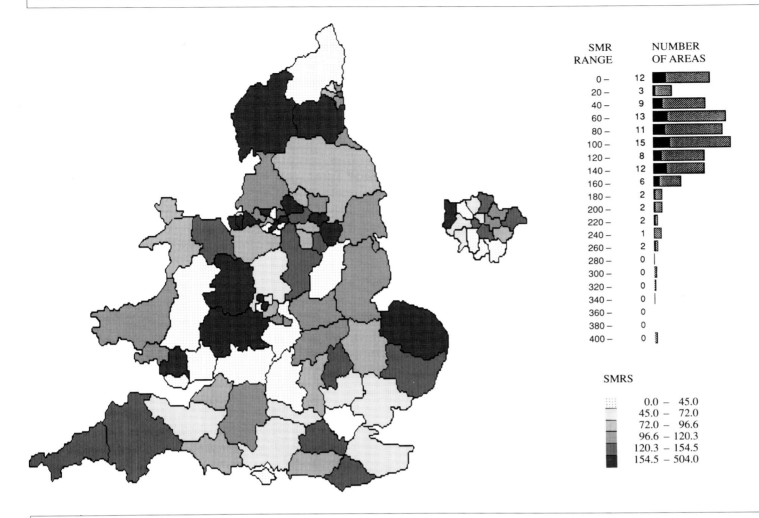

SMR RANGE	NUMBER OF AREAS
0 –	12
20 –	3
40 –	9
60 –	13
80 –	11
100 –	15
120 –	8
140 –	12
160 –	6
180 –	2
200 –	2
220 –	2
240 –	1
260 –	2
280 –	0
300 –	0
320 –	0
340 –	0
360 –	0
380 –	0
400 –	0

SMRS

	0.0 – 45.0
	45.0 – 72.0
	72.0 – 96.6
	96.6 – 120.3
	120.3 – 154.5
	154.5 – 504.0

ENGLAND AND WALES: PERINATAL MORTALITY

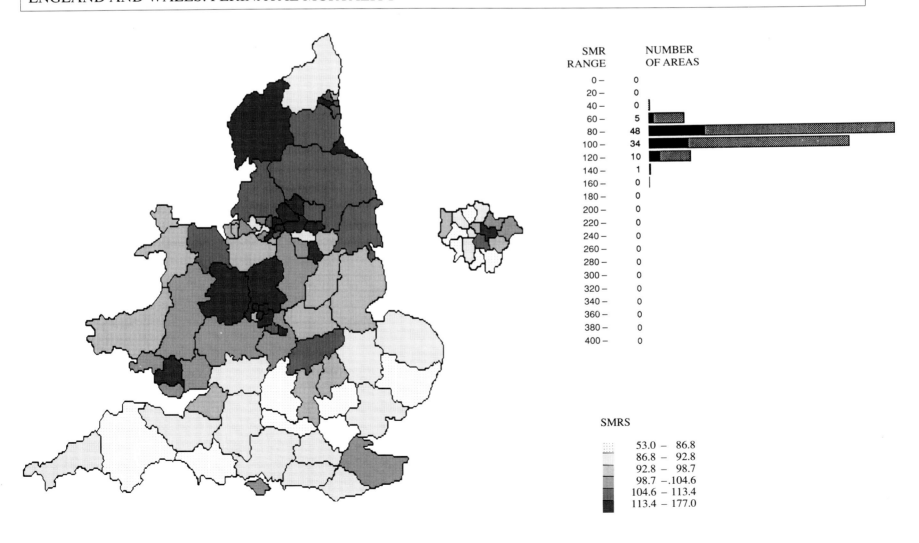

SMR RANGE	NUMBER OF AREAS
0 –	0
20 –	0
40 –	0
60 –	5
80 –	48
100 –	34
120 –	10
140 –	1
160 –	0
180 –	0
200 –	0
220 –	0
240 –	0
260 –	0
280 –	0
300 –	0
320 –	0
340 –	0
360 –	0
380 –	0
400 –	0

SMRS

	53.0 – 86.8
	86.8 – 92.8
	92.8 – 98.7
	98.7 – .104.6
	104.6 – 113.4
	113.4 – 177.0

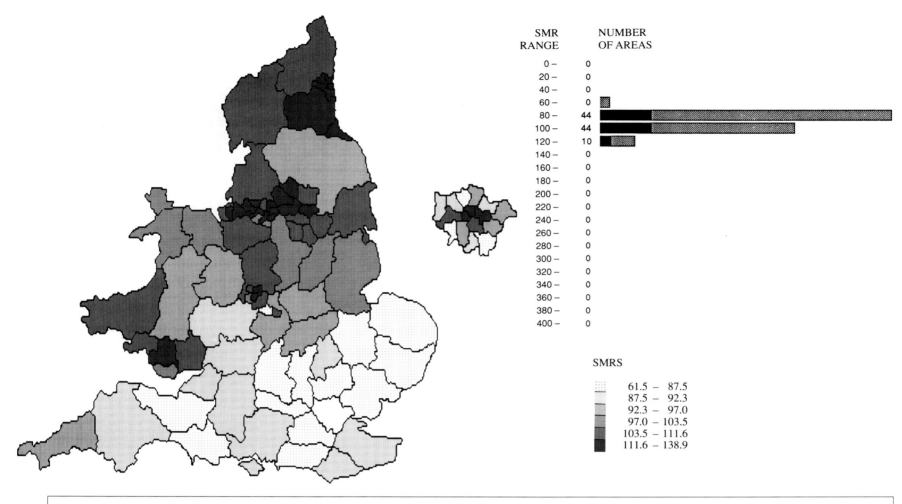

SMR RANGE	NUMBER OF AREAS
0 –	0
20 –	0
40 –	0
60 –	0
80 –	**44**
100 –	**44**
120 –	10
140 –	0
160 –	0
180 –	0
200 –	0
220 –	0
240 –	0
260 –	0
280 –	0
300 –	0
320 –	0
340 –	0
360 –	0
380 –	0
400 –	0

SMRS

| 61.5 – 87.5 |
| 87.5 – 92.3 |
| 92.3 – 97.0 |
| 97.0 – 103.5 |
| 103.5 – 111.6 |
| 111.6 – 138.9 |

ENGLAND AND WALES: ALL CAUSES MORTALITY ALL AGES

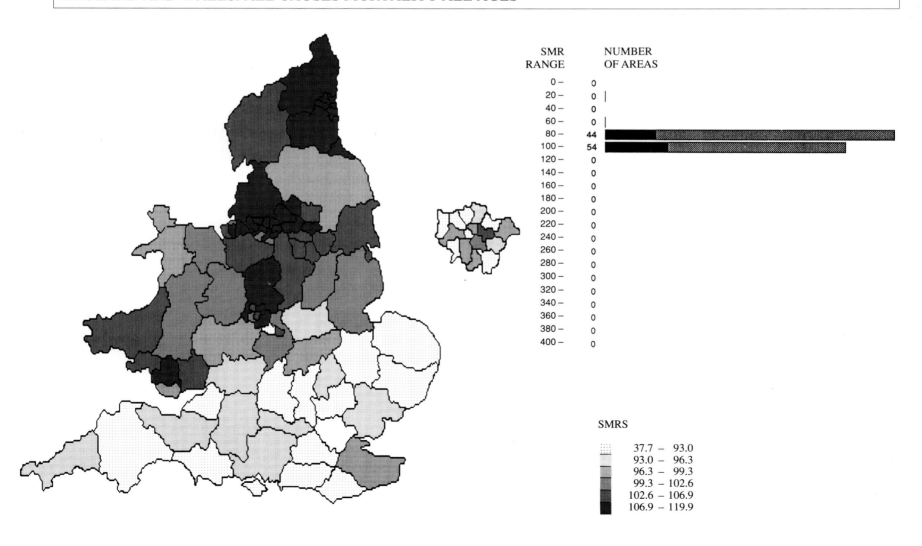

SMR RANGE	NUMBER OF AREAS
0 –	0
20 –	0
40 –	0
60 –	0
80 –	**44**
100 –	**54**
120 –	0
140 –	0
160 –	0
180 –	0
200 –	0
220 –	0
240 –	0
260 –	0
280 –	0
300 –	0
320 –	0
340 –	0
360 –	0
380 –	0
400 –	0

SMRS

| 37.7 – 93.0 |
| 93.0 – 96.3 |
| 96.3 – 99.3 |
| 99.3 – 102.6 |
| 102.6 – 106.9 |
| 106.9 – 119.9 |

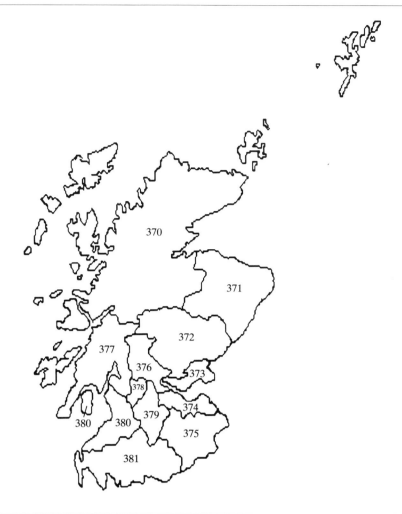

SCOTLAND: TUBERCULOSIS MORTALITY AGES 5–64

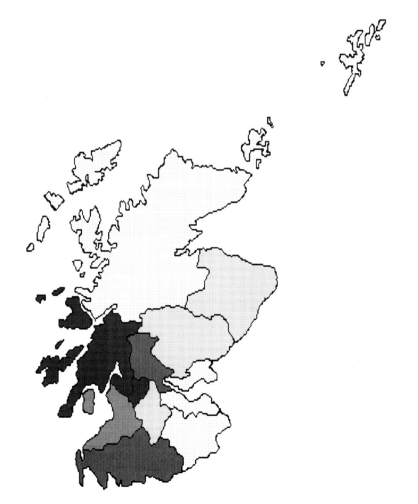

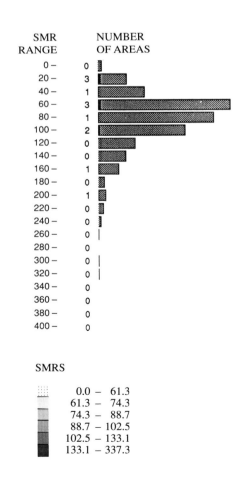

SMR RANGE	NUMBER OF AREAS
0 –	0
20 –	3
40 –	1
60 –	3
80 –	1
100 –	2
120 –	0
140 –	0
160 –	1
180 –	0
200 –	1
220 –	0
240 –	0
260 –	0
280 –	0
300 –	0
320 –	0
340 –	0
360 –	0
380 –	0
400 –	0

SMRS

0.0 – 61.3
61.3 – 74.3
74.3 – 88.7
88.7 – 102.5
102.5 – 133.1
133.1 – 337.3

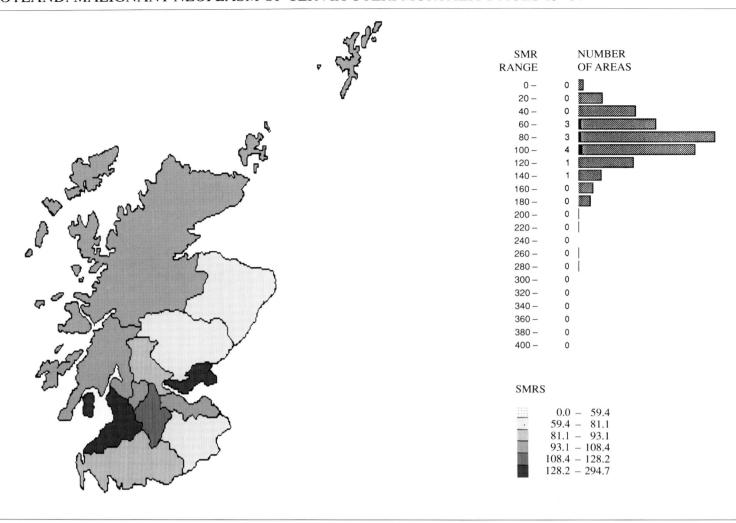

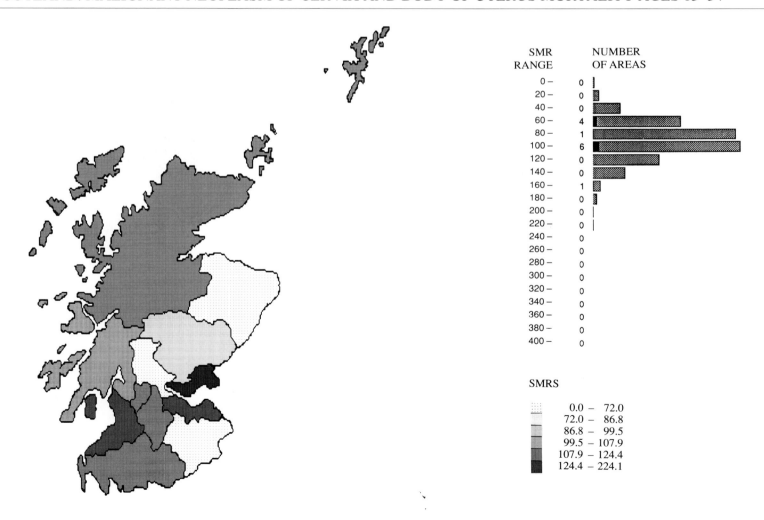

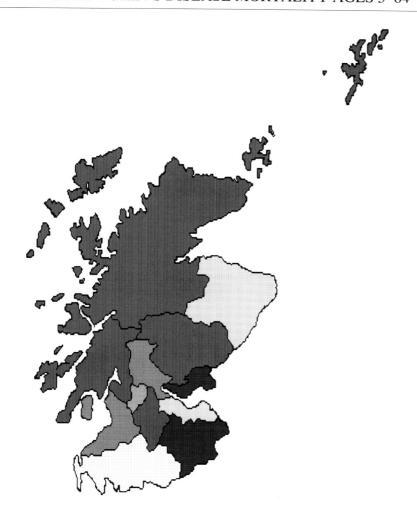

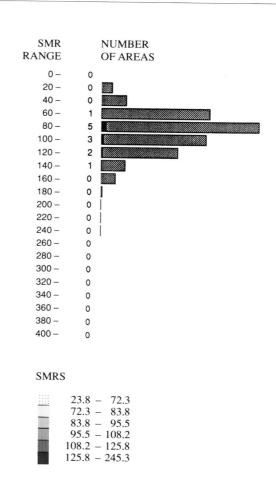

SMR RANGE	NUMBER OF AREAS
0 –	0
20 –	0
40 –	0
60 –	1
80 –	5
100 –	3
120 –	2
140 –	1
160 –	0
180 –	0
200 –	0
220 –	0
240 –	0
260 –	0
280 –	0
300 –	0
320 –	0
340 –	0
360 –	0
380 –	0
400 –	0

SMRS

	23.8 – 72.3
	72.3 – 83.8
	83.8 – 95.5
	95.5 – 108.2
	108.2 – 125.8
	125.8 – 245.3

SCOTLAND: CHRONIC RHEUMATIC HEART DISEASE MORTALITY AGES 5–44

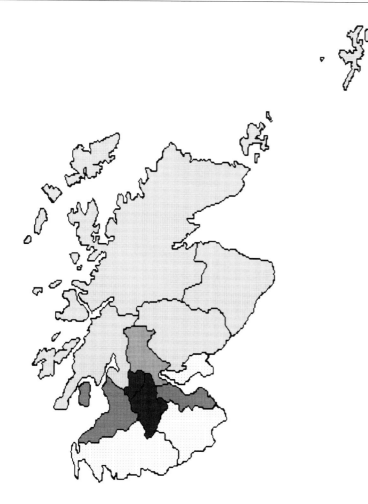

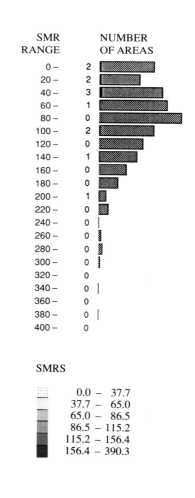

SMR RANGE	NUMBER OF AREAS
0 –	2
20 –	2
40 –	3
60 –	1
80 –	0
100 –	2
120 –	0
140 –	1
160 –	0
180 –	0
200 –	1
220 –	0
240 –	0
260 –	0
280 –	0
300 –	0
320 –	0
340 –	0
360 –	0
380 –	0
400 –	0

SMRS

	0.0 – 37.7
	37.7 – 65.0
	65.0 – 86.5
	86.5 – 115.2
	115.2 – 156.4
	156.4 – 390.3

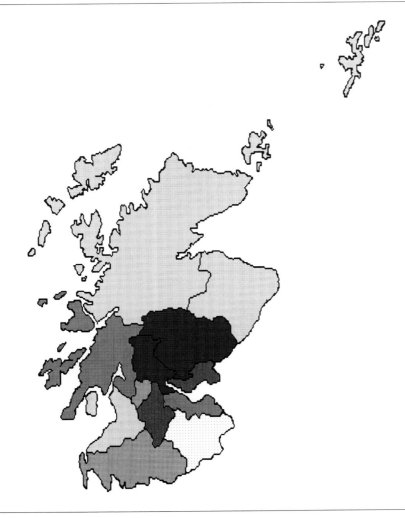

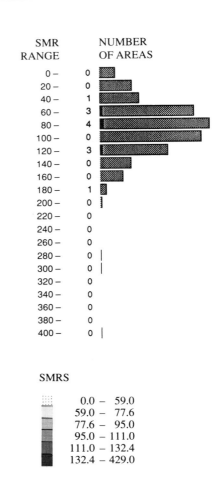

SMR RANGE	NUMBER OF AREAS
0 –	0
20 –	0
40 –	1
60 –	3
80 –	4
100 –	0
120 –	3
140 –	0
160 –	0
180 –	1
200 –	0
220 –	0
240 –	0
260 –	0
280 –	0
300 –	0
320 –	0
340 –	0
360 –	0
380 –	0
400 –	0

SMRS

	0.0 – 59.0
	59.0 – 77.6
	77.6 – 95.0
	95.0 – 111.0
	111.0 – 132.4
	132.4 – 429.0

SCOTLAND: ASTHMA MORTALITY AGES 5–44

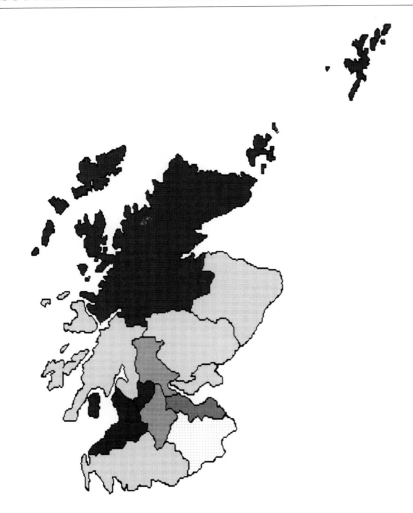

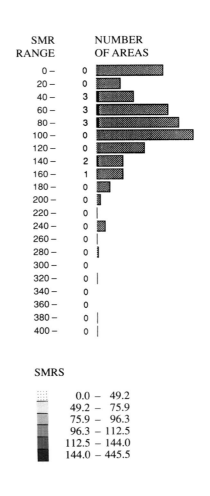

SMR RANGE	NUMBER OF AREAS
0 –	0
20 –	0
40 –	3
60 –	3
80 –	3
100 –	0
120 –	0
140 –	2
160 –	1
180 –	0
200 –	0
220 –	0
240 –	0
260 –	0
280 –	0
300 –	0
320 –	0
340 –	0
360 –	0
380 –	0
400 –	0

SMRS

	0.0 – 49.2
	49.2 – 75.9
	75.9 – 96.3
	96.3 – 112.5
	112.5 – 144.0
	144.0 – 445.5

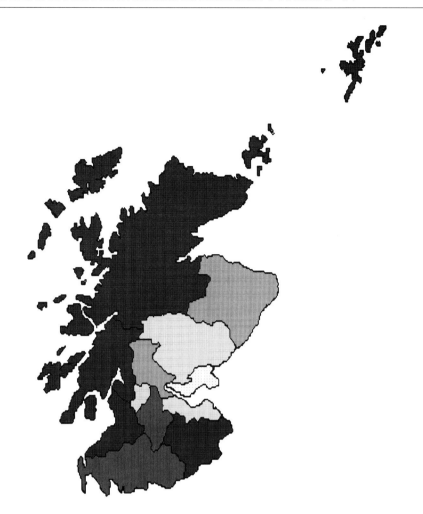

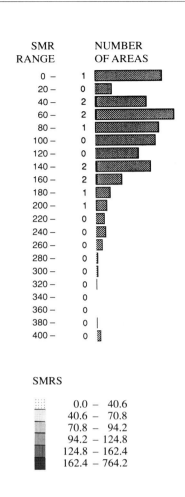

SMR RANGE	NUMBER OF AREAS
0 –	1
20 –	0
40 –	2
60 –	2
80 –	1
100 –	0
120 –	0
140 –	2
160 –	2
180 –	1
200 –	1
220 –	0
240 –	0
260 –	0
280 –	0
300 –	0
320 –	0
340 –	0
360 –	0
380 –	0
400 –	0

SMRS

0.0 –	40.6
40.6 –	70.8
70.8 –	94.2
94.2 –	124.8
124.8 –	162.4
162.4 –	764.2

SCOTLAND: ABDOMINAL HERNIA MORTALITY AGES 5–64

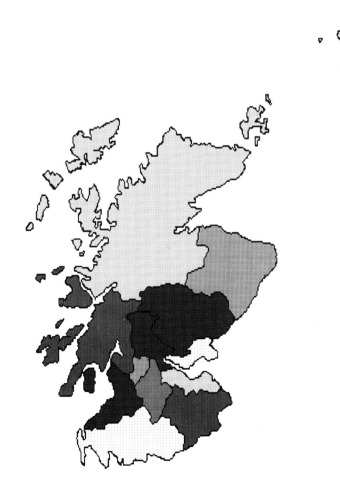

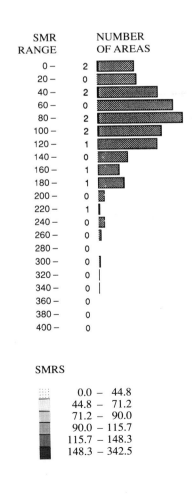

SMR RANGE	NUMBER OF AREAS
0 –	2
20 –	0
40 –	2
60 –	0
80 –	2
100 –	2
120 –	1
140 –	0
160 –	1
180 –	1
200 –	0
220 –	1
240 –	0
260 –	0
280 –	0
300 –	0
320 –	0
340 –	0
360 –	0
380 –	0
400 –	0

SMRS

0.0 –	44.8
44.8 –	71.2
71.2 –	90.0
90.0 –	115.7
115.7 –	148.3
148.3 –	342.5

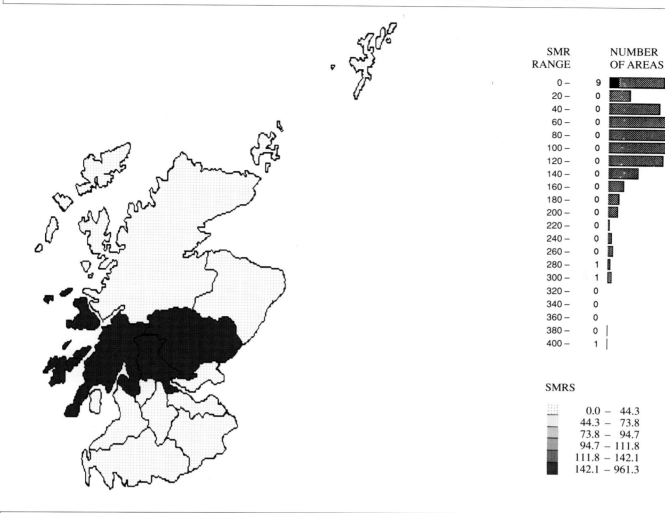

SMR RANGE	NUMBER OF AREAS
0 –	9
20 –	0
40 –	0
60 –	0
80 –	0
100 –	0
120 –	0
140 –	0
160 –	0
180 –	0
200 –	0
220 –	0
240 –	0
260 –	0
280 –	1
300 –	1
320 –	0
340 –	0
360 –	0
380 –	0
400 –	1

SMRS

	0.0 – 44.3
	44.3 – 73.8
	73.8 – 94.7
	94.7 – 111.8
	111.8 – 142.1
	142.1 – 961.3

SCOTLAND: HYPERTENSIVE AND CEREBROVASCULAR DISEASES MORTALITY AGES 35–64

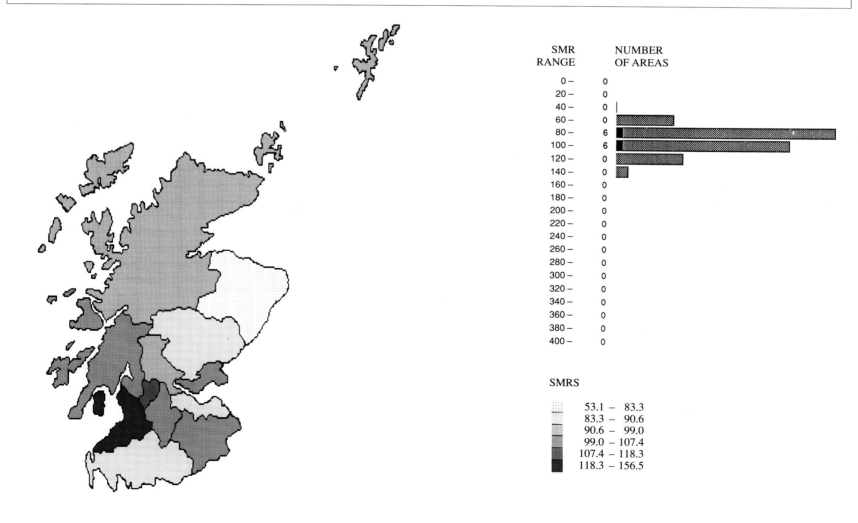

SMR RANGE	NUMBER OF AREAS
0 –	0
20 –	0
40 –	0
60 –	0
80 –	6
100 –	6
120 –	0
140 –	0
160 –	0
180 –	0
200 –	0
220 –	0
240 –	0
260 –	0
280 –	0
300 –	0
320 –	0
340 –	0
360 –	0
380 –	0
400 –	0

SMRS

	53.1 – 83.3
	83.3 – 90.6
	90.6 – 99.0
	99.0 – 107.4
	107.4 – 118.3
	118.3 – 156.5

SCOTLAND: MATERNAL MORTALITY ALL AGES

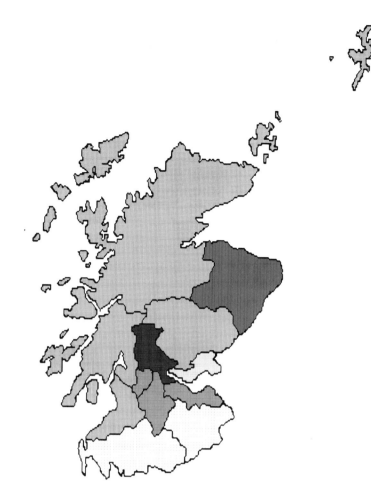

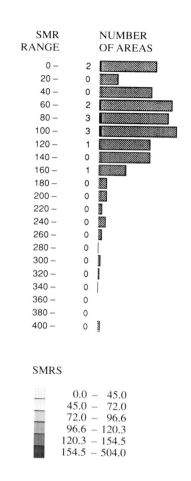

SMR RANGE	NUMBER OF AREAS
0 –	2
20 –	0
40 –	0
60 –	2
80 –	3
100 –	3
120 –	1
140 –	0
160 –	1
180 –	0
200 –	0
220 –	0
240 –	0
260 –	0
280 –	0
300 –	0
320 –	0
340 –	0
360 –	0
380 –	0
400 –	0

SMRS

- 0.0 – 45.0
- 45.0 – 72.0
- 72.0 – 96.6
- 96.6 – 120.3
- 120.3 – 154.5
- 154.5 – 504.0

SCOTLAND: PERINATAL MORTALITY

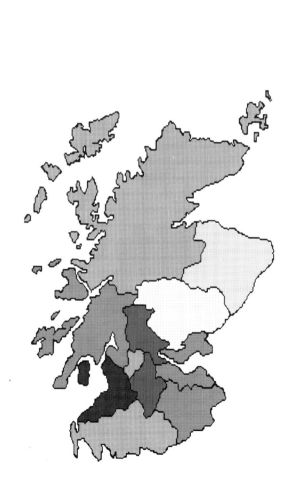

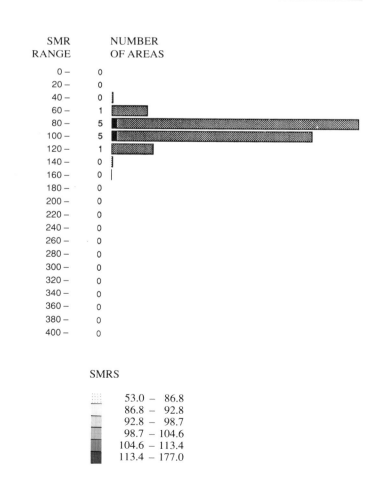

SMR RANGE	NUMBER OF AREAS
0 –	0
20 –	0
40 –	0
60 –	1
80 –	5
100 –	5
120 –	1
140 –	0
160 –	0
180 –	0
200 –	0
220 –	0
240 –	0
260 –	0
280 –	0
300 –	0
320 –	0
340 –	0
360 –	0
380 –	0
400 –	0

SMRS

- 53.0 – 86.8
- 86.8 – 92.8
- 92.8 – 98.7
- 98.7 – 104.6
- 104.6 – 113.4
- 113.4 – 177.0

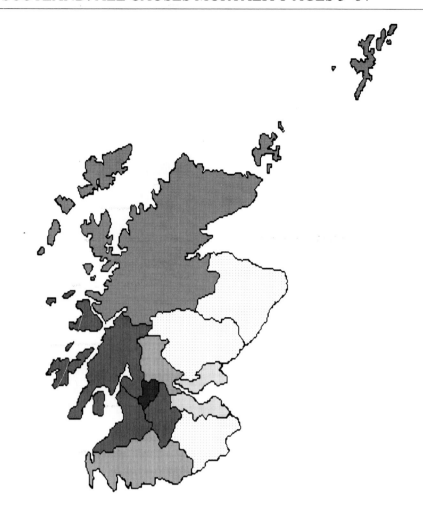

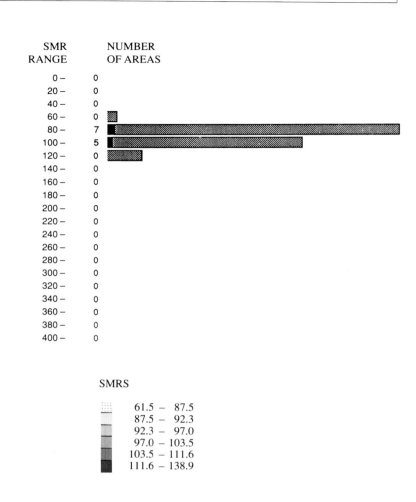

SMR RANGE	NUMBER OF AREAS
0 –	0
20 –	0
40 –	0
60 –	0
80 –	7
100 –	5
120 –	0
140 –	0
160 –	0
180 –	0
200 –	0
220 –	0
240 –	0
260 –	0
280 –	0
300 –	0
320 –	0
340 –	0
360 –	0
380 –	0
400 –	0

SMRS

61.5 – 87.5
87.5 – 92.3
92.3 – 97.0
97.0 – 103.5
103.5 – 111.6
111.6 – 138.9

SCOTLAND: ALL CAUSES MORTALITY ALL AGES

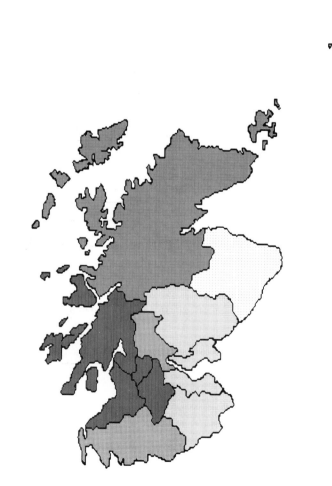

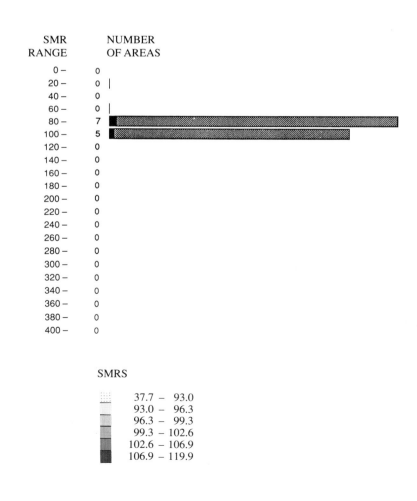

SMR RANGE	NUMBER OF AREAS
0 –	0
20 –	0
40 –	0
60 –	0
80 –	7
100 –	5
120 –	0
140 –	0
160 –	0
180 –	0
200 –	0
220 –	0
240 –	0
260 –	0
280 –	0
300 –	0
320 –	0
340 –	0
360 –	0
380 –	0
400 –	0

SMRS

37.7 – 93.0
93.0 – 96.3
96.3 – 99.3
99.3 – 102.6
102.6 – 106.9
106.9 – 119.9

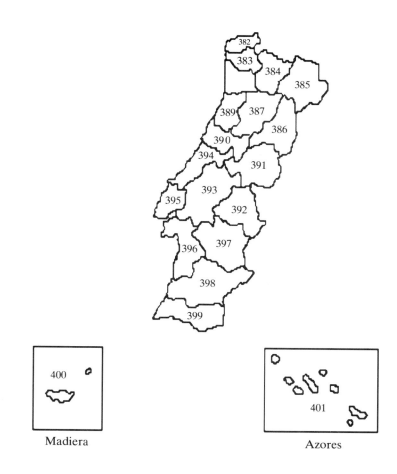

Madiera

Azores

PORTUGAL: TUBERCULOSIS MORTALITY AGES 5–64

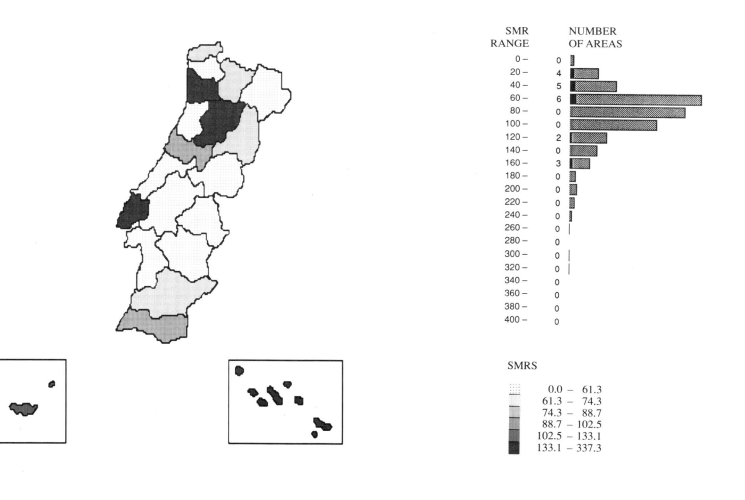

SMR RANGE	NUMBER OF AREAS
0 –	0
20 –	4
40 –	5
60 –	6
80 –	0
100 –	0
120 –	2
140 –	0
160 –	3
180 –	0
200 –	0
220 –	0
240 –	0
260 –	0
280 –	0
300 –	0
320 –	0
340 –	0
360 –	0
380 –	0
400 –	0

SMRS

0.0 – 61.3
61.3 – 74.3
74.3 – 88.7
88.7 – 102.5
102.5 – 133.1
133.1 – 337.3

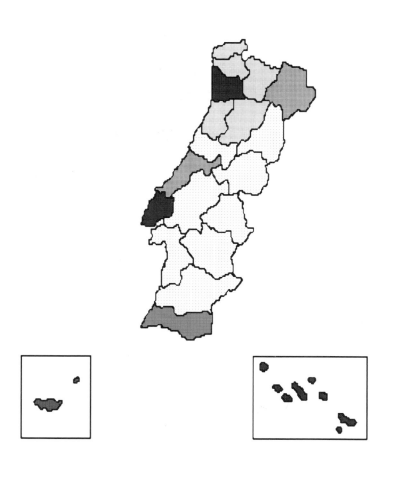

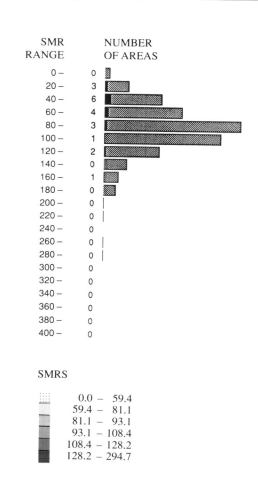

SMR RANGE	NUMBER OF AREAS
0 –	0
20 –	3
40 –	6
60 –	4
80 –	3
100 –	1
120 –	2
140 –	0
160 –	1
180 –	0
200 –	0
220 –	0
240 –	0
260 –	0
280 –	0
300 –	0
320 –	0
340 –	0
360 –	0
380 –	0
400 –	0

SMRS

	0.0 – 59.4
	59.4 – 81.1
	81.1 – 93.1
	93.1 – 108.4
	108.4 – 128.2
	128.2 – 294.7

PORTUGAL: MALIGNANT NEOPLASM OF CERVIX AND BODY OF UTERUS MORTALITY AGES 15–54

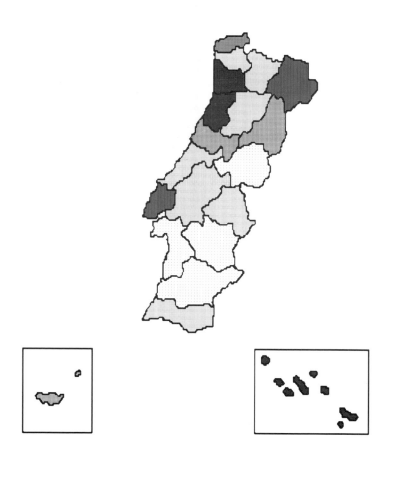

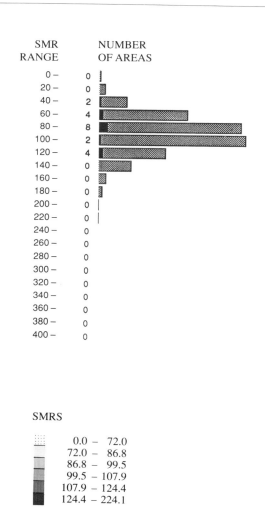

SMR RANGE	NUMBER OF AREAS
0 –	0
20 –	0
40 –	2
60 –	4
80 –	8
100 –	2
120 –	4
140 –	0
160 –	0
180 –	0
200 –	0
220 –	0
240 –	0
260 –	0
280 –	0
300 –	0
320 –	0
340 –	0
360 –	0
380 –	0
400 –	0

SMRS

	0.0 – 72.0
	72.0 – 86.8
	86.8 – 99.5
	99.5 – 107.9
	107.9 – 124.4
	124.4 – 224.1

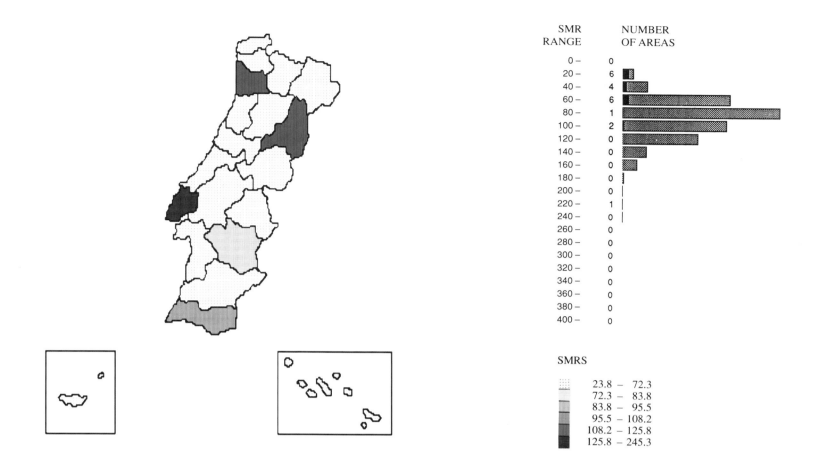

SMR RANGE — NUMBER OF AREAS

SMR RANGE	NUMBER OF AREAS
0 –	0
20 –	6
40 –	4
60 –	6
80 –	1
100 –	2
120 –	0
140 –	0
160 –	0
180 –	0
200 –	0
220 –	1
240 –	0
260 –	0
280 –	0
300 –	0
320 –	0
340 –	0
360 –	0
380 –	0
400 –	0

SMRS

	23.8 – 72.3
	72.3 – 83.8
	83.8 – 95.5
	95.5 – 108.2
	108.2 – 125.8
	125.8 – 245.3

PORTUGAL: CHRONIC RHEUMATIC HEART DISEASE MORTALITY AGES 5–44

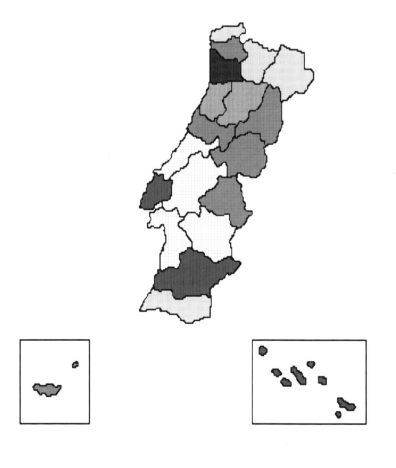

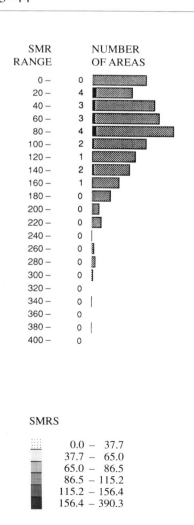

SMR RANGE	NUMBER OF AREAS
0 –	0
20 –	4
40 –	3
60 –	3
80 –	4
100 –	2
120 –	1
140 –	2
160 –	1
180 –	0
200 –	0
220 –	0
240 –	0
260 –	0
280 –	0
300 –	0
320 –	0
340 –	0
360 –	0
380 –	0
400 –	0

SMRS

	0.0 – 37.7
	37.7 – 65.0
	65.0 – 86.5
	86.5 – 115.2
	115.2 – 156.4
	156.4 – 390.3

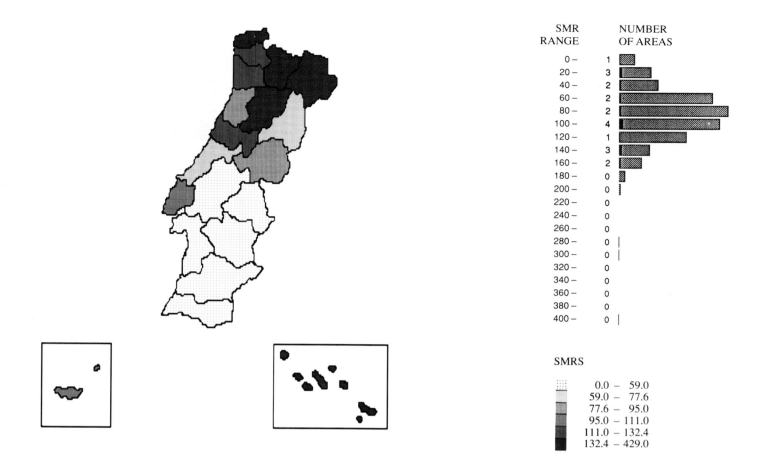

SMR RANGE	NUMBER OF AREAS
0 –	1
20 –	3
40 –	2
60 –	2
80 –	2
100 –	4
120 –	1
140 –	3
160 –	2
180 –	0
200 –	0
220 –	0
240 –	0
260 –	0
280 –	0
300 –	0
320 –	0
340 –	0
360 –	0
380 –	0
400 –	0

SMRS

	0.0 – 59.0
	59.0 – 77.6
	77.6 – 95.0
	95.0 – 111.0
	111.0 – 132.4
	132.4 – 429.0

PORTUGAL: ASTHMA MORTALITY AGES 5–44

DATA FOR THIS MAP ARE NOT AVAILABLE FOR PORTUGAL

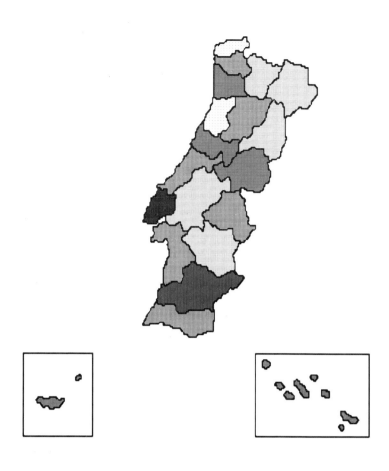

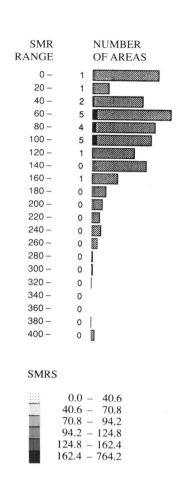

SMR RANGE	NUMBER OF AREAS
0 –	1
20 –	1
40 –	2
60 –	5
80 –	4
100 –	5
120 –	1
140 –	0
160 –	1
180 –	0
200 –	0
220 –	0
240 –	0
260 –	0
280 –	0
300 –	0
320 –	0
340 –	0
360 –	0
380 –	0
400 –	0

SMRS

	0.0 – 40.6
	40.6 – 70.8
	70.8 – 94.2
	94.2 – 124.8
	124.8 – 162.4
	162.4 – 764.2

PORTUGAL: ABDOMINAL HERNIA MORTALITY AGES 5–64

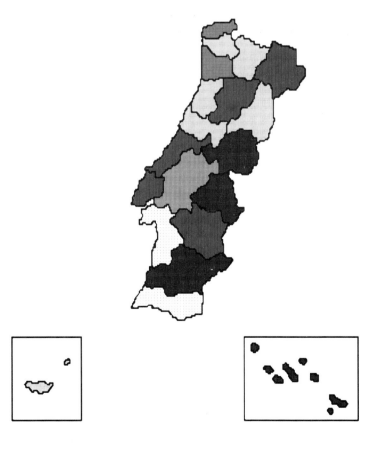

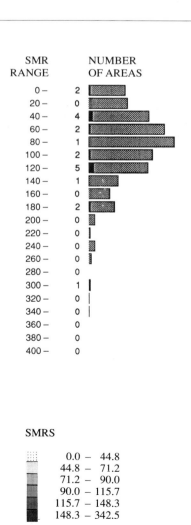

SMR RANGE	NUMBER OF AREAS
0 –	2
20 –	0
40 –	4
60 –	2
80 –	1
100 –	2
120 –	5
140 –	1
160 –	0
180 –	2
200 –	0
220 –	0
240 –	0
260 –	0
280 –	0
300 –	1
320 –	0
340 –	0
360 –	0
380 –	0
400 –	0

SMRS

	0.0 – 44.8
	44.8 – 71.2
	71.2 – 90.0
	90.0 – 115.7
	115.7 – 148.3
	148.3 – 342.5

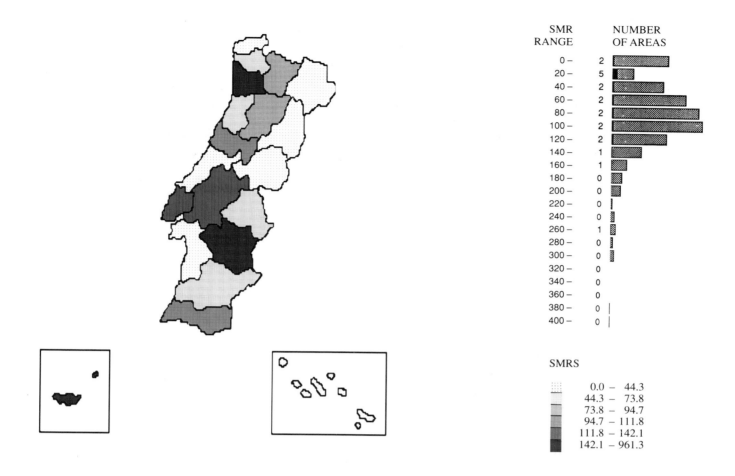

SMR RANGE	NUMBER OF AREAS
0 –	2
20 –	5
40 –	2
60 –	2
80 –	2
100 –	2
120 –	2
140 –	1
160 –	1
180 –	0
200 –	0
220 –	0
240 –	0
260 –	1
280 –	0
300 –	0
320 –	0
340 –	0
360 –	0
380 –	0
400 –	0

SMRS

	0.0 – 44.3
	44.3 – 73.8
	73.8 – 94.7
	94.7 – 111.8
	111.8 – 142.1
	142.1 – 961.3

PORTUGAL: HYPERTENSIVE AND CEREBROVASCULAR DISEASES MORTALITY AGES 35–64

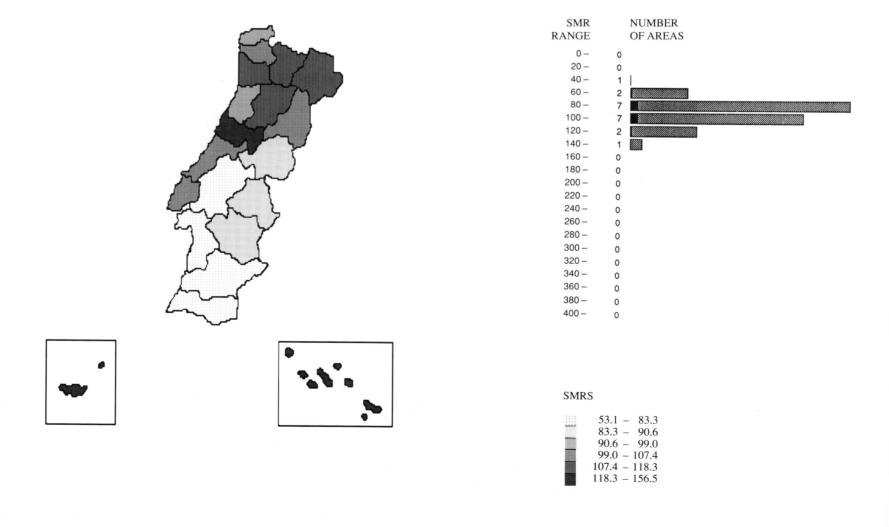

SMR RANGE	NUMBER OF AREAS
0 –	0
20 –	0
40 –	1
60 –	2
80 –	7
100 –	7
120 –	2
140 –	1
160 –	0
180 –	0
200 –	0
220 –	0
240 –	0
260 –	0
280 –	0
300 –	0
320 –	0
340 –	0
360 –	0
380 –	0
400 –	0

SMRS

	53.1 – 83.3
	83.3 – 90.6
	90.6 – 99.0
	99.0 – 107.4
	107.4 – 118.3
	118.3 – 156.5

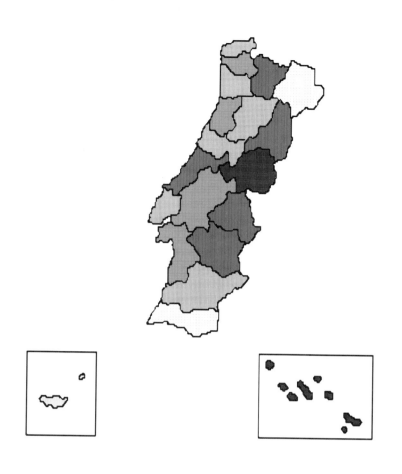

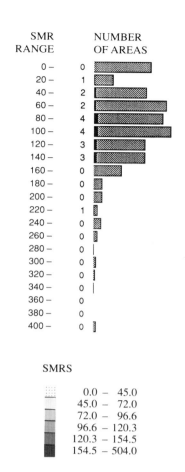

SMR RANGE	NUMBER OF AREAS
0 –	0
20 –	1
40 –	2
60 –	2
80 –	4
100 –	4
120 –	3
140 –	3
160 –	0
180 –	0
200 –	0
220 –	1
240 –	0
260 –	0
280 –	0
300 –	0
320 –	0
340 –	0
360 –	0
380 –	0
400 –	0

SMRS

	0.0 – 45.0
	45.0 – 72.0
	72.0 – 96.6
	96.6 – 120.3
	120.3 – 154.5
	154.5 – 504.0

PORTUGAL: PERINATAL MORTALITY

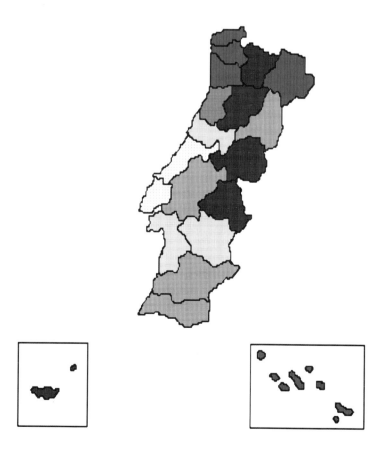

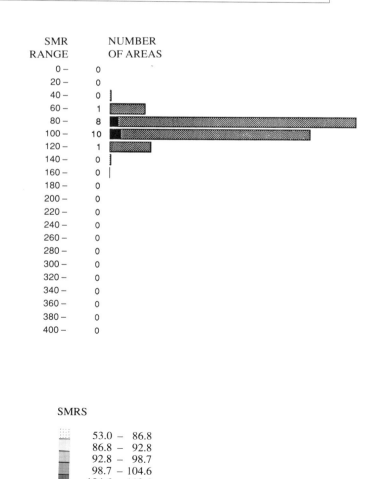

SMR RANGE	NUMBER OF AREAS
0 –	0
20 –	0
40 –	0
60 –	1
80 –	8
100 –	10
120 –	1
140 –	0
160 –	0
180 –	0
200 –	0
220 –	0
240 –	0
260 –	0
280 –	0
300 –	0
320 –	0
340 –	0
360 –	0
380 –	0
400 –	0

SMRS

	53.0 – 86.8
	86.8 – 92.8
	92.8 – 98.7
	98.7 – 104.6
	104.6 – 113.4
	113.4 – 177.0

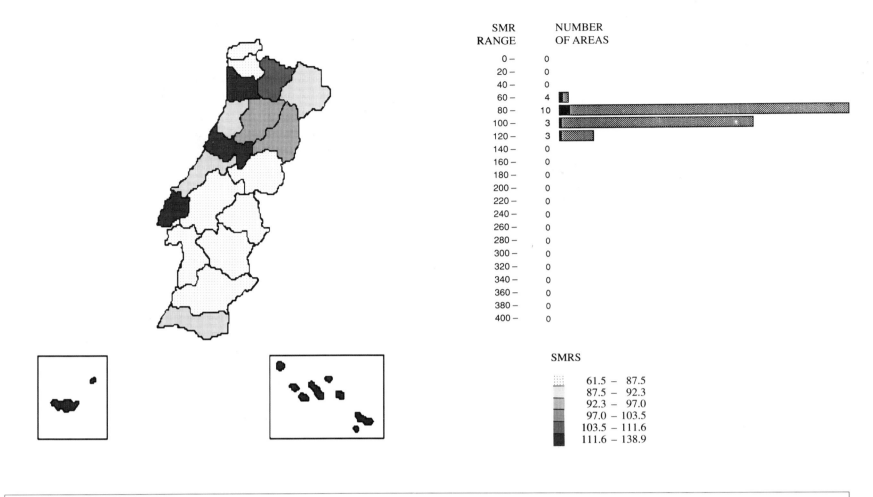

PORTUGAL: ALL CAUSES MORTALITY ALL AGES

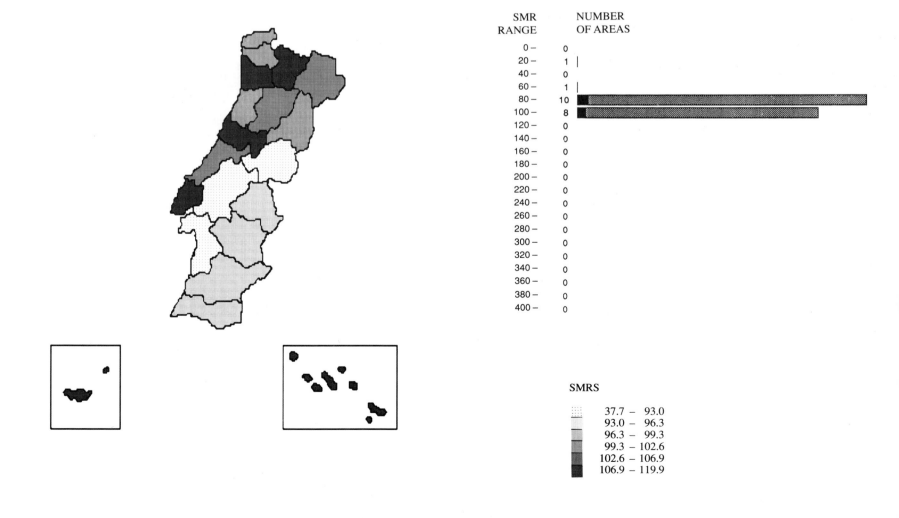

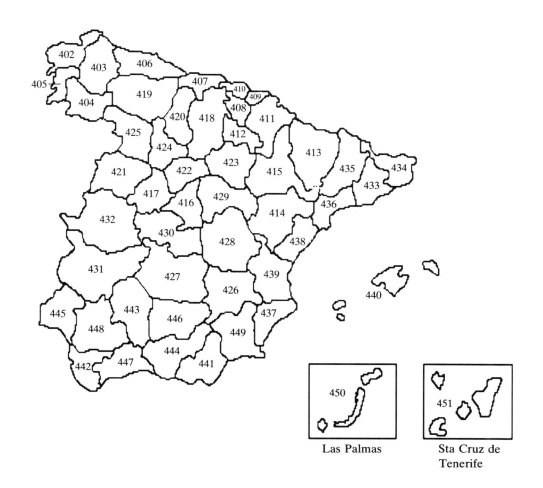

Las Palmas   Sta Cruz de
              Tenerife

SPAIN: TUBERCULOSIS MORTALITY AGES 5–64

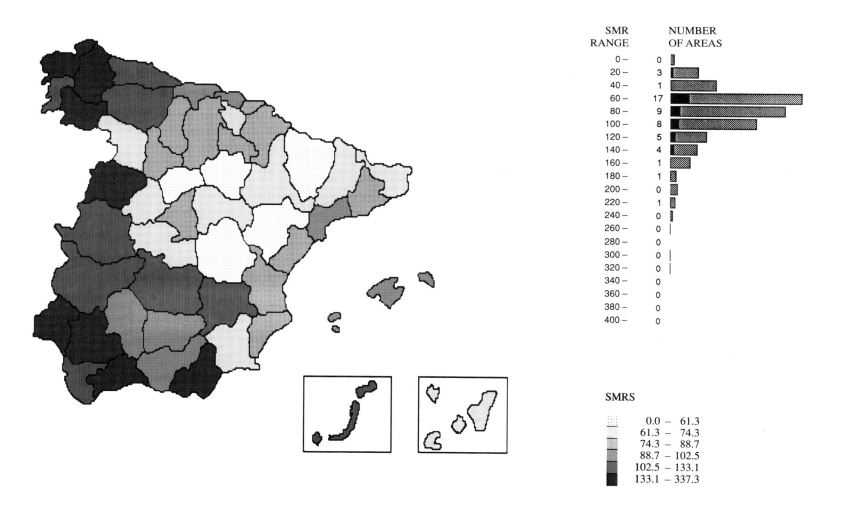

SMR RANGE	NUMBER OF AREAS
0 –	0
20 –	3
40 –	1
60 –	17
80 –	9
100 –	8
120 –	5
140 –	4
160 –	1
180 –	1
200 –	0
220 –	1
240 –	0
260 –	0
280 –	0
300 –	0
320 –	0
340 –	0
360 –	0
380 –	0
400 –	0

SMRS

0.0 – 61.3
61.3 – 74.3
74.3 – 88.7
88.7 – 102.5
102.5 – 133.1
133.1 – 337.3

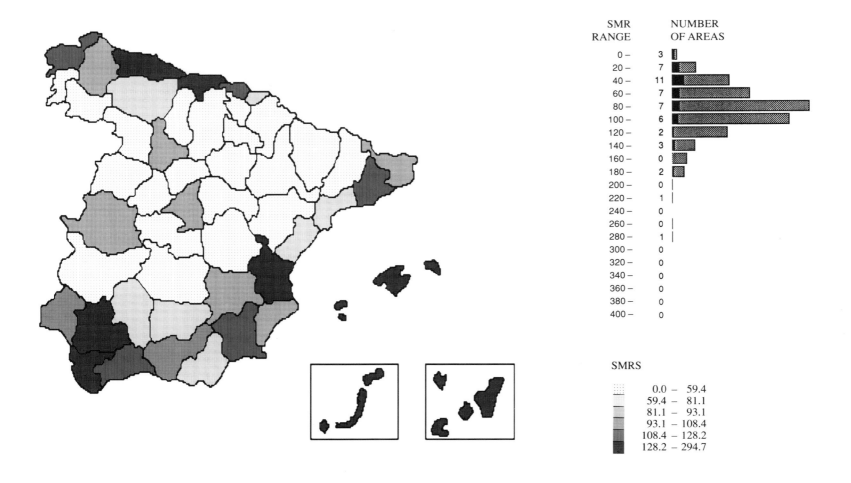

SMR RANGE	NUMBER OF AREAS	
0 –	3	
20 –	7	
40 –	11	
60 –	7	
80 –	7	
100 –	6	
120 –	2	
140 –	3	
160 –	0	
180 –	2	
200 –	0	
220 –	1	
240 –	0	
260 –	0	
280 –	1	
300 –	0	
320 –	0	
340 –	0	
360 –	0	
380 –	0	
400 –	0	

SMRS

	0.0 – 59.4
	59.4 – 81.1
	81.1 – 93.1
	93.1 – 108.4
	108.4 – 128.2
	128.2 – 294.7

SPAIN: MALIGNANT NEOPLASM OF CERVIX AND BODY OF UTERUS MORTALITY AGES 15–54

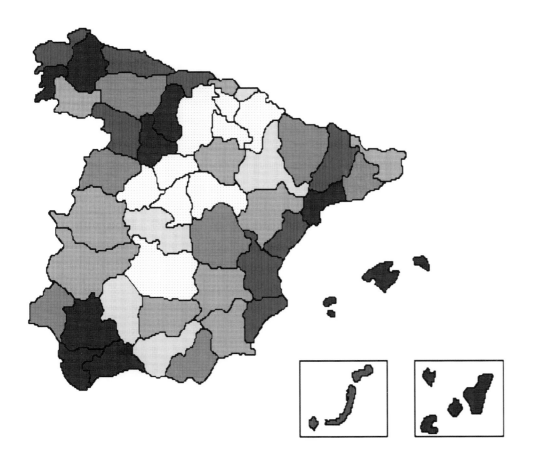

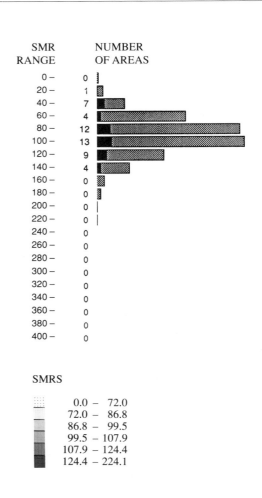

SMR RANGE	NUMBER OF AREAS	
0 –	0	
20 –	1	
40 –	7	
60 –	4	
80 –	12	
100 –	13	
120 –	9	
140 –	4	
160 –	0	
180 –	0	
200 –	0	
220 –	0	
240 –	0	
260 –	0	
280 –	0	
300 –	0	
320 –	0	
340 –	0	
360 –	0	
380 –	0	
400 –	0	

SMRS

	0.0 – 72.0
	72.0 – 86.8
	86.8 – 99.5
	99.5 – 107.9
	107.9 – 124.4
	124.4 – 224.1

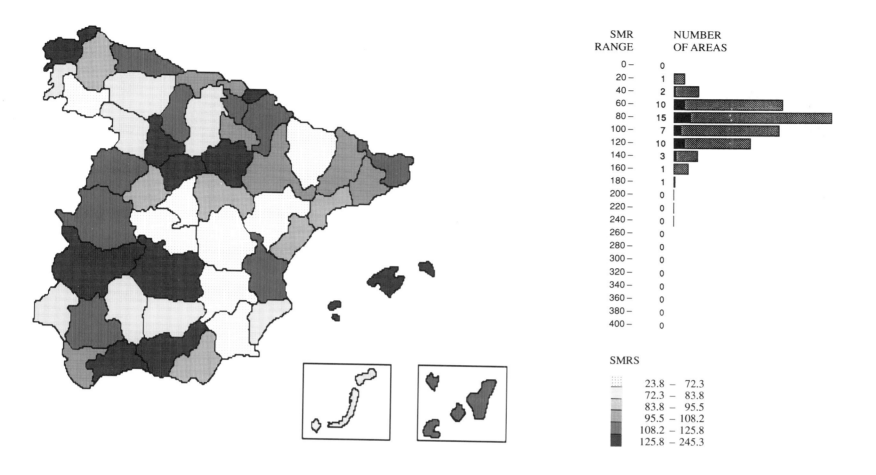

SMR RANGE	NUMBER OF AREAS
0 –	0
20 –	1
40 –	2
60 –	10
80 –	15
100 –	7
120 –	10
140 –	3
160 –	1
180 –	1
200 –	0
220 –	0
240 –	0
260 –	0
280 –	0
300 –	0
320 –	0
340 –	0
360 –	0
380 –	0
400 –	0

SMRS

	23.8 – 72.3
	72.3 – 83.8
	83.8 – 95.5
	95.5 – 108.2
	108.2 – 125.8
	125.8 – 245.3

SPAIN: CHRONIC RHEUMATIC HEART DISEASE MORTALITY AGES 5–44

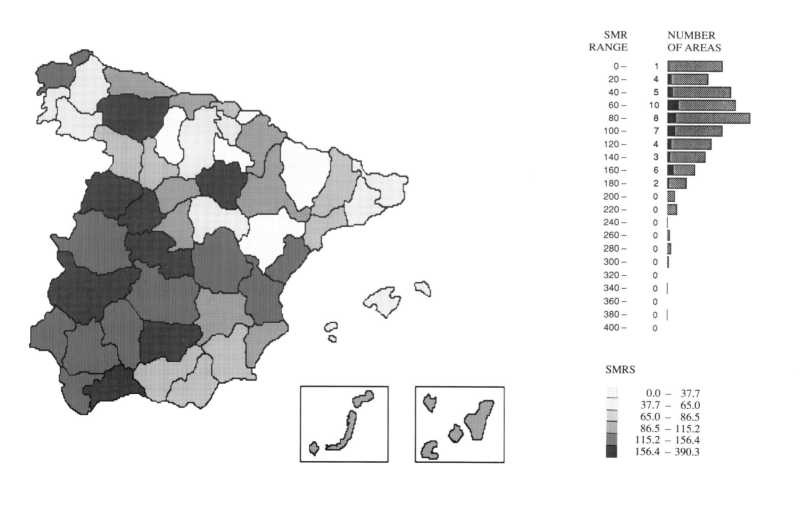

SMR RANGE	NUMBER OF AREAS
0 –	1
20 –	4
40 –	5
60 –	10
80 –	8
100 –	7
120 –	4
140 –	3
160 –	6
180 –	2
200 –	0
220 –	0
240 –	0
260 –	0
280 –	0
300 –	0
320 –	0
340 –	0
360 –	0
380 –	0
400 –	0

SMRS

	0.0 – 37.7
	37.7 – 65.0
	65.0 – 86.5
	86.5 – 115.2
	115.2 – 156.4
	156.4 – 390.3

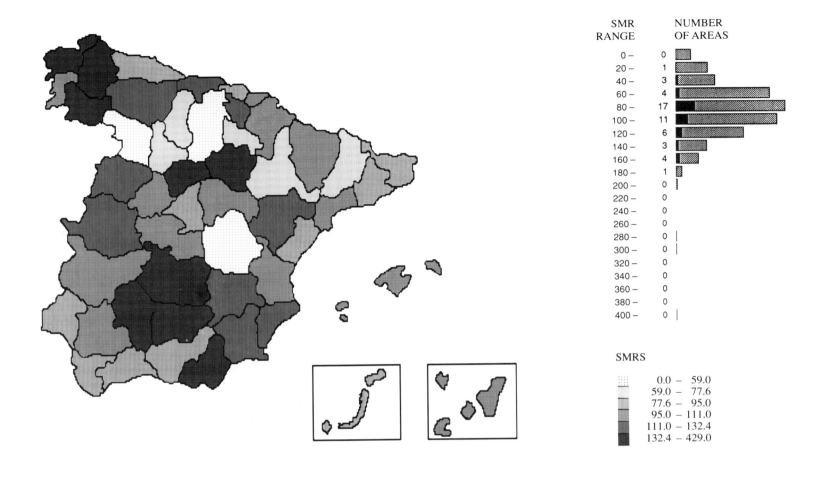

SMR RANGE	NUMBER OF AREAS
0 –	0
20 –	1
40 –	3
60 –	4
80 –	17
100 –	11
120 –	6
140 –	3
160 –	4
180 –	1
200 –	0
220 –	0
240 –	0
260 –	0
280 –	0
300 –	0
320 –	0
340 –	0
360 –	0
380 –	0
400 –	0

SMRS

	0.0 – 59.0
	59.0 – 77.6
	77.6 – 95.0
	95.0 – 111.0
	111.0 – 132.4
	132.4 – 429.0

SPAIN: ASTHMA MORTALITY AGES 5–44

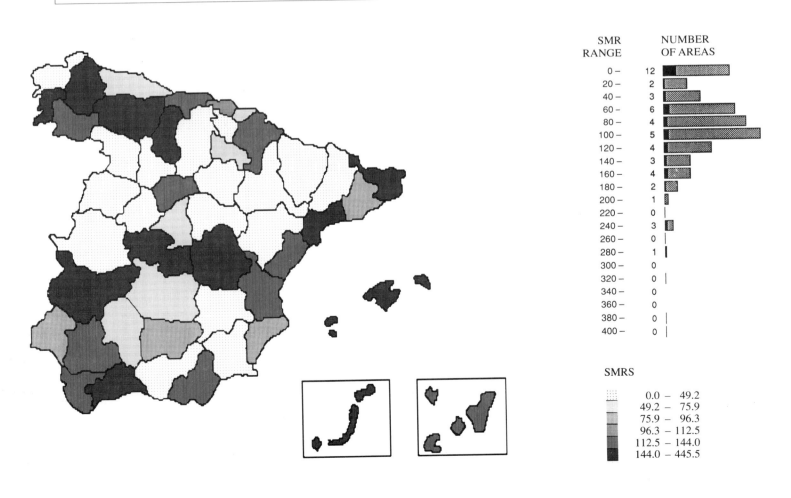

SMR RANGE	NUMBER OF AREAS
0 –	12
20 –	2
40 –	3
60 –	6
80 –	4
100 –	5
120 –	4
140 –	3
160 –	4
180 –	2
200 –	1
220 –	0
240 –	3
260 –	0
280 –	1
300 –	0
320 –	0
340 –	0
360 –	0
380 –	0
400 –	0

SMRS

	0.0 – 49.2
	49.2 – 75.9
	75.9 – 96.3
	96.3 – 112.5
	112.5 – 144.0
	144.0 – 445.5

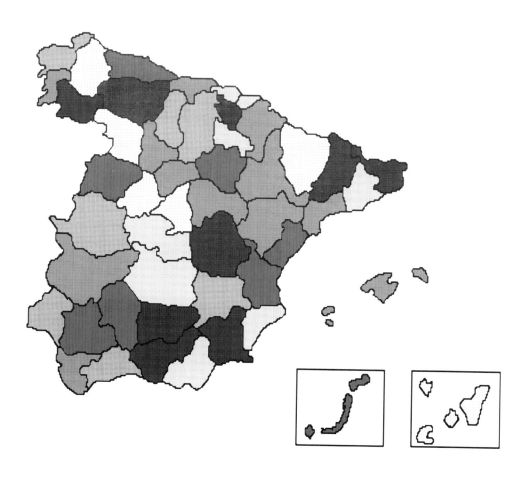

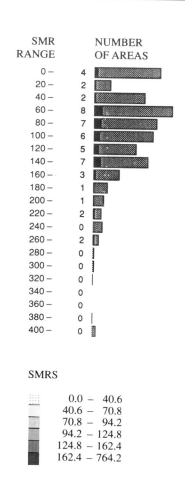

SMR RANGE	NUMBER OF AREAS
0 –	4
20 –	2
40 –	2
60 –	8
80 –	7
100 –	6
120 –	5
140 –	7
160 –	3
180 –	1
200 –	1
220 –	2
240 –	0
260 –	2
280 –	0
300 –	0
320 –	0
340 –	0
360 –	0
380 –	0
400 –	0

SMRS

	0.0 – 40.6
	40.6 – 70.8
	70.8 – 94.2
	94.2 – 124.8
	124.8 – 162.4
	162.4 – 764.2

SPAIN: ABDOMINAL HERNIA MORTALITY AGES 5–64

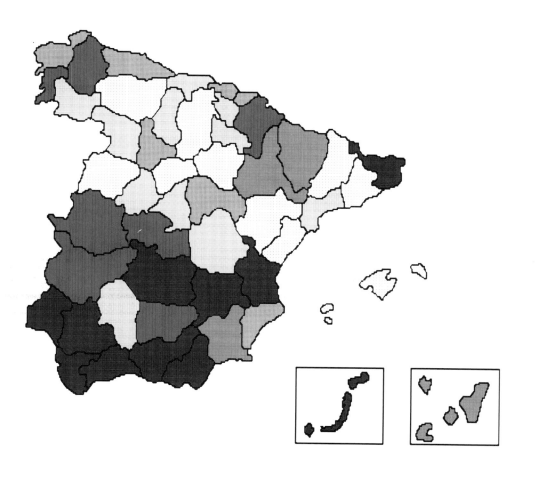

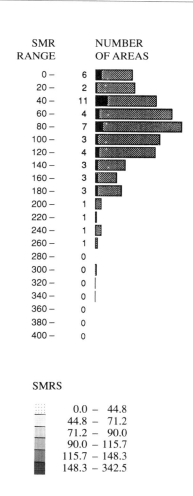

SMR RANGE	NUMBER OF AREAS
0 –	6
20 –	2
40 –	11
60 –	4
80 –	7
100 –	3
120 –	4
140 –	3
160 –	3
180 –	3
200 –	1
220 –	1
240 –	1
260 –	1
280 –	0
300 –	0
320 –	0
340 –	0
360 –	0
380 –	0
400 –	0

SMRS

	0.0 – 44.8
	44.8 – 71.2
	71.2 – 90.0
	90.0 – 115.7
	115.7 – 148.3
	148.3 – 342.5

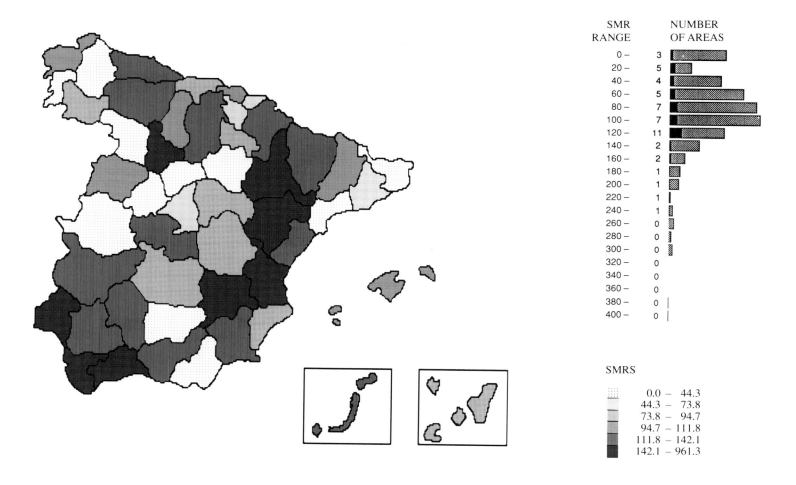

SPAIN: HYPERTENSIVE AND CEREBROVASCULAR DISEASES MORTALITY AGES 35–64

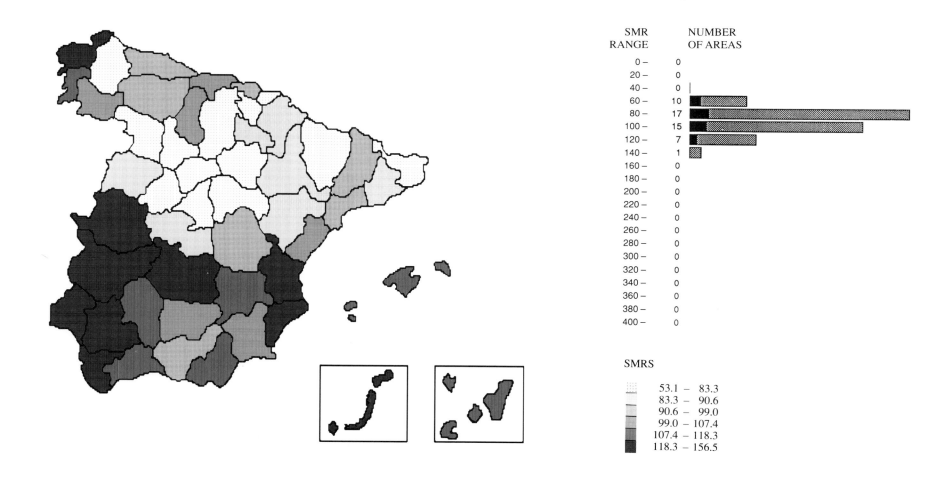

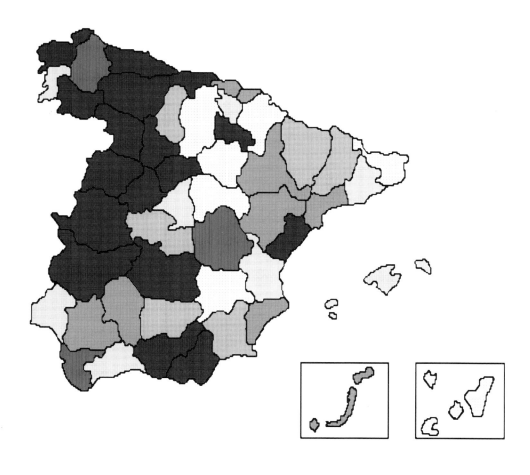

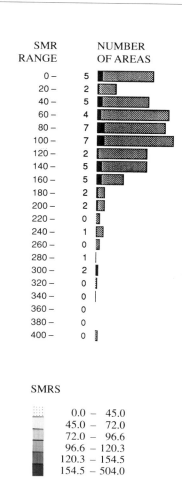

SMR RANGE	NUMBER OF AREAS
0 –	5
20 –	2
40 –	5
60 –	4
80 –	7
100 –	7
120 –	2
140 –	5
160 –	5
180 –	2
200 –	2
220 –	0
240 –	1
260 –	0
280 –	1
300 –	2
320 –	0
340 –	0
360 –	0
380 –	0
400 –	0

SMRS

0.0 –	45.0
45.0 –	72.0
72.0 –	96.6
96.6 –	120.3
120.3 –	154.5
154.5 –	504.0

SPAIN: PERINATAL MORTALITY

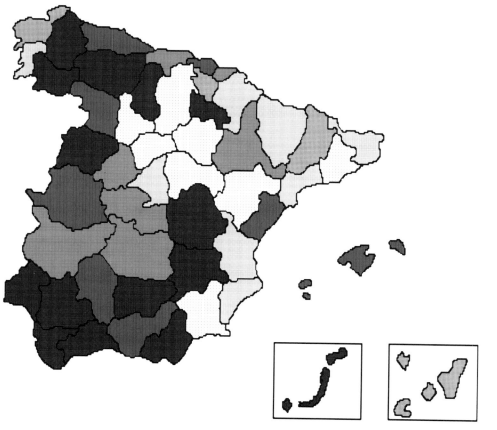

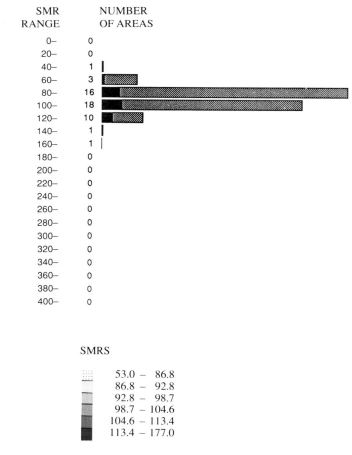

SMR RANGE	NUMBER OF AREAS
0–	0
20–	0
40–	1
60–	3
80–	16
100–	18
120–	10
140–	1
160–	1
180–	0
200–	0
220–	0
240–	0
260–	0
280–	0
300–	0
320–	0
340–	0
360–	0
380–	0
400–	0

SMRS

53.0 –	86.8
86.8 –	92.8
92.8 –	98.7
98.7 –	104.6
104.6 –	113.4
113.4 –	177.0

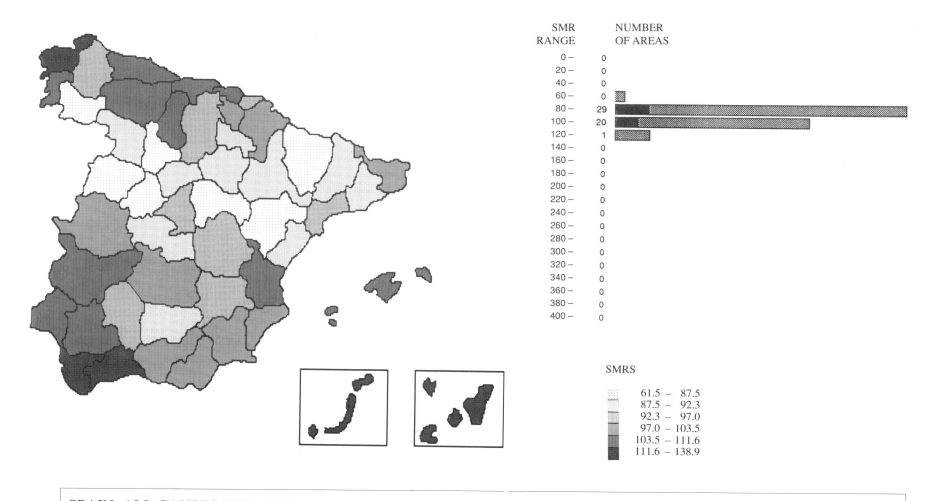

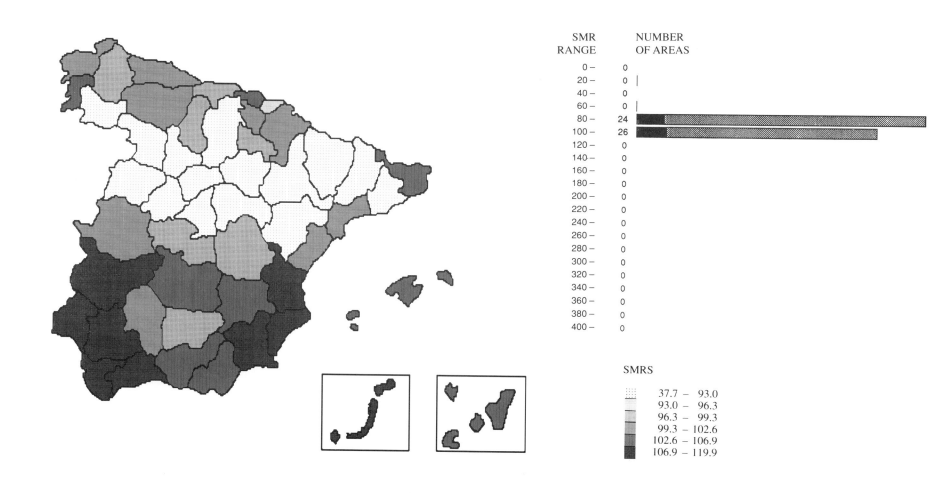

7. TABLES FOR THE PERIOD 1980–84

Mortality data for 1980–84 (except for Greece, 1980–82 and Spain, 1979–83) and population data for 1980–84 (except for France 1982; Greece, 1981; Ireland, 1981; and Spain, 1981). All data for Italy is for 1979–83.

Table 7.1.1. Population and total mortality by small area and country.

Table 7.1.2. Observed numbers of 'avoidable deaths' by small area and country.

Table 7.1.3(a)–(o). Total number of 'avoidable deaths', age-standardized mortality rates, range and heterogeneity of SMRs (chi square) by disease and country.

Table 7.1.4(a). 'Avoidable death' indicators by small area and country, standardized to the EC standard, for tuberculosis, malignant neoplasm of the cervix uteri, malignant neoplasm of the cervix and body of the uterus, Hodgkin's disease, chronic rheumatic heart disease, all respiratory diseases, and asthma.

Table 7.1.4(b). 'Avoidable death' indicators by small area and country, standardized to the EC standard, for appendicitis, abdominal hernia, cholelithiasis/cholecystitis, hypertensive/cerebrovascular diseases, maternal mortality, perinatal mortality, and all causes.

Table 7.1.5(a). 'Avoidable death' indicators by small area, standardized to own country's standard, for tuberculosis, malignant neoplasm of the cervix uteri, malignant neoplasm of the cervix and body of the uterus, Hodgkin's disease, chronic rheumatic heart disease, all respiratory diseases, and asthma.

Table 7.1.5(b). 'Avoidable death' indicators by small area, standardized to own country's standard, for appendicitis, abdominal hernia, cholelithiasis/cholecystitis, hypertensive/cerebrovascular diseases, maternal mortality, perinatal mortality, and all causes.

Table 7.1.6. Total 'avoidable deaths' and deaths from all causes by small area and country.

Tables 7.2.1–7.2.8. Observed numbers of deaths and mortality rates by country for infectious diseases, malignant neoplasm of trachea, bronchus, and lung, cirrhosis of the liver, and motor vehicle accidents.

Table 7.3.1. Health services resources and socio-economic indicators by small area or region.

Table 7.1.1. Population and total mortality by small area and country

Notes on the use of this table

1. This table shows 5-year average populations in thousands and total mortality expressed as SMRs, standardized to own country and EC standard death rates for all ages and ages 0–64.

2. The population and mortality data presented here are the totals for each small area.

3. The small area numbers are as in the key maps

4. The indicators have been tested for indicating significant excess mortality relative to national or EC rates. The *p*-values achieved for one-tail tests are indicated as follows: * *p*<0.05; ** *p*<0.01; *** *p*<0.001.

5. The mortality data are for 1980–84, except for Greece (1980–82) and Spain (1979–83). The population data are for 1980–84 except for France (1982), Greece (1981), Ireland (1981), and Spain (1981). All data for Italy are for 1979–83.

Table 7.1.1

Area		Total population (thousands)			Total (all causes) mortality (SMRs)			
					Ages 5–64		All ages	
		Total	Males	Females	Own standard	EC standard	Own standard	EC standard
BELGIUM		9855.1	4811.9	5043.2	100	105***	100	107***
1	Antwerpen	1576.0	776.6	799.4	89	94	96	102***
2	Brabant	2220.4	1069.1	1151.3	94	99	95	101***
3	West-Vlaanderen	1084.0	534.8	549.2	91	96	93	100
4	Oost-Vlaanderen	1331.7	655.6	676.1	95	100	99	106***
5	Hainaut	1291.6	623.4	668.1	119***	125***	109***	117***
6	Liège	995.8	479.7	516.1	114***	120***	110***	118***
7	Limburg	723.4	364.7	358.6	89	94	95	101*
8	Luxembourg(province)	223.1	109.6	113.6	114***	120***	104***	111***
9	Namur	409.1	198.4	210.8	120***	127***	111***	119***
LUXEMBOURG								
10	Luxembourg	364.6	177.9	186.7	100	122***	100	116***
FEDERAL REPUBLIC OF GERMANY		61495.1	29398.0	32097.1	100	104***	100	104***
11	Schleswig–Holstein	2613.0	1260.2	1352.8	99	103***	99	103***
12	Hamburg	1626.1	759.7	866.4	108***	112***	101***	105***
13	Braunschweig	1625.5	776.2	849.3	99	102**	99	103***
14	Hannover	2046.6	968.2	1078.4	102***	106***	98	102***
15	Luneburg	1463.0	712.8	750.2	100	104***	100	104***
16	Weser–Ems	2115.7	1021.5	1094.2	101	105***	100	104***
17	Bremen	684.2	321.9	362.3	110***	114***	100	104***
18	Düsseldorf	5163.7	2442.2	2721.5	106***	110***	103***	107***
19	Köln	3917.1	1892.1	2025.1	96	99	102***	106***
20	Münster	2414.8	1164.2	1250.7	104***	108***	104***	109***
21	Detmold	1808.2	859.4	948.8	98	101	96	100
22	Arnsberg	3652.7	1744.0	1908.7	107***	111***	105***	109***
23	Darmstadt	3430.0	1646.2	1783.8	96	99	97	101**
24	Giessen	971.8	471.9	500.0	93	96	99	103***

Table 7.1.1 cont

Area		Total population (thousands)			Total (all causes) mortality (SMRs)			
					Ages 5–64		All ages	
		Total	Males	Females	Own standard	EC standard	Own standard	EC standard
25	Kassel	1187.6	568.6	619.0	93	96	97	101*
26	Koblenz	1361.0	652.0	709.0	98	102*	101***	105***
27	Trier	472.2	224.3	247.8	104***	108***	103***	107***
28	Rheinhessen–Pfalz	1806.1	863.2	942.9	105***	108***	104***	108***
29	Stuttgart	3472.3	1681.7	1790.6	87	91	91	95
30	Karlsruhe	2401.0	1150.4	1250.6	96	99	97	101***
31	Freiburg	1868.1	892.7	975.4	89	92	91	95
32	Tübingen	1514.0	732.6	781.4	87	90	91	94
33	Oberbayern	3671.1	1773.6	1897.5	88	91	91	94
34	Niederbayern	1003.4	475.0	528.4	106***	110***	107***	111***
35	Oberpfalz	966.6	462.6	504.0	110***	115***	109***	113***
36	Oberfranken	1048.2	493.2	555.1	112***	116***	106***	111***
37	Mittelfranken	1522.6	724.6	798.0	101*	105***	102***	106***
38	Unterfranken	1197.5	574.6	622.8	95	98	101**	105***
39	Schwaben	1538.3	735.2	803.1	94	98	99	103***
40	Saarland	1058.0	501.7	556.3	112***	116***	110***	114***
41	Berlin (West)	1874.6	851.4	1023.2	135***	141***	114***	119***
DENMARK		5117.8	2523.1	2594.7	100	110***	100	102***
42	Kobenhavn and Frederiksberg (M)	576.6	267.5	309.1	139***	154***	110***	112***
43	Kobenhavns County	620.5	303.0	317.5	96	106***	97	100
44	Frederiksborg County	331.3	164.8	166.6	92	102	98	101
45	Roskilde County	205.1	102.7	102.4	92	101	100	102*
46	Vestsjaellands County	278.3	139.1	139.3	99	110***	101	103***
47	Storstroms County	258.8	128.8	130.0	102	113***	104***	106***
48	Bornholms County	47.4	23.8	23.6	92	101	101	103*
49	Fyns County	453.8	224.4	229.4	93	103*	98	101
50	Sonderjyllands County	250.2	124.7	125.5	89	98	96	98
51	Ribe County	214.2	107.9	106.3	93	102	95	97
52	Vejle County	326.6	161.9	164.7	96	105***	97	99
53	Ringkobing County	264.0	133.0	131.1	91	101	96	98
54	Arhus County	577.7	284.8	292.9	97	106***	99	101
55	Viborg County	231.1	116.2	114.9	89	98	95	97
56	Nordjyllands County	482.1	240.6	241.5	94	104***	97	99
FRANCE		54304.0	26492.9	27811.1	100	103***	100	92
57	Ain	420.6	209.0	211.7	93	96	97	89
58	Aisne	533.4	263.2	270.2	117***	121***	113***	103***
59	Allier	368.1	178.1	189.9	103**	106***	103***	94
60	Alpes-de-Haute-Provence	122.1	58.8	63.4	95	97	81	74
61	Hautes-Alpes	105.4	52.2	53.1	92	94	96	88
62	Alpes-Maritimes	880.0	412.2	467.8	88	90	87	79
63	Ardèche	267.6	131.3	136.3	94	96	99	90
64	Ardennes	302.5	150.0	152.5	117***	122***	110***	101
65	Ariège	136.9	67.6	69.3	84	86	95	86
66	Aube	288.8	142.4	146.4	103*	107***	99	91
67	Aude	280.9	137.4	143.4	83	84	92	84
68	Aveyron	277.9	136.4	141.6	78	79	92	83
69	Bouches-du-Rhône	1721.0	840.3	880.7	94	97	99	91
70	Calvados	589.3	285.6	303.7	106***	110***	102***	94
71	Cantal	163.1	80.5	82.6	102	104*	106***	97
72	Charente	340.4	165.9	174.5	89	92	96	87
73	Charente-Maritime	511.6	249.3	262.3	92	94	94	86
74	Cher	320.3	157.5	162.8	102	105**	100	91
75	Corrèze	242.8	118.3	124.5	92	94	100	91
76	Corse	240.0	121.5	118.5	97	100	98	89
77	Côte-d'Or	470.7	229.7	241.0	96	99	95	87
78	Côtes-du-Nord	539.7	261.9	277.7	118***	120***	110***	101
79	Creuse	139.2	68.0	71.2	104*	106**	100	91
80	Dordogne	377.6	183.7	193.9	92	94	98	89
81	Doubs	475.9	235.7	240.3	93	97	97	90

Table 7.1.1 cont

Area		Total population (thousands)			Total (all causes) mortality (SMRs)			
					Ages 5–64		All ages	
		Total	Males	Females	Own standard	EC standard	Own standard	EC standard
82	Drôme	388.7	190.5	198.2	91	94	95	87
83	Eure	463.3	228.6	234.8	110***	114***	104***	95
84	Eure-et-Loir	362.3	180.2	182.1	94	98	96	88
85	Finistère	829.6	402.5	427.2	121***	124***	111***	101**
86	Gard	528.6	257.9	270.8	92	95	97	88
87	Haute-Garonne	820.5	398.5	422.0	81	84	92	84
88	Gers	174.6	86.9	87.7	85	87	94	85
89	Gironde	1128.2	542.2	586.0	93	96	98	90
90	Hérault	708.8	342.4	366.4	85	87	94	86
91	Ille-et-Vilaine	748.3	361.9	386.4	103**	106***	108***	99
92	Indre	242.6	118.8	123.9	97	99	99	90
93	Indre-et-Loire	503.5	244.9	258.5	88	91	91	83
94	Isère	936.8	462.9	473.9	91	95	97	89
95	Jura	242.4	119.2	123.2	93	96	98	90
96	Landes	297.4	145.4	152.0	90	92	97	89
97	Loir-et-Cher	295.4	144.9	150.6	95	97	92	84
98	Loire	739.6	356.4	383.2	101	104***	102***	93
99	Haute-Loire	205.6	100.9	104.7	101	104*	101	92
100	Loire-Atlantique	995.7	482.0	513.7	111***	115***	105***	96
101	Loiret	535.8	263.8	272.0	92	95	95	86
102	Lot	154.5	75.2	79.3	80	82	95	87
103	Lot-et-Garonne	300.0	146.3	153.7	83	85	95	87
104	Lozère	74.1	37.2	36.9	92	94	101	92
105	Maine-et-Loire	676.8	329.5	347.3	93	96	96	88
106	Manche	464.9	227.1	237.9	100	102*	103***	94
107	Marne	542.4	266.4	276.0	106***	110***	101	93
108	Haute-Marne	210.5	105.0	105.5	108***	112***	105***	96
109	Mayenne	270.9	131.4	139.5	94	96	99	90
110	Meurthe-et-Moselle	716.5	351.2	365.3	110***	115***	107***	99
111	Meuse	200.4	99.1	101.3	117***	121***	109***	100
112	Morbihan	589.3	288.1	301.2	131***	135***	118***	108***
113	Moselle	1009.0	502.1	506.9	111***	116***	115***	106***
114	Nièvre	237.5	115.4	122.2	110***	113***	104***	94
115	Nord	2517.0	1228.5	1288.5	131***	136***	120***	110***
116	Oise	661.4	329.8	331.6	105***	109***	105***	96
117	Orne	295.7	145.2	150.5	102	105**	102**	93
118	Pas-de-Calais	1410.0	684.9	725.1	133***	137***	120***	110***
119	Puy-de-Dôme	595.8	291.8	304.0	104***	108***	104***	95
120	Pyrénées-Atlantiques	553.9	267.1	286.8	90	92	96	88
121	Hautes-Pyrénées	228.2	110.8	117.4	90	92	98	89
122	Pyrénées-Orientales	334.7	161.0	173.7	88	90	96	87
123	Bas-Rhin	913.3	445.4	467.9	107***	112***	110***	101
124	Haut-Rhin	648.9	318.6	330.2	107***	112***	112***	103***
125	Rhône	1441.7	701.0	740.7	91	95	95	87
126	Haute-Saône	231.9	114.7	117.2	102	105**	105***	96
127	Saône-et-Loire	571.5	280.0	291.5	99	102	99	90
128	Sarthe	504.8	247.1	257.6	88	91	93	85
129	Savoie	324.3	160.2	164.1	98	101	99	91
130	Haute-Savoie	494.3	244.8	249.5	97	101	98	91
131	Paris	2177.2	1008.7	1168.5	99	102***	88	80
132	Seine-Maritime	1193.4	583.1	610.3	114***	119***	106***	97
133	Seine-et-Marne	885.7	437.7	448.1	97	101	102***	94
134	Yvelines	1197.5	592.3	605.2	83	88	91	85
135	Deux-Sèvres	341.2	168.8	172.4	80	82	92	84
136	Somme	544.0	265.7	278.2	115***	119***	112***	103***
137	Tarn	338.8	165.0	173.8	80	81	93	85
138	Tarn-et-Garonne	189.5	92.7	96.9	83	85	93	85
139	Var	711.8	347.3	364.6	93	95	96	87
140	Vaucluse	427.9	210.6	217.2	93	95	98	90
141	Vendée	483.2	237.9	245.3	90	93	98	89
142	Vienne	371.7	181.6	190.1	84	87	88	80

Table 7.1.1 cont

Area		Total population (thousands)			Total (all causes) mortality (SMRs)			
		Total	Males	Females	Ages 5–64		All ages	
					Own standard	EC standard	Own standard	EC standard
143	Haute-Vienne	354.7	171.1	183.6	87	89	93	84
144	Vosges	394.1	191.9	202.2	113***	117***	107***	98
145	Yonne	311.3	153.5	157.8	111***	114***	102**	93
146	Territoire-de-Belfort	131.9	65.0	66.8	104	108***	106***	98
147	Essonne	988.0	491.5	496.6	87	92	92	85
148	Hauts-de-Seine	1386.3	668.4	717.8	91	94	92	84
149	Seine-Saint-Denis	1327.1	656.2	670.9	104***	109***	99	92
150	Val-de-Marne	1192.7	578.4	614.2	93	97	95	88
151	Val-d'Oise	918.4	453.6	464.8	93	97	99	92
GREECE		9739.5	4779.5	4960.0	100	79	100	95
152	Greater Athens	3027.3	1452.1	1575.2	101	80	103***	98
153	Rest of Central Greece and Eubea	1100.0	551.1	548.9	97	77	96	91
154	Peloponnisos	1012.8	508.1	504.7	92	73	93	89
155	Ionian Islands	182.5	88.0	94.5	97	77	107***	103**
156	Epirus	324.7	158.6	166.1	100	79	95	90
157	Thessaly	695.2	339.7	355.5	106***	84	102***	98
158	Macedonia	2121.6	1046.2	1075.4	102**	81	104***	99
159	Thrace	345.0	174.8	170.2	124***	97	113***	107***
160	Aegean Islands	428.3	214.1	214.2	95	76	100	96
161	Crete	502.1	246.8	255.3	89	71	88	84
ITALY		56784.9	27662.9	29122.0	100	96	100	102***
162	Torino	2307.4	1130.1	1177.3	103***	98	105***	106***
163	Vercelli	431.0	200.3	230.6	113***	108***	105***	107***
164	Novara	506.9	243.9	262.9	114***	109***	106***	108***
165	Cuneo	546.3	269.7	276.6	110***	105***	106***	108***
166	Asti	223.5	107.8	115.7	96	92	103***	106***
167	Alessandria	458.4	221.6	236.8	100	96	99	101
168	Aosta	127.5	61.7	65.9	128***	122***	104***	107***
169	Imperia	220.8	105.6	115.2	100	96	98	100
170	Savona	298.1	142.8	155.3	97	93	100	102*
171	Genova	1027.5	489.8	537.6	102**	98	102***	103***
172	La Spezia	265.8	124.0	141.7	93	89	97	99
173	Varese	780.7	377.7	403.0	103**	98	103***	105***
174	Como/Sondrio	947.4	459.2	488.2	113***	108***	107***	109***
175	Milano	3984.1	1928.1	2056.0	108***	103***	105***	106***
176	Bergamo	949.5	454.4	495.1	127***	120***	107***	109***
177	Brescia	1014.3	495.3	519.0	130***	124***	115***	117***
178	Pavia	515.4	246.9	268.5	122***	117***	111***	113***
179	Cremona	339.9	163.2	176.7	131***	125***	114***	117***
180	Mantova	376.4	181.7	194.7	109***	104**	107***	109***
181	Bolzano	434.0	212.7	221.3	111***	105***	101*	103***
182	Trento	440.7	215.2	225.5	118***	112***	103***	105***
183	Verona	769.9	375.4	394.5	111***	106***	103***	105***
184	Vicenza	728.8	354.9	373.9	115***	109***	106***	108***
185	Belluno	229.0	108.5	120.4	138***	132***	108***	110***
186	Treviso	710.9	347.5	363.3	109***	104***	98	100
187	Venezia	840.4	408.8	431.6	114***	109***	100	101**
188	Padova	812.0	395.4	416.6	112***	107***	101**	103***
189	Rovigo	262.4	126.3	136.1	113***	109***	105***	108***
190	Udine/Gorizia	665.1	322.6	342.5	129***	123***	108***	109***
191	Trieste	292.1	134.6	157.5	117***	112***	102***	105***
192	Pordenone	279.0	135.0	144.0	122***	116***	102*	104***
193	Piacenza	277.7	135.0	142.6	114***	109***	100	101*
194	Parma	396.0	192.2	203.8	98	94	97	99
195	Reggio Emilia	413.8	201.8	212.0	94	90	94	96
196	Modena	591.6	288.8	302.7	97	93	96	97
197	Bologna	920.9	444.2	476.7	94	90	95	96
198	Ferrara	396.6	189.0	207.6	104**	99	97	100
199	Ravenna	359.1	174.5	184.6	87	83	89	90

Table 7.1.1 cont

Area		Total population (thousands)			Total (all causes) mortality (SMRs)			
		Total	Males	Females	Ages 5–64		All ages	
					Own standard	EC standard	Own standard	EC standard
200	Forli	596.9	292.6	304.3	88	84	92	93
201	Pesaro	339.0	166.3	172.7	86	83	91	93
202	Ancona	431.6	208.9	222.7	82	78	90	91
203	Macerata	296.0	143.7	152.3	82	78	91	93
204	Ascoli Piceno	353.7	172.6	181.0	79	76	91	93
205	Massa-Carrara	206.1	99.5	106.6	101	97	98	100
206	Lucca	381.5	183.4	198.0	100	96	98	100
207	Pistoia	269.5	129.4	140.0	90	86	94	96
208	Firenze	1180.2	570.8	609.4	85	81	89	91
209	Livorno	369.3	175.9	193.4	93	89	95	98
210	Pisa	386.5	187.5	198.9	87	84	95	97
211	Arezzo	316.2	154.7	161.5	86	83	92	94
212	Siena	256.4	125.2	131.2	82	79	90	92
213	Grosseto	224.1	109.4	114.8	95	91	95	97
214	Perugia	573.6	282.5	291.1	88	84	92	93
215	Terni	235.6	114.4	121.2	81	78	96	98
216	Viterbo/Rieti	408.3	201.9	206.4	96	93	100	102**
217	Roma	3673.0	1781.3	1891.7	92	88	99	100
218	Latina	489.2	235.3	254.0	91	87	99	102***
219	Frosinone	460.6	228.1	232.5	90	86	95	97
220	Caserta	758.8	375.9	382.9	108***	103*	110***	111***
221	Benevento	295.6	144.5	151.1	85	82	96	98
222	Napoli	2942.4	1452.5	1489.9	117***	112***	119***	120***
223	Avellino	462.8	224.9	237.9	102	97	108***	111***
224	Salerno	1014.3	502.4	512.0	92	88	93	94
225	L'Aquila	305.5	147.9	157.6	97	93	98	101
226	Teramo	273.1	134.9	138.1	86	82	93	95
227	Pescara	288.9	140.9	148.0	79	76	90	91
228	Chieti	370.6	181.7	188.8	82	78	90	92
229	Isernia/Campobasso	331.6	162.2	169.4	88	84	93	95
230	Foggia	684.3	337.3	347.0	87	83	92	94
231	Bari	1461.9	717.3	744.6	88	84	93	95
232	Taranto	591.6	290.2	301.4	88	83	98	100
233	Brindisi	397.9	193.8	204.1	92	88	101	103***
234	Lecce	765.6	370.5	395.1	86	82	98	99
235	Potenza/Matera	615.8	304.8	311.0	85	81	93	95
236	Cosenza	742.5	367.6	374.9	86	82	91	93
237	Catanzaro	748.9	372.4	376.5	87	83	91	93
238	Reggio Calabria	584.9	288.3	296.6	91	87	91	93
239	Trapani	427.8	209.3	218.4	87	83	97	99
240	Palermo	1193.8	583.3	610.5	92	88	99	101*
241	Messina	683.9	331.5	352.4	80	77	94	96
242	Agrigento	482.9	238.5	244.4	83	79	95	97
243	Caltanisetta	294.7	144.8	149.9	92	88	102**	104***
244	Enna	197.7	96.8	101.0	89	85	102	104***
245	Catania	1002.0	493.0	509.0	92	88	103***	104***
246	Ragusa	286.7	139.5	147.3	84	80	106***	108***
247	Siracusa	396.4	196.3	200.1	86	82	98	100
248	Sassari	433.9	214.9	219.0	95	91	95	96
249	Nuoro	278.9	137.7	141.2	102	98	94	96
250	Cagliari/Oristano	881.3	437.3	444.0	96	92	94	96
IRELAND		3430.2	1722.9	1707.3	100	115***	100	122***
251	Eastern	1193.2	579.1	614.1	102*	115***	97	117***
252	Midland	200.7	104.1	96.6	100	115***	104***	127***
253	Mid-Western	306.4	156.4	150.0	104**	120***	107***	130***
254	North Eastern	287.3	147.2	140.1	102	117***	102*	124***
255	North Western	206.4	106.0	100.4	95	111***	98	120***
256	South Eastern	372.6	189.6	183.0	100	115***	103***	125***
257	Southern	523.6	265.1	258.5	103*	119***	103***	125***
258	Western	340.0	175.4	164.6	89	103*	94	116***

Table 7.1.1 cont

Area		Total population (thousands)			Total (all causes) mortality (SMRs)			
					Ages 5–64		All ages	
		Total	Males	Females	Own standard	EC standard	Own standard	EC standard
NETHERLANDS		14298.4	7084.8	7213.6	100	85	100	92
259	Groningen	559.2	277.8	281.4	104**	89	99	91
260	Friesland	592.4	294.8	297.6	99	85	99	91
261	Drenthe	424.1	212.3	211.8	101	86	99	91
262	Overijssel	1034.6	516.6	518.0	102*	87	101*	93
263	Gelderland	1722.3	854.5	867.8	101*	86	101**	93
264	Utrecht	918.5	449.9	468.7	96	82	99	90
265	Noord Holland	2310.6	1135.1	1175.6	100	86	100	92
266	Zuid Holland	3122.9	1534.1	1588.8	98	84	98	90
267	Zeeland	353.6	175.9	177.7	93	79	95	87
268	Noord Brabant	2087.3	1047.3	1039.9	99	84	103***	93
269	Limburg	1078.3	538.7	539.7	107***	91	107***	97
270	Zuidelijke Ijsselmeerpolders	94.4	47.9	46.6	85	72	86	76
UK:ENGLAND AND WALES		49652.1	24176.2	25475.8	100	104***	100	105***
271	Cleveland	567.5	278.5	289.0	123***	127***	114***	120***
272	Cumbria	482.3	234.2	248.1	108***	112***	105***	110***
273	Durham	608.7	297.6	311.1	117***	121***	111***	117***
274	Northumberland	299.8	146.3	153.5	107***	112***	111***	116***
275	Gateshead	211.9	103.0	108.9	127***	132***	114***	120***
276	Newcastle upon Tyne	283.1	136.5	146.6	120***	126***	108***	113***
277	Northern Tyneside	196.8	94.3	102.5	114***	120***	110***	116***
278	Southern Tyneside	160.6	78.2	82.4	125***	131***	113***	119***
279	Sunderland	298.5	144.9	153.6	120***	124***	113***	118***
280	Bradford	464.3	226.1	238.2	114***	119***	110***	116***
281	Calderdale	192.1	92.4	99.7	114***	118***	109***	114***
282	Humberside	855.7	417.4	438.3	104***	107***	103***	109***
283	Kirklees	377.3	182.8	194.5	113***	117***	112***	118***
284	Leeds	716.3	347.0	369.3	111***	116***	103***	109***
285	North Yorkshire	681.8	331.8	350.0	93	96	98	103***
286	Wakefield	312.9	153.6	159.3	114***	118***	114***	120***
287	Barnsley	225.1	110.9	114.2	111***	115***	107***	112***
288	Derbyshire	912.2	448.5	463.8	102*	106***	103***	109***
289	Doncaster	289.5	143.1	146.5	107***	111***	105***	111***
290	Leicestershire	860.6	424.8	435.8	94	97	96	101*
291	Lincolnshire	553.0	271.9	281.1	98	102	101*	106***
292	Nottinghamshire	994.0	488.4	505.6	103**	106***	103***	108***
293	Rotherham	252.7	124.2	128.5	109***	113***	106***	112***
294	Sheffield	545.2	264.5	280.7	106***	111***	103***	108***
295	Cambridgeshire	597.2	297.1	300.1	86	88	93	97
296	Norfolk	705.9	343.4	362.5	83	86	91	96
297	Suffolk	608.0	299.5	308.5	83	86	91	96
298	Barnet	295.5	140.7	154.8	80	83	90	94
299	Bedfordshire	511.0	255.3	255.7	90	92	96	101
300	Brent and Harrow	454.0	219.9	234.1	88	91	88	93
301	Ealing/Hammersmith/Hounslow	637.4	309.3	328.1	104***	107***	99	104***
302	Hertfordshire	970.0	475.8	494.2	84	87	93	97
303	Hillingdon	233.0	114.5	118.5	90	93	92	97
304	Kensington/Chelsea/Westminster	324.4	153.3	171.2	113***	116***	93	98
305	Barking and Havering	392.6	190.8	201.8	95	99	99	104***
306	Camden and Islington	342.7	164.6	178.2	114***	118***	98	103***
307	City and East London	548.2	268.2	280.0	120***	124***	106***	112***
308	Enfield and Haringey	468.3	225.6	242.7	94	97	96	101
309	Essex	1486.0	725.1	760.9	87	90	95	100
310	Redbridge and Waltham Forest	444.9	214.1	230.8	92	95	93	97
311	Bromley	298.5	143.7	154.8	81	85	90	95
312	East Sussex	670.3	308.3	362.1	89	93	91	96
313	Greenwich and Bexley	433.5	209.7	223.8	93	96	96	101
314	Kent	1485.3	721.2	764.1	91	94	97	102***
315	Lambeth/Southwark/Lewisham	700.5	335.6	364.8	112***	116***	102***	107***
316	Croydon	320.9	155.2	165.7	89	92	98	102***

Table 7.1.1 cont

Area		Total population (thousands)			Total (all causes) mortality (SMRs)			
					Ages 5–64		All ages	
		Total	Males	Females	Own standard	EC standard	Own standard	EC standard
317	Kingston and Richmond	295.3	140.8	154.5	86	89	90	95
318	Merton/Sutton/Wandsworth	596.8	284.6	312.2	97	100	97	102***
319	Surrey	1014.8	492.8	522.0	82	85	91	96
320	West Sussex	672.2	315.9	356.3	83	86	89	94
321	Dorset	604.6	286.0	318.7	86	90	87	92
322	Hampshire	1491.8	740.7	751.0	88	91	93	98
323	Isle of Wight	119.1	56.2	62.9	88	93	91	96
324	Wiltshire	529.1	260.8	268.3	89	91	94	99
325	Berkshire	700.8	350.4	350.4	86	88	95	100
326	Buckinghamshire	577.9	285.4	292.4	83	85	92	97
327	Northamptonshire	535.5	262.5	273.0	93	96	97	102**
328	Oxfordshire	546.8	275.0	271.8	84	86	90	94
329	Avon	932.5	451.9	480.6	88	92	93	98
330	Cornwall and Scilly Isles	430.4	205.9	224.5	92	97	96	101*
331	Devon	969.2	467.1	502.1	92	96	93	98
332	Gloucestershire	506.0	246.1	259.8	89	93	94	99
333	Somerset	433.2	210.6	222.6	87	90	94	99
334	Birmingham	1017.1	500.1	517.0	111***	116***	108***	114***
335	Coventry	317.9	157.8	160.1	107***	111***	103***	108***
336	Dudley	300.7	148.3	152.4	98	102	102*	107***
337	Hereford and Worcester	638.6	313.4	325.2	91	94	99	104***
338	Salop	381.6	188.9	192.7	94	97	100	105***
339	Sandwell	308.4	151.0	157.4	114***	119***	107***	113***
340	Solihull	199.3	97.8	101.5	82	85	90	94
341	Staffordshire	1018.2	502.7	515.5	108***	111***	107***	113***
342	Walsall	266.5	131.7	134.7	112***	116***	109***	115***
343	Warwickshire	477.2	235.5	241.6	96	100	102**	107***
344	Wolverhampton	255.9	126.7	129.2	109***	114***	104***	109***
345	Bolton	261.9	127.3	134.6	122***	126***	114***	120***
346	Bury	175.7	85.0	90.7	106**	110***	109***	115***
347	Lancashire	1382.6	665.9	716.6	112***	116***	109***	114***
348	Manchester	459.7	225.7	234.0	137***	143***	117***	123***
349	Oldham	220.9	107.4	113.5	116***	120***	114***	120***
350	Rochdale	207.6	101.2	106.4	121***	125***	111***	117***
351	Salford	245.8	119.7	126.1	132***	138***	117***	123***
352	Stockport	289.7	139.4	150.3	98	101	102*	107***
353	Tameside	217.2	105.0	112.1	118***	123***	111***	117***
354	Trafford	220.2	105.9	114.3	102	106***	100	106***
355	Wigan	309.1	150.7	158.5	120***	124***	115***	121***
356	Cheshire	933.2	456.0	477.2	104***	108***	105***	111***
357	Liverpool	509.8	244.8	264.9	130***	135***	114***	120***
358	St Helens and Knowsley	362.3	176.8	185.5	127***	132***	116***	122***
359	Sefton	299.9	142.5	157.4	108***	112***	103***	108***
360	Wirral	339.3	161.5	177.8	111***	115***	105***	111***
361	Clwyd	394.5	189.9	204.6	103**	107***	101	106***
362	Dyfed	334.2	161.9	172.3	104**	109***	105***	111***
363	Gwent	440.7	215.3	225.4	109***	114***	106***	112***
364	Gwynedd	231.8	111.3	120.5	102	106***	98	103***
365	Mid Glamorgan	538.6	261.9	276.7	118***	122***	113***	119***
366	Powys	110.5	55.0	55.5	96	100	102*	108***
367	South Glamorgan	391.4	189.6	201.8	101	105***	99	104***
368	West Glamorgan	368.6	178.4	190.2	111***	115***	106***	112***
UK:NORTHERN IRELAND								
369	Northern Ireland	1540.4	755.6	784.8	100	122***	100	119***
UK:SCOTLAND		5159.2	2486.7	2672.5	100	129***	100	119***
370	Highlands and Islands	269.1	132.9	136.3	102	132***	100	119***
371	Grampian	487.8	237.8	249.9	85	109***	93	110***
372	Tayside	396.5	189.4	207.1	87	113***	94	112***
373	Fife	342.2	166.3	175.9	92	119***	96	115***

Table 7.1.1 cont

Area		Total population (thousands)			Total (all causes) mortality (SMRs)			
					Ages 5–64		All ages	
		Total	Males	Females	Own standard	EC standard	Own standard	EC standard
374	Lothian	747.2	357.3	389.9	90	116***	94	112***
375	Borders	100.8	48.2	52.7	84	109***	93	111***
376	Forth Valley	272.7	132.6	140.1	96	124***	99	118***
377	Argyll and Clyde	453.1	218.7	234.4	109***	141***	106***	127***
378	Greater Glasgow	996.0	473.7	522.3	115***	149***	106***	126***
379	Lanarkshire	572.2	278.6	293.7	106***	136***	106***	127***
380	Ayrshire and Arran	376.5	180.9	195.5	104**	134***	106***	126***
381	Dumfries and Galloway	145.2	70.5	74.7	96	125***	97	116***
PORTUGAL		9995.3	4795.2	5200.1	100	113***	100	105***
382	Viana do Castelo	259.0	117.8	141.1	87	98	99	103***
383	Braga	725.2	350.7	374.5	84	97	99	107***
384	Vila Real	265.5	130.7	134.8	104**	117***	110***	116***
385	Braganca	185.3	92.3	93.0	90	101	102*	107***
386	Guarda	204.6	98.1	106.5	96	107***	96	100
387	Viseu	426.1	205.0	221.2	94	105***	102**	107***
388	Porto	1590.3	766.6	823.7	115***	132***	116***	125***
389	Aveiro	632.0	305.4	326.6	88	100	99	106***
390	Coimbra	439.3	207.8	231.6	132***	148***	118***	123***
391	Castelo Branco	279.5	112.1	167.4	86	95	38	38
392	Portalegre	142.1	69.0	73.1	80	88	94	97
393	Santarem	455.9	220.2	235.7	78	87	92	96
394	Leiria	424.6	207.3	217.2	89	100	100	105***
395	Lisboa	2086.3	994.8	1091.5	118***	134***	118***	125***
396	Setubal	678.2	333.9	344.3	62	70	78	83
397	Evora	180.0	87.7	92.3	74	82	95	98
398	Beja	187.2	93.2	94.1	84	93	95	99
399	Faro	326.8	160.8	165.9	89	99	96	100
400	Madeira	259.1	119.1	140.0	123***	141***	108***	114***
401	Azores	248.1	122.5	125.6	124***	141***	116***	123***
SPAIN		37698.1	18501.8	19196.3	100	87	100	89
402	La Coruña	1095.4	528.7	566.7	112***	98	102***	91
403	Lugo	404.9	199.3	205.6	95	82	99	89
404	Orense	429.8	210.0	219.8	86	74	90	81
405	Pontevedra	886.9	426.8	460.1	107***	93	104***	93
406	Asturias	1132.3	550.0	582.3	111***	96	102***	91
407	Cantabria	514.8	252.4	262.4	106***	93	99	89
408	Alava	260.1	130.8	129.3	102	89	100	89
409	Guipuzcoa	697.2	346.1	351.1	96	84	93	83
410	Vizcaya	1194.5	590.2	604.3	109***	95	104***	93
411	Navarra	510.7	254.3	256.4	102	89	101*	91
412	Rioja	255.2	127.4	127.8	90	78	99	89
413	Huesca	214.7	108.7	106.0	81	70	82	74
414	Teruel	152.8	77.0	75.8	87	75	89	80
415	Zaragoza	831.2	407.6	423.6	91	79	93	83
416	Madrid Centro	4721.0	2278.6	2442.4	94	82	92	82
417	Avila	182.6	92.4	90.2	85	74	83	75
418	Burgos	363.5	182.7	180.8	96	83	83	75
419	Leon	522.3	258.1	264.2	105***	91	100	90
420	Palencia	187.8	92.9	94.9	110***	96	99	89
421	Salamanca	363.8	178.1	185.7	87	76	85	76
422	Segovia	149.2	74.5	74.7	92	79	93	84
423	Soria	100.3	49.9	50.4	88	76	81	74
424	Valladolid	483.8	238.6	245.2	86	75	85	76
425	Zamora	226.8	111.7	115.1	88	76	89	80
426	Albacete	339.5	168.8	170.7	93	81	105***	94
427	Ciudad Real	473.9	231.2	242.7	100	87	106***	95
428	Cuenca	214.8	106.9	107.9	95	82	97	88
429	Guadalajara	143.0	72.7	70.3	85	73	80	72
430	Toledo	474.7	235.5	239.2	89	77	98	87

Table 7.1.1 cont

Area		Total population (thousands)			Total (all causes) mortality (SMRs)			
					Ages 5–64		All ages	
		Total	Males	Females	Own standard	EC standard	Own standard	EC standard
431	Badajoz	641.5	315.9	325.6	109***	95	108***	97
432	Caceres	420.0	207.6	212.4	100	87	100	90
433	Barcelona	4648.7	2271.4	2377.3	90	78	91	81
434	Gerona	469.0	232.0	237.0	99	86	104***	93
435	Lerida	353.4	176.8	176.6	89	77	93	83
436	Tarragona	516.1	255.8	260.3	96	84	101	90
437	Alicante	1157.8	568.8	589.0	101	88	108***	97
438	Castellon de la Plana	433.6	213.5	220.1	88	77	101	90
439	Valencia	2075.9	1015.4	1060.5	109***	95	113***	101***
440	Baleares	660.8	325.9	334.9	107***	93	103***	92
441	Almeria	411.8	203.4	208.4	100	87	107***	95
442	Cadiz	992.3	493.5	498.8	118***	103**	117***	104***
443	Cordoba	720.4	351.9	368.5	94	82	102***	91
444	Granada	759.3	372.8	386.5	100	87	106***	95
445	Huelva	419.1	206.5	212.6	108***	94	111***	99
446	Jaen	639.0	314.7	324.3	89	77	99	89
447	Malaga	1032.0	508.6	523.4	118***	103**	116***	103***
448	Sevilla	1483.5	727.4	756.1	111***	97	114***	101**
449	Murcia	960.1	471.6	488.5	103**	90	109***	97
450	Las Palmas	714.6	359.9	354.7	130***	114***	118***	105***
451	Sta Cruz de Tenerife	661.7	326.5	335.2	112***	98	107***	95

Table 7.1.2. Observed numbers of 'avoidable deaths' by small area and country

Notes on the use of this table

1. This table shows observed numbers of deaths (5-year totals) for each disease group. Asthma data for Greece and Portugal are not available.

2. The mortality data presented here are the totals for each small area.

3. All countries supplied data classified according to the 9th revision of the International Classification of Diseases except for Denmark where 8th revision coding rules still apply.

4. Key for the abbreviations used for columns of the table:
   TUB   — tuberculosis (ICD8 010–019; ICD9 010–018,137), ages 5–64;
   CERV   — malignant neoplasm of the cervix uteri (ICD8 180; ICD9 180), ages 15–64;
   UTER   — malignant neoplasm of the cervix and body of the uterus (ICD8 180, 182; ICD9 179,180, 182), ages 15–54;
   HODG   — Hodgkin's disease (ICD8 201; ICD9 201), ages 5–64;
   CRHD   — chronic rheumatic heart disease (ICD8 393–398; ICD9 393–398), ages 5–44;
   RESP   — all respiratory diseases (ICD8 460–519; ICD9 460–519), ages 1–14;
   ASTH   — asthma (ICD8 493; ICD9 493), ages 5–44;
   APP   — appendicitis (ICD8 540–543; ICD9 540–543), ages 5–64;
   HERN   — abdominal hernia (ICD8 550–553; ICD9 550–553), ages 5–64;
   CHOLY— cholelithiasis and cholecystitis (ICD8 574–575; ICD9 574–575.1, 576.1)), ages 5–64;
   HYP/S — hypertensive and cerebrovascular diseases (ICD8 400–404, 430–438; ICD9 401–405, 430–438),ages 35–64;
   MAT   — maternal deaths (ICD8 630–678; ICD9 630–676), all ages;
   PER   — perinatal mortality (all causes), aged under 1 week plus stillbirths.

5. The small area numbers are as in the key maps

6. The data are for 1980–84 (except for Greece, 1980–82; Italy, 1979–83; and Spain, 1979–83).

Table 7.1.2

Area

Observed number of deaths

Area		TUB	CERV	UTER	HODG	CRHD	RESP	ASTH	APP	HERN	CHOLY	HYP/S	MAT	PER
BELGIUM		331	524	471	428	11	159	261	29	41	139	6385	44	7713
1	Antwerpen	19	92	68	92	1	21	35	2	3	16	1016	9	1271
2	Brabant	116	97	114	71	3	39	54	9	12	33	1381	11	1644
3	West-Vlaanderen	23	57	46	44	1	13	34	1	4	16	512	3	919
4	Oost-Vlaanderen	18	78	61	81	1	29	23	8	5	9	748	3	1014
5	Hainaut	74	101	62	51	3	17	52	3	10	28	1065	3	928
6	Liège	40	37	56	37	2	21	31	2	3	15	774	5	686
7	Limburg	16	33	34	30	0	10	10	1	1	8	370	6	720
8	Luxembourg (province)	3	9	9	9	0	2	2	0	1	8	172	2	194
9	Namur	22	20	21	13	0	7	20	3	2	6	347	2	337
LUXEMBOURG														
10	Luxembourg	5	19	23	10	5	4	8	4	2	7	322	0	236
FEDERAL REPUBLIC OF GERMANY		2828	4980	3763	2617	314	829	1886	465	398	1080	43928	487	30320
11	Schleswig–Holstein	89	228	169	106	3	27	84	21	15	45	1516	15	1137
12	Hamburg	65	152	115	41	10	21	50	14	8	24	1123	9	577
13	Braunschweig	68	132	99	106	4	23	55	19	11	32	1225	9	773
14	Hannover	91	208	153	151	9	33	72	19	12	47	1472	6	859
15	Luneburg	52	103	75	73	1	20	52	16	12	26	945	3	646
16	Weser–Ems	67	182	143	99	8	36	60	21	11	29	1336	16	1276
17	Bremen	26	68	53	19	2	6	28	7	4	12	568	1	267
18	Düsseldorf	227	504	343	195	23	60	166	29	23	63	3840	51	2792
19	Köln	187	340	244	159	21	31	125	18	16	54	2741	36	1871
20	Münster	86	175	138	78	18	26	72	18	12	44	1816	26	1619
21	Detmold	68	129	95	68	10	35	58	11	6	30	1204	13	949
22	Arnsberg	169	304	232	138	23	65	114	37	28	72	3064	37	2078
23	Darmstadt	150	233	178	159	35	34	130	23	39	65	2353	32	1474
24	Giessen	44	51	45	38	9	13	35	11	13	17	658	8	461

Table 7.1.2

Area		Observed number of deaths												
		TUB	CERV	UTER	HODG	CRHD	RESP	ASTH	APP	HERN	CHOLY	HYP/S	MAT	PER
25	Kassel	38	81	67	46	11	17	46	14	6	30	823	8	559
26	Koblenz	53	90	63	87	7	16	42	11	12	14	1220	10	669
27	Trier	21	46	39	27	2	5	11	1	5	5	420	4	232
28	Rheinhessen–Pfalz	71	154	116	91	18	25	72	18	9	26	1618	22	940
29	Stuttgart	131	227	180	136	29	41	90	19	25	56	2056	26	1624
30	Karlsruhe	152	179	123	76	22	33	57	19	14	48	1757	17	1098
31	Freiburg	105	114	110	58	9	25	53	10	15	39	1090	13	732
32	Tübingen	57	79	62	50	7	33	36	7	9	18	883	9	730
33	Oberbayern	150	248	185	139	3	62	92	17	12	36	2092	18	1550
34	Niederbayern	64	90	80	41	0	13	25	11	12	27	771	15	535
35	Oberpfalz	81	86	74	55	1	17	24	10	12	23	806	13	573
36	Oberfranken	128	94	66	55	3	13	31	10	14	35	929	9	499
37	Mittelfranken	114	121	106	91	1	14	49	12	15	36	1081	12	723
38	Unterfranken	60	81	56	42	1	16	35	7	6	38	709	10	676
39	Schwaben	44	106	86	74	3	23	35	16	7	14	1006	22	812
40	Saarland	60	84	59	45	13	21	36	5	6	24	1078	5	581
41	Berlin (West)	110	291	209	74	8	25	51	14	9	51	1728	12	1008
DENMARK		97	753	462	165	25	62	62	31	27	52	2991	15	2357
42	Kobenhavn and Frederiksberg (M)	26	120	64	21	3	2	9	3	3	6	477	2	222
43	Kobenhavns County	13	75	42	29	3	7	5	3	2	6	370	2	193
44	Frederiksborg County	5	29	21	10	2	1	3	2	1	3	158	2	131
45	Roskilde County	2	27	19	11	1	3	1	1	0	0	95	0	85
46	Vestsjaellands County	5	38	24	15	2	3	0	1	1	2	151	2	138
47	Storstroms County	3	34	25	7	2	9	1	3	2	3	164	0	92
48	Bornholms County	1	8	4	1	0	0	0	0	0	0	24	0	27
49	Fyns County	9	74	47	10	1	6	8	3	3	9	235	0	189
50	Sonderjyllands County	2	35	23	6	1	7	5	3	4	2	138	0	140
51	Ribe County	6	33	19	5	4	3	4	0	1	2	116	0	107
52	Vejle County	5	56	31	10	0	5	7	3	3	4	195	0	139
53	Ringkobing County	1	29	17	7	0	4	3	2	1	6	165	1	157
54	Arhus County	8	82	56	14	3	5	7	3	3	4	283	1	342
55	Viborg County	3	41	18	5	0	0	3	1	2	2	145	1	131
56	Nordjyllands County	8	72	52	14	3	7	6	3	1	3	275	4	264
FRANCE		2732	2352	2882	1487	263	683	581	353	558	152	31290	545	46876
57	Ain	11	14	14	7	2	2	3	6	8	1	204	6	330
58	Aisne	32	20	28	11	2	9	7	7	6	3	354	8	531
59	Allier	13	13	27	12	0	6	2	4	4	1	265	3	270
60	Alpes-de-Haute-Provence	5	5	3	2	1	1	0	1	0	0	70	1	95
61	Hautes-Alpes	8	1	1	1	0	0	5	1	1	1	55	1	92
62	Alpes-Maritimes	45	36	46	29	4	7	12	4	5	1	418	5	642
63	Ardèche	17	11	14	10	1	3	0	2	5	2	174	3	225
64	Ardennes	19	17	23	7	1	8	4	0	8	2	189	3	319
65	Ariège	7	9	6	4	0	1	4	1	0	0	70	0	101
66	Aube	19	22	23	5	0	1	1	3	4	3	168	3	241
67	Aude	9	7	7	11	0	4	2	0	4	0	150	2	166
68	Aveyron	11	8	8	8	1	5	4	0	6	1	150	3	192
69	Bouches-du-Rhône	90	65	85	60	12	14	12	9	14	5	957	23	1476
70	Calvados	33	31	33	21	2	6	8	4	8	1	348	4	484
71	Cantal	10	8	7	6	1	3	1	3	2	0	133	1	147
72	Charente	12	24	30	11	1	5	2	2	4	1	179	4	285
73	Charente-Maritime	19	22	30	11	2	4	3	2	2	1	275	2	347
74	Cher	18	16	17	7	2	4	4	4	5	2	194	2	225
75	Corrèze	12	6	14	6	0	2	3	3	5	0	170	0	142
76	Corse	12	5	10	5	1	2	2	0	1	0	149	1	203
77	Côte-d'Or	11	35	27	15	3	6	6	3	5	1	224	6	456
78	Côtes-du-Nord	26	21	29	9	3	6	3	2	9	1	468	3	318
79	Creuse	5	2	10	9	1	0	0	2	2	1	138	1	362
80	Dordogne	24	18	26	7	0	6	5	5	6	0	297	3	73
81	Doubs	17	22	23	6	5	8	1	2	3	0	242	4	233
82	Drôme	15	25	22	11	3	5	3	6	4	1	183	1	495
83	Eure	19	26	32	10	2	5	8	2	4	2	252	4	355
84	Eure-et-Loir	12	16	27	8	0	7	1	2	0	0	174	2	307
85	Finistère	48	27	36	16	3	1	9	3	9	3	663	8	586
86	Gard	26	12	17	16	3	1	3	9	6	2	267	7	479
87	Haute-Garonne	32	32	59	16	2	10	11	1	4	4	365	7	587
88	Gers	3	7	12	4	0	5	2	0	1	0	99	1	103

Table 7.1.2 cont

Area   Observed number of deaths

		TUB	CERV	UTER	HODG	CRHD	RESP	ASTH	APP	HERN	CHOLY	HYP/S	MAT	PER
89	Gironde	52	44	63	30	4	11	16	8	8	3	628	7	836
90	Hérault	23	20	29	20	5	7	8	4	11	4	381	8	607
91	Ille-et-Vilaine	42	33	30	13	1	6	9	5	7	3	505	6	621
92	Indre	8	9	9	8	1	1	6	2	7	1	161	0	169
93	Indre-et-Loire	15	24	22	17	2	6	6	5	5	2	187	3	336
94	Isère	46	52	41	21	3	11	4	7	6	7	416	7	744
95	Jura	7	11	10	10	4	2	4	1	0	0	159	2	207
96	Landes	7	10	6	5	1	3	1	0	0	1	181	0	203
97	Loir-et-Cher	11	20	21	8	1	4	5	0	2	1	196	1	168
98	Loire	39	31	35	16	4	7	9	7	11	3	408	5	575
99	Haute-Loire	7	2	6	11	2	0	1	2	4	1	143	2	152
100	Loire-Atlantique	68	34	41	21	1	19	12	8	11	0	595	6	842
101	Loiret	10	26	26	15	2	8	5	1	3	1	251	1	466
102	Lot	4	8	11	1	0	1	0	0	2	0	110	0	96
103	Lot-et-Garonne	11	12	16	10	1	1	2	3	0	0	187	2	217
104	Lozère	6	2	3	2	0	1	2	1	1	0	52	1	67
105	Maine-et-Loire	34	21	27	25	1	10	8	4	5	2	317	3	642
106	Manche	16	15	19	13	6	3	3	0	4	2	303	3	358
107	Marne	20	23	23	16	4	9	4	6	5	0	262	8	489
108	Haute-Marne	11	5	11	12	1	4	1	2	1	0	115	7	214
109	Mayenne	13	8	8	8	1	4	2	5	4	1	159	1	221
110	Meurthe-et-Moselle	52	48	41	16	2	8	8	1	10	1	435	6	625
111	Meuse	4	7	9	7	2	1	1	4	4	0	142	5	223
112	Morbihan	63	16	16	15	4	10	7	3	4	1	552	4	490
113	Moselle	54	55	58	28	7	15	14	9	11	2	715	27	1008
114	Nièvre	16	8	14	5	0	2	2	4	5	0	175	2	171
115	Nord	207	131	149	84	14	43	42	33	41	14	1883	26	3040
116	Oise	28	36	40	14	4	7	8	3	8	1	338	4	620
117	Orne	10	12	16	12	0	3	0	2	1	1	181	2	188
118	Pas-de-Calais	116	74	79	51	11	20	30	11	27	5	1144	17	1781
119	Puy-de-Dôme	30	15	23	24	4	4	7	3	5	1	381	4	551
120	Pyrénées-Atlantiques	30	13	26	12	1	2	9	0	5	0	296	7	367
121	Hautes-Pyrénées	7	8	12	7	0	4	2	1	4	0	157	1	170
122	Pyrénées-Orientales	13	9	19	5	1	5	2	3	2	1	194	9	253
123	Bas-Rhin	56	65	60	26	6	15	6	0	11	5	591	4	606
124	Haut-Rhin	30	30	40	18	5	17	7	6	6	0	436	9	578
125	Rhône	51	64	60	32	10	25	8	5	16	4	648	17	1258
126	Haute-Saône	12	11	3	6	2	4	2	4	2	0	160	4	196
127	Saône-et-Loire	20	28	27	18	1	7	3	7	4	3	351	6	476
128	Sarthe	12	22	21	12	1	3	9	6	4	2	210	7	387
129	Savoie	20	18	16	7	3	2	2	1	6	1	180	1	207
130	Haute-Savoie	25	30	25	16	4	6	4	3	8	2	236	4	388
131	Paris	154	116	155	60	13	17	22	9	23	3	1124	30	2011
132	Seine-Maritime	107	76	91	53	9	25	14	4	14	1	691	9	1215
133	Seine-et-Marne	38	28	52	19	5	23	9	7	7	3	370	10	765
134	Yvelines	38	48	69	29	3	20	16	7	7	3	484	22	1033
135	Deux-Sévres	9	3	10	3	1	1	3	5	5	3	174	4	283
136	Somme	31	19	32	25	3	8	4	3	4	3	309	7	520
137	Tarn	5	9	13	8	1	4	5	1	4	1	185	2	229
138	Tarn-et-Garonne	6	11	10	4	0	1	1	0	0	0	116	0	151
139	Var	39	32	40	12	5	7	10	2	6	6	412	4	598
140	Vaucluse	11	12	17	11	4	2	5	2	2	2	222	3	398
141	Vendée	15	14	20	12	1	10	3	3	4	1	290	0	374
142	Vienne	15	14	22	11	0	0	5	2	3	1	173	2	283
143	Haute-Vienne	12	13	20	7	0	5	5	0	2	0	224	3	176
144	Vosges	16	13	21	9	1	6	1	3	6	0	274	10	342
145	Yonne	11	18	18	10	1	5	6	3	4	1	202	2	227
146	Territoire-de-Belfort	4	7	11	3	1	0	2	1	2	1	79	1	111
147	Essonne	35	39	39	20	8	20	12	6	6	1	436	15	777
148	Hauts-de-Seine	74	56	76	43	6	17	9	7	4	2	718	17	1287
149	Seine-Saint-Denis	74	48	80	33	4	21	17	6	14	2	680	18	1500
150	Val-de-Marne	49	55	76	28	5	15	9	7	8	1	571	16	1023
151	Val-d'Oise	43	28	53	29	7	8	11	2	7	1	391	9	893
GREECE		367	165	323	214	51	157	-	14	19	40	4558	58	12251
152	Greater Athens	120	79	112	68	7	35	-	4	8	12	1458	11	4373
153	Rest of Central Greece and Eubea	34	14	23	27	4	19	-	1	2	6	543	9	1120
154	Peloponnisos	33	13	28	17	4	12	-	1	1	3	465	3	1241

Table 7.1.2 cont

Area		TUB	CERV	UTER	HODG	CRHD	RESP	ASTH	APP	HERN	CHOLY	HYP/S	MAT	PER
155	Ionian Islands	3	3	4	3	1	1	-	2	1	0	99	1	157
156	Epirus	11	3	4	7	0	8	-	0	0	1	133	4	409
157	Thessaly	30	7	28	13	1	11	-	2	2	6	350	0	763
158	Macedonia	81	28	74	43	18	28	-	3	4	7	908	10	2742
159	Thrace	31	3	7	13	5	25	-	0	0	0	196	11	478
160	Aegean Islands	17	7	20	11	4	8	-	0	1	2	193	6	428
161	Crete	7	8	23	12	7	10	-	1	0	3	213	3	540
ITALY		3132	1161	3588	2845	1515	1416	245	324	558	1476	50342	355	49514
162	Torino	156	84	164	131	62	42	13	20	36	101	2202	14	1776
163	Vercelli	19	17	29	30	11	3	0	2	1	12	515	1	277
164	Novara	36	10	36	33	11	10	4	0	6	10	574	2	285
165	Cuneo	41	20	36	27	13	5	5	5	15	18	577	3	362
166	Asti	11	4	13	9	7	7	1	1	1	7	236	3	115
167	Alessandria	26	10	29	22	11	3	3	6	7	16	489	1	237
168	Aosta	14	1	9	5	2	3	0	1	1	3	97	0	70
169	Imperia	18	14	27	20	5	1	1	6	2	7	196	0	91
170	Savona	19	8	14	17	4	6	0	1	2	6	289	0	140
171	Genova	73	30	58	74	18	10	8	6	14	48	983	4	438
172	La Spezia	10	7	17	16	4	1	0	0	4	7	226	1	104
173	Varese	32	13	30	50	21	16	7	2	5	24	718	3	566
174	Como/Sondrio	61	19	48	42	20	20	7	1	5	27	914	1	587
175	Milano	193	69	217	229	97	67	12	20	34	79	3722	13	2354
176	Bergamo	89	8	58	54	23	16	5	4	7	22	924	4	696
177	Brescia	116	23	42	64	25	18	5	7	3	18	1067	3	679
178	Pavia	32	11	41	47	6	6	2	3	5	12	700	2	245
179	Cremona	27	12	18	14	8	2	2	3	3	9	445	2	190
180	Mantova	20	4	19	27	3	6	2	1	4	5	455	1	189
181	Bolzano	34	10	21	15	5	8	2	4	2	12	303	5	330
182	Trento	52	17	25	16	14	5	2	0	4	17	345	1	282
183	Verona	41	16	38	38	8	7	2	4	1	22	781	5	571
184	Vicenza	38	17	30	33	12	14	1	5	6	23	702	4	450
185	Belluno	31	5	15	11	3	3	1	1	1	6	260	2	114
186	Treviso	37	19	33	43	10	7	3	0	7	16	545	2	420
187	Venezia	44	31	42	54	8	7	6	4	5	17	631	0	505
188	Padova	50	14	31	52	12	26	4	2	7	12	646	3	536
189	Rovigo	11	9	10	12	3	1	1	1	5	8	242	2	139
190	Udine/Gorizia	54	31	39	27	10	5	3	3	7	21	680	2	348
191	Trieste	28	9	18	20	7	2	2	3	1	12	243	1	67
192	Pordenone	12	10	12	10	6	0	0	1	2	7	214	1	146
193	Piacenza	13	7	13	15	7	1	0	2	0	10	311	1	128
194	Parma	26	7	24	22	4	5	3	3	4	14	392	2	228
195	Reggio Emilia	13	8	19	37	3	3	0	1	0	8	352	0	228
196	Modena	25	10	30	40	8	5	1	1	5	16	490	2	324
197	Bologna	50	20	50	43	18	10	3	6	8	29	848	5	399
198	Ferrara	15	10	17	16	3	6	0	1	2	8	356	2	173
199	Ravenna	7	5	24	10	3	2	1	1	2	8	262	0	164
200	Forli	24	13	26	30	4	7	0	0	3	8	406	5	325
201	Pesaro	8	2	13	8	4	10	1	3	2	10	256	3	206
202	Ancona	17	12	20	15	5	9	1	1	4	9	355	1	252
203	Macerata	15	2	17	13	3	3	1	2	1	9	245	2	210
204	Ascoli Piceno	21	5	22	17	5	3	0	1	3	8	298	1	270
205	Massa-Carrara	22	6	18	12	6	2	1	3	2	6	197	1	133
206	Lucca	32	7	22	19	2	3	4	4	3	7	327	1	221
207	Pistoia	16	4	13	15	8	3	3	1	2	5	181	0	134
208	Firenze	45	22	67	69	19	16	1	2	7	27	893	2	660
209	Livorno	13	4	15	14	4	5	1	8	3	12	293	3	200
210	Pisa	9	12	21	23	5	5	3	1	1	16	254	3	224
211	Arezzo	20	9	21	12	8	3	0	2	1	10	257	1	197
212	Siena	15	3	19	12	4	5	2	5	6	8	227	0	150
213	Grosseto	10	7	11	5	5	0	1	0	1	6	218	4	120
214	Perugia	25	6	20	46	15	9	1	0	8	12	533	2	313
215	Terni	8	10	16	10	11	4	1	0	2	4	196	0	171
216	Viterbo/Rieti	24	5	26	25	11	12	2	2	6	15	408	3	326
217	Roma	210	109	273	202	96	75	16	21	39	92	2752	20	2767
218	Latina	20	8	40	23	19	11	1	1	3	13	346	2	465
219	Frosinone	20	9	34	20	19	2	1	1	4	9	470	4	482
220	Caserta	21	3	45	23	43	33	4	5	21	17	881	11	1208

Table 7.1.2 cont

Area   Observed number of deaths

		TUB	CERV	UTER	HODG	CRHD	RESP	ASTH	APP	HERN	CHOLY	HYP/S	MAT	PER
221	Benevento	19	4	17	13	9	6	1	0	2	4	281	6	332
222	Napoli	174	41	254	133	137	182	20	25	52	87	2873	27	4744
223	Avellino	12	2	25	13	16	20	2	1	1	12	363	2	457
224	Salerno	61	9	63	47	56	38	4	11	7	23	922	14	1352
225	L'Aquila	28	10	22	8	12	6	2	1	3	8	289	2	271
226	Teramo	20	1	19	12	4	4	1	1	2	7	223	2	217
227	Pescara	13	5	18	9	11	8	2	3	2	6	240	4	230
228	Chieti	22	6	19	18	10	6	1	4	1	15	287	1	344
229	Isernia/Campobasso	20	6	14	17	18	9	1	1	4	11	336	3	312
230	Foggia	39	15	44	23	21	36	0	1	8	7	510	5	957
231	Bari	80	31	118	51	65	54	7	12	10	28	1032	6	1981
232	Taranto	21	5	40	24	19	25	1	5	8	14	382	11	797
233	Brindisi	21	7	39	20	23	20	0	5	2	6	313	3	580
234	Lecce	45	15	50	39	25	29	4	3	9	14	557	5	987
235	Potenza/Matera	34	11	38	21	21	25	3	5	7	14	545	3	711
236	Cosenza	30	13	64	18	28	32	2	3	9	27	671	5	944
237	Catanzaro	34	9	42	32	40	33	4	7	4	13	532	10	1000
238	Reggio Calabria	29	10	33	27	16	17	2	2	5	9	455	1	854
239	Trapani	18	8	56	20	13	11	7	0	4	8	438	3	433
240	Palermo	32	15	108	58	33	69	4	9	14	20	1082	13	1638
241	Messina	19	5	59	29	20	29	1	6	9	21	571	7	821
242	Agrigento	14	5	37	24	20	23	2	2	8	6	385	2	567
243	Caltanisetta	12	1	21	9	8	8	3	3	4	5	247	4	452
244	Enna	9	3	18	9	8	7	2	1	4	5	211	3	245
245	Catania	33	17	96	48	30	53	1	10	7	35	955	16	1545
246	Ragusa	14	7	31	12	13	14	2	2	2	8	263	10	331
247	Siracusa	14	3	30	14	12	8	0	0	6	8	332	5	512
248	Sassari	33	4	11	21	9	16	0	0	5	10	323	4	445
249	Nuoro	13	1	6	14	7	11	3	2	3	8	205	4	300
250	Cagliari/Oristano	50	15	41	24	20	38	6	4	10	37	594	7	1168
IRELAND		232	167	114	149	24	130	95	17	14	39	2406	24	4857
251	Eastern	64	47	33	39	8	33	39	5	1	11	789	5	1768
252	Midland	15	12	7	11	1	8	4	0	1	2	131	3	247
253	Mid-Western	37	12	12	10	4	14	4	4	2	1	245	2	428
254	North Eastern	13	16	12	12	1	17	8	2	3	5	221	3	444
255	North Western	6	9	8	15	0	7	4	2	1	3	167	1	287
256	South Eastern	28	24	12	24	2	15	11	1	2	5	264	4	579
257	Southern	36	35	19	27	5	22	13	1	1	9	375	2	727
258	Western	33	12	11	11	3	14	12	2	3	3	214	4	377
NETHERLANDS		188	780	538	428	75	177	151	67	78	220	6509	67	9159
259	Groningen	6	26	10	18	1	5	2	4	1	3	258	1	336
260	Friesland	6	34	24	15	3	7	9	3	4	6	264	4	415
261	Drenthe	9	24	21	8	4	4	0	1	1	8	193	3	262
262	Overijssel	23	43	35	38	8	13	7	7	8	15	493	6	708
263	Gelderland	16	84	61	52	12	21	18	7	7	23	797	3	1120
264	Utrecht	18	42	33	25	3	10	9	1	5	7	419	5	617
265	Noord Holland	24	149	85	81	10	18	31	9	15	46	946	13	1397
266	Zuid Holland	33	190	130	96	14	44	37	12	16	49	1441	18	1967
267	Zeeland	3	29	15	12	2	5	1	4	1	4	146	0	245
268	Noord Brabant	24	102	81	49	13	36	20	10	16	41	961	11	1355
269	Limburg	26	56	43	32	5	13	16	8	4	18	565	3	663
270	Zuidelijke Ijsselmeerpolders	0	1	0	2	0	1	1	1	0	0	26	0	74
UK:ENGLAND AND WALES		1417	5333	3455	1657	391	1275	1312	201	420	498	40556	271	36429
271	Cleveland	21	77	47	33	7	17	16	6	5	8	572	4	554
272	Cumbria	7	61	27	22	2	13	12	0	1	2	514	5	366
273	Durham	28	78	47	20	5	20	28	4	4	5	655	5	471
274	Northumberland	9	36	17	12	3	7	6	0	2	3	280	0	186
275	Gateshead	10	25	12	5	0	4	11	1	1	2	265	1	171
276	Newcastle upon Tyne	12	36	17	9	0	4	6	2	2	4	282	1	212
277	Northern Tyneside	6	33	17	7	0	6	1	1	2	3	190	1	129
278	Southern Tyneside	6	23	10	5	1	1	4	0	3	1	192	1	124
279	Sunderland	15	36	23	8	4	7	7	5	1	8	309	2	266
280	Bradford	28	62	29	15	6	20	13	1	1	2	487	3	519
281	Calderdale	13	30	19	10	3	3	2	1	2	1	206	3	181
282	Humberside	24	116	65	38	5	29	17	3	9	8	730	5	685

Table 7.1.2 cont

Area   Observed number of deaths

		TUB	CERV	UTER	HODG	CRHD	RESP	ASTH	APP	HERN	CHOLY	HYP/S	MAT	PER
283	Kirklees	9	53	31	16	3	9	10	4	4	3	358	3	365
284	Leeds	19	99	68	30	9	15	14	2	5	8	624	4	536
285	North Yorkshire	12	60	46	24	4	13	11	2	4	2	542	3	473
286	Wakefield	5	43	32	16	4	15	8	0	1	3	257	3	283
287	Barnsley	0	32	24	5	2	5	7	0	2	3	185	1	148
288	Derbyshire	17	91	67	33	10	25	18	3	8	5	840	7	672
289	Doncaster	8	54	30	10	5	4	7	1	4	2	270	4	217
290	Leicestershire	25	90	64	39	4	27	21	5	5	7	649	6	634
291	Lincolnshire	11	62	39	22	2	16	14	2	4	4	454	3	363
292	Nottinghamshire	32	114	75	25	14	25	30	6	8	11	885	1	668
293	Rotherham	3	31	23	4	2	6	7	1	1	3	233	2	248
294	Sheffield	10	50	34	15	9	9	10	0	6	5	510	2	344
295	Cambridgeshire	10	37	27	16	4	7	15	1	7	5	353	3	399
296	Norfolk	16	68	41	11	6	23	19	2	7	7	444	6	427
297	Suffolk	10	58	31	23	4	16	26	3	10	4	365	5	367
298	Barnet	4	15	12	11	0	3	8	1	2	3	161	1	176
299	Bedfordshire	8	58	30	18	4	14	18	1	3	6	344	5	420
300	Brent and Harrow	19	35	23	17	2	9	20	2	1	3	281	1	330
301	Ealing/Hammersmith/Hounslow	40	57	36	15	8	22	22	1	9	1	462	2	454
302	Hertfordshire	20	53	41	31	2	22	26	0	11	8	619	3	529
303	Hillingdon	1	24	18	7	3	4	3	1	2	2	135	2	161
304	Kensington/Chelsea/Westminster	30	36	26	16	5	5	7	2	5	3	281	2	193
305	Barking and Havering	11	44	29	21	0	15	13	2	1	3	283	3	271
306	Camden and Islington	19	34	15	11	2	4	11	3	6	4	265	1	239
307	City and East London	46	61	43	13	6	25	27	1	4	9	502	5	662
308	Enfield and Haringey	15	52	32	10	12	14	12	1	2	8	313	4	335
309	Essex	33	119	71	50	4	29	30	8	8	18	899	5	984
310	Redbridge and Waltham Forest	12	38	22	8	3	14	14	1	2	2	322	3	339
311	Bromley	6	15	14	13	2	5	12	1	0	1	213	0	135
312	East Sussex	12	80	53	21	4	14	17	0	4	6	474	4	338
313	Greenwich and Bexley	12	26	22	15	4	11	15	3	3	7	296	2	323
314	Kent	31	151	101	47	11	37	27	7	8	19	1035	4	1068
315	Lambeth/Southwark/Lewisham	51	63	42	24	6	15	16	8	11	6	653	6	632
316	Croydon	8	28	22	6	1	6	6	2	1	4	238	0	208
317	Kingston and Richmond	4	21	15	13	2	5	10	3	1	2	201	1	151
318	Merton/Sutton/Wandsworth	22	58	39	17	4	14	21	1	3	4	438	1	406
319	Surrey	22	84	54	34	6	26	27	4	9	5	607	6	580
320	West Sussex	13	46	31	20	2	12	14	2	2	4	416	3	391
321	Dorset	14	50	33	16	4	17	19	3	9	6	394	2	272
322	Hampshire	27	138	93	45	9	53	39	1	10	6	864	5	960
323	Isle of Wight	3	8	6	2	0	2	5	2	0	0	90	0	69
324	Wiltshire	5	48	21	22	2	16	10	3	5	3	333	3	345
325	Berkshire	18	40	32	21	3	11	11	2	3	3	404	2	448
326	Buckinghamshire	8	29	16	17	2	19	14	2	2	5	336	3	439
327	Northamptonshire	11	38	25	16	2	11	14	3	1	4	396	3	433
328	Oxfordshire	4	31	27	14	2	13	15	1	4	4	294	1	262
329	Avon	15	65	41	29	5	14	25	5	8	12	622	4	624
330	Cornwall and Scilly Isles	8	49	34	8	2	10	9	0	4	9	322	3	259
331	Devon	19	101	71	23	1	23	27	4	12	5	686	7	535
332	Gloucestershire	10	57	36	12	3	19	14	3	6	6	415	0	314
333	Somerset	13	40	29	14	2	7	14	1	6	2	338	1	261
334	Birmingham	50	96	66	38	13	29	39	3	11	15	1058	5	1027
335	Coventry	17	39	24	19	1	13	8	1	1	5	316	2	319
336	Dudley	9	34	25	14	5	6	3	3	1	5	293	0	201
337	Hereford and Worcester	13	70	54	18	7	13	14	4	7	3	511	6	460
338	Salop	3	42	31	11	1	7	11	1	6	2	330	5	345
339	Sandwell	14	39	26	13	1	16	6	2	4	2	383	4	352
340	Solihull	1	14	14	7	0	4	9	1	3	0	123	1	136
341	Staffordshire	23	131	91	48	11	34	32	3	10	21	895	4	907
342	Walsall	14	32	25	7	2	12	6	2	8	3	270	1	260
343	Warwickshire	14	53	36	19	3	16	22	0	6	5	382	1	335
344	Wolverhampton	11	39	21	13	5	9	11	3	2	7	250	4	259
345	Bolton	13	41	23	7	6	13	7	1	0	5	252	3	218
346	Bury	4	19	9	4	0	5	3	1	4	2	147	0	149
347	Lancashire	33	190	113	33	14	34	36	7	29	15	1340	8	1139
348	Manchester	35	85	48	14	8	10	11	3	5	6	525	5	451
349	Oldham	6	30	19	8	4	8	5	0	2	3	258	3	211
350	Rochdale	4	39	18	7	1	6	5	0	2	6	200	2	226

Table 7.1.2 cont

Area | Observed number of deaths

		TUB	CERV	UTER	HODG	CRHD	RESP	ASTH	APP	HERN	CHOLY	HYP/S	MAT	PER
351	Salford	8	36	23	4	3	7	5	2	2	2	298	1	165
352	Stockport	6	20	18	11	1	4	6	2	2	1	258	0	199
353	Tameside	6	24	13	10	0	8	4	3	0	2	248	0	182
354	Trafford	7	23	16	6	5	6	5	0	0	4	197	0	164
355	Wigan	6	39	24	7	4	3	7	0	0	3	294	2	223
356	Cheshire	20	137	94	25	4	19	28	2	7	15	765	4	663
357	Liverpool	28	96	62	16	5	9	14	2	5	7	574	5	378
358	St Helens and Knowsley	10	69	53	10	1	7	4	1	2	8	398	4	298
359	Sefton	9	50	34	12	2	8	7	2	1	3	300	1	190
360	Wirral	13	55	43	10	2	7	3	1	1	3	307	3	242
361	Clwyd	3	57	36	18	4	14	3	0	4	4	353	3	309
362	Dyfed	9	50	33	15	6	5	5	2	4	7	384	2	216
363	Gwent	12	41	33	22	3	14	12	2	3	4	426	1	337
364	Gwynedd	10	26	14	9	2	5	4	1	1	1	225	1	151
365	Mid Glamorgan	18	68	43	20	13	15	26	3	4	11	606	5	515
366	Powys	1	13	6	5	0	3	3	0	1	1	103	0	77
367	South Glamorgan	15	48	28	11	2	12	7	1	4	3	323	1	301
368	West Glamorgan	12	41	22	16	4	8	9	1	1	2	381	2	270
UK:NORTHERN IRELAND														
369	Northern Ireland	37	124	89	67	11	59	45	8	13	20	1287	12	1895
UK:SCOTLAND		220	576	373	170	49	121	119	24	41	4	5713	45	3897
370	Highlands and Islands	4	29	20	10	1	5	9	2	1	0	260	2	209
371	Grampian	13	40	22	13	2	7	8	2	3	0	408	6	331
372	Tayside	12	29	21	14	2	12	6	1	6	1	397	3	214
373	Fife	3	58	40	15	1	10	4	0	0	0	397	2	264
374	Lothian	13	80	59	21	8	16	17	2	3	0	718	7	537
375	Borders	1	7	5	5	0	1	1	1	1	0	122	0	65
376	Forth Valley	12	28	13	9	2	12	6	1	5	2	291	4	226
377	Argyll and Clyde	31	52	30	18	2	11	6	4	5	1	532	3	363
378	Greater Glasgow	91	115	75	28	18	18	34	3	7	0	1302	9	732
379	Lanarkshire	17	68	44	22	9	19	12	4	5	0	638	6	500
380	Ayrshire and Arran	16	55	33	12	4	7	14	3	5	0	502	3	356
381	Dumfries and Galloway	7	15	11	3	0	3	2	1	0	0	146	0	100
PORTUGAL		1586	486	760	269	422	712	-	79	70	123	14491	134	16418
382	Viana do Castelo	27	10	21	2	4	31	-	0	2	1	378	3	476
383	Braga	47	17	39	7	32	79	-	5	2	4	838	14	1631
384	Vila Real	27	8	13	2	6	31	-	1	1	3	459	5	645
385	Braganca	14	8	16	3	3	20	-	1	2	0	322	1	319
386	Guarda	23	5	13	6	8	8	-	1	1	1	358	3	283
387	Viseu	90	16	24	4	11	50	-	3	4	5	732	5	886
388	Porto	370	95	157	45	120	146	-	14	10	30	2088	21	3221
389	Aveiro	42	22	59	6	20	42	-	1	2	5	776	11	1148
390	Coimbra	56	13	34	8	17	32	-	4	2	6	888	4	611
391	Castelo Branco	23	4	10	3	8	11	-	2	3	0	361	6	355
392	Portalegre	14	3	9	2	5	4	-	1	4	1	225	2	214
393	Santarem	29	11	31	4	4	16	-	2	3	8	636	6	616
394	Leiria	21	19	28	6	4	19	-	3	4	2	649	8	526
395	Lisboa	584	183	197	137	130	138	-	28	21	35	3389	21	2462
396	Setubal	40	20	30	12	9	12	-	4	0	3	522	9	907
397	Evora	13	4	11	4	2	4	-	1	2	4	288	3	225
398	Beja	21	5	10	2	10	2	-	2	3	2	255	2	257
399	Faro	43	16	21	8	7	7	-	2	0	5	414	1	461
400	Madeira	43	13	16	4	9	23	-	2	1	7	464	2	556
401	Azores	59	14	21	4	13	37	-	2	3	1	449	7	619
SPAIN		3442	908	1949	1128	992	1213	233	235	290	512	26728	273	33771
402	La Coruña	187	34	73	51	36	54	2	6	7	15	955	13	868
403	Lugo	59	10	30	11	6	14	4	0	5	2	300	3	353
404	Orense	67	7	24	5	7	15	3	5	2	6	381	3	422
405	Pontevedra	104	12	69	19	12	32	9	6	9	5	668	3	755
406	Asturias	136	40	69	41	31	26	5	11	8	20	860	12	877
407	Cantabria	44	18	32	15	12	19	4	4	2	6	379	6	464
408	Alava	15	2	6	9	4	10	0	4	1	2	116	1	216
409	Guipuzcoa	49	12	27	29	4	21	3	2	4	6	372	4	530
410	Vizcaya	108	31	62	38	25	30	8	5	7	18	784	8	1018

Table 7.1.2 cont

Area   Observed number of deaths

		TUB	CERV	UTER	HODG	CRHD	RESP	ASTH	APP	HERN	CHOLY	HYP/S	MAT	PER
411	Navarra	41	4	11	18	12	15	4	4	5	8	320	1	378
412	Rioja	20	2	6	8	2	5	1	1	1	3	180	5	255
413	Huesca	5	3	12	3	1	6	0	0	2	5	150	1	140
414	Teruel	5	0	8	3	1	4	0	1	0	5	113	1	85
415	Zaragoza	61	9	38	26	21	16	0	6	8	19	598	5	628
416	Madrid Centro	326	94	145	100	131	140	21	8	17	29	2265	20	3763
417	Avila	13	2	5	5	7	5	0	0	1	1	116	2	133
418	Burgos	29	5	8	9	5	5	1	2	1	7	222	0	181
419	Leon	59	10	30	12	24	17	5	8	2	10	400	7	563
420	Palencia	15	2	13	7	1	3	2	1	1	3	151	1	177
421	Salamanca	56	5	20	13	14	12	1	3	0	6	243	4	325
422	Segovia	7	1	4	6	3	8	1	1	0	0	100	2	93
423	Soria	3	0	5	6	4	4	0	1	0	0	69	0	53
424	Valladolid	32	9	32	21	11	12	1	3	3	14	227	6	221
425	Zamora	15	2	14	6	4	2	0	0	1	0	146	4	172
426	Albacete	37	7	16	7	9	14	0	2	4	12	273	1	428
427	Ciudad Real	47	2	18	18	14	21	2	2	8	6	439	9	447
428	Cuenca	13	3	12	3	6	3	2	4	1	3	169	2	195
429	Guadalajara	10	1	2	4	2	4	0	1	1	2	84	0	92
430	Toledo	33	5	18	9	20	15	4	2	5	9	327	3	450
431	Badajoz	66	5	28	30	27	22	8	5	6	12	646	8	663
432	Caceres	44	9	21	14	14	15	0	2	5	2	390	9	402
433	Barcelona	325	132	260	141	84	120	29	18	16	46	2991	15	2167
434	Gerona	31	11	24	16	6	13	7	7	7	3	284	0	342
435	Lerida	24	5	23	11	6	7	0	4	0	6	289	2	258
436	Tarragona	45	8	37	15	10	16	9	4	3	3	377	4	396
437	Alicante	77	24	63	25	34	45	6	5	7	13	988	11	1027
438	Castellon de la Plana	36	7	26	12	13	12	3	4	0	8	341	6	399
439	Valencia	165	73	124	78	85	66	15	20	31	48	1996	10	1633
440	Baleares	56	37	48	29	8	20	10	4	2	10	533	3	661
441	Almeria	51	7	21	11	7	20	3	1	5	2	284	6	588
442	Cadiz	101	28	58	26	30	37	7	6	15	17	740	13	1684
443	Cordoba	65	13	30	16	21	40	3	7	3	12	546	7	794
444	Granada	68	18	28	28	15	21	2	9	15	13	487	10	851
445	Huelva	59	10	21	9	12	12	2	2	6	9	365	2	640
446	Jaen	57	10	32	15	29	36	3	7	7	3	460	4	807
447	Malaga	123	26	63	41	45	32	12	5	14	28	780	6	1349
448	Sevilla	287	63	111	52	60	57	13	13	24	23	1197	15	2241
449	Murcia	59	24	43	17	19	40	0	12	7	16	665	7	904
450	Las Palmas	69	25	36	16	21	24	12	6	7	10	542	7	1038
451	Sta Cruz de Tenerife	38	41	43	23	17	26	6	1	4	6	420	1	645

Tables 7.1.3(a)–(o). Total number of 'avoidable deaths', age-standardized mortality rates, range and heterogeneity of SMRs (chi square) by disease and country

Notes on the use of these tables

1. These tables show the total number of 'avoidable deaths', age-standardized mortality rates (based on the EC standard), and range and heterogeneity of SMRs (based on the country's own standard) by disease and country. Asthma data for Greece and Portugal are not available.

2. The maximum and minimum SMRs (based on the country's own standard) show the range of SMRs found in the small areas in a particular country. The chi-square value provides a test of whether the degree of heterogeneity between different small areas within one country is greater than could be expected by chance.

3. The mortality data are for 1980–84, except for Greece (1980–82), Italy (1979–83), and Spain (1979–83).

Table 7.1.3(a). Tuberculosis ICD9 010–018, 137 (ages 5–64)

Country	Total deaths	Rates and SMRs based on EC standard		Within-country variation of SMRs based on own country standard			
		Age-standardized mortality rate (100 000)	National SMR	Minimum	Maximum	χ^2 heterogeneity	df
Belgium	331	0.80	61	35.9	165.3	91.2**	8
Luxembourg	5	0.34	26	-	-	-	-
Fed. Rep. Germany	2828	1.10	84	63.6	258.0	281.2**	30
Denmark	97	0.48	36	21.6	213.8	24.2*	14
France	2732	1.28	97	26.3	207.9	367.1**	94
Greece	367	1.59	121	37.4	254.2	42.5**	9
Italy	3132	1.36	103	31.6	239.1	385.1**	88
Ireland	232	2.10	160	39.4	174.1	23.6**	7
Netherlands	188	0.35	27	0.0	174.6	28.4**	11
UK : England and Wales	1417	0.70	53	0.0	337.3	455.8**	97
: N. Ireland	37	0.68	52	-	-	-	-
: Scotland	220	1.06	81	20.8	205.1	89.2**	11
Portugal	1586	4.11	313	30.0	168.5	481.2**	19
Spain	3442	2.38	181	21.7	230.8	512.5**	49

*p=<0.05.
**p=<0.01.

Table 7.1.3 (b). Malignant neoplasm of the cervix uteri ICD9 180 (ages 15–64)

Country	Total deaths	Rates and SMRs based on EC standard		Within-country variation of SMRs based on own country standard			
		Age-standardized mortality rate (100 000)	National SMR	Minimum	Maximum	χ^2 heterogeneity	df
Belgium	524	3.16	90	66.8	142.4	26.7**	8
Luxembourg	19	3.12	88	-	-	-	-
Fed. Rep. Germany	4980	4.58	130	67.0	193.9	232.5**	30
Denmark	753	9.12	258	62.5	131.0	29.9**	14
France	2352	2.73	77	20.7	182.0	220.4**	94
Greece	165	1.73	49	53.8	146.5	19.3*	9
Italy	1161	1.22	34	18.5	263.4	206.6**	88
Ireland	167	3.82	108	71.6	134.5	10.1	7
Netherlands	780	3.60	102	25.0	149.2	17.3	11
UK : England and Wales	5333	6.56	186	42.8	183.8	445.4**	97
: N. Ireland	124	5.54	157	-	-	-	-
: Scotland	576	6.77	192	60.4	153.2	25.9**	11
Portugal	486	3.02	85	31.7	163.0	100.2**	19
Spain	908	1.54	44	0.0	294.7	223.1**	49

*p=<0.05.
**p=<0.01.

Table 7.1.3(c). Malignant neoplasm of the cervix and body of the uterus ICD9 179, 180, 182 (ages 15–54)

Country	Total deaths	Rates and SMRs based on EC standard		Within-country variation of SMRs based on own country standard			
		Age-standardized mortality rate (100 000)	National SMR	Minimum	Maximum	χ^2 heterogeneity	df
Belgium	471	3.47	80	88.4	116.3	3.6	8
Luxembourg	23	4.31	99	-	-	-	-
Fed. Rep. Germany	3763	4.23	97	70.6	185.7	163.1**	30
Denmark	462	6.93	159	64.3	140.9	25.2*	14
France	2882	4.03	92	18.8	168.2	162.0**	94
Greece	323	3.66	84	37.6	160.5	20.4*	9
Italy	3588	4.37	100	39.1	224.1	360.0**	88
Ireland	114	3.19	73	78.6	131.8	3.9	7
Netherlands	538	2.95	68	0.0	131.0	12.2	11
UK : England and Wales	3455	5.39	124	37.8	208.9	289.0**	97
: N. Ireland	89	4.87	112	-	-	-	-
: Scotland	373	5.49	126	63.1	164.4	22.1*	11
Portugal	760	5.62	129	52.9	137.7	49.9**	19
Spain	1949	3.84	88	28.6	155.8	159.6**	49

*p=<0.05.
**p=<0.01.

Table 7.1.3 (d). Hodgkin's disease ICD9 201 (ages 5–64)

Country	Total deaths	Rates and SMRs based on EC standard		Within-country variation of SMRs based on own country standard			
		Age-standardized mortality rate (100 000)	National SMR	Minimum	Maximum	χ^2 heterogeneity	df
Belgium	428	1.05	115	72.4	141.7	28.0**	8
Luxembourg	10	0.66	72	-	-	-	-
Fed. Rep. Germany	2617	1.02	111	57.9	173.4	161.3**	30
Denmark	165	0.80	87	66.8	168.4	14.8	14
France	1487	0.68	74	23.8	245.2	126.0*	94
Greece	214	0.93	101	72.7	176.7	7.2	9
Italy	2845	1.24	135	41.6	172.8	145.9**	88
Ireland	149	1.26	137	74.2	167.9	14.3*	7
Netherlands	428	0.75	82	63.3	127.0	9.4	11
UK : England and Wales	1657	0.83	90	47.0	178.1	112.4	97
: N. Ireland	67	1.19	129	-	-	-	-
: Scotland	170	0.83	90	63.0	154.2	6.2	11
Portugal	269	0.70	76	29.6	225.2	140.1**	19
Spain	1128	0.78	85	36.3	193.7	85.9**	49

*p=<0.05.
**p=<0.01.

Table 7.1.3(e). Chronic rheumatic heart disease ICD9 393–398 (ages 5–44)

Country	Total deaths	Rates and SMRs based on EC standard		Within-country variation of SMRs based on own country standard			
		Age-standardized mortality rate (100 000)	National SMR	Minimum	Maximum	χ^2 heterogeneity	df
Belgium	11	0.04	9	0.0	215.9	4.8	8
Luxembourg	5	0.45	99	-	-	-	-
Fed. Rep. Germany	314	0.16	36	0.0	251.6	117.3**	30
Denmark	25	0.16	35	0.0	390.2	14.6	14
France	263	0.17	38	0.0	354.1	80.1	94
Greece	51	0.31	68	0.0	288.8	30.2**	9
Italy	1515	0.91	201	19.8	227.4	374.2**	88
Ireland	24	0.27	60	0.0	189.4	4.6	7
Netherlands	75	0.17	38	0.0	184.9	7.7	11
UK : England and Wales	391	0.28	61	0.0	314.8	171.2**	97
: N. Ireland	11	0.27	58	-	-	-	-
: Scotland	49	0.34	75	0.0	203.6	20.2*	11
Portugal	422	1.57	345	21.6	169.8	103.0**	19
Spain	992	0.99	218	19.9	191.4	160.5**	49

*p=<0.05.
**p=<0.01.

Table 7.1.3 (f). All respiratory diseases ICD9 460–519 (ages 14)

Country	Total deaths	Rates and SMRs based on EC standard		Within-country variation of SMRs based on own country standard			
		Age-standardized mortality rate (100 000)	National SMR	Minimum	Maximum	χ^2 heterogeneity	df
Belgium	159	1.74	78	51.0	136.5	9.8	8
Luxembourg	4	1.27	57	-	-	-	-
Fed. Rep. Germany	829	1.75	78	60.5	154.9	47.8*	30
Denmark	62	1.32	59	0.0	301.3	25.1*	14
France	683	1.18	53	0.0	290.7	112.0	94
Greece	157	2.32	104	36.2	428.6	70.9**	9
Italy	1416	2.51	112	0.0	188.5	309.2**	88
Ireland	130	2.57	115	74.5	146.9	6.4	7
Netherlands	177	1.26	57	56.2	133.8	8.3	11
UK : England and Wales	1275	2.74	123	25.5	195.5	110.8	97
: N. Ireland	59	3.02	135	-	-	-	-
: Scotland	121	2.42	108	45.6	183.7	11.6	11
Portugal	712	6.15	275	17.8	168.7	105.0**	19
Spain	1213	2.62	117	38.2	200.0	79.1**	49

*p=<0.05.
**p=<0.01.

Table 7.1.3(g). Asthma ICD9 483 (ages 5–44)

Country	Total deaths	Rates and SMRs based on EC standard		Within-country variation of SMRs based on own country standard			
		Age-standardized mortality rate (100 000)	National SMR	Minimum	Maximum	χ^2 heterogeneity	df
Belgium	261	0.93	170	35.8	189.5	35.6**	8
Luxembourg	8	0.74	134	-	-	-	-
Fed. Rep. Germany	1886	1.01	185	75.3	135.4	46.1*	30
Denmark	62	0.41	75	0.0	177.2	15.2	14
France	581	0.37	68	0.0	445.4	127.8*	94
Greece	-	-	-	-	-	-	-
Italy	245	0.15	27	0.0	394.9	98.0	88
Ireland	95	0.99	180	48.1	137.3	4.7	7
Netherlands	151	0.34	62	0.0	151.6	15.7	11
UK : England and Wales	1312	0.93	170	20.2	201.4	131.9**	97
: N. Ireland	45	1.03	187	-	-	-	-
: Scotland	119	0.81	148	46.1	161.0	17.9	11
Portugal	-	-	-	-	-	-	-
Spain	233	0.22	41	0.0	290.8	95.4**	49

*p=<0.05.
**p=<0.01.

Table 7.1.3 (h). Appendicitis ICD9 540–543 (ages 5–64)

Country	Total deaths	Rates and SMRs based on EC standard		Within-country variation of SMRs based on own country standard			
		Age-standardized mortality rate (100 000)	National SMR	Minimum	Maximum	χ^2 heterogeneity	df
Belgium	29	0.07	49	0.0	247.4	12.6	8
Luxembourg	4	0.28	188	-	-	-	-
Fed. Rep. Germany	465	0.19	128	27.4	153.4	43.6	30
Denmark	31	0.15	104	0.0	200.1	5.7	14
France	353	0.16	112	0.0	308.7	144.6**	94
Greece	14	0.06	41	0.0	764.2	14.6	9
Italy	324	0.14	96	0.0	447.5	142.0**	88
Ireland	17	0.14	94	0.0	259.9	7.6	7
Netherlands	67	0.12	83	23.6	251.1	11.4	11
UK : England and Wales	201	0.10	69	0.0	409.0	103.1	97
: N. Ireland	8	0.14	94	-	-	-	-
: Scotland	24	0.12	79	0.0	211.7	7.8	11
Portugal	79	0.20	136	0.0	164.7	15.5	19
Spain	235	0.16	108	0.0	279.5	80.2**	49

*p=<0.05.
**p=<0.01.

Table 7.1.3 (i). Abdominal hernia ICD9 550–553 (ages 5–64)

Country	Total deaths	Rates and SMRs based on EC standard		Within-country variation of SMRs based on own country standard			
		Age-standardized mortality rate (100 000)	National SMR	Minimum	Maximum	χ^2 heterogeneity	df
Belgium	41	0.10	49	38.3	177.1	7.5	8
Luxembourg	2	0.14	69	-	-	-	-
Fed. Rep. Germany	398	0.16	79	51.4	208.9	65.3**	30
Denmark	27	0.13	65	0.0	313.6	11.0	14
France	558	0.26	130	0.0	271.5	124.9*	94
Greece	19	0.08	42	0.0	240.5	4.6	9
Italy	558	0.24	122	0.0	333.2	170.3**	88
Ireland	14	0.13	63	22.8	251.4	8.0	7
Netherlands	78	0.15	74	0.0	148.3	8.7	11
UK : England and Wales	420	0.20	102	0.0	342.5	130.7*	97
: N. Ireland	13	0.23	117	-	-	-	-
: Scotland	41	0.19	96	0.0	230.0	14.2	11
Portugal	70	0.18	90	0.0	314.7	22.7	19
Spain	290	0.20	101	0.0	264.8	128.8**	49

*p=<0.05.
**p=<0.01.

Table 7.1.3 (j). Cholelithiasis and cholecystitis ICD9 574–575.1, 576.1 (ages 5–64)

Country	Total deaths	Rates and SMRs based on EC standard		Within-country variation of SMRs based on own country standard			
		Age-standardized mortality rate (100 000)	National SMR	Minimum	Maximum	χ^2 heterogeneity	df
Belgium	139	0.33	97	49.2	260.4	18.3*	8
Luxembourg	7	0.48	140	-	-	-	-
Fed. Rep. Germany	1080	0.43	123	52.4	183.9	105.8**	30
Denmark	52	0.25	73	0.0	241.9	13.2	14
France	152	0.07	21	0.0	381.3	91.5	94
Greece	40	0.18	51	0.0	203.6	6.8	9
Italy	1476	0.65	187	45.7	192.1	139.6**	88
Ireland	39	0.35	102	28.0	152.6	4.8	7
Netherlands	220	0.42	120	0.0	135.0	15.6	11
UK : England and Wales	498	0.24	70	0.0	300.8	126.0*	97
: N. Ireland	20	0.36	105	-	-	-	-
: Scotland	4	0.02	5	0.0	961.3	21.3*	11
Portugal	123	0.32	92	0.0	263.2	38.7**	19
Spain	512	0.36	103	0.0	259.0	127.1**	49

*p=<0.05.
**p=<0.01.

Table 7.1.3 (k). Hypertensive and cerebrovascular diseases ICD9 410–405, 430–438 (ages 35–64)

Country	Total deaths	Rates and SMRs based on EC standard		Within-country variation of SMRs based on own country standard			
		Age-standardized mortality rate (100 000)	National SMR	Minimum	Maximum	χ^2 heterogeneity	df
Belgium	6385	35.10	82	75.4	131.9	146.8**	8
Luxembourg	322	51.13	119	-	-	-	-
Fed. Rep. Germany	43928	39.53	92	81.4	138.5	793.9**	30
Denmark	2991	33.05	77	82.8	127.8	46.6**	14
France	31290	33.53	78	66.4	156.4	1223.0**	94
Greece	4558	46.09	107	85.7	135.5	30.4**	9
Italy	50342	50.44	117	65.2	156.1	1562.6**	88
Ireland	2406	50.10	117	81.7	111.0	16.8*	7
Netherlands	6509	28.31	66	83.3	109.0	36.8**	11
UK : England and Wales	40556	44.91	104	66.7	146.5	1630.1**	97
: N. Ireland	1287	53.57	125	-	-	-	-
: Scotland	5713	61.67	143	80.0	119.3	84.2**	11
Portugal	14491	85.42	199	53.2	148.1	536.9**	19
Spain	26728	42.65	99	71.6	145.3	1084.0**	49

*p=<0.05.
**p=<0.01.

Table 7.1.3 (l). Maternal deaths ICD9 630–676 (all ages)

Country	Total deaths	Rates and SMRs based on EC standard		Within-country variation of SMRs based on own country standard			
		Age-standardized mortality rate (100 000)	National SMR	Minimum	Maximum	χ^2 heterogeneity	df
Belgium	44	7.27	62	52.3	185.2	6.2	8
Luxembourg	0	0.00	0	-	-	-	-
Fed. Rep. Germany	487	15.97	136	21.7	162.1	49.6*	30
Denmark	15	5.62	48	0.0	270.0	13.3	14
France	545	13.85	118	0.0	348.4	147.8**	94
Greece	58	8.40	72	0.0	503.1	54.2**	9
Italy	355	11.39	97	0.0	445.9	128.4**	88
Ireland	24	6.83	58	56.5	203.0	6.1	7
Netherlands	67	7.60	65	0.0	154.5	9.9	11
UK : England and Wales	271	8.52	73	0.0	279.2	81.3	97
: N. Ireland	12	8.64	74	-	-	-	-
: Scotland	45	13.38	114	0.0	172.4	4.8	11
Portugal	134	17.71	151	25.7	238.9	14.7	19
Spain	273	10.64	91	0.0	316.7	94.6**	49

*p=<0.05.
**p=<0.01.

Table 7.3.1 (m). Perinatal deaths

Country	Total deaths	Rates and SMRs based on EC standard		Within-country variation of SMRs based on own country standard			
		Age-standardized mortality rate (100 000)	National SMR	Minimum	Maximum	χ^2 heterogeneity	df
Belgium	7713	12.74	99	91.9	109.7	19.5*	8
Luxembourg	236	11.04	86	-	-	-	-
Fed. Rep. Germany	30320	9.94	77	82.6	124.3	376.0**	30
Denmark	2357	8.83	69	74.1	121.1	50.1**	14
France	46876	11.92	93	73.8	128.6	608.0**	94
Greece	12251	17.73	138	80.1	107.8	117.3**	9
Italy	49514	15.89	124	53.1	139.3	1273.5**	88
Ireland	4857	13.83	108	82.1	107.8	31.3**	7
Netherlands	9159	10.39	81	75.6	105.8	12.4	11
UK : England and Wales	36429	11.45	89	65.7	147.8	664.4**	97
: N. Ireland	1895	13.64	106	-	-	-	-
: Scotland	3897	11.59	90	76.5	123.4	43.1**	11
Portugal	16418	21.70	169	77.1	138.9	330.5**	19
Spain	33771	13.16	102	53.2	176.0	1626.3**	49

*p=<0.05.
**p=<0.01.

Table 7.1.3 (n). All causes (ages 5–64)

Country	Total deaths	Rates and SMRs based on EC standard		Within-country variation of SMRs based on own country standard			
		Age-standardized mortality rate (100 000)	National SMR	Minimum	Maximum	χ^2 heterogeneity	df
Belgium	123752	300.60	105	89.3	120.4	1671.1**	8
Luxembourg	5096	348.10	122	-	-	-	-
Fed. Rep. Germany	753470	296.44	104	86.9	135.2	6440.5**	30
Denmark	64659	315.18	110	88.5	138.8	1409.6**	14
France	633730	295.27	103	77.7	133.0	11348.6**	94
Greece	51676	226.21	79	89.2	123.6	196.6**	9
Italy	625425	272.85	96	79.1	137.6	10858.0**	88
Ireland	37293	327.80	115	88.6	104.1	72.6**	7
Netherlands	131427	243.46	85	85.5	106.6	116.7**	11
UK : England and Wales	602565	296.16	104	80.3	137.2	10380.6**	97
: N. Ireland	19434	348.92	122	-	-	-	-
: Scotland	77203	368.92	129	83.8	115.1	898.2**	11
Portugal	125725	323.24	113	61.5	132.1	4779.0**	19
Spain	360103	248.47	87	80.7	130.1	3586.7**	49

*p=<0.05.
**p=<0.01.

Table 7.1.3 (o). All causes (all ages)

Country	Total deaths	Rates and SMRs based on EC standard		Within-country variation of SMRs based on own country standard			
		Age-standardized mortality rate (100 000)	National SMR	Minimum	Maximum	χ^2 heterogeneity	df
Belgium	563017	1084.75	107	93.3	111.4	2515.4**	8
Luxembourg	20704	1176.29	116	-	-	-	-
Fed. Rep. Germany	3566537	1058.93	104	90.6	114.0	10949.1**	30
Denmark	280635	1039.80	102	95.2	109.6	656.3**	14
France	2728240	931.01	92	80.9	119.9	19779.3**	94
Greece	258776	969.04	95	87.6	113.1	857.1**	9
Italy	2718889	1033.70	102	88.7	118.8	12947.0**	88
Ireland	163916	1238.80	122	94.3	106.7	236.6**	7
Netherlands	584573	931.05	92	85.7	107.0	420.9**	11
UK : England and Wales	2878384	1069.67	105	87.4	117.0	16669.7**	97
: N. Ireland	80740	1208.76	119	-	-	-	-
: Scotland	317948	1212.01	119	92.8	106.3	1007.6**	11
Portugal	477008	1070.00	105	37.7	118.1	21753.8**	19
Spain	1440845	909.42	89	80.2	118.2	11925.7**	49

*p=<0.05.
**p=<0.01.

Table 7.1.4(a). 'Avoidable death' indicators by small area and country, standardized to the EC standard, for tuberculosis, malignant neoplasm of the cervix uteri, malignant neoplasm of the cervix and body of the uterus, Hodgkin's disease, chronic rheumatic heart disease, all respiratory diseases, and asthma

Notes on the use of this table

1. This table shows within-EC variations, the value for the whole EC being 100. Asthma data for Greece and Portugal are not available.

2. Key for the abbreviations used for columns of the table:
   TUB   —   tuberculosis (ICD8 010–019; ICD9 010–018, 137), ages 5–64;
   CERV —   malignant neoplasm of the cervix uteri (ICD8 180; ICD9 180), ages 15–64;
   UTER —   malignant neoplasm of the cervix and body of the uterus (ICD8 180, 182; ICD9 179, 180, 182), ages 15–54;
   HODG —   Hodgkin's disease (ICD8 201; ICD9 201), ages 5–64;
   CRHD —   chronic rheumatic heart disease (ICD8 393–398; ICD9 393–398), ages 5–44;
   RESP —   all respiratory diseases (ICD8 460–519; ICD9 460–519), ages 1–14;
   ASTH —   asthma (ICD8 493; ICD9 493), ages 5–44.

3. The small area numbers are as in the key maps.

4. The indicators have been tested for indicating significant excess mortality relative to EC rates. The *p*-values achieved for one-tail tests are indicated as follows: *$p<0.05$; **$p<0.01$; ***$p<0.001$.

5. The indicators are based on mortality data for 1980–84, except for Greece (1980–82) and Spain (1979–83). The population data are for 1980–84 except for France (1982), Greece (1981), Ireland (1981), and Spain (1981). All data for Italy are for 1979–83.

Table 7.1.4(a)

Area	Indicators (SMRs)						
	TUB	CERV	UTER	HODG	CRHD	RESP	ASTH
BELGIUM	61	90	80	115**	9	78	170***
1 Antwerpen	22	99	71	153***	5	66	141*
2 Brabant	93	71	83	83	10	89	157***
3 West-Vlaanderen	40	91	71	109	7	57	201***
4 Oost-Vlaanderen	25	101	76	162***	6	105	111
5 Hainaut	101	128**	82	104	19	64	269***
6 Liège	70	60	93	97	16	106	205***
7 Limburg	45	88	81	112	0	57	81
8 Luxembourg (province)	26	71	73	111	0	40	60
9 Namur	100	83	90	85	0	78	320***
LUXEMBOURG							
10 Luxembourg	26	88	99	72	99	57	134
FEDERAL REPUBLIC OF GERMANY	84	130***	97	111***	36	78	185***
11 Schleswig–Holstein	65	144***	105	109	8	60	190***
12 Hamburg	70	141***	108	65	42	94	187***
13 Braunschweig	76	129**	99	172***	18	86	210***
14 Hannover	80	159***	117*	193***	31	100	217***
15 Luneburg	67	117	84	134**	5	75	214***
16 Weser–Ems	62	148***	114	129**	28	84	172***
17 Bremen	68	153***	122	72	21	58	251***
18 Düsseldorf	76	149***	99	96	31	72	196***
19 Köln	86	139***	96	104	36	47	186***
20 Münster	66	119**	91	85	54	57	180***
21 Detmold	69	115	84	101	41	108	200***
22 Arnsberg	81	129***	98	98	46	103	194***
23 Darmstadt	79	108	80	118*	67	61	222***
24 Giessen	84	87	78	103	67	76	219***
25 Kassel	57	107	93	103	69	83	246***
26 Koblenz	69	103	75	168***	39	67	195***
27 Trier	80	154**	137*	153*	34	57	150

Table 7.1.4(a) cont

Area		Indicators (SMRs)						
		TUB	CERV	UTER	HODG	CRHD	RESP	ASTH
28	Rheinhessen–Pfalz	71	135***	101	131**	72	81	244***
29	Stuttgart	70	108	82	103	56	65	152***
30	Karlsruhe	116*	119**	81	82	63	82	140**
31	Freiburg	107	101	95	83	34	73	170***
32	Tübingen	74	90	68	90	33	111	141*
33	Oberbayern	75	108	79	97	5	107	142***
34	Niederbayern	120	145***	132**	111	0	64	156*
35	Oberpfalz	156***	144***	125*	152***	8	90	153*
36	Oberfranken	217***	138***	99	139**	22	69	189***
37	Mittelfranken	136***	126**	110	155***	5	55	194***
38	Unterfranken	94	111	78	94	6	70	179***
39	Schwaben	53	112	93	129*	14	79	139*
40	Saarland	98	121*	85	108	90	121	209***
41	Berlin (West)	115	252***	181***	108	29	88	167***
DENMARK		36	258***	159***	87	35	59	75
42	Kobenhavn and Frederiksberg (M)	81	339***	224***	96	42	27	106
43	Kobenhavns County	37	190***	103	118	32	57	47
44	Frederiksborg County	30	160**	102	81	37	13	50
45	Roskilde County	20	249***	151*	145	29	64	26
46	Vestsjaellands County	34	243***	155*	146	52	52	0
47	Storstroms County	21	222***	170**	72	59	178*	25
48	Bornholms County	39	299***	155	58	0	0	0
49	Fyns County	38	287***	184***	60	16	64	111
50	Sonderjyllands County	16	256***	161*	66	30	127	125
51	Ribe County	56	289***	161*	65	137	61	114
52	Vejle County	30	308***	169**	84	0	70	133
53	Ringkobing County	8	209***	118	74	0	63	70
54	Arhus County	28	262***	176***	66	37	40	72
55	Viborg County	25	323***	143	60	0	0	84
56	Nordjyllands County	32	265***	193***	79	47	68	78
FRANCE		97	77	92	74	38	53	68
57	Ain	52	62	60	46	35	19	45
58	Aisne	119	69	96	57	31	65	86
59	Allier	63	58	127	88	0	80	39
60	Alpes-de-Haute-Provence	76	72	44	45	65	42	0
61	Hautes-Alpes	140	16	17	25	0	0	305**
62	Alpes-Maritimes	89	64	87	88	37	45	96
63	Ardèche	117	72	95	102	31	51	0
64	Ardennes	127	107	140	65	27	101	85
65	Ariège	88	109	79	79	0	40	220
66	Aube	131	140	144*	48	0	14	22
67	Aude	55	40	44	106	0	75	52
68	Aveyron	71	49	51	79	32	90	104
69	Bouches-du-Rhône	98	65	83	93	52	36	43
70	Calvados	115	99	101	100	27	39	85
71	Cantal	111	85	78	100	53	86	43
72	Charente	66	124	156**	89	25	66	40
73	Charente-Maritime	68	73	105	59	33	35	40
74	Cher	106	89	96	60	52	58	85
75	Corrèze	85	40	102	66	0	43	90
76	Corse	89	36	75	55	31	42	54
77	Côte-d'Or	47	139*	104	88	49	52	79
78	Côtes-du-Nord	87	65	99	45	48	48	39
79	Creuse	61	24	134	178*	72	0	0
80	Dordogne	108	77	122	49	0	82	98
81	Doubs	74	89	88	35	79	63	13
82	Drôme	74	114	98	77	60	53	50
83	Eure	85	108	128	61	33	41	108
84	Eure-et-Loir	68	85	138*	62	0	74	18
85	Finistère	108	55	78	53	31	5	74
86	Gard	88	38	55	80	46	9	38
87	Haute-Garonne	75	68	121	52	18	59	82
88	Gers	30	67	120	62	0	155	82

Table 7.1.4(a) cont

Area		TUB	CERV	UTER	HODG	CRHD	RESP	ASTH
89	Gironde	88	68	97	72	28	44	91
90	Hérault	60	48	72	76	57	47	74
91	Ille-et-Vilaine	113	81	72	48	11	31	76
92	Indre	60	64	66	91	36	20	176
93	Indre-et-Loire	60	88	79	94	32	51	76
94	Isère	99	104	76	61	23	47	26
95	Jura	55	80	75	114	134	35	110
96	Landes	42	57	35	45	28	49	23
97	Loir-et-Cher	72	124	132	76	28	60	116
98	Loire	100	73	81	59	43	39	79
99	Haute-Loire	62	17	53	147	84	0	34
100	Loire-Atlantique	138**	62	73	59	8	71	76
101	Loiret	38	90	88	78	29	60	59
102	Lot	45	84	128	17	0	34	0
103	Lot-et-Garonne	64	65	91	89	28	16	46
104	Lozère	149	49	80	74	0	63	192
105	Maine-et-Loire	107	60	75	107	12	51	76
106	Manche	65	57	73	77	112	26	44
107	Marne	78	83	78	83	57	64	45
108	Haute-Marne	106	45	99	161*	39	74	31
109	Mayenne	94	54	54	83	32	55	50
110	Meurthe-et-Moselle	145**	124	100	61	22	45	69
111	Meuse	39	65	83	98	85	20	33
112	Morbihan	203***	48	49	70	58	68	80
113	Moselle	105	100	99	75	53	59	84
114	Nièvre	123	57	109	58	0	41	61
115	Nord	169***	98	108	94	45	61	106
116	Oise	91	110	112	60	45	38	73
117	Orne	65	73	98	112	0	40	0
118	Pas-de-Calais	163***	95	101	101	66	52	139*
119	Puy-de-Dôme	95	44	67	108	52	30	74
120	Pyrénées-Atlantiques	99	40	80	59	15	17	110
121	Hautes-Pyrénées	54	57	88	81	0	88	60
122	Pyrénées-Orientales	67	42	98	40	26	76	43
123	Bas-Rhin	124	130*	116	78	49	70	40
124	Haut-Rhin	91	84	105	75	58	108	66
125	Rhône	69	80	69	60	51	71	34
126	Haute-Saône	104	89	25	73	70	67	57
127	Saône-et-Loire	66	86	85	87	15	53	36
128	Sarthe	48	81	75	67	17	24	117
129	Savoie	119	100	86	58	70	26	38
130	Haute-Savoie	102	113	87	87	56	48	47
131	Paris	128**	84	115*	69	42	47	62
132	Seine-Maritime	184***	120	136**	123	59	81	73
133	Seine-et-Marne	93	63	102	60	39	96	59
134	Yvelines	65	75	92	65	17	62	76
135	Deux-Sèvres	51	16	54	25	25	12	60
136	Somme	117	67	110	130	46	57	47
137	Tarn	26	44	65	63	26	57	104
138	Tarn-et-Garonne	57	98	92	57	0	26	37
139	Var	97	73	97	45	56	48	94
140	Vaucluse	48	49	68	69	71	21	74
141	Vendée	61	54	79	70	18	78	42
142	Vienne	80	70	112	83	0	0	89
143	Haute-Vienne	61	62	98	53	0	73	98
144	Vosges	80	60	96	64	21	61	17
145	Yonne	68	106	112	91	28	70	135
146	Territoire-de-Belfort	61	98	143	62	58	0	94
147	Essonne	74	76	63	55	54	77	68
148	Hauts-de-Seine	96	66	86	78	31	57	39
149	Seine-Saint-Denis	111	66	99	66	21	61	76
150	Val-de-Marne	78	79	100	61	30	54	45
151	Val-d'Oise	97	58	95	85	53	32	69

Table 7.1.4(a) cont

Area		Indicators (SMRs)						
		TUB	CERV	UTER	HODG	CRHD	RESP	ASTH
GREECE		121***	49	84	101	68	104	-
152	Greater Athens	125**	72	89	99	28	79	-
153	Rest of Central Greece and Eubea	99	38	55	116	49	105	-
154	Peloponnisos	103	38	76	80	57	76	-
155	Ionian Islands	48	44	57	76	82	38	-
156	Epirus	108	26	32	102	0	153	-
157	Thessaly	135	29	101	86	18	98	-
158	Macedonia	127*	39	85	95	106	84	-
159	Thrace	306***	27	53	178*	185	444***	-
160	Aegean Islands	128	50	135	123	134	123	-
161	Crete	46	48	126	115	195*	119	-
ITALY		103*	34	100	135***	201***	112***	27
162	Torino	119*	58	101	143***	180***	91	33
163	Vercelli	81	65	108	196***	214**	45	0
164	Novara	128	32	107	172***	161	105	51
165	Cuneo	131*	59	104	129	181*	50	61
166	Asti	87	29	94	111	265**	198*	33
167	Alessandria	92	32	94	123	187*	43	45
168	Aosta	217**	14	121	113	125	141	0
169	Imperia	133	92	176**	230***	172	28	30
170	Savona	103	39	68	144	102	129	0
171	Genova	111	41	79	177***	131	62	52
172	La Spezia	66	42	106	167*	130	26	0
173	Varese	76	28	58	168***	185**	96	53
174	Como/Sondrio	123	34	79	119	150*	98	45
175	Milano	87	27	77	146***	161***	84	18
176	Bergamo	197***	16	103	163***	180**	78	33
177	Brescia	215***	38	65	167***	172**	80	29
178	Pavia	104	32	116	235***	89	72	26
179	Cremona	139*	56	82	108	178	33	39
180	Mantova	91	17	78	185***	61	85	35
181	Bolzano	161**	42	83	97	85	78	28
182	Trento	222***	65	93	98	237***	55	28
183	Verona	98	34	78	130	75	43	16
184	Vicenza	102	41	67	124	119	87	8
185	Belluno	248***	36	110	131	103	72	29
186	Treviso	100	46	76	163***	101	45	26
187	Venezia	97	62	78	170***	68	40	43
188	Padova	118	30	61	173***	107	148*	30
189	Rovigo	76	57	62	124	94	20	26
190	Udine/Gorizia	140**	72	91	104	107	41	28
191	Trieste	155**	44	94	177**	187*	51	49
192	Pordenone	82	62	72	98	158	0	0
193	Piacenza	76	38	70	136	193*	23	0
194	Parma	106	26	91	140	77	77	51
195	Reggio Emilia	53	30	71	229***	55	40	0
196	Modena	71	26	76	170***	98	46	11
197	Bologna	85	31	76	113	141	70	21
198	Ferrara	63	38	65	105	60	93	0
199	Ravenna	33	21	99	71	63	33	18
200	Forli	71	35	67	130	49	59	0
201	Pesaro	42	10	62	63	92	149	20
202	Ancona	66	43	70	89	88	106	15
203	Macerata	86	11	88	114	79	55	23
204	Ascoli Piceno	103	22	95	124	108	42	0
205	Massa-Carrara	184**	46	137	153	229*	53	33
206	Lucca	143*	28	89	129	40	42	69
207	Pistoia	104	24	75	147	225**	61	74
208	Firenze	63	28	83	147***	115	76	5
209	Livorno	63	18	66	104	87	79	19
210	Pisa	39	48	82	153*	97	70	51
211	Arezzo	106	45	104	98	197*	53	0

Table 7.1.4(a) cont

Area		Indicators (SMRs)						
		TUB	CERV	UTER	HODG	CRHD	RESP	ASTH
212	Siena	92	17	111	117	124	124	56
213	Grosseto	73	47	74	57	173	0	30
214	Perugia	71	16	52	201***	198**	81	11
215	Terni	56	65	104	110	369***	97	30
216	Viterbo/Rieti	99	19	101	158*	213**	143	33
217	Roma	103	47	108	141***	182***	94	26
218	Latina	94	34	156**	147*	319***	96	14
219	Frosinone	82	34	124	119	328***	18	14
220	Caserta	60	8	106	89	454***	148*	33
221	Benevento	123	24	98	125	265**	86	23
222	Napoli	132***	28	156***	133***	362***	201***	41
223	Avellino	53	8	97	84	305***	187**	30
224	Salerno	121	16	104	131*	442***	142*	25
225	L'Aquila	166**	53	120	72	341***	97	46
226	Teramo	138	6	116	121	116	65	24
227	Pescara	83	29	98	84	295***	125	45
228	Chieti	105	26	82	129	216**	73	18
229	Isernia/Campobasso	112	31	70	141	458***	123	21
230	Foggia	123	43	117	100	252***	182***	0
231	Bari	120	41	143***	102	348***	130*	30
232	Taranto	79	17	120	121	250***	149*	11
233	Brindisi	110	33	169***	145*	457***	180**	0
234	Lecce	120	35	106	145**	258***	136*	33
235	Potenza/Matera	111	33	105	98	284***	158*	32
236	Cosenza	85	33	152***	70	305***	162**	17
237	Catanzaro	100	24	104	128	446***	156**	34
238	Reggio Calabria	103	32	103	136	232***	111	23
239	Trapani	84	34	225***	135	245***	103	108
240	Palermo	55	23	154***	139**	219***	213***	21
241	Messina	53	13	146**	119	245***	182***	10
242	Agrigento	61	20	134*	147*	347***	180**	27
243	Caltanisetta	87	6	127	91	228**	100	67
244	Enna	92	27	158*	132	342***	140	67
245	Catania	67	31	164***	136*	239***	193***	6
246	Ragusa	99	44	189***	122	377***	199**	47
247	Siracusa	73	14	132	101	233**	75	0
248	Sassari	162**	18	44	140	158	141	0
249	Nuoro	102	7	39	150	204*	149	69
250	Cagliari/Oristano	124	34	83	79	173**	157**	41
IRELAND		160***	108	73	137***	60	115	180***
251	Eastern	134**	87	57	102	54	86	198***
252	Midland	170*	135	80	173*	45	116	135
253	Mid-Western	280***	88	88	103	113	136	87
254	North Eastern	107	127	97	133	30	169*	185*
255	North Western	65	97	92	232***	0	104	138
256	South Eastern	175**	144*	73	205***	47	117	197*
257	Southern	158**	146*	80	162**	83	130	165*
258	Western	217***	78	76	103	82	130	248***
NETHERLANDS		27	102	68	82	38	57	62
259	Groningen	22	89	34	89	13	42	22
260	Friesland	22	114	79	73	39	49	93
261	Drenthe	42	104	89	52	69	42	0
262	Overijssel	46	80	63	103	58	52	41
263	Gelderland	19	93	64	84	50	54	62
264	Utrecht	41	87	65	75	23	50	57
265	Noord Holland	21	116*	65	93	31	39	79
266	Zuid Holland	21	111	75	83	32	67	71
267	Zeeland	17	153*	80	95	43	63	18
268	Noord Brabant	24	94	68	64	43	75	54
269	Limburg	46	92	67	78	32	59	85
270	Zuidelijke Ijsselmeerpolders	0	25	0	61	0	33	56

Table 7.1.4(a) cont

Area		Indicators (SMRs)						
		TUB	CERV	UTER	HODG	CRHD	RESP	ASTH
	UK:ENGLAND AND WALES	53	186***	124***	90	61	123***	170***
271	Cleveland	70	240***	146**	157**	95	127	177*
272	Cumbria	26	210***	98	122	33	133	165*
273	Durham	83	216***	134*	87	64	156*	297***
274	Northumberland	54	203***	99	107	77	110	131
275	Gateshead	83	193***	97	62	0	93	342***
276	Newcastle upon Tyne	78	217***	111	86	0	74	140
277	Northern Tyneside	52	264***	147	93	0	151	34
278	Southern Tyneside	63	227***	108	81	52	31	169
279	Sunderland	94	209***	134	72	106	102	150
280	Bradford	118	244***	117	91	105	178**	184*
281	Calderdale	127	270***	182**	144	124	72	69
282	Humberside	52	235***	135**	121	46	156**	129
283	Kirklees	46	251***	150*	118	62	105	171*
284	Leeds	49	240***	170***	114	100	103	127
285	North Yorkshire	33	151***	119	96	46	99	105
286	Wakefield	30	238***	179***	137	96	220***	160
287	Barnsley	0	242***	186**	60	68	103	200*
288	Derbyshire	34	170***	129*	97	84	130	127
289	Doncaster	51	322***	180***	92	134	62	154
290	Leicestershire	56	190***	134**	124	35	142*	152*
291	Lincolnshire	37	192***	125	108	28	138	164*
292	Nottinghamshire	60	200***	133**	68	108	119	191***
293	Rotherham	22	213***	160*	43	59	104	174
294	Sheffield	33	156***	115	74	132	89	120
295	Cambridgeshire	33	115	82	74	49	53	153*
296	Norfolk	42	164***	104	43	67	162**	180**
297	Suffolk	32	169***	94	105	51	122	278***
298	Barnet	25	86	71	100	0	52	174
299	Bedfordshire	31	212***	104	96	56	114	212***
300	Brent and Harrow	80	136*	87	101	33	97	274***
301	Ealing/Hammersmith/Hounslow	120	159***	101	63	92	174**	212***
302	Hertfordshire	37	92	70	84	15	107	168**
303	Hillingdon	8	175**	133	79	98	85	81
304	Kensington/Chelsea/Westminster	178***	195***	141*	126	106	127	122
305	Barking and Havering	48	177***	124	138	0	186**	220**
306	Camden and Islington	107	176***	80	84	43	74	191*
307	City and East London	162***	205***	151**	65	89	204***	320***
308	Enfield and Haringey	61	195***	119	58	191*	150	160*
309	Essex	42	138***	83	91	20	90	128
310	Redbridge and Waltham Forest	50	146**	88	49	52	154	205**
311	Bromley	34	79	76	112	51	88	261***
312	East Sussex	34	200***	150**	90	53	125	187**
313	Greenwich and Bexley	51	102	89	93	70	120	220***
314	Kent	40	177***	121*	87	57	117	117
315	Lambeth/Southwark/Lewisham	136*	156***	111	92	69	111	147
316	Croydon	47	150*	117	50	23	89	116
317	Kingston and Richmond	25	116	87	116	49	95	216**
318	Merton/Sutton/Wandsworth	69	166***	115	76	51	123	224***
319	Surrey	38	135**	87	88	45	131	171**
320	West Sussex	36	114	83	83	25	94	146
321	Dorset	42	137*	101	74	57	159*	226***
322	Hampshire	35	166***	112	83	45	168***	161**
323	Isle of Wight	45	108	92	47	0	94	307**
324	Wiltshire	18	162***	71	114	29	139	118
325	Berkshire	50	104	80	81	31	71	93
326	Buckinghamshire	27	92	47	80	24	139	145
327	Northamptonshire	40	129	85	83	28	89	163*
328	Oxfordshire	15	107	91	70	27	115	163*
329	Avon	30	120	78	84	41	75	172**
330	Cornwall and Scilly Isles	33	185***	138*	51	37	117	144
331	Devon	37	177***	136**	66	9	126	191***
332	Gloucestershire	37	193***	126	64	46	183**	179*

Table 7.1.4(a) cont

Area		TUB	CERV	UTER	HODG	CRHD	RESP	ASTH
333	Somerset	56	157**	121	89	37	80	216**
334	Birmingham	92	167***	123*	102	105	130	251***
335	Coventry	98	214***	140*	161*	25	189**	161
336	Dudley	53	189***	138	121	120	94	62
337	Hereford and Worcester	38	191***	148**	76	81	93	137
338	Salop	15	197***	145*	79	19	83	179*
339	Sandwell	80	212***	152*	113	26	240***	130
340	Solihull	9	117	112	92	0	91	276***
341	Staffordshire	42	223***	153***	125	78	152**	194***
342	Walsall	94	203***	157*	69	57	204**	143
343	Warwickshire	54	191***	129	106	46	157*	285***
344	Wolverhampton	77	262***	147*	137	161	158	285***
345	Bolton	95	277***	162**	73	175	217**	171
346	Bury	44	190**	90	62	0	129	108
347	Lancashire	45	237***	148***	66	81	116	174***
348	Manchester	148*	340***	212***	85	151	109	156
349	Oldham	52	241***	158*	100	139	158	145
350	Rochdale	37	339***	159*	93	37	120	154
351	Salford	59	250***	174**	44	101	140	135
352	Stockport	38	117	104	102	26	64	132
353	Tameside	51	189***	108	124	0	170	119
354	Trafford	58	176**	124	73	176	131	146
355	Wigan	37	222***	140	62	94	42	140
356	Cheshire	40	253***	172***	72	32	92	188***
357	Liverpool	102	323***	226***	86	84	87	183*
358	St Helens and Knowsley	53	336***	257***	75	22	81	70
359	Sefton	54	275***	191***	108	53	130	155
360	Wirral	71	272***	222***	81	47	96	59
361	Clwyd	15	251***	167***	127	80	166*	50
362	Dyfed	47	246***	177***	120	146	74	101
363	Gwent	49	156**	131	133	53	148	177*
364	Gwynedd	81	193***	112	109	72	105	119
365	Mid Glamorgan	61	215***	144**	100	186*	124	312***
366	Powys	16	199**	98	123	0	133	183
367	South Glamorgan	72	214***	131	77	41	145	115
368	West Glamorgan	58	183***	105	116	87	105	163
UK:NORTHERN IRELAND								
369	Northern Ireland	52	157***	112	129*	58	135*	187***
UK:SCOTLAND		81	192***	126***	90	75	108	148***
370	Highlands and Islands	29	198***	136	104	29	78	216**
371	Grampian	53	147**	80	73	32	66	103
372	Tayside	56	123	92	97	41	149	100
373	Fife	17	294***	208***	120	23	132	75
374	Lothian	33	185***	138**	76	83	107	143
375	Borders	18	115	88	136	0	50	68
376	Forth Valley	83	176**	82	89	56	200**	138
377	Argyll and Clyde	130	198***	114	109	35	108	84
378	Greater Glasgow	167***	191***	131**	76	153*	87	226***
379	Lanarkshire	58	209***	130*	105	120	138	129
380	Ayrshire and Arran	80	247***	150**	87	83	83	239***
381	Dumfries and Galloway	87	171*	130	56	0	99	92
PORTUGAL		313***	85	129***	76	345***	275***	-
382	Viana do Castelo	208***	65	138	23	147	443***	-
383	Braga	160***	51	109	31	392***	335***	-
384	Vila Real	203***	56	93	22	218*	415***	-
385	Braganca	141	75	158*	46	157	428***	-
386	Guarda	204***	40	114	83	384***	172	-
387	Viseu	420***	67	104	28	247***	421***	-
388	Porto	520***	116	177***	83	592***	323***	-
389	Aveiro	143*	66	168***	28	258***	237***	-
390	Coimbra	235***	48	126	50	324***	306***	-

Table 7.1.4(a) cont

Area		Indicators (SMRs)						
		TUB	CERV	UTER	HODG	CRHD	RESP	ASTH
391	Castelo Branco	169**	27	72	35	329***	227**	-
392	Portalegre	160*	32	101	37	332**	139	-
393	Santarem	111	38	108	23	74	156*	-
394	Leiria	93	77	111	39	77	177**	-
395	Lisboa	510***	140***	141***	171***	444***	281***	-
396	Setubal	112	51	68	47	92	69	-
397	Evora	118	34	93	58	98	102	-
398	Beja	189**	43	90	29	496***	49	-
399	Faro	229***	80	108	66	179	97	-
400	Madeira	386***	98	113	49	321***	293***	-
401	Azores	521***	115	175**	50	488***	470***	-
SPAIN		181***	44	88	85	218***	117***	41
402	La Coruña	330***	53	107	130*	266***	190***	12
403	Lugo	238***	37	117	71	132	178*	73
404	Orense	267***	26	88	31	133	172*	48
405	Pontevedra	242***	25	133**	62	111	123	67
406	Asturias	214***	58	98	97	235***	96	30
407	Cantabria	165***	62	107	81	200**	141	52
408	Alava	124	15	41	98	114	133	0
409	Guipuzcoa	142**	32	65	116	44	112	27
410	Vizcaya	178***	47	84	87	164**	95	42
411	Navarra	156**	14	38	98	192*	115	51
412	Rioja	144	14	39	85	66	79	27
413	Huesca	39	22	95	37	44	129	0
414	Teruel	55	0	87	53	64	132	0
415	Zaragoza	132*	18	74	84	210***	81	0
416	Madrid Centro	143***	36	51	60	214***	103	28
417	Avila	124	18	48	75	363***	124	0
418	Burgos	148*	24	38	68	120	59	19
419	Leon	195***	31	90	61	417***	146	68
420	Palencia	145	18	117	102	49	70	75
421	Salamanca	285***	24	93	100	357***	149	19
422	Segovia	84	11	45	111	189	236**	48
423	Soria	52	0	84	164	389**	200	0
424	Valladolid	139*	36	118	125	182*	87	13
425	Zamora	111	14	97	71	168	45	0
426	Albacete	216***	38	82	60	239**	149	0
427	Ciudad Real	186***	7	64	107	273***	173**	30
428	Cuenca	108	24	95	39	271**	63	69
429	Guadalajara	128	12	25	79	136	117	0
430	Toledo	129	19	65	53	386***	123	60
431	Badajoz	202***	14	77	136*	388***	129	87
432	Caceres	201***	39	86	102	312***	146	0
433	Barcelona	137***	50	92	84	141***	95	40
434	Gerona	121	40	86	93	109	108	103
435	Lerida	117	23	107	83	152	87	0
436	Tarragona	165***	27	124	81	164	116	119
437	Alicante	136**	39	96	62	243***	132*	34
438	Castellon de la Plana	155**	28	103	77	255***	106	48
439	Valencia	158***	63	102	106	332***	113	47
440	Baleares	164***	100	125	122	98	116	101
441	Almeria	267***	34	92	80	148	156*	49
442	Cadiz	240***	61	114	82	255***	109	45
443	Cordoba	181***	33	73	65	262***	197***	28
444	Granada	184***	45	65	109	176*	97	18
445	Huelva	290***	46	91	64	255***	95	33
446	Jaen	181***	29	87	69	411***	201***	32
447	Malaga	255***	49	110	118	361***	101	75
448	Sevilla	420***	83	137***	105	341***	120	57
449	Murcia	130*	48	78	53	170**	134*	0
450	Las Palmas	243***	80	98	71	236***	103	102
451	Sta Cruz de Tenerife	133*	128	119	106	210***	126	57

Table 7.1.4(b). 'Avoidable death' indicators by small area and country, standardized to the EC standard, for appendicitis, abdominal hernia, cholelithiasis/cholecystitis, hypertensive/cerebrovascular diseases, maternal mortality, perinatal mortality, and all causes

Notes on the use of this table

1. This table shows within-EC variations, the value for the whole EC being 100.

2. Key for the abbreviations used for columns of the table:
   APP   — appendicitis (ICD8 540–543; ICD9 540–543), ages 5–64;
   HERN   — abdominal hernia (ICD8 550–553; ICD9 550–553), ages 5–64;
   CHOLY— cholelithiasis and cholecystitis diseases (ICD8 574–575; ICD9 574–575.1, 576.1), ages 5–64;
   HYP/S   — hypertensive and cerebrovascular diseases (ICD8 400–404, 430–438; ICD9 401–405, 430–438), ages 35–64;
   MAT   — maternal deaths (ICD8 630–678; ICD9 630–676), all ages;
   PER   — perinatal mortality (all causes) deaths aged under 1 week plus stillbirths;
   ALL   — mortality from all causes (all ICD8/ICD9 codes), all ages.

3. The small area numbers are as in the key maps.

4. The indicators have been tested for indicating significant excess mortality relative to EC rates. The *p*-values achieved for one-tail tests are indicated as follows: *$p<0.05$;**$p<0.01$;***$p<0.001$.

5. The indicators are based on mortality data for 1980–84, except for Greece (1980–82) and Spain (1979–83). The population data are for 1980–84 except for France (1982), Greece (1981), Ireland (1981), and Spain (1981). All data for Italy are for 1979–83.

Table 7.1.4(b)

Area	Indicators (SMRs)						
	APP	HERN	CHOLY	HYP/S	MAT	PER	ALL
BELGIUM	49	49	97	82	62	99	107***
1 Antwerpen	21	23	70	82	79	101	102***
2 Brabant	67	62	99	76	71	96	101***
3 West-Vlaanderen	16	45	105	62	38	106*	100
4 Oost-Vlaanderen	101	45	47	72	32	100	106***
5 Hainaut	38	87	141*	99	33	94	117***
6 Liège	33	34	98	93	73	91	118***
7 Limburg	24	19	89	76	99	109*	101*
8 Luxembourg (province)	0	54	254**	100	115	102	111***
9 Namur	122	58	101	108	64	99	119***
LUXEMBOURG							
10 Luxembourg	188	69	140	119***	0	86	116***
FEDERAL REPUBLIC OF GERMANY	128***	79	123***	92	136***	77	104***
11 Schleswig–Holstein	140	73	126	78	106	73	103***
12 Hamburg	145	57	99	85	117	68	105***
13 Braunschweig	196**	81	135*	95	102	80	103***
14 Hannover	156*	70	158***	90	56	74	102***
15 Luneburg	187**	103	128	85	37	72	104***
16 Weser–Ems	173**	68	104	88	117	85	104***
17 Bremen	172	69	120	104	30	72	104***
18 Düsseldorf	92	51	81	90	181***	90	107***
19 Köln	77	50	96	90	162**	77	106***
20 Münster	125	62	130*	99	169**	96	109***
21 Detmold	103	40	117	86	123	82	100
22 Arnsberg	166***	89	132**	103	174***	89	109***
23 Darmstadt	113	137*	132*	88	171**	72	101**
24 Giessen	192*	164*	124	88	138	73	103***
25 Kassel	196**	59	170**	85	124	79	101*
26 Koblenz	133	102	69	110***	125	76	105***
27 Trier	35	124	72	111*	134	71	107***

Table 7.1.4(b) cont

Area		APP	HERN	CHOLY	HYP/S	MAT	PER	ALL
		\multicolumn{7}{Indicators (SMRs)}						
28	Rheinhessen–Pfalz	166*	60	99	113***	209***	81	108***
29	Stuttgart	93	91	117	79	120	68	95
30	Karlsruhe	134	71	141**	95	121	71	101***
31	Freiburg	92	103	154**	79	125	64	95
32	Tübingen	81	79	91	83	88	65	94
33	Oberbayern	79	41	70	75	87	68	94
34	Niederbayern	186*	148	193***	101	221***	72	111***
35	Oberpfalz	174*	152	169**	109**	202**	81	113***
36	Oberfranken	157	155*	224***	109**	142	72	111***
37	Mittelfranken	133	118	164**	90	133	73	106***
38	Unterfranken	99	62	227***	78	124	76	105***
39	Schwaben	177*	56	65	85	220***	74	103***
40	Saarland	77	65	149*	123***	83	88	114***
41	Berlin (West)	137	63	205***	128***	111	85	119***
DENMARK		104	65	73	77	48	69	102***
42	Kobenhavn and Frederiksberg (M)	89	57	67	97	65	66	112***
43	Kobenhavns County	78	37	64	72	58	51	100
44	Frederiksborg County	106	42	72	70	103	61	101
45	Roskilde County	88	0	0	72	0	66	102*
46	Vestsjaellands County	61	44	51	71	122	77	103***
47	Storstroms County	192	88	77	77	0	59	106***
48	Bornholms County	0	0	0	63	0	80	103*
49	Fyns County	113	81	141	68	0	64	101
50	Sonderjyllands County	209	205	60	75	0	76	98
51	Ribe County	0	61	71	75	0	64	97
52	Vejle County	159	116	90	80	0	60	99
53	Ringkobing County	134	51	176	89	53	76	98
54	Arhus County	92	69	53	70	27	83	101
55	Viborg County	75	107	63	83	65	77	97
56	Nordjyllands County	106	25	44	74	130	78	99
FRANCE		112*	130***	21	78	118***	93	92
57	Ain	249*	249**	18	68	170	85	89
58	Aisne	226*	145	42	92	163	99	103***
59	Allier	179	122	18	86	126	103	94
60	Alpes-de-Haute-Provence	140	0	0	72	124	107	74
61	Hautes-Alpes	159	112	65	65	120	101	88
62	Alpes-Maritimes	76	63	7	56	86	101	79
63	Ardèche	125	218*	51	81	156	107	90
64	Ardennes	0	353***	51	90	110	107	101
65	Ariège	118	0	0	58	0	113	86
66	Aube	182	180	78	81	127	93	91
67	Aude	0	153	0	61	112	85	84
68	Aveyron	0	243*	24	65	168	98	83
69	Bouches-du-Rhône	88	100	21	73	169**	99	91
70	Calvados	120	183*	13	86	73	81	94
71	Cantal	305*	141	0	100	89	119*	97
72	Charente	100	141	21	68	157	102	87
73	Charente-Maritime	65	45	13	66	53	84	86
74	Cher	214	190	44	79	88	90	91
75	Corrèze	201	221*	0	80	0	86	91
76	Corse	0	48	0	76	59	109	89
77	Côte-d'Or	112	141	16	68	142	99	87
78	Côtes-du-Nord	61	188*	12	105	74	71	101
79	Creuse	235	151	44	111	25	81	91
80	Dordogne	212*	167	0	88	412**	91	89
81	Doubs	75	88	0	76	171	91	90
82	Drôme	264**	129	19	63	22	98	87
83	Eure	77	118	34	80	122	99	95
84	Eure-et-Loir	98	0	0	69	61	86	88
85	Finistère	61	129	25	101	121	80	101**
86	Gard	279***	129	25	61	175	109*	88
87	Haute-Garonne	21	61	35	60	116	89	84
88	Gers	0	63	0	66	100	94	85

Table 7.1.4(b) cont

Area		Indicators (SMRs)						
		APP	HERN	CHOLY	HYP/S	MAT	PER	ALL
89	Gironde	121	87	19	73	80	87	90
90	Hérault	94	182*	38	67	153	106	86
91	Ille-et-Vilaine	116	123	31	95	90	85	99
92	Indre	139	336***	28	82	0	100	90
93	Indre-et-Loire	174	129	30	52	74	76	83
94	Isère	131	87	58	64	86	83	89
95	Jura	70	0	0	85	104	98	90
96	Landes	0	0	22	74	0	94	89
97	Loir-et-Cher	0	84	24	88	46	70	84
98	Loire	161	184*	29	73	81	85	93
99	Haute-Loire	163	226*	33	86	138	96	92
100	Loire-Atlantique	141	148	0	86	66	84	96
101	Loiret	33	74	14	66	21	91	86
102	Lot	0	138	0	81	0	90	87
103	Lot-et-Garonne	162	0	0	73	96	95	87
104	Lozère	227	155	0	86	185	113	92
105	Maine-et-Loire	107	104	24	71	45	88	88
106	Manche	0	104	30	84	74	81	94
107	Marne	199*	131	0	74	157	88	93
108	Haute-Marne	167	63	0	78	371***	103	96
109	Mayenne	318**	187	27	80	41	83	90
110	Meurthe-et-Moselle	24	186*	11	87	94	89	99
111	Meuse	345**	256*	0	98	286**	116*	100
112	Morbihan	86	82	12	121***	80	89	108***
113	Moselle	153	144	15	100	297***	101	106***
114	Nièvre	283*	241*	0	90	122	95	94
115	Nord	230***	220***	44	109***	100	107***	110***
116	Oise	82	177	13	80	65	92	96
117	Orne	114	41	24	80	80	68	93
118	Pas-de-Calais	134	246***	27	112***	123	117***	110***
119	Puy-de-Dôme	85	104	12	85	89	112**	95
120	Pyrénées-Atlantiques	0	106	0	67	180	86	88
121	Hautes-Pyrénées	71	195	0	82	68	106	89
122	Pyrénées-Orientales	144	64	19	66	399***	102	87
123	Bas-Rhin	0	164*	43	94	52	71	101
124	Haut-Rhin	161	123	0	96	158	93	103***
125	Rhône	60	146	21	63	127	86	87
126	Haute-Saône	301*	112	0	96	204	91	96
127	Saône-et-Loire	207*	84	37	79	137	99	90
128	Sarthe	207*	103	30	58	168	84	85
129	Savoie	53	236*	23	76	38	72	91
130	Haute-Savoie	107	221*	32	70	92	82	91
131	Paris	71	125	9	65	158**	97	80
132	Seine-Maritime	59	159*	7	84	78	96	97
133	Seine-et-Marne	145	118	29	67	126	88	94
134	Yvelines	103	84	21	62	194***	83	85
135	Deux-Sèvres	251*	182	64	68	150	96	84
136	Somme	97	98	43	82	145	98	103***
137	Tarn	48	130	19	64	86	90	85
138	Tarn-et-Garonne	0	0	0	74	0	109	85
139	Var	46	94	55	69	75	102	87
140	Vaucluse	79	57	33	68	88	106	90
141	Vendée	108	105	15	82	0	81	89
142	Vienne	94	103	20	64	70	91	80
143	Haute-Vienne	0	65	0	78	134	72	84
144	Vosges	132	197*	0	96	294***	91	98
145	Yonne	167	157	23	85	81	84	93
146	Territoire-de-Belfort	133	205	59	87	82	83	98
147	Essonne	109	91	9	70	170*	80	85
148	Hauts-de-Seine	84	34	10	66	134	92	84
149	Seine-Saint-Denis	79	144	12	75	132	100	92
150	Val-de-Marne	100	86	6	65	150	87	88
151	Val-d'Oise	39	110	9	66	101	91	92

Table 7.1.4(b) cont

Area		Indicators (SMRs)						
		APP	HERN	CHOLY	HYP/S	MAT	PER	ALL
GREECE		41	42	51	107***	72	138***	95
152	Greater Athens	38	56	49	109***	41	149***	98
153	Rest of Central Greece and Eubea	26	39	68	112**	106	120***	91
154	Peloponnisos	28	20	35	100	38	144***	89
155	Ionian Islands	300	102	0	107	77	110	103**
156	Epirus	0	0	38	92	154	144***	90
157	Thessaly	81	60	104	111*	0	118***	98
158	Macedonia	42	44	44	105	58	145***	99
159	Thrace	0	0	0	143***	361***	143***	107***
160	Aegean Islands	0	49	57	100	180	117***	96
161	Crete	58	0	74	97	68	112**	84
ITALY		96	122***	187***	117***	97	124***	102***
162	Torino	141	188***	303***	122***	117	135***	106***
163	Vercelli	82	28	195**	153***	57	144***	107***
164	Novara	0	142	136	144***	78	101	108***
165	Cuneo	150	314***	218***	128***	103	113*	108***
166	Asti	76	51	209*	128***	324*	113	106***
167	Alessandria	207*	161	213**	118***	56	120**	101
168	Aosta	144	103	179	106	0	114	107***
169	Imperia	426***	96	195*	100	0	91	100
170	Savona	52	70	121	106	0	115*	102*
171	Genova	89	138	274***	102	103	102	103***
172	La Spezia	0	169	171	101	105	99	99
173	Varese	43	81	225***	124***	67	116***	105***
174	Como/Sondrio	18	68	212***	133***	17	93	109***
175	Milano	82	104	139**	121***	63	103	106***
176	Bergamo	78	106	192***	149***	68	109*	109***
177	Brescia	116	38	131	143***	48	99	117***
178	Pavia	94	107	148	158***	94	105	113***
179	Cremona	146	102	177*	161***	121	105	117***
180	Mantova	43	119	86	143***	57	98	109***
181	Bolzano	164	64	223**	104	160	96	103***
182	Trento	0	114	280***	104	39	100	105***
183	Verona	86	16	202***	132***	111	116***	105***
184	Vicenza	118	108	240***	135***	92	94	108***
185	Belluno	74	52	181	144***	179	93	110***
186	Treviso	0	127	167*	105	48	91	100
187	Venezia	80	74	146	100	0	110*	101**
188	Padova	42	111	110	109*	65	105	103***
189	Rovigo	64	227*	211*	117**	149	95	108***
190	Udine/Gorizia	73	119	206***	122***	65	103	109***
191	Trieste	163	35	245***	90	107	66	105***
192	Pordenone	62	91	184	103	70	93	104***
193	Piacenza	112	0	218**	123***	89	104	101*
194	Parma	118	105	213**	109*	122	127***	99
195	Reggio Emilia	38	0	122	98	0	106	96
196	Modena	27	93	173*	97	72	107	97
197	Bologna	99	88	185***	99	148	108	96
198	Ferrara	40	55	127	103	136	107	100
199	Ravenna	44	61	142	85	0	103	90
200	Forli	0	58	90	84	160	95	93
201	Pesaro	146	68	198*	93	162	101	93
202	Ancona	37	102	133	96	43	99	91
203	Macerata	109	37	195*	97	132	126***	93
204	Ascoli Piceno	45	96	148	101	47	116**	93
205	Massa-Carrara	236	109	189	113*	97	117*	100
206	Lucca	168	87	118	101	53	107	100
207	Pistoia	61	85	123	82	0	96	96
208	Firenze	27	65	144*	87	37	112**	91
209	Livorno	365***	93	217**	96	191	116	98
210	Pisa	41	29	264***	77	159	108	97
211	Arezzo	101	34	199*	93	64	115*	94

Table 7.1.4(b) cont

Area		Indicators (SMRs)						
		APP	HERN	CHOLY	HYP/S	MAT	PER	ALL
212	Siena	300**	235*	182*	94	0	125**	92
213	Grosseto	0	47	164	109	414**	113	97
214	Perugia	0	147	128	104	61	88	93
215	Terni	0	91	105	94	0	139***	98
216	Viterbo/Rieti	77	160	232***	115**	118	117**	102**
217	Roma	93	129	175***	96	91	115***	100
218	Latina	40	96	241***	119***	58	123***	102***
219	Frosinone	37	109	142	136***	111	121***	97
220	Caserta	119	406***	191**	183***	143	143***	111***
221	Benevento	0	84	98	126***	254**	128***	98
222	Napoli	155*	268***	260***	159***	91	145***	120***
223	Avellino	39	29	203**	113**	57	118***	111***
224	Salerno	189*	93	178**	132***	155*	137***	94
225	L'Aquila	55	114	177	117**	102	125***	101
226	Teramo	62	91	185*	108	103	101	95
227	Pescara	173	84	147	108	217	114*	91
228	Chieti	176	31	271***	95	40	127***	92
229	Isernia/Campobasso	51	146	233**	130***	132	125***	95
230	Foggia	26	168	86	115***	81	141***	94
231	Bari	149	101	164**	112***	47	141***	95
232	Taranto	157	203*	206**	104	213**	141***	100
233	Brindisi	223*	70	121	117**	78	138***	103***
234	Lecce	69	161	145	106	74	133***	99
235	Potenza/Matera	142	153	177*	127***	61	131***	95
236	Cosenza	72	170	296***	136***	79	135***	93
237	Catanzaro	171	79	149	113**	144	131***	93
238	Reggio Calabria	61	117	122	114**	19	150***	93
239	Trapani	0	124	144	144***	87	115**	99
240	Palermo	133	161*	133	133***	150	172***	101*
241	Messina	151	165	223***	111**	140	150***	96
242	Agrigento	75	232**	101	119***	48	123***	97
243	Caltanisetta	184	191	139	127***	155	160***	104***
244	Enna	89	268*	195	151***	175	130***	104***
245	Catania	174*	95	275***	138***	169*	149***	104***
246	Ragusa	125	93	215*	130***	434***	131***	108***
247	Siracusa	0	208*	161	123***	150	140***	100
248	Sassari	0	165	191*	114**	130	131***	96
249	Nuoro	133	159	245**	116*	186	127***	96
250	Cagliari/Oristano	83	168*	360***	107*	99	150***	96
IRELAND		94	63	102	117***	58	108***	122***
251	Eastern	82	14	90	121***	35	112***	117***
252	Midland	0	72	85	102	118	89	127***
253	Mid-Western	245*	98	29	129***	54	105	130***
254	North Eastern	132	159	155	127***	82	111*	124***
255	North Western	180	68	120	122**	42	109	120***
256	South Eastern	51	81	119	115**	88	116***	125***
257	Southern	36	28	148	114**	33	109**	125***
258	Western	109	124	73	95	103	88	116***
NETHERLANDS		83	74	120**	66	65	81	92
259	Groningen	128	24	42	67	26	79	91
260	Friesland	92	95	83	68	85	80	91
261	Drenthe	41	30	142	63	100	80	91
262	Overijssel	121	107	116	71	73	78	93
263	Gelderland	73	56	107	69	24	82	93
264	Utrecht	20	76	62	69	74	83	90
265	Noord Holland	68	84	150**	57	84	83	92
266	Zuid Holland	68	67	120	65	79	79	90
267	Zeeland	200	37	86	58	0	84	87
268	Noord Brabant	85	109	161**	70	73	82	93
269	Limburg	126	48	124	72	42	86	97
270	Zuidelijke Ijsselmeerpolders	212	0	0	55	0	61	76

Table 7.1.4(b) cont

Area		APP	HERN	CHOLY	HYP/S	MAT	PER	ALL
		Indicators (SMRs)						
UK:ENGLAND AND WALES		69	102	70	104***	73	89	105***
271	Cleveland	178	108	100	132***	82	103	120***
272	Cumbria	0	24	28	130***	152	101	110***
273	Durham	108	76	55	132***	113	97	117***
274	Northumberland	0	77	67	115**	0	79	116***
275	Gateshead	76	53	61	148***	66	103	120***
276	Newcastle upon Tyne	119	82	96	124***	49	95	113***
277	Northern Tyneside	81	109	95	110	73	86	116***
278	Southern Tyneside	0	198	38	135***	89	100	119***
279	Sunderland	281**	41	189*	134***	81	99	118***
280	Bradford	37	27	32	141***	69	109*	115***
281	Calderdale	88	124	36	136***	203	112	114***
282	Humberside	59	126	65	109*	78	98	109***
283	Kirklees	183	132	58	126***	98	108	118***
284	Leeds	47	83	78	111**	77	94	109***
285	North Yorkshire	50	71	21	102	68	98	103***
286	Wakefield	0	38	67	105	124	106	120***
287	Barnsley	0	104	91	102	59	80	112***
288	Derbyshire	55	102	37	114***	106	92	109***
289	Doncaster	57	163	47	117**	172	85	111***
290	Leicestershire	100	73	60	102	87	84	101*
291	Lincolnshire	61	86	50	103	79	87	107***
292	Nottinghamshire	101	96	77	113***	14	84	108***
293	Rotherham	66	48	83	118**	100	113*	112***
294	Sheffield	0	127	62	115***	57	90	108***
295	Cambridgeshire	30	154	64	83	65	79	97
296	Norfolk	48	117	68	79	127	82	96
297	Suffolk	85	203*	47	79	112	75	96
298	Barnet	58	81	71	70	45	73	94
299	Bedfordshire	34	77	89	94	109	83	101
300	Brent and Harrow	76	28	48	82	27	80	92
301	Ealing/Hammersmith/Hounslow	27	177*	11	97	37	76	104***
302	Hertfordshire	0	132	56	79	43	69	98
303	Hillingdon	72	101	59	73	113	83	97
304	Kensington/Chelsea/Westminster	109	195	68	118**	88	78	98
305	Barking and Havering	80	27	48	82	108	89	104***
306	Camden and Islington	153	219*	85	104	38	83	103***
307	City and East London	31	90	118	121***	87	104	112***
308	Enfield and Haringey	37	53	123	88	108	82	101
309	Essex	91	65	85	78	46	82	100
310	Redbridge and Waltham Forest	38	53	31	91	86	89	97
311	Bromley	54	0	21	83	0	65	95
312	East Sussex	0	70	62	89	101	77	95
313	Greenwich and Bexley	116	82	112	87	59	87	101
314	Kent	81	66	92	91	37	90	102***
315	Lambeth/Southwark/Lewisham	193*	186*	59	118***	100	96	107***
316	Croydon	106	38	88	96	0	74	102**
317	Kingston and Richmond	172	40	46	84	49	68	95
318	Merton/Sutton/Wandsworth	29	61	47	94	22	81	102***
319	Surrey	65	101	33	72	92	81	96
320	West Sussex	52	35	41	78	69	82	94
321	Dorset	85	171	66	79	56	69	92
322	Hampshire	12	86	30	79	44	78	98
323	Isle of Wight	284	0	0	90	0	90	96
324	Wiltshire	98	119	41	84	75	78	99
325	Berkshire	49	56	32	80	35	72	100
326	Buckinghamshire	60	45	65	81	65	86	97
327	Northamptonshire	98	24	56	101	71	94	102**
328	Oxfordshire	32	97	57	77	25	59	94
329	Avon	91	103	90	85	61	87	98
330	Cornwall and Scilly Isles	0	106	138	90	103	81	101*
331	Devon	71	147	36	89	111	77	98
332	Gloucestershire	100	141	82	103	0	81	99

Table 7.1.4(b) cont

Area		APP	HERN	CHOLY	HYP/S	MAT	PER	ALL
		Indicators (SMRs)						
333	Somerset	39	165	32	99	34	82	99
334	Birmingham	49	128	102	131***	56	104	114***
335	Coventry	52	37	107	124***	77	111*	109***
336	Dudley	163	38	111	119**	0	83	107***
337	Hereford and Worcester	107	134	33	104	129	90	104***
338	Salop	45	199*	39	117**	181	114**	105***
339	Sandwell	105	145	42	147***	164	132***	113***
340	Solihull	82	177	0	77	76	94	95
341	Staffordshire	49	118	144*	113***	51	105	113***
342	Walsall	122	349***	76	125***	49	115*	116***
343	Warwickshire	0	150	72	101	30	91	107***
344	Wolverhampton	191	89	182	119**	200	118**	109***
345	Bolton	65	0	136	126***	137	91	120***
346	Bury	98	284*	82	111	0	101	115***
347	Lancashire	86	251***	75	123***	77	99	114***
348	Manchester	112	133	93	150***	130	107	123***
349	Oldham	0	111	97	153***	160	102	120***
350	Rochdale	0	121	211*	129***	109	112*	117***
351	Salford	135	93	55	148***	54	81	123***
352	Stockport	116	83	24	113*	0	86	107***
353	Tameside	231	0	63	143***	0	97	117***
354	Trafford	0	0	124	112	0	92	106***
355	Wigan	0	0	70	127***	81	83	121***
356	Cheshire	36	91	113	106	58	87	111***
357	Liverpool	66	116	95	142***	124	85	120***
358	St Helens and Knowsley	47	68	159	145***	131	89	122***
359	Sefton	111	39	68	124***	49	84	108***
360	Wirral	50	35	61	114*	117	86	111***
361	Clwyd	0	124	72	117**	106	99	106***
362	Dyfed	98	133	136	135***	87	85	111***
363	Gwent	74	78	61	118***	30	92	112***
364	Gwynedd	74	51	30	123***	62	86	103***
365	Mid Glamorgan	93	87	139	140***	112	106	119***
366	Powys	0	103	60	113	0	93	108***
367	South Glamorgan	43	123	54	106	32	88	104***
368	West Glamorgan	44	30	35	123***	73	90	112***
UK:NORTHERN IRELAND								
369	Northern Ireland	94	117	105	125***	74	106**	119***
UK:SCOTLAND		79	96	5	143***	114	90	119***
370	Highlands and Islands	130	48	0	132***	92	88	119***
371	Grampian	72	79	0	115**	158	79	110***
372	Tayside	42	179	17	126***	106	69	112***
373	Fife	0	0	0	151***	75	90	115***
374	Lothian	46	49	0	126***	131	92	112***
375	Borders	166	113	0	147***	0	91	111***
376	Forth Valley	62	224*	52	139***	197	101	118***
377	Argyll and Clyde	150	136	16	154***	84	93	127***
378	Greater Glasgow	50	81	0	161***	118	87	126***
379	Lanarkshire	119	111	0	151***	126	96	127***
380	Ayrshire and Arran	134	160	0	171***	103	111*	126***
381	Dumfries and Galloway	113	0	0	122**	0	89	116***
PORTUGAL		136**	90	92	199***	151***	169***	105***
382	Viana do Castelo	0	97	28	196***	126	182***	103***
383	Braga	132	45	53	205***	170*	180***	107***
384	Vila Real	64	47	84	233***	200	235***	116***
385	Braganca	89	125	0	216***	64	185***	107***
386	Guarda	81	55	32	209***	187	161***	100
387	Viseu	121	117	86	230***	121	195***	107***
388	Porto	161*	94	165**	213***	133	186***	125***
389	Aveiro	28	45	65	187***	180*	171***	106***
390	Coimbra	152	54	94	254***	111	154***	123***

Table 7.1.4(b) cont

Area		Indicators (SMRs)						
		APP	HERN	CHOLY	HYP/S	MAT	PER	ALL
391	Castelo Branco	137	136	0	175***	361***	195***	38
392	Portalegre	109	283*	41	169***	199	194***	97
393	Santarem	70	73	113	164***	173	162***	96
394	Leiria	118	115	33	199***	217*	130***	105***
395	Lisboa	221***	122	118	209***	129	137***	125***
396	Setubal	99	0	33	105	161	148***	83
397	Evora	86	115	135	176***	219	149***	98
398	Beja	168	168	66	152***	142	167***	99
399	Faro	99	0	98	148***	39	163***	100
400	Madeira	144	59	241**	294***	76	193***	114***
401	Azores	147	169	33	272***	237**	191***	123***
SPAIN		108	101	103	99	91	102***	89
402	La Coruña	94	82	102	119***	158*	96	91
403	Lugo	0	127	30	81	121	129***	89
404	Orense	187	51	89	103	141	180***	81
405	Pontevedra	120	139	45	110**	41	94	93
406	Asturias	158	82	119	94	162*	108*	91
407	Cantabria	133	49	86	99	147	104	89
408	Alava	279*	57	66	71	49	96	89
409	Guipuzcoa	50	78	68	78	88	106	83
410	Vizcaya	72	78	116	93	95	111***	93
411	Navarra	134	125	116	86	27	93	91
412	Rioja	65	47	82	90	275**	128***	89
413	Huesca	0	97	142	77	74	95	74
414	Teruel	104	0	203	83	106	82	80
415	Zaragoza	118	113	156*	90	90	103	83
416	Madrid Centro	30	50	50	72	52	89	82
417	Avila	0	60	35	74	171	103	75
418	Burgos	92	33	135	78	0	70	75
419	Leon	244**	43	125	91	190*	139***	90
420	Palencia	88	62	108	100	73	118*	89
421	Salamanca	137	0	115	85	158	117**	76
422	Segovia	109	0	0	82	197	83	84
423	Soria	162	0	0	81	0	85	74
424	Valladolid	111	87	236***	71	162	54	76
425	Zamora	0	47	0	73	288*	113	80
426	Albacete	101	153	267***	111*	34	133***	94
427	Ciudad Real	70	203*	89	119***	229**	104	95
428	Cuenca	304**	53	92	95	138	123**	88
429	Guadalajara	117	81	95	73	0	84	72
430	Toledo	70	126	132	88	77	105	87
431	Badajoz	134	120	140	138***	140	106	97
432	Caceres	81	149	35	124***	267**	109*	90
433	Barcelona	67	45	75	90	50	66	81
434	Gerona	247**	177	44	76	0	89	93
435	Lerida	180	0	108	95	86	101	83
436	Tarragona	131	72	42	96	99	89	90
437	Alicante	76	82	88	124***	107	91	97
438	Castellon de la Plana	155	0	130	101	181	110*	90
439	Valencia	167*	196***	176***	135***	60	89	101***
440	Baleares	104	38	111	108*	56	111**	92
441	Almeria	44	175	41	106	142	126***	95
442	Cadiz	114	242***	160*	129***	117	138***	104***
443	Cordoba	168	55	128	107	106	110**	91
444	Granada	207*	266***	135	93	145	112***	95
445	Huelva	84	194	169	126***	49	144***	99
446	Jaen	191*	146	36	102	69	127***	89
447	Malaga	87	193**	225***	115***	62	126***	103***
448	Sevilla	158*	233***	130	125***	99	135***	101**
449	Murcia	223**	103	137	105	73	86	97
450	Las Palmas	163	171	142	144***	97	131***	105***
451	Sta Cruz de Tenerife	28	95	83	107	16	95	95

Table 7.1.5(a). 'Avoidable death' indicators by small area , standardized to own country's standard, for tuberculosis, malignant neoplasm of the cervix uteri, malignant neoplasm of the cervix and body of the uterus, Hodgkin's disease, chronic rheumatic heart disease, all respiratory diseases, and asthma

---

Notes on the use of this table

1. This table shows within-country variations, the value for the whole country being 100. Asthma data for Greece and Portugal are not available.

2. Key for the abbreviations used for columns of the table:
   TUB   — tuberculosis (ICD8 010–019; ICD9 010–018, 137), ages 5–64;
   CERV — malignant neoplasm of the cervix uteri (ICD8 180; ICD9 180), ages 15–64;
   UTER — malignant neoplasm of the cervix and body of the uterus (ICD8 180, 182; ICD9 179, 180, 182), ages 15–54;
   HODG — Hodgkin's disease (ICD8 201; ICD9 201), ages 5–64;
   CRHD — chronic rheumatic heart disease (ICD8 393–398; ICD9 393–398), ages 5–44;
   RESP — all respiratory diseases (ICD8 460–519; ICD9 460–519), ages 1–14;
   ASTH — asthma (ICD8 493; ICD9 493), ages 5–44.

3. The small area numbers are as in the key maps

4. The indicators have been tested for indicating significant excess mortality relative to EC rates. The *p*-values achieved for one-tail tests are indicated as follows:
   *$p<0.05$;**$p<0.01$;***$p<001$.

5. The indicators are based on mortality data for 1980–84, except for Greece (1980–82) and Spain (1979–83). The population data are for 1980–84 except for France (1982), Greece (1981), Ireland (1981), and Spain (1981). All data for Italy are for 1979–83.

Table 7.1.5(a)

Area	Indicators (SMRs)						
	TUB	CERV	UTER	HODG	CRHD	RESP	ASTH
BELGIUM							
1 Antwerpen	36	111	89	134**	56	84	82
2 Brabant	152***	79	104	72	120	114	91
3 West-Vlaanderen	65	101	88	95	83	73	119
4 Oost-Vlaanderen	41	112	95	142***	67	135	65
5 Hainaut	165***	142***	103	90	216	83	158***
6 Liège	115	67	116	84	184	137	120
7 Limburg	74	99	102	97	0	73	48
8 Luxembourg (province)	42	79	92	97	0	51	36
9 Namur	163*	93	113	74	0	101	189**
LUXEMBOURG							
10 Luxembourg	100	100	100	100	100	100	100
FEDERAL REPUBLIC OF GERMANY							
11 Schleswig–Holstein	77	111	108	98	22	77	103
12 Hamburg	84	109	112	58	115	121	101
13 Braunschweig	90	99	102	154***	50	110	113
14 Hannover	95	123**	121**	173***	86	127	117
15 Luneburg	79	90	87	120	13	96	115
16 Weser–Ems	74	114*	117*	116	79	107	93
17 Bremen	81	118	126*	65	58	74	135
18 Düsseldorf	90	115***	102	86	86	92	106
19 Köln	102	107	99	93	101	60	101
20 Münster	79	92	95	76	154*	72	97
21 Detmold	83	89	87	90	115	138*	108
22 Arnsberg	96	100	102	87	127	131*	104
23 Darmstadt	93	83	83	106	187***	78	120*
24 Giessen	100	67	80	92	190*	97	118
25 Kassel	68	83	96	92	194*	106	133*
26 Koblenz	82	80	77	150***	108	86	105
27 Trier	96	119	142*	137	96	73	80

Table 7.1.5(a) cont

Area		Indicators (SMRs)						
		TUB	CERV	UTER	HODG	CRHD	RESP	ASTH
28	Rheinhessen–Pfalz	84	104	104	117	201**	104	132**
29	Stuttgart	84	83	84	93	157**	83	82
30	Karlsruhe	138***	92	83	73	176**	105	76
31	Freiburg	128**	78	98	75	97	94	91
32	Tübingen	88	69	71	81	92	142*	76
33	Oberbayern	89	84	81	87	14	137**	77
34	Niederbayern	143**	112	136**	99	0	82	84
35	Oberpfalz	186***	111	129*	136*	22	116	83
36	Oberfranken	258***	107	102	124	61	89	102
37	Mittelfranken	161***	97	113	139***	13	70	105
38	Unterfranken	112	86	80	84	18	90	97
39	Schwaben	64	86	96	116	39	101	75
40	Saarland	117	93	88	97	252***	155*	113
41	Berlin (West)	136***	194***	186***	98	80	113	91

DENMARK

42	Kobenhavn and Frederiksberg (M)	214***	131**	141**	113	121	46	148
43	Kobenhavns County	102	74	65	136*	94	97	63
44	Frederiksborg County	88	62	64	92	105	23	66
45	Roskilde County	61	97	95	164*	81	108	35
46	Vestsjaellands County	94	94	97	168*	148	87	0
47	Storstroms County	56	86	107	84	166	301***	34
48	Bornholms County	106	116	98	67	0	0	0
49	Fyns County	104	111	116	69	47	109	149
50	Sonderjyllands County	44	99	101	76	86	214*	166
51	Ribe County	156	112	101	74	390**	102	153
52	Vejle County	82	119	106	97	0	118	177
53	Ringkobing County	22	81	74	85	0	107	93
54	Arhus County	79	101	111	76	103	68	97
55	Viborg County	69	125	90	69	0	0	112
56	Nordjyllands County	87	103	122	91	133	114	105

FRANCE

57	Ain	53	81	65	61	94	35	66
58	Aisne	122	90	104	77	83	123	127
59	Allier	64	75	136	120	0	151	57
60	Alpes-de-Haute-Provence	78	93	48	61	171	79	0
61	Hautes-Alpes	143	21	19	34	0	0	445***
62	Alpes-Maritimes	91	83	93	120	98	85	140
63	Ardèche	119	93	102	138	80	96	0
64	Ardennes	131	139	151*	88	73	190*	127
65	Ariège	90	141	85	109	0	75	323**
66	Aube	134	182**	156*	65	0	27	33
67	Aude	57	52	47	145	0	142	77
68	Aveyron	72	63	55	107	84	169	153
69	Bouches-du-Rhône	101	85	90	125*	136	68	63
70	Calvados	119	128	110	134	72	73	125
71	Cantal	114	110	84	137	140	163	63
72	Charente	68	161**	168**	120	66	125	59
73	Charente-Maritime	70	95	113	80	88	67	60
74	Cher	109	115	103	82	137	109	125
75	Corrèze	87	52	109	91	0	82	132
76	Corse	92	46	81	74	81	79	78
77	Côte-d'Or	49	181***	113	118	130	99	116
78	Côtes-du-Nord	89	85	106	62	128	90	58
79	Creuse	62	31	143	245**	191	0	0
80	Dordogne	110	99	130	68	0	154	144
81	Doubs	77	116	95	47	208*	119	19
82	Drôme	76	148*	106	104	158	101	73
83	Eure	87	141*	139*	81	89	77	160
84	Eure-et-Loir	70	110	150*	84	0	141	26
85	Finistère	111	72	83	72	82	10	109
86	Gard	90	49	59	109	121	17	55
87	Haute-Garonne	77	88	132*	69	49	111	120
88	Gers	31	87	129	84	0	291**	120

Table 7.1.5(a) cont

Area		Indicators (SMRs)						
		TUB	CERV	UTER	HODG	CRHD	RESP	ASTH
89	Gironde	90	88	106	96	74	83	133
90	Hérault	61	62	77	103	150	88	108
91	Ille-et-Vilaine	116	105	78	65	28	58	112
92	Indre	62	83	71	124	95	38	260**
93	Indre-et-Loire	61	114	86	127	84	96	112
94	Isère	102	135*	83	81	61	89	38
95	Jura	56	104	81	155	354**	65	162
96	Landes	43	73	38	62	75	93	34
97	Loir-et-Cher	74	160*	143*	103	75	113	171
98	Loire	103	95	87	80	114	74	117
99	Haute-Loire	64	22	56	200**	221	0	50
100	Loire-Atlantique	143**	81	79	79	21	135	113
101	Loiret	39	118	96	104	77	113	87
102	Lot	45	109	137	24	0	64	0
103	Lotet-Garonne	65	84	97	121	74	31	68
104	Lozère	152	64	87	101	0	120	282
105	Maine-et-Loire	111	78	82	144*	32	98	113
106	Manche	66	73	79	105	297**	48	65
107	Marne	80	108	85	110	151	120	67
108	Haute-Marne	109	59	107	217**	104	139	46
109	Mayenne	97	70	58	112	83	104	74
110	Meurthe-et-Moselle	150**	160***	108	81	57	85	101
111	Meuse	41	84	89	132	225	38	49
112	Morbihan	208***	62	53	95	152	128	118
113	Moselle	108	130*	107	100	138	112	123
114	Nièvre	126	74	117	80	0	78	89
115	Nord	174***	127**	117*	126*	120	116	156**
116	Oise	94	144*	123	79	119	73	107
117	Orne	66	94	106	152	0	76	0
118	Pas-de-Calais	168***	123*	109	137*	175*	98	206***
119	Puy-de-Dôme	98	58	72	145*	137	57	109
120	Pyrénées-Atlantiques	102	51	86	80	40	33	162
121	Hautes-Pyrénées	55	74	94	110	0	166	88
122	Pyrénées-Orientales	68	55	105	55	70	142	64
123	Bas-Rhin	128*	169***	125*	104	130	132	58
124	Haut-Rhin	94	108	114	100	152	205**	97
125	Rhône	72	103	75	80	135	135	49
126	Haute-Saône	107	115	27	99	187	127	84
127	Saône-et-Loire	67	112	91	118	39	100	53
128	Sarthe	49	104	81	91	44	45	174*
129	Savoie	123	129	93	78	186	49	56
130	Haute-Savoie	106	147*	95	116	148	91	70
131	Paris	132***	110	125**	92	113	90	88
132	Seine-Maritime	189***	155***	147***	165***	156	153*	107
133	Seine-et-Marne	96	82	112	79	104	181**	88
134	Yvelines	67	98	101	86	44	117	112
135	Deux-Sèvres	52	21	58	33	66	23	89
136	Somme	120	86	119	175**	121	107	70
137	Tarn	26	56	69	86	67	107	154
138	Tarn-et-Garonne	58	126	99	78	0	48	55
139	Var	99	95	104	61	148	90	138
140	Vaucluse	50	63	73	93	186	39	109
141	Vendée	63	70	85	95	47	148	62
142	Vienne	82	91	121	112	0	0	131
143	Haute-Vienne	63	80	106	72	0	138	143
144	Vosges	83	78	103	86	55	114	25
145	Yonne	70	138	121	124	73	131	199*
146	Territoire-de-Belfort	62	127	155	83	153	0	138
147	Essonne	77	98	69	72	142	146*	100
148	Hauts-de-Seine	98	86	93	104	83	108	57
149	Seine-Saint-Denis	114	86	107	87	57	115	110
150	Val-de-Marne	80	102	109	81	78	102	65
151	Val-d'Oise	101	75	103	113	140	61	101

Table 7.1.5(a) cont

Area	Indicators (SMRs)						
	TUB	CERV	UTER	HODG	CRHD	RESP	ASTH
GREECE							
152 Greater Athens	104	146***	106	98	41	76	–
153 Rest of Central Greece and Eubea	82	78	66	114	73	101	–
154 Peloponnisos	84	79	90	78	86	74	–
155 Ionian Islands	39	91	68	73	121	36	–
156 Epirus	89	54	38	99	0	148	–
157 Thessaly	112	59	121	85	27	94	–
158 Macedonia	106	79	101	94	158*	81	–
159 Thrace	254***	54	63	177*	278**	429***	–
160 Aegean Islands	105	104	161*	120	197	118	–
161 Crete	37	99	150*	113	289**	114	–
ITALY							
162 Torino	116*	170***	101	106	90	81	122
163 Vercelli	78	187**	106	144*	107	40	0
164 Novara	124	92	106	127	80	93	187
165 Cuneo	126	170**	103	95	91	44	224*
166 Asti	84	83	93	81	132	176	121
167 Alessandria	89	92	93	90	94	38	167
168 Aosta	210**	41	120	83	62	126	0
169 Imperia	129	263***	174**	169**	86	25	111
170 Savona	99	111	67	106	51	116	0
171 Genova	107	117	78	130*	66	56	191*
172 La Spezia	63	119	104	123	65	23	0
173 Varese	74	81	58	125	93	86	196*
174 Como/Sondrio	119	99	79	88	75	87	165
175 Milano	84	80	77	108	81	75	65
176 Bergamo	192***	47	104	121	90	69	121
177 Brescia	209***	111	65	124*	86	71	108
178 Pavia	101	93	115	173***	45	64	97
179 Cremona	135	161*	81	80	89	29	143
180 Mantova	88	47	77	137	30	76	129
181 Bolzano	157**	124	83	72	42	70	102
182 Trento	215***	190**	93	72	118	49	104
183 Verona	95	100	77	96	38	38	59
184 Vicenza	99	119	67	92	59	77	31
185 Belluno	239***	103	109	97	51	64	108
186 Treviso	97	134	76	121	51	40	94
187 Venezia	95	179***	78	126*	34	36	158
188 Padova	115	87	61	128*	53	132	110
189 Rovigo	74	163	61	92	47	18	96
190 Udine/Gorizia	135*	207***	91	77	54	37	104
191 Trieste	149*	124	94	129	94	46	179
192 Pordenone	80	180*	73	72	79	0	0
193 Piacenza	73	107	69	100	97	20	0
194 Parma	102	74	90	103	38	69	188
195 Reggio Emilia	51	86	71	168***	27	36	0
196 Modena	69	75	76	126	49	42	40
197 Bologna	82	88	75	83	71	63	78
198 Ferrara	61	110	64	77	30	83	0
199 Ravenna	32	62	98	52	32	29	67
200 Forli	68	102	67	96	24	52	0
201 Pesaro	40	28	62	46	46	132	72
202 Ancona	64	122	69	66	44	95	56
203 Macerata	83	30	87	84	40	49	84
204 Ascoli Piceno	99	65	94	92	54	38	0
205 Massa-Carrara	177**	130	136	113	115	47	121
206 Lucca	138*	81	88	95	20	38	253*
207 Pistoia	101	68	75	108	113	55	273*
208 Firenze	61	81	82	108	58	68	20
209 Livorno	60	50	65	76	43	70	70
210 Pisa	38	138	82	113	48	63	188
211 Arezzo	102	127	103	72	98	47	0

Table 7.1.5(a) cont

Area		TUB	CERV	UTER	HODG	CRHD	RESP	ASTH
212	Siena	88	49	109	86	62	111	205
213	Grosseto	70	135	73	42	86	0	112
214	Perugia	68	45	51	148**	99	72	42
215	Terni	54	185*	103	81	185*	86	109
216	Viterbo/Rieti	95	55	100	116	106	127	121
217	Roma	100	138***	107	105	91	84	95
218	Latina	92	101	156**	110	159*	85	50
219	Frosinone	80	99	124	88	163*	16	52
220	Caserta	58	23	106	67	225***	131	120
221	Benevento	118	67	97	92	132	76	86
222	Napoli	128***	82	157***	99	179***	178***	150*
223	Avellino	51	23	97	62	151*	166*	111
224	Salerno	117	47	104	97	219***	126	91
225	L'Aquila	159**	152	119	53	169*	86	171
226	Teramo	133	18	115	89	58	58	88
227	Pescara	80	84	97	62	147	112	163
228	Chieti	102	76	82	95	108	65	66
229	Isernia/Campobasso	108	87	69	104	227***	109	76
230	Foggia	119	125	117	74	125	162**	0
231	Bari	116	122	144***	76	172***	116	108
232	Taranto	76	50	121	90	124	132	39
233	Brindisi	106	95	169***	108	227***	159*	0
234	Lecce	116	103	106	108	128	120	120
235	Potenza/Matera	108	96	105	72	141	140*	117
236	Cosenza	82	97	151***	52	151*	144*	63
237	Catanzaro	97	70	104	95	220***	138*	125
238	Reggio Calabria	99	92	103	101	115	99	83
239	Trapani	82	98	224***	99	122	91	395***
240	Palermo	53	67	154***	103	108	189***	78
241	Messina	51	36	145**	88	121	162**	36
242	Agrigento	59	57	133*	109	172**	160*	100
243	Caltanisetta	84	19	127	67	113	89	243
244	Enna	89	79	157*	97	170	125	247
245	Catania	65	90	163***	101	118	171***	23
246	Ragusa	95	128	188***	90	187*	176*	173
247	Siracusa	70	41	133	75	116	67	0
248	Sassari	157**	52	45	104	79	125	0
249	Nuoro	99	21	39	112	101	133	251*
250	Cagliari/Oristano	121	99	83	59	86	140*	151
IRELAND								
251	Eastern	86	81	79	75	90	75	111
252	Midland	105	125	108	125	76	101	75
253	Mid-Western	174***	81	120	75	189	118	48
254	North Eastern	66	117	132	97	51	147	103
255	North Western	39	88	125	168*	0	90	76
256	South Eastern	109	133	100	149*	79	102	109
257	Southern	98	134*	110	118	138	113	91
258	Western	132	72	103	74	136	113	137
NETHERLANDS								
259	Groningen	82	87	50	109	36	75	34
260	Friesland	81	111	117	90	103	86	152
261	Drenthe	155	101	131	63	185	74	0
262	Overijssel	173**	79	93	127	154	92	66
263	Gelderland	73	91	95	103	134	95	99
264	Utrecht	154*	86	97	92	62	88	91
265	Noord Holland	76	114	97	114	81	69	126
266	Zuid Holland	78	109	110	102	86	117	113
267	Zeeland	62	149*	118	116	114	111	29
268	Noord Brabant	92	93	100	78	114	134*	88
269	Limburg	175**	91	99	95	85	105	138
270	Zuidelijke Ijsselmeerpolders	0	25	0	74	0	56	88

Table 7.1.5(a) cont

Area		Indicators (SMRs)						
		TUB	CERV	UTER	HODG	CRHD	RESP	ASTH
UK:ENGLAND AND WALES								
271	Cleveland	131	129*	118	174***	158	104	103
272	Cumbria	49	114	80	136	54	109	97
273	Durham	156**	117	109	97	105	127	175**
274	Northumberland	102	109	80	119	126	89	77
275	Gateshead	154	105	80	69	0	76	201**
276	Newcastle upon Tyne	145	117	90	95	0	60	82
277	Northern Tyneside	96	143*	120	103	0	123	20
278	Southern Tyneside	117	124	89	90	86	26	99
279	Sunderland	177*	112	109	80	176	83	88
280	Bradford	221***	131*	95	100	176	146*	107
281	Calderdale	237***	146*	147*	159	203	59	41
282	Humberside	98	127**	110	134*	76	127	76
283	Kirklees	86	135*	121	130	101	85	100
284	Leeds	93	130**	138**	126	165	84	74
285	North Yorkshire	62	82	97	106	75	81	62
286	Wakefield	56	128	145*	151*	157	179*	94
287	Barnsley	0	131	151*	66	112	84	118
288	Derbyshire	63	92	105	107	136	106	75
289	Doncaster	95	173***	146*	102	221*	51	90
290	Leicestershire	106	102	108	136*	58	116	89
291	Lincolnshire	69	104	102	119	45	113	97
292	Nottinghamshire	112	107	108	75	178*	97	113
293	Rotherham	42	115	129	47	97	85	102
294	Sheffield	62	84	93	82	219**	72	71
295	Cambridgeshire	63	62	66	81	81	43	90
296	Norfolk	78	89	84	47	109	132	106
297	Suffolk	59	91	76	116	83	99	164**
298	Barnet	47	46	57	111	0	42	103
299	Bedfordshire	59	113	83	106	93	93	125
300	Brent and Harrow	151*	73	70	111	54	80	162*
301	Ealing/Hammersmith/Hounslow	227***	85	80	69	153	142*	126
302	Hertfordshire	70	49	57	93	25	87	99
303	Hillingdon	15	94	108	88	162	69	48
304	Kensington/Chelsea/Westminster	337***	103	111	137	180	104	73
305	Barking and Havering	89	96	102	154*	0	152	130
306	Camden and Islington	201***	94	63	92	73	60	113
307	City and East London	302***	110	121	72	152	167**	186***
308	Enfield and Haringey	115	104	95	63	315***	122	95
309	Essex	78	74	67	101	33	73	76
310	Redbridge and Waltham Forest	94	78	71	54	85	126	121
311	Bromley	65	43	62	125	82	72	155
312	East Sussex	63	109	122	100	86	102	111
313	Greenwich and Bexley	96	55	72	102	116	98	130
314	Kent	75	95	98	96	93	95	69
315	Lambeth/Southwark/Lewisham	253***	84	89	101	116	91	86
316	Croydon	88	80	94	55	38	73	69
317	Kingston and Richmond	46	63	70	128	80	78	129
318	Merton/Sutton/Wandsworth	130	89	92	84	84	101	133
319	Surrey	72	73	71	98	72	107	102
320	West Sussex	67	62	67	93	40	77	86
321	Dorset	79	74	82	82	93	130	134
322	Hampshire	67	89	90	91	74	137*	95
323	Isle of Wight	84	59	76	52	0	76	182
324	Wiltshire	34	87	58	126	47	113	70
325	Berkshire	96	56	64	89	51	58	55
326	Buckinghamshire	52	49	38	88	39	113	86
327	Northamptonshire	76	69	68	91	45	72	96
328	Oxfordshire	28	57	73	77	45	94	96
329	Avon	56	65	63	93	68	61	101
330	Cornwall and Scilly Isles	62	100	113	56	61	96	85
331	Devon	68	96	110	73	14	103	113
332	Gloucestershire	69	104	103	71	75	149*	105

Table 7.1.5(a) cont

Area		TUB	CERV	UTER	HODG	CRHD	RESP	ASTH
333	Somerset	105	85	98	99	60	65	127
334	Birmingham	171***	90	100	113	175*	106	147**
335	Coventry	184**	116	114	178**	42	154	94
336	Dudley	100	102	112	135	194	77	37
337	Hereford and Worcester	72	103	119	84	131	76	81
338	Salop	29	106	117	88	32	68	106
339	Sandwell	149	115	124	125	44	196**	76
340	Solihull	17	63	91	102	0	74	164
341	Staffordshire	79	120*	124*	138*	128	124	115
342	Walsall	177*	110	129	77	93	166*	84
343	Warwickshire	101	103	105	117	74	128	169**
344	Wolverhampton	144	142*	120	152	267*	129	166*
345	Bolton	178*	149**	131	81	288**	177*	101
346	Bury	82	102	72	69	0	105	64
347	Lancashire	83	128***	120*	73	132	95	102
348	Manchester	274***	184***	171***	93	261**	89	90
349	Oldham	97	129	127	110	227*	129	86
350	Rochdale	70	182***	128	103	62	98	90
351	Salford	110	136*	142*	49	168	114	79
352	Stockport	72	63	85	113	42	52	78
353	Tameside	95	102	87	138	0	139	70
354	Trafford	109	95	101	81	288**	107	86
355	Wigan	70	119	112	68	153	35	83
356	Cheshire	75	136***	139***	80	52	75	111
357	Liverpool	191***	175***	184***	95	142	71	106
358	St Helens and Knowsley	99	181***	209***	83	36	66	41
359	Sefton	102	149**	157**	121	87	106	91
360	Wirral	132	147**	181***	90	78	78	35
361	Clwyd	27	136*	135*	141	131	135	30
362	Dyfed	88	134*	145*	134	239*	61	60
363	Gwent	92	84	107	148*	87	121	104
364	Gwynedd	152	104	91	121	119	86	70
365	Mid Glamorgan	115	116	116	111	306***	101	183***
366	Powys	30	108	80	136	0	108	108
367	South Glamorgan	135	115	106	85	69	119	67
368	West Glamorgan	108	99	86	129	143	86	96

UK:NORTHERN IRELAND

369	Northern Ireland	100	100	100	100	100	100	100

UK:SCOTLAND

370	Highlands and Islands	37	103	107	115	38	73	146
371	Grampian	66	76	63	80	42	61	70
372	Tayside	69	64	73	108	55	137	68
373	Fife	21	153***	164***	134	31	122	51
374	Lothian	41	96	109	84	111	99	98
375	Borders	22	60	70	154	0	46	46
376	Forth Valley	103	92	65	99	75	184*	93
377	Argyll and Clyde	162**	103	91	121	46	100	57
378	Greater Glasgow	205***	100	105	86	204**	80	152**
379	Lanarkshire	72	109	103	116	158	127	87
380	Ayrshire and Arran	99	129*	119	97	109	77	161*
381	Dumfries and Galloway	106	89	104	63	0	91	62

PORTUGAL

382	Viana do Castelo	68	77	107	30	43	161**	-
383	Braga	51	59	85	41	112	122*	-
384	Vila Real	66	66	72	30	63	152**	-
385	Braganca	46	89	123	62	45	156*	-
386	Guarda	67	48	89	111	111	63	-
387	Viseu	137**	80	81	37	71	153**	-
388	Porto	163***	136**	138***	109	170***	117*	-
389	Aveiro	45	78	130*	37	74	86	-
390	Coimbra	76	57	98	66	94	111	-

Table 7.1.5(a) cont

Area		Indicators (SMRs)						
		TUB	CERV	UTER	HODG	CRHD	RESP	ASTH
391	Castelo Branco	56	32	56	46	95	83	-
392	Portalegre	53	38	78	49	97	51	-
393	Santarem	36	45	84	31	22	57	-
394	Leiria	30	90	86	51	22	64	-
395	Lisboa	161***	163***	109	225***	130**	102	-
396	Setubal	35	59	53	61	27	25	-
397	Evora	39	39	72	77	29	37	-
398	Beja	62	51	69	38	145	18	-
399	Faro	75	94	84	86	52	35	-
400	Madeira	123	114	88	65	92	107	-
401	Azores	168***	136	136	66	140	169***	-
SPAIN								
402	La Coruña	182***	123	122*	153**	122	163***	29
403	Lugo	133*	85	132	84	61	152	177
404	Orense	148***	59	99	36	61	146	115
405	Pontevedra	133**	57	151***	73	51	105	163
406	Asturias	119*	134*	110	114	107	82	75
407	Cantabria	91	143	122	96	92	121	130
408	Alava	68	36	47	116	52	114	0
409	Guipuzcoa	78	74	74	137*	20	95	65
410	Vizcaya	98	108	95	103	75	81	103
411	Navarra	87	33	43	116	88	98	125
412	Rioja	80	31	45	100	30	68	65
413	Huesca	22	51	107	43	20	111	0
414	Teruel	31	0	97	62	29	113	0
415	Zaragoza	73	41	84	100	96	69	0
416	Madrid Centro	78	83	58	71	98	88	67
417	Avila	69	42	54	88	167	105	0
418	Burgos	83	55	43	80	55	50	46
419	Leon	109	70	101	72	191***	124	169
420	Palencia	81	41	131	120	22	60	190
421	Salamanca	159***	54	105	119	164*	126	49
422	Segovia	47	26	50	132	87	200*	121
423	Soria	29	0	94	194	179	170	0
424	Valladolid	76	82	136*	148*	83	74	32
425	Zamora	62	32	109	84	77	38	0
426	Albacete	120	87	93	71	110	127	0
427	Ciudad Real	103	17	72	127	126	147*	75
428	Cuenca	60	53	107	46	125	53	174
429	Guadalajara	72	28	29	93	62	100	0
430	Toledo	72	42	74	63	177**	105	149
431	Badajoz	112	33	87	160**	179**	110	219*
432	Caceres	112	88	97	121	144	124	0
433	Barcelona	75	115	105	99	64	81	96
434	Gerona	67	92	98	110	50	92	251**
435	Lerida	65	53	121	98	70	74	0
436	Tarragona	92	63	140*	95	75	99	291***
437	Alicante	75	89	109	73	111	113	84
438	Castellon de la Plana	86	64	116	91	117	91	116
439	Valencia	87	144***	116	125*	152***	97	115
440	Baleares	90	230***	143**	144*	45	99	244**
441	Almeria	147**	77	105	94	68	133	122
442	Cadiz	131**	141*	131*	96	117	93	113
443	Cordoba	101	76	82	76	120	168***	71
444	Granada	102	102	73	128	81	82	45
445	Huelva	160***	105	103	75	117	81	82
446	Jaen	100	67	98	82	189***	171***	81
447	Malaga	140***	112	126*	139*	166***	86	186*
448	Sevilla	231***	191***	156***	124	156***	102	142
449	Murcia	72	110	89	62	78	114	0
450	Las Palmas	131*	185***	113	82	108	87	257***
451	Sta Cruz de Tenerife	72	295***	136*	125	96	107	142

Table 7.1.5(b). 'Avoidable death' indicators by small area, standardized to own country's standard, for appendicitis, abdominal hernia, cholelithiasis/cholecystitis, hypertensive/cerebrovascular diseases, maternal mortality, perinatal mortality, and all causes

Notes on the use of this table

1. This table shows within-country variations, the value for the whole country being 100.

2. Key for the abbreviations used for columns of the table:
   APP — appendicitis (ICD8 540–543; ICD9 540–543), ages 5–64;
   HERN — abdominal hernia (ICD8 550–553; ICD9 550–553), ages 5–64;
   CHOLY— cholelithiasis and cholecystitis diseases (ICD8 574–575; ICD9 574–575.1, 576.1), ages 5–64;
   HYP/S — hypertensive and cerebrovascular diseases (ICD8 400–404, 430–438; ICD9 401–405, 430–438), ages 35–64;
   MAT — maternal deaths (ICD8 630–678; ICD9 630–676), all ages;
   PER — perinatal mortality (all causes), deaths aged under 1 week plus stillbirths;
   ALL — mortality from all causes (all ICD8/ICD9 codes), all ages.

3. The small area numbers are as in the key maps

4. The indicators have been tested for indicating significant excess mortality relative to national rates. The *p*-values achieved for one-tail tests are indicated as follows: *p<0.05; ** p<0.01;***p<0.001.

5. The indicators are based on mortality data for 1980–84, except for Greece (1980–82) and Spain (1979–83). The population data are for 1980–84 except for France (1982), Greece (1981), Ireland (1981), and Spain (1981). All data for Italy are for 1979–83.

Table 7.1.5(b)

Area	Indicators (SMRs)						
	APP	HERN	CHOLY	HYP/S	MAT	PER	ALL
BELGIUM							
1 Antwerpen	43	46	72	100	127	102	96
2 Brabant	136	126	102	93	114	97	95
3 West-Vlaanderen	32	92	109	75	61	107*	93
4 Oost-Vlaanderen	209*	92	49	89	52	101	99
5 Hainaut	75	177*	144*	121***	54	95	109***
6 Liège	66	69	101	114***	117	92	110***
7 Limburg	52	38	94	93	160	110**	95
8 Luxembourg (province)	0	111	260**	123**	185	102	104***
9 Namur	247	118	104	132***	103	99	111***
LUXEMBOURG							
10 Luxembourg	100	100	100	100	100	100	100
FEDERAL REPUBLIC OF GERMANY							
11 Schleswig–Holstein	109	93	103	85	78	95	99
12 Hamburg	112	72	80	92	86	88	101*
13 Braunschweig	153*	102	109	103	75	104	99
14 Hannover	122	89	128 *	98	41	95	98
15 Luneburg	147	130	104	93	27	93	100
16 Weser–Ems	137	87	85	96	86	110	100***
17 Bremen	134	88	97	113**	22	93	100
18 Düsseldorf	72	65	66	98	133*	117***	103***
19 Köln	60	63	78	98	119	99	102***
20 Münster	99	78	106	108***	124	124***	104***
21 Detmold	81	51	95	93	90	106*	96
22 Arnsberg	130	113	107	112***	128	115***	105***
23 Darmstadt	88	174***	107	95	125	93	97
24 Giessen	151	209**	100	96	102	94	99
25 Kassel	153	75	137*	93	91	102	97
26 Koblenz	104	130	56	120***	92	99	101***
27 Trier	27	158	58	121***	98	91	103***

Table 7.1.5(b) cont

Area		APP	HERN	CHOLY	HYP/S	MAT	PER	ALL
		Indicators (SMRs)						

Area		APP	HERN	CHOLY	HYP/S	MAT	PER	ALL
28	Rheinhessen–Pfalz	130	76	80	123***	153	105	104***
29	Stuttgart	73	115	95	86	88	88	91
30	Karlsruhe	105	90	114	103	89	92	97
31	Freiburg	73	131	125	86	91	83	91
32	Tübingen	64	101	74	90	64	84	91
33	Oberbayern	62	52	57	81	64	88	91
34	Niederbayern	147	188*	156*	110**	162*	93	107***
35	Oberpfalz	137	194**	137	118***	148	105	109***
36	Oberfranken	123	197**	181***	118***	104	93	106***
37	Mittelfranken	104	150	133*	98	98	95	102***
38	Unterfranken	78	79	184***	85	91	99	101**
39	Schwaben	139	71	52	93	162*	96	99
40	Saarland	60	82	121	134***	61	114***	110***
41	Berlin (West)	107	80	167***	138***	81	110**	114***

DENMARK

Area		APP	HERN	CHOLY	HYP/S	MAT	PER	ALL
42	Kobenhavn and Frederiksberg (M)	85	90	92	128***	136	96	110***
43	Kobenhavns County	74	56	87	94	121	74	97
44	Frederiksborg County	103	63	100	90	215	89	98
45	Roskilde County	85	0	0	92	0	97	100
46	Vestsjaellands County	59	68	70	92	254	111	101
47	Storstroms County	185	135	105	100	0	85	104***
48	Bornholms County	0	0	0	83	0	117	101
49	Fyns County	109	124	193*	88	0	93	98
50	Sonderjyllands County	200	314**	81	98	0	111	96
51	Ribe County	0	93	97	98	0	93	95
52	Vejle County	153	178	123	104	0	88	97
53	Ringkobing County	129	77	242*	116*	111	111	96
54	Arhus County	89	106	74	90	56	121***	99
55	Viborg County	72	165	85	108	135	113	95
56	Nordjyllands County	102	39	60	97	270*	113*	97

FRANCE

Area		APP	HERN	CHOLY	HYP/S	MAT	PER	ALL
57	Ain	222*	192*	88	87	144	92	97
58	Aisne	203*	111	204	118**	138	106	113***
59	Allier	162	94	87	111*	107	112*	103***
60	Alpes-de-Haute-Provence	126	0	0	93	104	115	81
61	Hautes-Alpes	143	86	316	84	102	109	96
62	Alpes-Maritimes	69	48	36	72	73	109*	87
63	Ardèche	113	168	247	104	132	115*	99
64	Ardennes	0	271**	250	115*	93	115**	110***
65	Ariège	109	0	0	75	0	122*	95
66	Aube	163	138	381**	104	108	101	99
67	Aude	0	117	0	79	95	91	92
68	Aveyron	0	186	115	83	142	106	92
69	Bouches-du-Rhne	79	77	101	93	143*	107**	99
70	Calvados	107	141	65	110*	62	87	102***
71	Cantal	277*	108	0	129**	75	129**	106***
72	Charente	90	109	100	87	133	110	96
73	Charente-Maritime	59	35	64	86	45	91	94
74	Cher	193	146	215	101	74	97	100
75	Corrèze	184	170	0	104	0	93	100
76	Corse	0	37	0	98	50	118**	98
77	Côte-d'Or	100	109	80	87	120	106	95
78	Côtes-du-Nord	55	145	60	135***	63	77	110***
79	Creuse	216	116	215	143***	21	88	100
80	Dordogne	194	128	0	114*	348*	99	98
81	Doubs	66	68	0	97	144	98	97
82	Drôme	237*	99	91	80	18	106	95
83	Eure	68	91	167	102	103	106	104***
84	Eure-et-Loir	88	0	0	89	52	93	96
85	Finistère	55	99	122	131***	102	87	111***
86	Gard	253**	99	122	79	148	118***	97
87	Haute-Garonne	19	47	172	77	98	96	92
88	Gers	0	48	0	86	85	102	94

Table 7.1.5(b) cont

Area		Indicators (SMRs)						
		APP	HERN	CHOLY	HYP/S	MAT	PER	ALL
89	Gironde	109	67	92	94	67	93	98
90	Hérault	85	140	187	87	129	114***	94
91	Ille-et-Vilaine	104	95	149	122***	76	92	108***
92	Indre	126	258**	136	106	0	108	99
93	Indre-et-Loire	156	99	146	66	63	82	91
94	Isère	116	67	284**	82	73	90	97
95	Jura	63	0	0	110	88	105	98
96	Landes	0	0	109	96	0	101	97
97	Loir-et-Cher	0	64	119	113*	38	75	92
98	Loire	144	141	142	93	69	92	102***
99	Haute-Loire	148	173	160	111	117	103	101
100	Loire-Atlantique	126	114	0	110*	56	91	105***
101	Loiret	30	57	70	85	18	98	95
102	Lot	0	106	0	105	0	97	95
103	Lot-et-Garonne	147	0	0	94	81	102	95
104	Lozère	207	119	0	111	156	122	101
105	Maine-et-Loire	95	80	117	91	38	95	96
106	Manche	0	80	147	108	63	87	103***
107	Marne	177	101	0	94	133	94	101
108	Haute-Marne	149	48	0	100	313***	111	105***
109	Mayenne	286**	143	132	102	35	90	99
110	Meurthe-et-Moselle	22	143	52	111*	80	96	107***
111	Meuse	309**	197	0	125**	242*	126***	109***
112	Morbihan	77	63	58	156***	67	96	118***
113	Moselle	135	110	74	128***	251***	109**	115***
114	Nièvre	258*	185	0	116*	104	103	104***
115	Nord	205***	169***	212**	139***	85	115***	120***
116	Oise	73	136	62	102	55	99	105***
117	Orne	103	32	117	103	68	74	102**
118	Pas-de-Calais	120	189***	129	144***	104	127***	120***
119	Puy-de-Dôme	76	80	59	109	75	120***	104***
120	Pyrénées-Atlantiques	0	82	0	86	152	93	96
121	Hautes-Pyrénées	64	150	0	105	58	114*	98
122	Pyrénées-Orientales	132	49	91	85	337***	110	96
123	Bas-Rhin	0	126	210*	120***	44	77	110***
124	Haut-Rhin	142	94	0	122***	134	100	112***
125	Rhône	53	112	103	81	107	92	95
126	Haute-Saône	271*	86	0	123**	173	98	105***
127	Saône-et-Loire	187*	65	179	102	116	107	99
128	Sarthe	186	80	146	75	142	91	93
129	Savoie	47	181	111	97	32	78	99
130	Haute-Savoie	95	170	155	89	78	88	98
131	Paris	63	96	46	84	134	104*	88
132	Seine-Maritime	53	123	32	108*	66	103	106***
133	Seine-et-Marne	128	91	142	85	107	95	102***
134	Yvelines	91	65	101	79	164**	89	91
135	Deux-Sèvres	227*	140	309*	87	126	104	92
136	Somme	87	76	208	105	122	106	112***
137	Tarn	43	100	92	83	73	97	93
138	Tarn-et-Garonne	0	0	0	95	0	117*	93
139	Var	42	73	268**	89	63	110*	96
140	Vaucluse	71	44	162	87	74	115**	98
141	Vendée	97	81	74	105	0	87	98
142	Vienne	85	79	97	82	60	98	88
143	Haute-Vienne	0	50	0	100	114	77	93
144	Vosges	118	151	0	124***	248**	99	107***
145	Yonne	151	121	112	109	69	91	102**
146	Territoire-de-Belfort	117	157	287	110	69	90	106***
147	Essonne	96	70	42	89	144	86	92
148	Hauts-de-Seine	74	26	48	84	113	100	92
149	Seine-Saint-Denis	70	111	58	95	112	108**	99
150	Val-de-Marne	89	66	30	83	126	94	95
151	Val-d'Oise	34	85	44	83	85	99	99

Table 7.1.5(b) cont

Area		Indicators (SMRs)						
		APP	HERN	CHOLY	HYP/S	MAT	PER	ALL
GREECE								
152	Greater Athens	87	135	94	102	57	108***	103***
153	Rest of Central Greece and Eubea	65	92	132	104	148	87	96
154	Peloponnisos	72	48	69	93	53	105	93
155	Ionian Islands	764***	241	0	99	108	80	107***
156	Epirus	0	0	74	86	215	104	95
157	Thessaly	201	142	204*	104	0	86	102***
158	Macedonia	100	104	87	99	81	105**	104***
159	Thrace	0	0	0	136***	503***	103	113***
160	Aegean Islands	0	116	109	92	251**	85	100
161	Crete	145	0	142	89	95	81	88
ITALY								
162	Torino	147*	154**	161***	104*	120	109***	105***
163	Vercelli	86	23	104	130***	59	116**	105***
164	Novara	0	116	73	122***	80	82	106***
165	Cuneo	157	255***	116	109*	105	91	106***
166	Asti	80	42	112	109	333*	92	103***
167	Alessandria	217*	130	114	101	57	97	99
168	Aosta	150	84	95	90	0	92	104***
169	Imperia	448***	78	105	85	0	74	98
170	Savona	55	57	65	90	0	93	100
171	Genova	93	112	147**	87	106	83	102***
172	La Spezia	0	136	92	85	108	80	97
173	Varese	45	67	120	106	69	94	103***
174	Como/Sondrio	19	56	113	113***	18	76	107***
175	Milano	86	86	74	103*	64	84	105***
176	Bergamo	81	87	102	128***	70	88	107***
177	Brescia	121	31	70	122***	49	80	115***
178	Pavia	98	87	79	134***	97	85	111***
179	Cremona	153	84	95	137***	125	85	114***
180	Mantova	45	96	46	121***	59	79	107***
181	Bolzano	170	53	119	89	164	78	101*
182	Trento	0	93	149*	89	40	81	103***
183	Verona	90	13	108	112***	114	94	103***
184	Vicenza	123	89	128	115***	94	76	106***
185	Belluno	78	42	97	122***	184	75	108***
186	Treviso	0	104	89	90	49	74	98
187	Venezia	83	61	78	85	0	89	100
188	Padova	44	91	59	93	66	85	101**
189	Rovigo	67	185	113	99	153	76	105***
190	Udine/Gorizia	76	96	110	104	66	83	108***
191	Trieste	173	28	132	76	110	53	102***
192	Pordenone	65	74	98	88	72	75	102*
193	Piacenza	118	0	117	105	92	84	100
194	Parma	124	85	114	92	126	103	97
195	Reggio Emilia	40	0	65	83	0	86	94
196	Modena	28	76	92	82	74	86	96
197	Bologna	104	72	99	84	152	87	95
198	Ferrara	42	44	68	87	140	87	97
199	Ravenna	47	50	76	72	0	83	89
200	Forli	0	48	48	71	165	77	92
201	Pesaro	152	56	106	79	166	82	91
202	Ancona	38	83	71	81	44	80	90
203	Macerata	114	30	104	82	135	102	91
204	Ascoli Piceno	47	78	79	86	49	94	91
205	Massa-Carrara	247	88	101	96	99	95	98
206	Lucca	176	71	63	86	54	86	98
207	Pistoia	64	69	66	69	0	78	94
208	Firenze	28	53	77	74	38	91	89
209	Livorno	382***	76	116	82	196	94	95
210	Pisa	43	23	142	65	163	87	95
211	Arezzo	106	28	107	79	66	93	92

Table 7.1.5(b) cont

Area		Indicators (SMRs)						
		APP	HERN	CHOLY	HYP/S	MAT	PER	ALL
212	Siena	316**	191	98	80	0	101	90
213	Grosseto	0	38	88	92	425***	91	95
214	Perugia	0	120	69	88	63	71	92
215	Terni	0	74	56	80	0	113	96
216	Viterbo/Rieti	81	130	124	98	121	94	100
217	Roma	97	105	93	82	93	93	99
218	Latina	42	79	128	102	60	100	99
219	Frosinone	38	89	76	116***	114	98	95
220	Caserta	122	333***	102	156***	147	116***	110***
221	Benevento	0	69	52	107	261**	104	96
222	Napoli	158*	220***	138**	136***	93	117***	119***
223	Avellino	41	24	109	96	58	96	108***
224	Salerno	195*	76	95	112***	109*	110***	93
225	L'Aquila	57	92	95	99	104	101	98
226	Teramo	65	74	99	92	105	82	93
227	Pescara	180	69	78	92	223	92	90
228	Chieti	183	25	145	81	42	103	90
229	Isernia/Campobasso	53	119	125	111*	136	101	93
230	Foggia	27	138	46	98	83	114***	92
231	Bari	153	83	87	95	48	114***	93
232	Taranto	161	167	110	89	219**	114***	98
233	Brindisi	229*	57	65	99	80	111**	101
234	Lecce	70	132	77	91	76	108**	98
235	Potenza/Matera	146	125	94	108*	62	106	93
236	Cosenza	74	139	158**	116***	81	109**	91
237	Catanzaro	175	64	79	96	148	106*	91
238	Reggio Calabria	63	95	65	97	20	121***	91
239	Trapani	0	101	77	123***	90	93	97
240	Palermo	137	132	71	113***	154	139***	99
241	Messina	156	134	120	95	144	121***	94
242	Agrigento	77	190*	54	102	49	99	95
243	Caltanisetta	189	156	74	108	160	129***	102**
244	Enna	92	219	104	129***	179	105	102
245	Catania	179*	78	147*	118***	174*	120***	103***
246	Ragusa	129	76	115	111	446***	106	106***
247	Siracusa	0	170	86	105	155	114**	98
248	Sassari	0	135	102	97	133	106	95
249	Nuoro	136	130	131	99	191	103	94
250	Cagliari/Oristano	85	138	192***	91	102	121***	94
IRELAND								
251	Eastern	88	23	88	104	60	104*	97
252	Midland	0	114	83	88	203	83	104***
253	Mid-Western	260*	155	28	111	92	97	107***
254	North Eastern	139	251*	153	109	141	103	102*
255	North Western	190	107	116	105	72	102	98
256	South Eastern	53	128	116	99	151	108*	103***
257	Southern	38	45	145	98	57	102	103***
258	Western	116	196	71	82	176	82	94
NETHERLANDS								
259	Groningen	155	33	35	102	40	97	99
260	Friesland	111	128	69	103	130	99	99
261	Drenthe	49	41	117	95	154	99	99
262	Overijssel	146	145	97	107	112	97	101*
263	Gelderland	88	76	89	104	37	101	101**
264	Utrecht	24	103	52	104	114	103	99
265	Noord Holland	82	115	124	87	130	102	100
266	Zuid Holland	82	92	99	99	122	97	98
267	Zeeland	241*	50	71	87	0	105	95
268	Noord Brabant	103	148	135*	106*	112	101	103***
269	Limburg	153	65	103	109*	65	106	107***
270	Zuidelijke Ijsselmeerpolders	251	0	0	83	0	76	86

Table 7.1.5(b) cont

Area		Indicators (SMRs)						
		APP	HERN	CHOLY	HYP/S	MAT	PER	ALL
	UK:ENGLAND AND WALES							
271	Cleveland	259**	106	143	126***	113	116***	114***
272	Cumbria	0	23	39	124***	208*	113**	105***
273	Durham	157	75	79	127***	155	108*	111***
274	Northumberland	0	76	96	110	0	89	111***
275	Gateshead	110	52	87	142***	91	115*	114***
276	Newcastle upon Tyne	173	81	137	118**	67	106	108***
277	Northern Tyneside	116	108	136	105	100	96	110***
278	Southern Tyneside	0	195	55	129***	122	112	113***
279	Sunderland	409***	40	268**	128***	112	111*	113***
280	Bradford	54	27	45	135***	95	122***	110***
281	Calderdale	128	123	52	130***	279*	125**	109***
282	Humberside	86	124	93	104	108	110**	103***
283	Kirklees	267*	130	82	120***	134	122***	112***
284	Leeds	69	82	111	106	105	105	103***
285	North Yorkshire	73	69	29	97	94	110*	98
286	Wakefield	0	38	96	101	170	119**	114***
287	Barnsley	0	102	129	98	81	90	107***
288	Derbyshire	79	100	53	109**	145	104	103***
289	Doncaster	83	160	68	112*	237*	96	105***
290	Leicestershire	148	72	85	97	120	96	96
291	Lincolnshire	89	84	71	99	109	98	101*
292	Nottinghamshire	147	94	109	108**	19	94	103***
293	Rotherham	97	47	119	113*	137	126***	106***
294	Sheffield	0	125	88	110*	79	101	103***
295	Cambridgeshire	44	151	91	79	89	88	93
296	Norfolk	70	116	97	75	175	92	91
297	Suffolk	125	200*	68	76	154	84	91
298	Barnet	85	80	101	67	62	82	90
299	Bedfordshire	51	75	127	90	150	94	96
300	Brent and Harrow	112	27	68	79	37	90	88
301	Ealing/Hammersmith/Hounslow	40	173*	16	93	51	86	99
302	Hertfordshire	0	130	79	76	59	78	93
303	Hillingdon	105	99	84	69	156	93	92
304	Kensington/Chelsea/Westminster	165	191	96	113*	121	87	93
305	Barking and Havering	116	27	68	78	149	100.	99
306	Camden and Islington	229	215*	120	99	53	93	98
307	City and East London	46	88	168	116***	119	117***	106***
308	Enfield and Haringey	54	52	175	85	148	92	96
309	Essex	133	64	122	75	63	92	95
310	Redbridge and Waltham Forest	56	53	44	88	119	100	93
311	Bromley	78	0	30	79	0	73	90
312	East Sussex	0	70	88	85	138	87	91
313	Greenwich and Bexley	170	81	160	83	81	97	96
314	Kent	119	65	131	87	51	101	97
315	Lambeth/Southwark/Lewisham	283**	183*	84	113***	137	107*	102***
316	Croydon	155	37	126	92	0	83	98
317	Kingston and Richmond	252*	39	66	81	68	76	90
318	Merton/Sutton/Wandsworth	42	60	67	90	30	91	97
319	Surrey	94	100	47	69	127	91	91
320	West Sussex	75	35	59	75	95	92	89
321	Dorset	122	169	95	76	76	77	87
322	Hampshire	17	84	43	76	61	87	93
323	Isle of Wight	408*	0	0	86	0	101	91
324	Wiltshire	144	117	59	81	103	88	94
325	Berkshire	73	54	46	77	49	81	95
326	Buckinghamshire	89	44	93	78	89	97	92
327	Northamptonshire	144	24	79	97	98	105	97
328	Oxfordshire	48	95	81	73	34	66	90
329	Avon	133	101	128	81	84	97	93
330	Cornwall and Scilly Isles	0	105	198*	86	142	91	96
331	Devon	103	145	51	85	152	87	93
332	Gloucestershire	145	139	117	99	0	90	94

Table 7.1.5(b) cont

Area		Indicators (SMRs)						
		APP	HERN	CHOLY	HYP/S	MAT	PER	ALL
333	Somerset	57	163	46	95	47	92	94
334	Birmingham	72	126	145	126***	77	117***	108***
335	Coventry	76	36	153	119**	105	125***	103***
336	Dudley	237	38	159	114*	0	93	102*
337	Hereford and Worcester	156	132	48	100	178	101	99
338	Salop	67	196*	55	112*	248*	127***	100
339	Sandwell	151	143	60	141***	226*	148***	107***
340	Solihull	119	174	0	74	105	106	90
341	Staffordshire	72	116	206***	108*	70	118***	107***
342	Walsall	177	342***	108	120**	67	130***	110***
343	Warwickshire	0	148	104	97	41	102	102***
344	Wolverhampton	276*	88	260**	114*	275*	132***	104***
345	Bolton	95	0	195	121**	188	102	114***
346	Bury	144	280*	118	106	0	113	109***
347	Lancashire	125	247***	108	118***	105	111***	109***
348	Manchester	165	130	133	143***	179	120***	117***
349	Oldham	0	110	139	147***	219	115*	14***
350	Rochdale	0	119	301**	124**	150	126***	111***
351	Salford	195	92	78	142***	74	91	117***
352	Stockport	169	81	34	109	0	96	102*
353	Tameside	336*	0	90	137***	0	109	111***
354	Trafford	0	0	177	107	0	104	100
355	Wigan	0	0	101	121***	112	93	115***
356	Cheshire	53	89	161*	101	80	98	105***
357	Liverpool	96	114	135	136***	170	95	114***
358	St Helens and Knowsley	68	67	227**	139***	180	100	116***
359	Sefton	160	38	97	119**	67	95	103***
360	Wirral	72	34	87	109	161	97	105***
361	Clwyd	0	122	103	112*	145	111*	101
362	Dyfed	141	131	194*	130***	119	96	105***
363	Gwent	108	77	87	113**	41	104	106***
364	Gwynedd	107	51	43	118**	85	96	98
365	Mid Glamorgan	134	86	199*	134***	155	118***	113***
366	Powys	0	102	86	108	0	104	102*
367	South Glamorgan	63	121	77	101	44	99	99
368	West Glamorgan	64	30	51	118***	101	101	106***
	UK:NORTHERN IRELAND							
369	Northern Ireland	100	100	100	100	100	100	100
	UK:SCOTLAND							
370	Highlands and Islands	166	49	0	92	81	98	100
371	Grampian	91	81	0	80	138	88	93
372	Tayside	54	187	312	88	93	76	94
373	Fife	0	0	0	105	65	100	96
374	Lothian	58	51	0	88	115	102	94
375	Borders	212	119	0	102	0	101	93
376	Forth Valley	78	230*	961***	97	172	112*	99
377	Argyll and Clyde	190	140	291	107	73	103	106***
378	Greater Glasgow	64	85	0	112***	103	97	106***
379	Lanarkshire	151	113	0	106	111	107	106***
380	Ayrshire and Arran	171	165	0	119***	90	123***	106***
381	Dumfries and Galloway	145	0	0	85	0	98	97
	PORTUGAL							
382	Viana do Castelo	0	107	31	98	83	108*	99
383	Braga	92	50	58	103	112	107**	99
384	Vila Real	47	53	92	117***	132	139***	110***
385	Braganca	66	140	0	107	42	110*	102*
386	Guarda	61	61	35	104	124	95	96
387	Viseu	89	130	95	115***	80	116***	102**
388	Porto	115	105	178***	108***	88	110***	116***
389	Aveiro	20	50	71	94	119	101	99
390	Coimbra	114	60	103	127***	73	91	118***

Table 7.1.5(b) cont

Area		APP	HERN	CHOLY	HYP/S	MAT	PER	ALL
391	Castelo Branco	106	151	0	87	239*	115**	38
392	Portalegre	85	315**	45	84	132	115*	94
393	Santarem	54	81	124	82	114	96	92
394	Leiria	88	128	36	100	144	77	100
395	Lisboa	165**	137	127	106***	85	81	118***
396	Setubal	73	0	35	53	107	88	78
397	Evora	66	129	147	88	144	88	95
398	Beja	130	187	72	76	94	99	95
399	Faro	76	0	107	74	26	97	96
400	Madeira	102	65	263**	148***	50	115***	108***
401	Azores	106	185	36	136***	157	113**	116***

SPAIN

Area		APP	HERN	CHOLY	HYP/S	MAT	PER	ALL
402	La Coruña	87	80	98	119***	174*	94	102***
403	Lugo	0	124	29	81	133	126***	99
404	Orense	170	50	86	103	155	176***	90
405	Pontevedra	111	137	43	111**	45	92	104***
406	Asturias	146	81	115	94	178*	105	102***
407	Cantabria	123	48	83	100	162	101	99
408	Alava	260*	57	63	72	54	94	100
409	Guipuzcoa	46	78	65	79	97	104	93
410	Vizcaya	67	78	112	94	105	108**	104***
411	Navarra	124	124	113	86	30	91	101*
412	Rioja	60	46	79	90	302**	125***	99
413	Huesca	0	95	139	78	82	93	82
414	Teruel	95	0	198	84	116	80	89
415	Zaragoza	109	111	151*	90	100	101	93
416	Madrid Centro	28	50	48	72	57	87	92
417	Avila	0	59	34	75	188	101	83
418	Burgos	85	33	131	79	0	69	83
419	Leon	225**	42	121	92	209*	136***	100
420	Palencia	81	61	106	101	81	116*	99
421	Salamanca	126	0	112	85	174	114**	85
422	Segovia	101	0	0	83	216	81	93
423	Soria	149	0	0	82	0	83	81
424	Valladolid	103	87	228***	72	179	53	85
425	Zamora	0	46	0	73	317**	110	89
426	Albacete	94	151	259***	112*	58	130***	105***
427	Ciudad Real	65	201*	87	120***	252**	101	106***
428	Cuenca	279*	52	90	95	152	120**	97
429	Guadalajara	108	80	93	73	0	82	80
430	Toledo	65	124	129	88	85	103	98
431	Badajoz	124	119	136	139***	155	104	108***
432	Caceres	75	148	34	125***	294***	106	100
433	Barcelona	62	45	72	91	55	64	91
434	Gerona	228*	174	43	77	0	87	104***
435	Lerida	165	0	105	95	95	99	93
436	Tarragona	121	71	40	97	109	87	101
437	Alicante	71	81	86	125***	117	89	108***
438	Castellon de la Plana	144	0	126	102	199*	107	101
439	Valencia	155*	194***	170***	136***	66	87	113***
440	Baleares	96	37	107	109*	61	109*	103***
441	Almeria	41	175	39	108	156	124***	107***
442	Cadiz	107	241***	153*	130***	129	135***	117***
443	Cordoba	156	54	124	107*	117	107*	102***
444	Granada	192*	265***	131	93	159	110**	106***
445	Huelva	79	191	164	127***	54	140***	111***
446	Jaen	177	145	35	103	76	124***	99
447	Malaga	81	191**	217***	116***	68	123***	116***
448	Sevilla	148	232***	126	126***	109	132***	114***
449	Murcia	209**	103	133	106	80	84	109***
450	Las Palmas	153	172	136	145***	107	128***	118***
451	Sta Cruz de Tenerife	27	95	79	108	18	93	107***

> **Table 7.1.6.** Total 'avoidable deaths' and deaths from all causes by small area and country

Notes on the use of this table

1. This table shows total numbers (5-year) of all 'avoidable deaths', total numbers of deaths (5-year) from all causes (age group 0–64 and all ages), and the percentage of all deaths which are 'avoidable' in the 0–64 age group and for all ages.

2. The mortality data presented here are the totals for each small area.

3. The small area numbers are as in the key maps.

4. This table is based on mortality data for 1980–84, except for Greece (1980–82), Italy (1979–83), and Spain (1979–83).

Table 7.1.6

Area		Total avoidable deaths	Total deaths (all causes ages 0–64)	'Avoidable deaths' as a percentage of total deaths (ages 0–64)	Total deaths (all causes all ages)	'Avoidable deaths' as a percentage of total deaths (all ages)
		(1)	(2)	((1)/(2))×100	(3)	((1)/(3))×100
BELGIUM		16258	131774	12.3	563017	2.9
1	Antwerpen	2598	18874	13.8	83773	3.1
2	Brabant	3523	28695	12.3	127791	2.8
3	West-Vlaanderen	1646	13076	12.6	58023	2.8
4	Oost-Vlaanderen	2042	16787	12.2	77545	2.6
5	Hainaut	2351	20942	11.2	85129	2.8
6	Liège	1682	15577	10.8	65257	2.6
7	Limburg	1220	8023	15.2	26349	4.6
8	Luxembourg (province)	407	3335	12.2	13450	3.0
9	Namur	789	6465	12.2	25700	3.1
LUXEMBOURG						
10	Luxembourg	632	5384	11.7	20704	3.1
FEDERAL REPUBLIC OF GERMANY		91159	793553	11.5	3566537	2.6
11	Schleswig–Holstein	3326	32095	10.4	156601	2.1
12	Hamburg	2130	23085	9.2	115791	1.8
13	Braunschweig	2486	20784	12.0	101495	2.4
14	Hannover	3009	27038	11.1	128217	2.3
15	Luneburg	1969	18396	10.7	84694	2.3
16	Weser–Ems	3173	26105	12.2	111669	2.8
17	Bremen	1019	9788	10.4	44017	2.3
18	Düsseldorf	8050	74019	10.9	311712	2.6
19	Köln	5667	49131	11.5	209736	2.7
20	Münster	4031	32447	12.4	125684	3.2
21	Detmold	2604	22666	11.5	104871	2.5
22	Arnsberg	6192	52539	11.8	218439	2.8
23	Darmstadt	4773	42489	11.2	189875	2.5
24	Giessen	1375	11570	11.9	54919	2.5

Table 7.1.6 cont

Area		Total avoidable deaths	Total deaths (all causes ages 0–64)	'Avoidable deaths' as a percentage of total deaths (ages 0–64)	Total deaths (all causes all ages)	'Avoidable deaths' as a percentage of total deaths (all ages)
		(1)	(2)	((1)/(2))×100	(3)	((1)/(3))×100
25	Kassel	1697	14530	11.7	72961	2.3
26	Koblenz	2249	17751	12.7	83645	2.7
27	Trier	790	6493	12.2	27929	2.8
28	Rheinhessen–Pfalz	3094	24705	12.5	107187	2.9
29	Stuttgart	4511	38585	11.7	169941	2.7
30	Karlsruhe	3504	29576	11.8	130603	2.7
31	Freiburg	2299	20554	11.2	94033	2.4
32	Tübingen	1938	16008	12.1	71637	2.7
33	Oberbayern	4476	41104	10.9	187554	2.4
34	Niederbayern	1638	13465	12.2	58477	2.8
35	Oberpfalz	1731	13697	12.6	56182	3.1
36	Oberfranken	1843	15371	12.0	68921	2.7
37	Mittelfranken	2307	20015	11.5	91061	2.5
38	Unterfranken	1699	14475	11.7	66729	2.5
39	Schwaben	2188	18611	11.8	88123	2.5
40	Saarland	1969	16065	12.3	64527	3.1
41	Berlin (West)	3422	30396	11.3	169307	2.0
DENMARK		6696	67298	9.9	280635	2.4
42	Kobenhavn and Frederiksberg (M)	898	11139	8.1	53060	1.7
43	Kobenhavns County	717	8430	8.5	26793	2.7
44	Frederiksborg County	353	3773	9.4	12925	2.7
45	Roskilde County	229	2247	10.2	7561	3.0
46	Vestsjaellands County	361	3637	9.9	15568	2.3
47	Storstroms County	325	3671	8.9	16641	2.0
48	Bornholms County	61	595	10.3	2950	2.1
49	Fyns County	552	5560	9.9	25775	2.1
50	Sonderjyllands County	346	2901	11.9	13041	2.7
51	Ribe County	283	2536	11.2	10080	2.8
52	Vejle County	431	4048	10.6	16959	2.5
53	Ringkobing County	378	3025	12.5	12149	3.1
54	Arhus County	759	6999	10.8	28913	2.6
55	Viborg County	336	2687	12.5	12567	2.7
56	Nordjyllands County	667	6050	11.0	25653	2.6
FRANCE		89435	671964	13.3	2728240	3.3
57	Ain	600	4725	12.7	19596	3.1
58	Aisne	1012	7581	13.3	29037	3.5
59	Allier	611	4984	12.3	24876	2.5
60	Alpes-de-Haute-Provence	182	1482	12.3	6898	2.6
61	Hautes-Alpes	166	1240	13.4	5519	3.0
62	Alpes-Maritimes	1232	10231	12.0	56580	2.2
63	Ardèche	459	3224	14.2	15824	2.9
64	Ardennes	588	4259	13.8	15591	3.8
65	Ariège	202	1560	12.9	9818	2.1
66	Aube	480	3601	13.3	15480	3.1
67	Aude	358	3117	11.5	18490	1.9
68	Aveyron	392	2822	13.9	17234	2.3
69	Bouches-du-Rhône	2784	20450	13.6	83854	3.3
70	Calvados	968	7306	13.2	26514	3.7
71	Cantal	320	2136	15.0	10533	3.0
72	Charente	544	3840	14.2	19372	2.8
73	Charente-Maritime	708	6028	11.7	28798	2.5
74	Cher	493	4025	12.2	19427	2.5
75	Corrèze	357	2995	11.9	16839	2.1
76	Corse	387	3049	12.7	13393	2.9
77	Côte-d'Or	777	5331	14.6	21894	3.5
78	Côtes-du-Nord	887	8224	10.8	33650	2.6
79	Creuse	533	1924	27.7	11859	4.5
80	Dordogne	460	4733	9.7	25483	1.8
81	Doubs	555	5270	10.5	18669	3.0

Table 7.1.6 cont

Area		Total avoidable deaths	Total deaths (all causes ages 0–64)	'Avoidable deaths' as a percentage of total deaths (ages 0–64)	Total deaths (all causes all ages)	'Avoidable deaths' as a percentage of total deaths (all ages)
		(1)	(2)	((1)/(2))×100	(3)	((1)/(3))×100
82	Drôme	763	4417	17.3	19071	4.0
83	Eure	708	5976	11.8	21652	3.3
84	Eure-et-Loir	549	4028	13.6	17321	3.2
85	Finistère	1398	12662	11.0	49454	2.8
86	Gard	840	6375	13.2	29100	2.9
87	Haute-Garonne	1109	8274	13.4	37806	2.9
88	Gers	232	1993	11.6	11226	2.1
89	Gironde	1684	13087	12.9	59389	2.8
90	Hérault	1118	7775	14.4	37809	3.0
91	Ille-et-Vilaine	1264	9250	13.7	35675	3.5
92	Indre	378	2961	12.8	16181	2.3
93	Indre-et-Loire	614	5317	11.5	24162	2.5
94	Isère	1342	10231	13.1	39022	3.4
95	Jura	411	2854	14.4	13054	3.1
96	Landes	414	3506	11.8	18121	2.3
97	Loiret-Cher	424	3420	12.4	16792	2.5
98	Loire	1135	9213	12.3	39034	2.9
99	Haute-Loire	331	2631	12.6	13309	2.5
100	Loire-Atlantique	1637	13133	12.5	46504	3.5
101	Loiret	803	5917	13.6	25427	3.2
102	Lot	227	1688	13.4	10254	2.2
103	Lotet-Garonne	456	3368	13.5	17547	2.6
104	Lozère	138	885	15.6	4886	2.8
105	Maine-et-Loire	1085	7239	15.0	30126	3.6
106	Manche	736	5837	12.6	24452	3.0
107	Marne	858	6644	12.9	24257	3.5
108	Haute-Marne	380	2711	14.0	10989	3.5
109	Mayenne	429	3126	13.7	13465	3.2
110	Meurthe-et-Moselle	1224	9532	12.8	33770	3.6
111	Meuse	405	2856	14.2	11399	3.6
112	Morbihan	1177	9639	12.2	34599	3.4
113	Moselle	1973	13784	14.3	44391	4.4
114	Nièvre	399	3338	12.0	17145	2.3
115	Nord	5642	39287	14.4	129260	4.4
116	Oise	1096	7869	13.9	28719	3.8
117	Orne	423	3768	11.2	15414	2.7
118	Pas-de-Calais	3331	22767	14.6	74642	4.5
119	Puy-de-Dôme	1049	7759	13.5	31503	3.3
120	Pyrénées-Atlantiques	761	6434	11.8	31855	2.4
121	Hautes-Pyrénées	367	2722	13.5	13410	2.7
122	Pyrénées-Orientales	510	4010	12.7	20839	2.4
123	Bas-Rhin	1414	11643	12.1	45670	3.1
124	Haut-Rhin	1161	8433	13.8	32901	3.5
125	Rhône	2162	16121	13.4	61249	3.5
126	Haute-Saône	402	2865	14.0	12670	3.2
127	Saône-et-Loire	936	7114	13.2	32633	2.9
128	Sarthe	687	5387	12.8	23820	2.9
129	Savoie	454	3921	11.6	15277	3.0
130	Haute-Savoie	735	5783	12.7	20000	3.7
131	Paris	3670	28091	13.1	116970	3.1
132	Seine-Maritime	2264	16179	14.0	56088	4.0
133	Seine-et-Marne	1314	9760	13.5	37031	3.5
134	Yvelines	1747	11929	14.6	38183	4.6
135	Deux-Sèvres	502	3407	14.7	17758	2.8
136	Somme	957	7443	12.9	29672	3.2
137	Tarn	463	3600	12.9	19742	2.3
138	Tarn-et-Garonne	291	2065	14.1	11245	2.6
139	Var	1152	8766	13.1	40020	2.9
140	Vaucluse	683	4984	13.7	21480	3.2
141	Vendée	739	5282	14.0	24583	3.0
142	Vienne	523	3769	13.9	18796	2.8

Table 7.1.6 cont

Area		Total avoidable deaths	Total deaths (all causes ages 0–64)	'Avoidable deaths' as a percentage of total deaths (ages 0–64)	Total deaths (all causes all ages)	'Avoidable deaths' as a percentage of total deaths (all ages)
		(1)	(2)	((1)/(2))×100	(3)	((1)/(3))×100
143	Haute-Vienne	459	3898	11.8	21897	2.1
144	Vosges	696	5413	12.9	21593	3.2
145	Yonne	498	4245	11.7	20517	2.4
146	Territoire-de-Belfort	217	1634	13.3	6238	3.5
147	Essonne	1395	10084	13.8	31926	4.4
148	Hauts-de-Seine	2277	16729	13.6	60202	3.8
149	Seine-Saint-Denis	2470	16973	14.6	50072	4.9
150	Val-de-Marne	1832	13982	13.1	49261	3.7
151	Val-d'Oise	1460	10044	14.5	32487	4.5
GREECE		18102	59538	30.4	258776	7.0
152	Greater Athens	6234	19466	32.0	71777	8.7
153	Rest of Central Greece and Eubea	1792	6344	28.2	29207	6.1
154	Peloponnisos	1815	5782	31.4	31639	5.7
155	Ionian Islands	273	1144	23.9	7330	3.7
156	Epirus	579	2006	28.9	8770	6.6
157	Thessaly	1206	4423	27.3	18944	6.4
158	Macedonia	3924	12702	30.9	53679	7.3
159	Thrace	768	2593	29.6	9112	8.4
160	Aegean Islands	691	2408	28.7	14679	4.7
161	Crete	820	2670	30.7	13639	6.0
ITALY		115879	675606	17.2	2718889	4.3
162	Torino	4750	29146	16.3	91216	5.2
163	Vercelli	906	5660	16.0	45229	2.0
164	Novara	1012	6891	14.7	30587	3.3
165	Cuneo	1115	7441	15.0	34232	3.3
166	Asti	414	2605	15.9	19965	2.1
167	Alessandria	855	6002	14.2	30018	2.8
168	Aosta	206	1751	11.8	13259	1.6
169	Imperia	380	2883	13.2	12562	3.0
170	Savona	504	3838	13.1	18672	2.7
171	Genova	1751	14192	12.3	58435	3.0
172	La Spezia	395	3008	13.1	26659	1.5
173	Varese	1481	9270	16.0	32733	4.5
174	Como/Sondrio	1744	12207	14.3	44861	3.9
175	Milano	7071	51569	13.7	156191	4.5
176	Bergamo	1906	12493	15.3	65826	2.9
177	Brescia	2058	15016	13.7	46880	4.4
178	Pavia	1108	7948	13.9	37618	2.9
179	Cremona	730	5371	13.6	25176	2.9
180	Mantova	731	5113	14.3	22424	3.3
181	Bolzano	746	5150	14.5	19444	3.8
182	Trento	769	5940	12.9	22319	3.4
183	Verona	1527	10147	15.0	35700	4.3
184	Vicenza	1326	9302	14.3	35191	3.8
185	Belluno	451	3680	12.3	17692	2.5
186	Treviso	1135	8752	13.0	29205	3.9
187	Venezia	1338	11031	12.1	37467	3.6
188	Padova	1388	10299	13.5	36682	3.8
189	Rovigo	442	3533	12.5	18865	2.3
190	Udine/Gorizia	1217	10540	11.5	35715	3.4
191	Trieste	410	4394	9.3	24704	1.7
192	Pordenone	417	3810	10.9	16588	2.5
193	Piacenza	504	4123	12.2	17233	2.9
194	Parma	731	5144	14.2	23215	3.1
195	Reggio Emilia	668	5007	13.3	22617	3.0
196	Modena	954	7346	13.0	28358	3.4
197	Bologna	1483	11635	12.7	46751	3.2
198	Ferrara	605	5198	11.6	28264	2.1
199	Ravenna	487	3980	12.2	18699	2.6

Table 7.1.6 cont

Area		Total avoidable deaths	Total deaths (all causes ages 0–64)	'Avoidable deaths' as a percentage of total deaths (ages 0–64)	Total deaths (all causes all ages)	'Avoidable deaths' as a percentage of total deaths (all ages)
		(1)	(2)	((1)/(2))×100	(3)	((1)/(3))×100
200	Forli	844	6491	13.0	26100	3.2
201	Pesaro	525	3577	14.7	18628	2.8
202	Ancona	695	4541	15.3	20374	3.4
203	Macerata	522	3105	16.8	16545	3.2
204	Ascoli Piceno	651	3590	18.1	16198	4.0
205	Massa-Carrara	407	2631	15.5	12763	3.2
206	Lucca	651	4807	13.5	20676	3.1
207	Pistoia	381	3002	12.7	16792	2.3
208	Firenze	1821	12990	14.0	52626	3.5
209	Livorno	574	4172	13.8	29850	1.9
210	Pisa	571	4338	13.2	21433	2.7
211	Arezzo	534	3521	15.2	18367	2.9
212	Siena	455	2892	15.7	15841	2.9
213	Grosseto	387	2787	13.9	13496	2.9
214	Perugia	988	6709	14.7	26007	3.8
215	Terni	427	2516	17.0	16000	2.7
216	Viterbo/Rieti	861	5143	16.7	20845	4.1
217	Roma	6615	41240	16.0	126083	5.2
218	Latina	948	4455	21.3	41582	2.3
219	Frosinone	1070	5058	21.2	19970	5.4
220	Caserta	2314	9174	25.2	29699	7.8
221	Benevento	691	3060	22.6	16255	4.3
222	Napoli	8727	37274	23.4	100149	8.7
223	Avellino	923	5362	17.2	36497	2.5
224	Salerno	2601	11005	23.6	36271	7.2
225	L'Aquila	655	3686	17.8	21008	3.1
226	Teramo	512	2784	18.4	13435	3.8
227	Pescara	549	2793	19.7	12536	4.4
228	Chieti	731	3856	19.0	16681	4.4
229	Isernia/Campobasso	750	3590	20.9	17167	4.4
230	Foggia	1657	6849	24.2	25361	6.5
231	Bari	3458	14444	23.9	50010	6.9
232	Taranto	1350	5658	23.9	27602	4.9
233	Brindisi	1037	4247	24.4	16321	6.4
234	Lecce	1774	7752	22.9	27402	6.5
235	Potenza/Matera	1432	6156	23.3	26364	5.4
236	Cosenza	1837	7304	25.2	28152	6.5
237	Catanzaro	1756	7190	24.4	28497	6.2
238	Reggio Calabria	1454	6149	23.6	26717	5.4
239	Trapani	1012	4396	23.0	21924	4.6
240	Palermo	3089	12841	24.1	46501	6.6
241	Messina	1594	6741	23.6	35713	4.5
242	Agrigento	1092	4561	23.9	23390	4.7
243	Caltanisetta	777	3170	24.5	14770	5.3
244	Enna	523	2094	25.0	10100	5.2
245	Catania	2837	11114	25.5	37362	7.6
246	Ragusa	704	2823	24.9	19150	3.7
247	Siracusa	942	4006	23.5	15634	6.0
248	Sassari	878	4459	19.7	17629	5.0
249	Nuoro	575	3013	19.1	13454	4.3
250	Cagliari/Oristano	2006	9075	22.1	29710	6.8
IRELAND		8178	41700	19.6	163916	5.0
251	Eastern	2817	13983	20.1	45990	6.1
252	Midland	437	2507	17.4	10212	4.3
253	Mid-Western	769	3969	19.4	16044	4.8
254	North Eastern	746	3563	20.9	13656	5.5
255	North Western	505	2538	19.9	12491	4.0
256	South Eastern	961	4539	21.2	18710	5.1
257	Southern	1253	6782	18.5	27520	4.6
258	Western	690	3819	18.1	19293	3.6

Table 7.1.6 cont

Area	Total avoidable deaths	Total deaths (all causes ages 0–64)	'Avoidable deaths' as a percentage of total deaths (ages 0–64)	Total deaths (all causes all ages)	'Avoidable deaths' as a percentage of total deaths (all ages)
	(1)	(2)	((1)/(2))×100	(3)	((1)/(3))×100
NETHERLANDS	18015	140579	12.8	584573	3.1
259 Groningen	664	5617	11.8	25415	2.6
260 Friesland	773	5552	13.9	26551	2.9
261 Drenthe	523	4289	12.2	17601	3.0
262 Overijssel	1382	10229	13.5	41506	3.3
263 Gelderland	2170	16823	12.9	69104	3.1
264 Utrecht	1169	8450	13.8	35928	3.3
265 Noord Holland	2752	23446	11.7	102262	2.7
266 Zuid Holland	3946	30648	12.9	135202	2.9
267 Zeeland	453	3278	13.8	16472	2.8
268 Noord Brabant	2657	19801	13.4	71627	3.7
269 Limburg	1420	11780	12.1	41516	3.4
270 Zuidelijke Ijsselmeerpolders	106	666	15.9	1389	7.6
UK:ENGLAND AND WALES	90165	641865	14.0	2878384	3.1
271 Cleveland	1323	8950	14.8	30529	4.3
272 Cumbria	1007	6924	14.5	30813	3.3
273 Durham	1325	9419	14.1	37345	3.5
274 Northumberland	543	4234	12.8	19413	2.8
275 Gateshead	496	3641	13.6	13682	3.6
276 Newcastle upon Tyne	571	4435	12.9	18947	3.0
277 Northern Tyneside	379	3151	12.0	12771	3.0
278 Southern Tyneside	363	2814	12.9	10647	3.4
279 Sunderland	668	4572	14.6	17055	3.9
280 Bradford	1160	6781	17.1	28636	4.1
281 Calderdale	459	2842	16.2	13043	3.5
282 Humberside	1675	11444	14.6	49435	3.4
283 Kirklees	841	5395	15.6	23862	3.5
284 Leeds	1372	10291	13.3	43407	3.2
285 North Yorkshire	1161	8124	14.3	42532	2.7
286 Wakefield	643	4597	14.0	18293	3.5
287 Barnsley	390	3283	11.9	12843	3.0
288 Derbyshire	1737	12311	14.1	53901	3.2
289 Doncaster	591	4067	14.5	15529	3.8
290 Leicestershire	1525	10126	15.1	43925	3.5
291 Lincolnshire	956	7061	13.5	33107	2.9
292 Nottinghamshire	1832	13230	13.8	55328	3.3
293 Rotherham	540	3566	15.1	13204	4.1
294 Sheffield	976	7656	12.7	35123	2.8
295 Cambridgeshire	858	6191	13.9	28991	3.0
296 Norfolk	1038	7673	13.5	42429	2.4
297 Suffolk	889	6373	13.9	34183	2.6
298 Barnet	390	3077	12.7	16750	2.3
299 Bedfordshire	903	5667	15.9	22586	4.0
300 Brent and Harrow	722	5076	14.2	22534	3.2
301 Ealing/Hammersmith/Hounslow	1094	8272	13.2	35632	3.1
302 Hertfordshire	1332	10877	12.2	45911	2.9
303 Hillingdon	352	2760	12.8	11746	3.0
304 Kensington/Chelsea/Westminster	587	4567	12.9	18078	3.2
305 Barking and Havering	672	5294	12.7	21683	3.1
306 Camden and Islington	599	4890	12.2	19729	3.0
307 City and East London	1361	8461	16.1	32347	4.2
308 Enfield and Haringey	777	5551	14.0	26330	3.0
309 Essex	2190	16640	13.2	78913	2.8
310 Redbridge and Waltham Forest	762	5363	14.2	25741	3.0
311 Bromley	405	3367	12.0	16174	2.5
312 East Sussex	980	7614	12.9	54961	1.8
313 Greenwich and Bexley	722	5288	13.7	23037	3.1
314 Kent	2459	17152	14.3	87140	2.8
315 Lambeth/Southwark/Lewisham	1491	10290	14.5	42264	3.5
316 Croydon	512	3676	13.9	17076	3.0

Table 7.1.6 cont

Area		Total avoidable deaths	Total deaths (all causes ages 0–64)	'Avoidable deaths' as a percentage of total deaths (ages 0–64)	Total deaths (all causes all ages)	'Avoidable deaths' as a percentage of total deaths (all ages)
		(1)	(2)	$((1)/(2))\times100$	(3)	$((1)/(3))\times100$
317	Kingston and Richmond	414	3319	12.5	17665	2.3
318	Merton/Sutton/Wandsworth	989	7454	13.3	36446	2.7
319	Surrey	1420	11271	12.6	54503	2.6
320	West Sussex	933	7198	13.0	46542	2.0
321	Dorset	806	6874	11.7	42660	1.9
322	Hampshire	2171	16346	13.3	75893	2.9
323	Isle of Wight	183	1417	12.9	8882	2.1
324	Wiltshire	796	5906	13.5	27365	2.9
325	Berkshire	972	7394	13.1	31238	3.1
326	Buckinghamshire	873	5875	14.9	24711	3.5
327	Northamptonshire	933	6140	15.2	27841	3.4
328	Oxfordshire	652	5483	11.9	24817	2.6
329	Avon	1433	10747	13.3	52142	2.7
330	Cornwall and Scilly Isles	691	5322	13.0	28517	2.4
331	Devon	1457	11495	12.7	65867	2.2
332	Gloucestershire	867	5880	14.7	28420	3.1
333	Somerset	704	4851	14.5	26870	2.6
334	Birmingham	2398	15001	16.0	60939	3.9
335	Coventry	741	4583	16.2	16972	4.4
336	Dudley	578	3937	14.7	15835	3.7
337	Hereford and Worcester	1136	7435	15.3	34618	3.3
338	Salop	768	4450	17.3	20541	3.7
339	Sandwell	843	4892	17.2	18449	4.6
340	Solihull	303	2194	13.8	8221	3.7
341	Staffordshire	2129	14220	15.0	54508	3.9
342	Walsall	618	4008	15.4	14031	4.4
343	Warwickshire	862	5977	14.4	25204	3.4
344	Wolverhampton	614	3794	16.2	14190	4.3
345	Bolton	567	4033	14.1	16520	3.4
346	Bury	340	2348	14.5	10810	3.1
347	Lancashire	2886	19921	14.5	95138	3.0
348	Manchester	1164	8000	14.6	31212	3.7
349	Oldham	540	3277	16.5	13924	3.9
350	Rochdale	498	3176	15.7	12161	4.1
351	Salford	535	4312	12.4	17030	3.1
352	Stockport	518	3667	14.1	16536	3.1
353	Tameside	490	3354	14.6	13455	3.6
354	Trafford	418	2988	14.0	12520	3.3
355	Wigan	591	4578	12.9	18270	3.2
356	Cheshire	1702	12425	13.7	50753	3.4
357	Liverpool	1141	8549	13.3	34445	3.3
358	St Helens and Knowsley	820	5815	14.1	19448	4.2
359	Sefton	587	4206	14.0	18727	3.1
360	Wirral	656	4903	13.4	21738	3.0
361	Clwyd	774	5163	15.0	25104	3.1
362	Dyfed	710	4726	15.0	22013	3.2
363	Gwent	880	6481	13.6	25953	3.4
364	Gwynedd	439	3006	14.6	15675	2.8
365	Mid Glamorgan	1309	8364	15.7	32992	4.0
366	Powys	206	1427	14.4	7243	2.8
367	South Glamorgan	730	5150	14.2	22070	3.3
368	West Glamorgan	752	5500	13.7	23155	3.2
UK:NORTHERN IRELAND						
369	Northern Ireland	3589	21453	16.7	80740	4.4
UK:SCOTLAND		11018	81540	13.5	317948	3.5
370	Highlands and Islands	534	4165	12.8	17141	3.1
371	Grampian	834	6305	13.2	27917	3.0
372	Tayside	700	5530	12.7	25836	2.7
373	Fife	759	4991	15.2	20223	3.8

Table 7.1.6 cont

Area		Total avoidable deaths	Total deaths (all causes ages 0–64)	'Avoidable deaths' as a percentage of total deaths (ages 0–64)	Total deaths (all causes all ages)	'Avoidable deaths' as a percentage of total deaths (all ages)
		(1)	(2)	((1)/(2))×100	(3)	((1)/(3))×100
374	Lothian	1425	10626	13.4	44235	3.2
375	Borders	205	1407	14.6	7254	2.8
376	Forth Valley	599	4164	14.4	15546	3.9
377	Argyll and Clyde	1033	7738	13.3	28010	3.7
378	Greater Glasgow	2364	18697	12.6	68174	3.5
379	Lanarkshire	1307	9348	14.0	29937	4.4
380	Ayrshire and Arran	979	6235	15.7	24120	4.1
381	Dumfries and Galloway	279	2334	12.0	9555	2.9
PORTUGAL		35253	144546	24.4	477008	7.4
382	Viana do Castelo	949	3231	29.4	13640	7.0
383	Braga	2704	8188	33.0	26055	10.4
384	Vila Real	1197	4119	29.1	13281	9.0
385	Braganca	704	2669	26.4	9942	7.1
386	Guarda	707	2973	23.8	12665	5.6
387	Viseu	1821	5907	30.8	22476	8.1
388	Porto	6250	25445	24.6	67275	9.3
389	Aveiro	2119	7459	28.4	25505	8.3
390	Coimbra	1665	8584	19.4	28007	5.9
391	Castelo Branco	783	3152	24.8	14062	5.6
392	Portalegre	483	1853	26.1	8890	5.4
393	Santarem	1360	5450	25.0	23240	5.9
394	Leiria	1278	5374	23.8	19696	6.5
395	Lisboa	7218	36835	19.6	106506	6.8
396	Setubal	1559	5761	27.1	19936	7.8
397	Evora	559	2186	25.6	9686	5.8
398	Beja	567	2482	22.8	10948	5.2
399	Faro	976	4462	21.9	18543	5.3
400	Madeira	1134	4126	27.5	12680	8.9
401	Azores	1220	4290	28.4	13975	8.7
SPAIN		71156	382773	18.6	1440845	4.9
402	La Coruña	2285	12983	17.6	47318	4.8
403	Lugo	793	4635	17.1	23253	3.4
404	Orense	942	4255	22.1	20160	4.7
405	Pontevedra	1691	9396	18.0	34335	4.9
406	Asturias	2112	13802	15.3	49633	4.3
407	Cantabria	993	5696	17.4	20837	4.8
408	Alava	384	2462	15.6	7928	4.8
409	Guipuzcoa	1054	6635	15.9	21386	4.9
410	Vizcaya	2123	13192	16.1	41055	5.2
411	Navarra	820	5441	15.1	20833	3.9
412	Rioja	487	2512	19.4	10701	4.6
413	Huesca	326	2022	16.1	9329	3.5
414	Teruel	226	1527	14.8	8141	2.8
415	Zaragoza	1429	8368	17.1	33571	4.3
416	Madrid Centro	7008	43741	16.0	140796	5.0
417	Avila	289	1765	16.4	7959	3.6
418	Burgos	475	3776	12.6	13271	3.6
419	Leon	1140	6277	18.2	24115	4.7
420	Palencia	377	2248	16.8	8820	4.3
421	Salamanca	699	3429	20.4	15507	4.5
422	Segovia	225	1517	14.8	6926	3.2
423	Soria	145	988	14.7	4932	2.9
424	Valladolid	584	4036	14.5	14552	4.0
425	Zamora	366	2321	15.8	11305	3.2
426	Albacete	806	3248	24.8	14750	5.5
427	Ciudad Real	1031	5061	20.4	21794	4.7
428	Cuenca	415	2238	18.5	11397	3.6
429	Guadalajara	203	1307	15.5	6182	3.3
430	Toledo	897	4542	19.7	21188	4.2

Table 7.1.6 cont

Area		Total avoidable deaths	Total deaths (all causes ages 0–64)	'Avoidable deaths' as a percentage of total deaths (ages 0–64)	Total deaths (all causes all ages)	'Avoidable deaths' as a percentage of total deaths (all ages)
		(1)	(2)	((1)/(2))×100	(3)	((1)/(3))×100
431	Badajoz	1523	7207	21.1	30211	5.0
432	Caceres	923	4358	21.2	19400	4.8
433	Barcelona	6260	42314	14.8	152951	4.1
434	Gerona	744	4980	14.9	20641	3.6
435	Lerida	633	3580	17.7	15451	4.1
436	Tarragona	922	5193	17.8	22067	4.2
437	Alicante	2316	11404	20.3	45628	5.1
438	Castellon de la Plana	862	4012	21.5	19872	4.3
439	Valencia	4310	22969	18.8	87349	4.9
440	Baleares	1396	7286	19.2	28657	4.9
441	Almeria	1003	3918	25.6	15662	6.4
442	Cadiz	2744	10200	26.9	32897	8.3
443	Cordoba	1553	6950	22.3	28923	5.4
444	Granada	1556	7608	20.5	29646	5.2
445	Huelva	1145	4421	25.9	18461	6.2
446	Jaen	1465	5719	25.6	25429	5.8
447	Malaga	2514	11551	21.8	39264	6.4
448	Sevilla	4124	15719	26.2	55057	7.5
449	Murcia	1797	9601	18.7	37488	4.8
450	Las Palmas	1798	7713	23.3	21844	8.2
451	Sta Cruz de Tenerife	1243	6650	18.7	21973	5.7

Tables 7.2.1 – 7.2.8. Observed numbers of deaths and mortality rates of infectious diseases, malignant neoplasm of trachea, bronchus, and lung, cirrhosis of the liver, and motor vehicle accidents by country

Notes on the use of these tables

1. These tables show the observed numbers of deaths and mortality rates from infectious diseases; malignant neoplasm of the trachea, bronchus, and lung; cirrhosis of the liver; and motor vehicle accidents within each country.

2. The mortality data presented here are the totals for each country in specified age groups.

3. Mortality rates have been calculated per 100 000 population except for diseases for which relatively few deaths were recorded, where the rates have been calculated per 1 000 000 population.

4. The mortality data are for 1980–84, except for Greece (1980–82), Italy (1979–83), and Spain (1979–83).

Table 7.2.1. Deaths from typhoid 1980–84

Country	Age group (years)						
	5–14	15–24	25–34	35–44	45–54	55–64	Total
Belgium	0	0	0	0	0	0	0
Luxembourg	0	0	0	1	0	0	1
Fed. Rep. Germany	1	3	1	0	0	1	6
Denmark	0	0	0	0	0	0	0
France	1	2	4	4	7	10	28
Greece	0	0	0	0	0	0	0
Italy	0	2	2	3	5	2	14
Ireland	0	0	0	0	0	0	0
Netherlands	0	0	0	0	0	0	0
UK : England,Wales							
& N.Ireland	0	3	1	1	1	1	7
: Scotland	0	0	0	0	0	1	1
Portugal	0	2	1	5	11	6	25
Spain	1	7	8	6	7	8	37

Deaths from typhoid 1980–84 (rates per 1 000 000)

Country	Age group (years)						
	5–14	15–24	25–34	35–44	45–54	55–64	Total
Belgium	0.00	0.00	0.00	0.00	0.00	0.00	0.00
Luxembourg	0.00	0.00	0.00	4.09	0.00	0.00	0.68
Fed. Rep. Germany	0.03	0.06	0.02	0.00	0.00	0.03	0.02
Denmark	0.00	0.00	0.00	0.00	0.00	0.00	0.00
France	0.02	0.05	0.09	0.12	0.22	0.36	0.13
Greece	0.00	0.00	0.00	0.00	0.00	0.00	0.00
Italy	0.00	0.05	0.05	0.08	0.14	0.07	0.06
Ireland	0.00	0.00	0.00	0.00	0.00	0.00	0.00
Netherlands	0.00	0.00	0.00	0.00	0.00	0.00	0.00
UK : England,Wales							
& N.Ireland	0.00	0.07	0.03	0.03	0.04	0.04	0.03
: Scotland	0.00	0.00	0.00	0.00	0.00	0.36	0.05
Portugal	0.00	0.24	0.15	0.87	1.91	1.19	0.62
Spain	0.03	0.23	0.32	0.28	0.30	0.44	0.24

Table 7.2.2. Deaths from whooping cough 1980–84

Country	Age group (years)				
	<1	1–4	5–9	10–14	Total
Belgium	3	1	1	0	5
Luxembourg	1	0	0	0	1
Fed. Rep. Germany	24	11	2	0	37
Denmark	1	0	0	0	1
France	20	1	0	0	21
Greece	2	0	0	0	2
Italy	29	5	0	0	34
Ireland	3	2	0	0	5
Netherlands	1	0	0	0	1
UK : England,Wales					
& N.Ireland	23	7	0	1	31
: Scotland	2	1	0	0	3
Portugal	11	1	0	0	12
Spain	14	1	1	0	16

Deaths from whooping cough 1980–84 (rates per 1 000 000)

Country	Age group (years)				
	<1	1–4	5–9	10–14	Total
Belgium	5.04	0.41	0.32	0.00	0.52
Luxembourg	45.87	0.00	0.00	0.00	2.96
Fed. Rep. Germany	7.93	0.93	0.13	0.00	0.71
Denmark	3.71	0.00	0.00	0.00	0.20
France	5.07	0.06	0.00	0.00	0.35
Greece	4.39	0.00	0.00	0.00	0.29
Italy	9.10	0.35	0.00	0.00	0.56
Ireland	8.25	1.43	0.00	0.00	0.96
Netherlands	1.14	0.00	0.00	0.00	0.07
UK : England,Wales					
& N.Ireland	7.03	0.55	0.00	0.05	0.60
: Scotland	6.04	0.78	0.00	0.00	0.56
Portugal	15.28	0.33	0.00	0.00	0.98
Spain	4.81	0.08	0.06	0.00	0.33

Table 7.2.3. Deaths from tetanus 1980–84

Country	Age groups (years)								
	<1	1–4	5–14	15–24	25–34	35–44	45–54	55–64	Total
Belgium	0	0	0	0	0	1	4	7	12
Luxembourg	0	0	0	0	0	0	0	0	0
Fed. Rep. Germany	0	0	0	1	0	2	3	8	14
Denmark	0	0	0	0	0	0	0	0	0
France	0	0	0	2	0	1	7	38	48
Greece	1	0	1	0	2	2	5	13	24
Italy	4	1	2	7	11	34	85	98	242
Ireland	0	0	0	0	1	0	0	0	1
Netherlands	0	0	0	1	0	0	1	1	3
UK : England, Wales									
& N.Ireland	0	0	0	0	2	1	3	1	7
: Scotland	0	0	0	0	1	0	0	0	1
Portugal	12	1	2	1	7	11	32	37	103
Spain	250	62	26	30	30	47	104	157	706

Deaths from tetanus 1980–84 (rates per 1 000 000)

Country	Age group (years)								
	<1	1–4	5–14	15–24	25–34	35–44	45–54	55–64	Total
Belgium	0.00	0.00	0.00	0.00	0.00	0.17	0.66	1.28	0.28
Luxembourg	0.00	0.00	0.00	0.00	0.00	0.00	0.00	0.00	0.00
Fed. Rep. Germany	0.00	0.00	0.00	0.02	0.00	0.05	0.08	0.25	0.05
Denmark	0.00	0.00	0.00	0.00	0.00	0.00	0.00	0.00	0.00
France	0.00	0.00	0.00	0.05	0.00	0.03	0.22	1.37	0.20
Greece	2.20	0.00	0.22	0.00	0.51	0.55	1.25	4.82	0.94
Italy	1.26	0.07	0.05	0.16	0.28	0.92	2.37	3.35	0.98
Ireland	0.00	0.00	0.00	0.00	0.42	0.00	0.00	0.00	0.07
Netherlands	0.00	0.00	0.00	0.08	0.00	0.00	0.13	0.15	0.05
UK : England, Wales									
& N.Ireland	0.00	0.00	0.00	0.00	0.06	0.03	0.11	0.04	0.03
: Scotland	0.00	0.00	0.00	0.00	0.28	0.00	0.00	0.00	0.05
Portugal	16.67	0.33	0.23	0.12	1.03	1.92	5.54	7.36	2.34
Spain	85.84	5.01	0.79	0.97	1.20	2.20	4.48	8.62	4.22

Table 7.2.4. Deaths from measles 1980–84

Country	Age group (years) 1–4	5–9	10–14	Total
Belgium	8	6	1	15
Luxembourg	0	1	1	2
Fed. Rep. Germany	23	13	10	46
Denmark	6	0	0	6
France	60	22	11	93
Greece	6	2	6	14
Italy	29	16	5	50
Ireland	12	1	2	15
Netherlands	2	0	0	2
UK : England, Wales & N.Ireland	40	12	5	57
: Scotland	4	6	1	11
Portugal	46	9	3	58
Spain	58	20	8	86

Deaths from measles 1980–84 (rates per 1 000 000)

Country	Age group (years) 1–4	5–9	10–14	Total
Belgium	3.30	1.94	0.29	1.67
Luxembourg	0.00	9.41	7.88	6.34
Fed. Rep. Germany	1.94	0.84	0.47	0.94
Denmark	5.07	0.00	0.00	1.25
France	3.82	1.15	0.51	1.66
Greece	3.19	0.89	2.55	2.16
Italy	2.06	0.76	0.22	0.86
Ireland	8.60	0.57	1.17	3.10
Netherlands	0.57	0.00	0.00	0.14
UK : England, Wales & N.Ireland	3.16	0.75	0.26	1.18
: Scotland	3.11	3.59	0.48	2.19
Portugal	15.20	2.13	0.70	5.03
Spain	4.68	1.21	0.48	1.89

Table 7.2.5. Deaths from osteomyelitis 1980–84

| Country | Age group (years) | | | | | | | |
	1–4	5–14	15–24	25–34	35–44	45–54	55–64	Total
Belgium	0	0	0	0	0	5	4	9
Luxembourg	0	0	0	0	0	0	0	0
Fed. Rep. Germany	0	0	3	6	14	37	78	138
Denmark	0	0	0	1	0	0	4	5
France	0	2	1	1	8	7	27	46
Greece	0	0	0	0	0	1	3	4
Italy	1	0	1	2	2	11	8	25
Ireland	0	0	0	1	3	2	2	8
Netherlands	0	0	0	0	2	2	5	9
UK : England, Wales								
& N.Ireland	0	2	2	2	5	6	42	59
: Scotland	0	0	0	0	0	0	2	2
Portugal	0	1	1	1	4	0	1	8
Spain	0	1	4	3	1	3	9	21

Deaths from osteomyelitis 1980–84 (rates per 1 000 000)

| Country | Age group (years) | | | | | | | |
	1–4	5–14	15–24	25–34	35–44	45–54	55–64	Total
Belgium	0.00	0.00	0.00	0.00	0.00	0.83	0.73	0.22
Luxembourg	0.00	0.00	0.00	0.00	0.00	0.00	0.00	0.00
Fed. Rep. Germany	0.00	0.00	0.06	0.14	0.32	0.94	2.43	0.53
Denmark	0.00	0.00	0.00	0.26	0.00	0.00	1.48	0.23
France	0.00	0.05	0.02	0.02	0.25	0.22	0.97	0.20
Greece	0.00	0.00	0.00	0.00	0.00	0.25	1.11	0.16
Italy	0.07	0.00	0.02	0.05	0.05	0.31	0.27	0.10
Ireland	0.00	0.00	0.00	0.42	1.68	1.33	1.39	0.53
Netherlands	0.00	0.00	0.00	0.00	0.21	0.26	0.74	0.14
UK: England, Wales								
& N.Ireland	0.00	0.06	0.05	0.06	0.16	0.21	1.47	0.28
: Scotland	0.00	0.00	0.00	0.00	0.00	0.00	0.72	0.09
Portugal	0.00	0.12	0.12	0.15	0.70	0.00	0.20	0.19
Spain	0.00	0.03	0.13	0.12	0.05	0.13	0.49	0.13

Table 7.2.6. Deaths from cancer of the trachea, bronchus, and lung 1980–84

Country	Age group (years)												Total
	5–9	10–14	15–19	20–24	25–29	30–34	35–39	40–44	45–49	50–54	55–59	60–64	
Belgium	0	2	7	3	16	50	128	341	856	1854	3346	4178	10781
Luxembourg	0	0	0	0	0	0	2	8	32	86	115	127	370
Fed. Rep. Germany	2	4	15	21	57	207	630	2064	4000	7967	11737	14395	41099
Denmark	0	0	1	1	4	21	61	139	377	780	1430	2274	5088
France	10	8	14	19	58	200	629	1458	3586	7301	11130	11902	36315
Greece	3	4	8	5	18	42	61	171	358	764	1164	1377	3975
Italy	13	14	20	40	97	249	715	2040	5121	10619	16712	16345	51985
Ireland	0	0	0	4	5	10	38	70	172	395	728	1070	2492
Netherlands	1	0	1	10	17	54	170	378	984	2055	3446	5433	12549
UK : England, Wales													
& N.Ireland	0	3	4	16	63	175	560	1315	3279	7884	16983	26556	56838
: Scotland	0	0	1	7	9	25	75	180	441	1111	2205	3128	7182
Portugal	3	5	5	11	16	42	68	153	307	665	1007	1162	3444
Spain	11	19	31	39	83	183	353	802	1843	3426	5561	6702	19053

Deaths from cancer of the trachea, bronchus, and lung 1980–84 (rates per 100 000)

Country	Age group (years)												Total
	5–9	10–14	15–19	20–24	25–29	30–34	35–39	40–44	45–49	50–54	55–59	60–64	
Belgium	0.0	0.1	0.2	0.1	0.4	1.4	4.0	12.3	29.0	60.0	111.6	169.1	27.4
Luxembourg	0.0	0.0	0.0	0.0	0.0	0.0	1.6	6.7	27.1	69.5	115.3	164.9	25.2
Fed. Rep. Germany	0.0	0.0	0.1	0.1	0.3	1.0	3.2	8.5	19.0	42.9	66.3	100.3	16.7
Denmark	0.0	0.0	0.0	0.1	0.2	1.1	3.0	8.7	27.0	58.2	103.9	170.9	25.0
France	0.1	0.0	0.1	0.1	0.3	0.9	3.5	10.1	23.3	45.4	73.0	94.9	16.6
Greece	0.1	0.2	0.4	0.2	0.9	2.1	3.7	8.6	18.0	38.0	79.3	112.0	17.2
Italy	0.1	0.1	0.1	0.2	0.5	1.3	3.9	10.8	28.4	59.4	98.2	133.6	22.7
Ireland	0.0	0.0	0.0	0.3	0.4	0.9	3.9	8.5	22.8	53.1	98.0	154.4	18.4
Netherlands	0.0	0.0	0.0	0.2	0.3	0.9	3.2	8.9	25.5	55.2	97.1	171.6	21.4
UK : England, Wales													
& N.Ireland	0.0	0.0	0.0	0.1	0.4	1.0	3.2	8.9	23.2	55.3	116.2	190.9	28.2
: Scotland	0.0	0.0	0.0	0.3	0.5	1.4	4.6	12.2	30.5	76.1	152.0	232.7	35.0
Portugal	0.1	0.1	0.1	0.3	0.5	1.3	2.3	5.5	10.6	23.2	37.1	50.2	8.6
Spain	0.1	0.1	0.2	0.3	0.7	1.5	3.2	7.9	15.6	30.1	54.3	84.0	12.5

Table 7.2.7. Deaths from cirrhosis of the liver 1980–84

Country	Age group (years)												Total
	15–19	20–24	25–29	30–34	35–39	40–44	45–49	50–54	55–59	60–64	65–69	70–74	
Belgium	3	8	52	119	183	271	462	710	839	829	827	879	5182
Luxembourg	0	0	7	6	19	33	41	59	54	53	55	49	376
Fed. Rep. Germany	28	99	538	1418	2654	5475	7166	8475	9226	8646	8727	10581	63033
Denmark	0	4	18	71	151	191	273	305	424	412	318	266	2433
France	15	36	236	965	1861	3021	6059	9705	11127	10614	8360	9144	61143
Greece	2	5	9	16	33	72	168	257	346	375	551	494	2328
Italy	65	157	404	924	1852	3522	6088	9477	12417	11497	18051	11596	76050
Ireland	0	3	4	7	13	28	36	58	64	80	84	80	457
Netherlands	3	10	41	85	137	202	302	412	442	414	443	408	2899
UK : England, Wales													
& N. Ireland	19	37	68	204	364	573	829	1110	1627	1829	1593	1385	9638
: Scotland	1	4	17	37	80	131	191	264	338	357	287	204	1911
Portugal	5	24	91	239	413	838	1406	1929	2248	2233	2158	1945	13529
Spain	37	99	203	545	918	1555	3077	4721	5686	5966	5713	5214	33734

Deaths from cirrhosis of the liver 1980–84 (rates per 100 000)

Country	Age group (years)												Total
	15–19	20–24	25–29	30–34	35–39	40–44	45–49	50–54	55–59	60–64	65–69	70–74	
Belgium	0.1	0.2	1.4	3.3	5.7	9.8	15.7	23.0	28.0	33.6	42.5	44.0	14.1
Luxembourg	0.0	0.0	4.8	4.2	15.3	27.5	34.7	47.7	54.2	68.8	66.5	67.0	27.0
Fed. Rep. Germany	0.1	0.4	2.4	6.8	13.6	22.6	34.1	45.7	52.1	60.2	66.5	75.0	26.7
Denmark	0.0	0.2	1.0	3.6	7.5	12.0	19.6	22.8	30.8	31.0	26.6	25.5	12.8
France	0.1	0.2	1.1	4.4	10.3	21.0	39.4	60.3	73.0	84.6	92.0	84.9	31.0
Greece	0.1	0.2	0.5	0.8	2.0	3.6	8.4	12.8	23.6	30.5	42.9	46.2	11.1
Italy	0.3	0.8	2.1	4.6	10.2	18.7	33.8	53.0	72.9	94.0	118.9	134.8	36.3
Ireland	0.0	0.2	0.3	0.6	1.3	3.4	4.8	7.8	8.6	11.5	12.6	15.6	4.0
Netherlands	0.0	0.2	0.7	1.4	2.6	4.8	7.8	11.1	12.5	13.1	16.4	17.9	5.5
UK : England, Wales													
& N.Ireland	0.1	0.2	0.4	1.1	2.1	3.9	5.9	7.8	11.1	13.1	13.1	12.7	5.1
: Scotland	0.0	0.2	0.9	2.1	4.9	8.9	13.2	18.1	23.3	26.6	24.3	19.4	10.0
Portugal	0.1	0.6	2.6	7.3	14.0	30.1	48.3	67.3	82.8	96.5	108.6	112.2	38.2
Spain	0.2	0.7	1.6	4.4	8.2	15.2	26.1	41.4	55.5	74.8	78.9	85.4	25.5

Table 7.2.8. Deaths from motor vehicle accidents 1980–84

Country	Age groups (years)														Total
	0–4	5–9	10–14	15–19	20–24	25–29	30–34	35–39	40–44	45–49	50–54	55–59	60–64	65+	
Belgium	177	247	288	1315	1651	972	719	540	526	546	525	538	442	2188	10674
Luxembourg	7	7	8	69	72	52	27	20	30	19	24	20	15	87	457
Fed. Rep. Germany	887	1337	1352	10008	8987	4067	2765	2555	2981	2607	2404	2153	1863	11663	55629
Denmark	65	93	125	540	405	194	151	163	136	141	145	159	183	881	3381
France	949	1059	1228	6469	9145	5001	3853	3153	2591	2871	3039	2845	2277	9427	53907
Greece	126	126	130	509	609	439	302	273	320	332	336	288	246	1043	5079
Italy	266	1084	1557	6335	5224	3189	2480	2267	2683	3127	3276	3620	2948	12635	50691
Ireland	109	131	110	454	432	175	143	120	121	84	107	140	134	550	2810
Netherlands	150	308	400	1267	1221	583	454	460	365	308	350	396	398	2073	8733
UK: England,Wales & N.Ireland	508	803	961	4763	3700	1877	1386	1113	966	940	1049	1169	1218	6145	26598
: Scotland	53	141	125	532	446	260	202	160	163	154	155	169	166	739	3465
Portugal	488	567	438	1255	1841	1208	849	754	830	968	1007	1014	947	2881	15047
Spain	808	841	774	2857	3361	2277	1783	1594	1654	1824	1986	1828	1455	5307	28349

Deaths from motor vehicle accidents 1980–84 (rates per 100 000)

Country	Age group (years)														Total
	0–4	5–9	10–14	15–19	20–24	25–29	30–34	35–39	40–44	45–49	50–54	55–59	60–64	65+	
Belgium	5.9	8.0	8.3	34.3	41.5	25.5	19.8	16.7	18.9	18.5	17.0	17.9	17.9	31.7	21.7
Luxembourg	6.7	6.6	6.3	49.4	49.5	35.4	19.0	16.1	25.0	16.1	19.4	20.1	19.5	35.2	25.1
Fed. Rep. Germany	6.0	8.6	6.3	38.2	36.4	18.4	13.2	13.1	12.3	12.4	13.0	12.2	13.0	25.2	18.1
Denmark	4.5	5.4	6.7	26.6	21.5	10.4	7.8	8.1	8.5	10.1	10.8	11.5	13.8	23.5	13.2
France	4.8	5.6	5.7	29.7	43.0	23.9	17.6	17.4	18.0	18.7	18.9	18.7	18.2	25.0	19.6
Greece	5.4	5.6	5.5	23.6	28.6	22.1	15.4	16.4	16.2	16.7	16.7	19.6	20.0	28.1	17.4
Italy	1.5	5.2	6.8	27.3	25.1	16.4	12.5	12.5	14.2	17.3	18.3	21.3	24.1	33.8	17.9
Ireland	6.2	7.5	6.5	27.9	31.4	14.3	12.4	12.4	14.7	11.1	14.4	18.8	19.3	30.0	16.4
Netherlands	3.4	6.4	6.7	20.3	19.8	10.0	7.7	8.7	8.6	8.0	9.4	11.2	12.6	24.7	12.2
UK: England,Wales & N.Ireland	3.2	5.0	4.9	22.4	18.6	10.7	7.6	6.4	6.6	6.7	7.4	8.0	8.8	16.0	10.4
: Scotland	3.3	8.4	6.0	23.5	21.1	14.3	11.4	9.8	11.1	10.6	10.6	11.6	12.3	20.2	13.4
Portugal	13.0	13.4	10.2	29.2	45.6	34.1	26.1	25.5	29.8	33.3	35.1	37.4	40.9	47.7	30.1
Spain	5.3	5.1	4.7	17.5	22.8	17.9	14.5	14.3	16.2	15.4	17.4	17.9	18.2	24.9	15.0

Table 7.3.1. Health services resources and socio-economic indicators by small area or region

Notes on the use of this table

Between-country comparisons using the data in this table should not be made.

1. This table shows three health services resources and three socio-economic status indicators by small area and region.

2. Key for the abbreviations used for columns of the table:
   GP   — number of GPs per 100 000 population;
   BEDS — number of acute hospital beds per 1 000 population;
   CONS — number of consultants per 100 000 population (excluding psychiatry, dentistry, and long-stay specialities);
   BATH — percentage of households with fixed bath or shower;
   ROOM — average number of persons per room (excluding kitchen and bathroom);
   CAR   — number of private cars per 100 inhabitants.

3. The small area numbers are as in the key maps. In some instances data were not available by small area and so have been presented for the region.

4. The majority of the data is taken from Eurostat 'regional statistics' and from data supplied by the individual countries themselves. It must be stressed that in spite of efforts made by Eurostat to produce comparable data they are not necessarily so; therefore country to country comparisons are inadvisable.

5. The indicators are based on data for the following years:

Country	Health services resources			Socio-economic status		
	GP	BED	CONS	BATH	ROOM	CAR
Belgium	1981	1981	1981(a)	1981(b)	1981	1981
Luxembourg	1981	1981	1981	1981	1981	1981
Fed. Rep. Germany	1981	1981	1981	1982(c)	1981(d)	1981
Denmark	1982	1982	1982	1981	1981	1982
France	1982	1982(j)	1982	1982	1982	1982
Greece	1981(e)	1981	(e)	1981	1981(f)	1981
Italy	1984	1982	1982	1981	1981	1982
Ireland	1981	1981	1981	1981	1981	1981
Netherlands	1981	1980	1980(k)	1981	1981	1980
UK:England	1981	1981	1981	1981	1981	1981
: Wales & N. Ireland	1981	1981	1981	1981	1981	1981
: Scotland	1981	1981	1981(g)	1981	1981	1981
Portugal	1981	1981(h)	1981	1981	1981	1981(i)
Spain	1984	1984	1984	1981	1981	1984

(a) All consultants.
(b) Percentage of houses with fixed bath or shower.
(c) Derived from a 1% sample survey.
(d) Data include kitchens.
(e) GPs and consultants combined.
(f) Number of households members/number of households.
(g) Excluding: geriatric, dental, psychiatric, laboratory, occupational health, and call CSA employees.
(h) Excluding: paedopsychiatry and psychiatry.
(i) Average figures for 1980–82.
(j) Public hospitals only.
(k) The consultants in region 12 for the Netherlands are assigned to region 4.

Table 7.3.1

Area		Region	Indicators					
			GP	BED	CONS	BATH	ROOM	CAR
BELGIUM								
1	Antwerpen		106.2	5.6	78.0	82.5	0.56	33.0
2	Brabant		159.2	5.3	172.3	78.0	0.52	35.3
3	West-Vlaanderen		105.3	6.3	72.9	69.8	0.56	31.3
4	Oost-Vlaanderen		109.4	5.7	78.4	69.9	0.56	30.2
5	Hainaut		119.1	6.1	96.1	71.5	0.52	30.4
6	Liège		155.2	4.7	123.6	76.2	0.52	33.4
7	Limburg		91.2	5.3	52.9	83.1	0.61	32.5
8	Luxembourg (province)		135.2	3.0	70.3	75.9	0.50	32.4
9	Namur		150.0	4.4	97.3	80.0	0.51	31.7
LUXEMBOURG								
10	Luxembourg		50.9	7.6	96.3	86.0	0.51	70.0
FEDERAL REPUBLIC OF GERMANY								
11	Schleswig–Holstein		49.6	5.8	95.6	90.3	0.55	37.5
12	Hamburg		54.9	9.6	187.0	95.0	0.55	34.7
13	Braunschweig	)						
14	Hannover	)Niedersachen	44.3	7.2	82.1	94.7	0.55	38.2
15	Luneburg	)						
16	Weser–Ems	)						
17	Bremen		36.6	12.4	139.4	92.3	0.54	35.0
18	Düsseldorf	)						
19	Köln	)						
20	Münster	)Nordrhein–Westfalen	37.3	8.1	98.8	91.2	0.61	38.0
21	Detmold	)						
22	Arnsberg	)						
23	Darmstadt	)						
24	Giessen	)Hessen	46.9	6.7	96.0	91.6	0.56	40.6
25	Kassel	)						
26	Koblenz	)						
27	Trier	)Rheinland–Pfalz	48.0	8.2	94.4	92.2	0.53	40.3
28	Rheinhessen–Pfalz	)						
29	Stuttgart	)						
30	Karlsruhe	)Baden Wurttemberg	50.5	6.8	95.6	91.8	0.56	39.8
31	Freiburg	)						
32	Tübingen	)						
33	Oberbayern	)						
34	Niederbayern	)						
35	Oberpfalz	)						
36	Oberfranken	)Bayern	53.2	7.2	92.9	91.1	0.57	38.3
37	Mittelfranken	)						
38	Unterfranken	)						
39	Schwaben	)						
40	Saarland		37.4	9.1	110.2	91.7	0.54	39.5
41	Berlin (West)		39.0	12.6	189.7	86.9	0.51	30.8
DENMARK								
42	Kobenhavn and Frederiksberg (M)		53.0	16.0	79.0	60.0	0.64	17.0
43	Kobenhavns County		55.0	6.0	31.0	92.0	0.69	25.0
44	Frederiksborg County		54.0	5.0	28.0	90.0	0.68	27.0
45	Roskilde County		54.0	3.0	19.0	90.0	0.67	31.0
46	Vestsjaellands County		56.0	9.0	38.0	81.0	0.65	28.0

Table 7.3.1 cont

Area		Region	Indicators					
			GP	BED	CONS	BATH	ROOM	CAR
47	Storstroms County		56.0	7.0	35.0	79.0	0.62	25.0
48	Bornholms County		70.0	5.0	40.0	82.0	0.61	27.0
49	Fyns County		57.0	7.0	39.0	84.0	0.63	28.0
50	Sonderjyllands County		56.0	6.0	30.0	87.0	0.63	29.0
51	Ribe County		56.0	7.0	34.0	87.0	0.66	28.0
52	Vejle County		54.0	7.0	36.0	84.0	0.64	28.0
53	Ringkobing County		57.0	5.0	27.0	89.0	0.64	29.0
54	Arhus County		56.0	8.0	45.0	83.0	0.66	26.0
55	Viborg County		58.0	8.0	36.0	84.0	0.63	29.0
56	Nordjyllands County		57.0	7.0	33.0	83.0	0.65	29.0
FRANCE								
57	Ain		9.9	4.0	4.2	86.7	0.72	40.4
58	Aisne		10.7	4.3	3.6	75.1	0.73	35.3
59	Allier		12.2	4.4	6.8	79.5	0.70	42.0
60	Alpes-de-Haute-Provence		14.5	6.9	9.3	90.5	0.71	43.2
61	Hautes-Alpes		16.2	6.2	9.7	88.8	0.74	43.7
62	Alpes-Maritimes		16.6	3.3	13.8	94.4	0.79	40.2
63	Ardèche		9.9	4.6	5.2	79.9	0.72	40.6
64	Ardennes		7.8	4.8	5.7	79.0	0.72	35.3
65	Ariège		14.2	4.1	5.8	83.5	0.66	39.9
66	Aube		9.6	3.7	4.7	81.3	0.73	40.4
67	Aude		13.0	4.4	8.9	89.2	0.66	40.9
68	Aveyron		11.0	3.2	6.4	81.4	0.71	43.7
69	Bouches-du-Rhône		17.0	4.4	16.1	91.7	0.81	35.2
70	Calvados		13.0	5.0	7.6	82.5	0.74	37.3
71	Cantal		11.3	4.0	5.6	71.5	0.73	38.0
72	Charente		12.0	3.3	5.5	79.5	0.69	43.5
73	Charente-Maritime		13.2	4.0	5.8	83.2	0.69	42.8
74	Cher		8.3	3.6	4.2	79.0	0.73	39.7
75	Corrèze		11.5	4.7	5.8	80.0	0.68	41.9
76	Corse		12.4	4.6	8.0	0.0	0.00	38.9
77	Côte-d'Or		11.8	5.3	8.8	84.5	0.72	38.8
78	Côtes-du-Nord		11.1	4.2	5.6	77.3	0.71	38.1
79	Creuse		11.1	3.3	3.8	65.2	0.65	38.6
80	Dordogne		11.8	2.9	4.7	81.5	0.68	42.6
81	Doubs		13.0	4.3	8.2	87.1	0.73	37.6
82	Drôme		11.7	3.4	8.4	89.2	0.71	43.9
83	Eure		9.1	3.8	4.7	84.0	0.74	38.2
84	Eure-et-Loir		10.0	4.0	5.6	86.4	0.74	39.4
85	Finistère		11.5	3.6	7.7	83.8	0.68	38.3
86	Gard		13.7	3.4	8.7	90.9	0.72	41.3
87	Haute-Garonne		16.3	3.9	14.2	91.7	0.72	41.1
88	Gers		12.2	4.5	4.7	84.7	0.67	45.1
89	Gironde		12.5	4.3	11.3	88.6	0.71	41.4
90	Hérault		16.8	4.5	13.8	92.5	0.72	38.4
91	Ille-et-Vilaine		11.8	3.8	8.6	80.3	0.77	38.1
92	Indre		9.0	3.3	4.4	77.8	0.72	42.5
93	Indre-et-Loire		14.0	3.9	8.1	85.7	0.75	38.7
94	Isère		13.1	3.7	8.6	89.8	0.74	38.5
95	Jura		9.8	4.8	4.5	82.7	0.70	40.0
96	Landes		14.7	2.9	6.0	88.6	0.66	41.7
97	Loir-et-Cher		9.9	3.0	4.7	82.7	0.73	42.4
98	Loire		11.0	4.1	6.5	81.1	0.77	36.7
99	Haute-Loire		9.9	4.0	3.8	70.0	0.71	37.5
100	Loire-Atlantique		12.9	3.4	7.4	86.7	0.77	36.9
101	Loiret		9.2	3.9	6.7	88.5	0.73	42.1
102	Lot		11.5	4.7	6.2	82.9	0.68	45.9
103	Lot-et-Garonne		12.1	3.6	6.8	86.9	0.69	45.0
104	Lozère		11.3	6.0	3.9	75.0	0.69	41.6
105	Maine-et-Loire		11.1	3.9	7.3	85.4	0.76	33.9
106	Manche		8.4	4.2	5.5	73.3	0.72	39.7
107	Marne		11.3	4.7	7.2	87.0	0.71	36.6

Table 7.3.1 cont

Area		Region	Indicators					
			GP	BED	CONS	BATH	ROOM	CAR
108		Haute-Marne	9.4	5.6	5.4	80.9	0.72	38.3
109		Mayenne	8.8	3.9	4.9	78.4	0.74	40.0
110		Meurthe-et-Moselle	14.7	5.8	9.5	85.0	0.71	35.1
111		Meuse	9.1	4.6	4.7	79.3	0.71	36.1
112		Morbihan	10.6	3.8	5.9	78.9	0.68	36.4
113		Moselle	9.6	3.2	6.0	88.1	0.75	33.8
114		Nièvre	10.4	5.6	5.6	75.5	0.71	42.2
115		Nord	13.2	3.7	6.4	76.3	0.72	31.0
116		Oise	8.0	3.3	5.2	84.2	0.76	33.7
117		Orne	9.6	4.8	4.3	75.9	0.74	40.1
118		Pas-de-Calais	10.6	2.6	4.0	71.7	0.73	30.0
119		Puy-de-Dôme	14.3	3.9	8.5	80.8	0.73	40.9
120		Pyrénées-Atlantiques	13.6	2.5	10.1	91.8	0.68	41.0
121		Hautes-Pyrénées	16.0	3.2	8.1	87.2	0.71	42.6
122		Pyrénées-Orientales	16.1	2.0	9.2	92.1	0.72	41.7
123		Bas-Rhin	13.2	5.3	11.2	87.1	0.69	35.4
124		Haut-Rhin	11.3	5.7	7.2	84.8	0.69	37.6
125		Rhône	15.1	4.6	10.4	87.1	0.78	38.5
126		Haute-Saône	9.6	3.7	4.0	78.3	0.68	36.3
127		Saône-et-Loire	9.4	3.3	5.8	79.4	0.73	40.5
128		Sarthe	9.2	3.7	5.9	81.6	0.76	38.2
129		Savoie	13.9	5.5	7.9	89.1	0.74	42.0
130		Haute-Savoie	12.4	4.7	7.8	91.4	0.76	41.1
131		Paris	22.3	9.4	27.9	77.5	0.79	41.8
132		Seine-Maritime	10.6	4.1	8.7	84.4	0.76	36.7
133		Seine-et-Marne	9.9	3.0	6.7	90.8	0.76	33.6
134		Yvelines	10.3	2.4	9.1	93.8	0.79	35.0
135		Deux-Sèvres	9.7	3.1	5.1	81.1	0.71	42.5
136		Somme	11.4	4.1	5.1	73.7	0.72	34.5
137		Tarn	11.6	3.4	7.8	87.5	0.68	43.5
138		Tarn-et-Garonne	10.5	3.0	7.0	84.8	0.71	44.8
139		Var	13.7	3.6	9.3	94.2	0.76	40.4
140		Vaucluse	12.7	3.6	9.8	93.9	0.72	44.8
141		Vendée	9.9	2.9	4.9	86.1	0.74	38.4
142		Vienne	12.4	3.6	5.6	80.8	0.72	41.4
143		Haute-Vienne	14.3	4.7	8.9	80.1	0.70	41.8
144		Vosges	10.1	4.4	5.8	79.2	0.69	35.1
145		Yonne	11.7	4.9	5.3	81.5	0.71	40.6
146		Territoire-de-Belfort	11.7	3.9	6.6	86.5	0.70	38.0
147		Essonne	10.2	1.8	8.5	94.4	0.79	26.5
148		Hauts-de-Seine	14.3	1.2	11.1	87.3	0.82	42.9
149		Seine-Saint-Denis	10.5	1.6	6.3	87.8	0.88	31.1
150		Val-de-Marne	11.2	1.1	10.6	90.0	0.83	32.4
151		Val-d'Oise	11.0	2.9	6.6	92.9	0.81	31.2
GREECE								
152		Greater Athens	457.6	9.5	N/A	93.7	2.90	12.6
153		Rest of Central Greece and Eubea	79.1	2.3	N/A	57.3	3.40	4.7
154		Peloponnisos	139.0	3.6	N/A	49.8	3.30	4.7
155		Ionian Islands	139.1	5.8	N/A	48.4	3.10	5.7
156		Epirus	132.2	2.6	N/A	39.8	3.30	4.1
157		Thessaly	140.7	4.2	N/A	49.5	3.40	5.4
158		Macedonia	252.6	6.0	N/A	66.3	3.20	7.3
159		Thrace	128.6	3.9	N/A	41.5	3.30	4.7
160		Aegean Islands	107.6	7.6	N/A	44.5	2.90	5.1
161		Crete	133.2	5.7	N/A	44.9	3.00	5.5
ITALY								
162		Torino	151.0	7.8	6.8	86.8	0.80	46.0
163		Vercelli	132.7	8.1	7.1	84.3	0.60	35.6
164		Novara	128.0	8.5	7.9	86.7	0.70	40.5
165		Cuneo	111.9	10.1	9.9	81.4	0.70	42.4
166		Asti	130.5	6.7	8.2	83.6	0.60	35.8

Table 7.3.1 cont

Area		Region	Indicators					
			GP	BED	CONS	BATH	ROOM	CAR
167	Alessandria		137.0	11.1	14.5	85.6	0.60	42.1
168	Aosta		128.6	4.1	8.8	82.8	0.70	37.7
169	Imperia		156.3	10.4	8.0	87.0	0.70	39.8
170	Savona		153.6	11.8	12.6	88.5	0.60	36.5
171	Genova		223.6	11.0	7.9	86.3	0.60	38.5
172	La Spezia		206.5	5.6	6.0	88.1	0.70	29.0
173	Varese		120.1	9.4	10.3	91.5	0.70	40.7
174	Como/Sondrio		122.8	8.3	11.1	90.1	0.80	38.5
175	Milano		139.4	6.3	5.9	90.8	0.80	41.5
176	Bergamo		113.8	6.7	8.9	91.8	0.80	29.9
177	Brescia		127.2	8.2	11.4	90.6	0.70	38.2
178	Pavia		156.4	10.7	15.4	85.2	0.70	40.1
179	Cremona		141.6	9.6	11.1	87.2	0.70	35.3
180	Mantova		134.8	9.4	19.8	90.7	0.70	39.5
181	Bolzano		54.0	8.3	16.7	86.2	0.80	34.0
182	Trento		128.1	10.4	20.6	89.9	0.70	37.3
183	Verona		144.8	12.1	19.1	92.7	0.70	41.3
184	Vicenza		110.6	10.4	15.3	91.7	0.70	38.4
185	Belluno		113.7	14.0	23.6	86.8	0.60	33.2
186	Treviso		98.8	9.9	17.7	92.6	0.70	37.9
187	Venezia		112.0	11.0	13.3	92.9	0.70	30.7
188	Padova		133.5	11.1	15.4	93.0	0.70	38.1
189	Rovigo		111.2	8.2	12.0	88.7	0.70	32.9
190	Udine/Gorizia		119.5	11.8	17.6	90.7	0.60	40.0
191	Trieste		161.8	12.0	12.4	84.2	0.60	38.5
192	Pordenone		96.6	12.1	23.2	92.9	0.60	36.7
193	Piacenza		152.8	9.4	13.1	88.8	0.70	41.2
194	Parma		182.6	9.0	18.1	91.6	0.60	44.4
195	Reggio Emilia		144.6	7.2	17.3	93.7	0.60	43.1
196	Modena		131.3	8.1	11.7	94.5	0.70	45.0
197	Bologna		184.0	9.9	16.0	94.7	0.70	47.0
198	Ferrara		144.6	8.8	16.8	92.4	0.70	35.5
199	Ravenna		149.0	9.4	14.0	95.0	0.60	45.8
200	Forli		156.4	9.4	11.8	95.0	0.70	42.8
201	Pesaro		141.0	9.6	19.7	89.3	0.80	38.4
202	Ancona		171.4	13.9	23.8	94.3	0.70	41.1
203	Macerata		141.3	12.6	20.3	92.0	0.70	38.3
204	Ascoli Piceno		152.9	9.1	21.0	91.7	0.70	39.1
205	Massa-Carrara		193.4	9.4	13.0	82.9	0.70	33.4
206	Lucca		162.9	9.0	11.3	87.6	0.60	42.0
207	Pistoia		158.5	6.1	6.6	91.5	0.60	40.9
208	Firenze		197.3	9.3	8.4	93.5	0.70	48.0
209	Livorno		187.3	7.4	10.9	91.5	0.70	34.9
210	Pisa		229.7	10.3	13.8	90.2	0.70	42.1
211	Arezzo		153.4	8.7	15.3	91.6	0.70	41.0
212	Siena		199.1	11.9	19.6	89.8	0.70	45.2
213	Grosseto		156.3	7.7	11.5	90.0	0.70	39.7
214	Perugia		157.1	9.3	18.3	92.6	0.70	41.5
215	Terni		179.7	6.8	8.5	91.3	0.70	36.8
216	Viterbo/Rieti		156.5	7.1	8.5	84.7	0.70	37.0
217	Roma		185.7	9.3	7.1	95.8	0.80	41.9
218	Latina		142.8	5.6	9.2	90.1	0.80	24.5
219	Frosinone		149.2	8.1	9.0	82.1	0.80	30.6
220	Caserta		212.6	4.5	5.9	76.2	0.90	21.9
221	Benevento		204.4	4.2	3.3	72.8	0.80	22.6
222	Napoli		206.7	5.8	6.3	84.2	1.00	23.5
223	Avellino		184.9	2.5	2.9	75.2	0.90	12.1
224	Salerno		210.4	9.7	11.1	79.2	0.90	37.1
225	L'Aquila		236.4	9.5	16.1	81.0	0.70	29.4
226	Teramo		161.7	8.3	12.9	86.1	0.80	28.8
227	Pescara		185.6	7.0	7.6	89.3	0.80	30.0
228	Chieti		183.2	8.6	18.1	81.9	0.70	41.5
229	Isernia/Campobasso		173.4	3.6	8.2	72.2	0.80	16.7

Table 7.3.1 cont

Area		Region	Indicators					
			GP	BED	CONS	BATH	ROOM	CAR
230	Foggia		155.3	3.6	5.7	80.8	1.10	13.1
231	Bari		142.7	14.6	16.5	75.8	1.00	34.1
232	Taranto		131.2	6.8	9.8	77.7	0.90	28.3
233	Brindisi		118.0	6.5	7.2	73.0	0.90	16.8
234	Lecce		156.7	8.1	9.1	76.1	0.80	29.6
235	Potenza/Matera		160.7	5.1	10.4	67.9	1.00	20.8
236	Cosenza		158.6	5.8	6.3	70.9	0.90	21.8
237	Catanzaro		163.5	6.3	10.3	69.2	0.90	23.9
238	Reggio Calabria		222.8	8.6	14.3	72.1	0.90	27.3
239	Trapani		160.5	2.8	3.2	80.2	0.80	16.0
240	Palermo		206.6	8.7	11.3	79.9	0.90	39.2
241	Messina		235.2	8.5	7.1	77.8	0.80	31.7
242	Agrigento		195.8	4.1	5.9	65.3	0.90	27.8
243	Caltanisetta		169.5	7.8	7.3	68.4	0.90	27.5
244	Enna		150.0	2.1	2.4	66.9	0.90	7.0
245	Catania		175.3	10.7	10.6	78.3	0.90	48.2
246	Ragusa		167.3	6.8	7.1	81.0	0.80	24.6
247	Siracusa		164.5	4.8	9.4	82.9	0.90	28.9
248	Sassari		167.3	10.3	18.0	84.7	0.80	36.2
249	Nuoro		141.1	2.6	4.5	79.6	0.80	10.8
250	Cagliari/Oristano		183.9	3.6	4.4	83.9	0.80	15.8
IRELAND								
251	Eastern		46.0	6.3	35.0	92.1	0.73	2.2
252	Midland		50.0	3.3	10.0	75.9	0.77	2.3
253	Mid-Western		42.0	4.1	17.0	76.1	0.76	2.3
254	North Eastern		46.0	3.7	13.0	79.3	0.74	2.3
255	North Western		55.0	3.8	15.0	69.8	0.77	2.1
256	South Eastern		48.0	4.4	12.0	76.2	0.74	2.4
257	Southern		48.0	5.8	27.0	78.7	0.73	2.4
258	Western		57.0	5.2	27.0	75.2	0.74	2.1
NETHERLANDS								
259	Groningen		40.9	4.6	35.3	94.2	0.68	31.5
260	Friesland		40.9	3.9	26.6	94.4	0.69	30.5
261	Drenthe		41.0	3.5	35.7	96.9	0.68	33.8
262	Overijssel		34.6	4.8	33.5	97.1	0.71	32.2
263	Gelderland		38.3	4.2	37.3	97.2	0.71	32.1
264	Utrecht		39.0	5.5	55.1	96.8	0.71	32.0
265	Noord Holland		39.9	5.3	48.0	93.4	0.70	31.8
266	Zuid Holland		36.1	4.4	37.5	94.8	0.70	30.9
267	Zeeland		39.2	4.3	27.7	95.3	0.66	33.2
268	Noord Brabant		36.1	4.2	35.8	98.4	0.70	33.7
269	Limburg		38.6	4.7	35.6	98.0	0.68	31.1
270	Zuidelijke Ijsselmeerpolders		42.3	0.0		100.0	0.79	27.7
UNITED KINGDOM England and Wales								
271	Cleveland	)	44.1	3.7		98.9	0.60	23.4
272	Cumbria	)	52.3	2.9		97.6	0.50	29.6
273	Durham	)	43.9	2.8		98.2	0.60	23.8
274	Northumberland	)	51.5	2.5		98.9	0.50	27.8
275	Gateshead	)Northern	49.1	2.4	22.2	98.8	0.60	19.0
276	Newcastle upon Tyne	)	54.6	7.9		99.4	0.60	19.6
277	Northern Tyneside	)	43.4	2.3		99.2	0.60	21.5
278	Southern Tyneside	)	45.3	2.6		97.8	0.60	18.0
279	Sunderland	)	42.8	3.8		98.4	0.60	19.4
280	Bradford	)	47.6	3.8		98.3	0.60	23.0
281	Calderdale	)	43.5	3.1		97.7	0.60	25.2
282	Humberside	)	46.3	3.1		97.5	0.50	26.0
283	Kirklees	)Yorkshire	46.6	2.8	20.0	97.0	0.60	25.5
284	Leeds	)	50.7	3.9		99.4	0.50	24.9
285	North Yorkshire	)	52.9	3.2		98.5	0.50	31.9

Table 7.3.1 cont

Area		Region	Indicators					
			GP	BED	CONS	BATH	ROOM	CAR
286	Wakefield	)	50.3	3.6		99.3	0.60	24.4
287	Barnsley	)	45.3	2.4		98.5	0.60	21.7
288	Derbyshire	)	45.2	2.0		97.9	0.50	28.4
289	Doncaster	)	46.1	2.1		98.9	0.60	22.7
290	Leicestershire	)Trent	47.1	2.4	17.8	98.2	0.50	30.1
291	Lincolnshire	)	48.3	2.8		97.5	0.50	33.0
292	Nottinghamshire	)	44.0	2.9		98.8	0.50	27.2
293	Rotherham	)	38.1	2.7		99.1	0.60	23.4
294	Sheffield	)	47.9	4.0		98.0	0.50	22.7
295	Cambridgeshire	)East	48.7	2.9		98.0	0.50	33.9
296	Norfolk	)Anglia	49.9	3.3	21.5	97.3	0.50	33.6
297	Suffolk	)	49.0	2.4		97.2	0.50	33.3
298	Barnet	)	58.0	3.9		99.3	0.50	34.0
299	Bedfordshire	)	46.9	1.9		98.4	0.60	32.5
300	Brent and Harrow	)North	57.4	2.5		99.2	0.60	29.1
301	Ealing/Hammersmith/Hounslow)West		58.5	3.5	24.5	97.5	0.60	26.9
302	Hertfordshire	)Thames	49.6	2.0		99.0	0.50	36.7
303	Hillingdon	)	50.3	5.1		99.6	0.60	35.6
304	Kensington/Chelsea/Westminster)		87.1	9.0		98.0	0.60	22.8
305	Barking and Havering	)	45.0	3.6		99.4	0.60	29.8
306	Camden and Islington	)North	63.8	8.1		97.9	0.60	19.5
307	City and East London	)East	55.6	5.6	24.2	92.3	0.70	16.8
308	Enfield and Haringey	)Thames	55.4	3.1		98.0	0.60	28.0
309	Essex	)	46.3	2.3		98.7	0.50	34.3
310	Redbridge and Waltham Forest	)	51.2	3.1		96.9	0.50	29.0
311	Bromley	)	48.8	2.8		99.0	0.50	36.2
312	East Sussex	)South	53.2	3.2		98.3	0.50	31.8
313	Greenwich and Bexley	)East	46.1	3.2	24.2	98.2	0.60	28.7
314	Kent	)Thames	48.1	2.8		97.6	0.50	32.2
315	Lambeth/Southwark/Lewisham	)	57.8	4.9		97.5	0.60	20.7
316	Croydon	)	51.4	2.0		98.3	0.50	31.9
317	Kingston and Richmond	)South	53.7	1.9		98.2	0.50	35.5
318	Merton/Sutton/Wandsworth	)West	52.8	4.1	21.3	97.7	0.60	23.4
319	Surrey	)Thames	50.0	2.9		98.9	0.50	41.3
320	West Sussex	)	50.1	2.3		99.3	0.50	36.8
321	Dorset	)	52.0	2.7		98.9	0.50	35.6
322	Hampshire	)Wessex	51.5	2.4	19.5	98.8	0.50	33.6
323	Isle of Wight	)	52.1	2.7		96.9	0.50	31.8
324	Wiltshire	)	47.7	4.5		98.5	0.50	33.7
325	Berkshire	)	51.5	2.9		98.8	0.50	36.4
326	Buckinghamshire	)Oxford	47.6	1.9	19.0	98.8	0.50	38.1
327	Northamptonshire	)	45.3	2.5		98.4	0.50	31.0
328	Oxfordshire	)	51.6	3.3		98.8	0.50	35.3
329	Avon	)	49.9	2.9		98.8	0.50	33.3
330	Cornwall and Scilly Isles	)South	57.0	2.0		96.0	0.50	34.2
331	Devon	)Western	51.6	3.4	18.9	98.1	0.50	31.7
332	Gloucestershire	)	52.4	2.8		98.0	0.50	34.9
333	Somerset	)	51.7	2.5		98.3	0.50	36.1
334	Birmingham	)	52.3	4.5		98.9	0.60	22.8
335	Coventry	)	49.5	3.5		98.8	0.60	25.5
336	Dudley	)	43.4	2.8		99.0	0.60	30.2
337	Hereford and Worcester	)	47.9	2.9		97.7	0.50	36.3
338	Salop	)	48.2	3.4		97.6	0.50	33.3

Table 7.3.1 cont

Area		Region	Indicators					
			GP	BED	CONS	BATH	ROOM	CAR
339	Sandwell	)West	49.7	1.7	19.6	98.4	0.60	21.2
340	Solihull	)Midlands	44.3	1.5		99.8	0.50	35.5
341	Staffordshire	)	43.4	2.0		97.2	0.50	30.9
342	Walsall	)	47.4	1.9		98.9	0.60	26.5
343	Warwickshire	)	46.1	2.3		98.7	0.50	33.9
344	Wolverhampton	)	47.1	3.4		98.8	0.60	24.5
345	Bolton	)	45.6	2.5		97.4	0.60	24.9
346	Bury	)	45.7	2.4		98.4	0.50	28.8
347	Lancashire	)	46.8	3.1		97.5	0.50	27.9
348	Manchester	)	57.4	8.6		98.6	0.60	18.0
349	Oldham	)North	43.5	2.2		97.2	0.60	22.9
350	Rochdale	)Western	42.5	2.3	23.0	97.3	0.60	23.3
351	Salford	)	53.6	4.2		99.0	0.60	21.0
352	Stockport	)	46.7	2.8		98.8	0.50	32.2
353	Tameside	)	44.0	2.2		97.6	0.60	23.8
354	Trafford	)	48.3	2.2		99.4	0.50	30.5
355	Wigan	)	44.7	2.0		97.6	0.60	25.0
356	Cheshire	)	46.9	2.2		98.3	0.50	31.9
357	Liverpool	)	53.6	4.7		96.5	0.60	16.6
358	St Helens and Knowsley	)Mersey	46.5	2.0	20.6	97.8	0.60	21.2
359	Sefton	)	44.2	5.3		98.5	0.50	26.6
360	Wirral	)	50.0	4.8		98.7	0.50	27.0
361	Clwyd	)	47.0	4.1		98.1	0.50	31.6
362	Dyfed	)	54.0	3.4		95.5	0.50	32.7
363	Gwent	)	47.6	4.0		97.2	0.50	27.2
364	Gwynedd	)Wales	60.7	3.5	20.5	95.3	0.50	32.8
365	Mid Glamorgan	)	49.0	4.0		93.9	0.50	24.0
366	Powys	)	65.1	2.5		94.7	0.50	36.2
367	South Glamorgan	)	54.8	5.3		98.1	0.50	28.0
368	West Glamorgan	)	48.8	4.5		97.5	0.50	26.6
	UNITED KINGDOM Northern Ireland							
369	Northern Ireland		51.4	4.7	34.3	90.4	0.63	23.2
	UNITED KINGDOM Scotland							
370	Highlands and Islands		74.3	4.5	21.0	95.3	0.66	28.3
371	Grampian		55.5	4.2	29.7	96.8	0.69	28.8
372	Tayside		56.9	4.9	40.2	96.8	0.70	25.2
373	Fife		52.1	3.6	16.3	98.7	0.72	24.8
374	Lothian		61.0	4.5	43.5	97.7	0.70	23.2
375	Borders		63.2	5.1	14.8	97.8	0.64	30.9
376	Forth Valley		57.8	3.5	19.2	99.0	0.72	25.6
377	Argyll and Clyde		58.7	4.2	17.3	97.6	0.76	21.6
378	Greater Glasgow		59.3	4.5	55.0	97.0	0.79	16.5
379	Lanarkshire		48.2	4.1	17.6	99.0	0.81	20.7
380	Ayrshire and Arran		56.1	3.6	18.1	99.1	0.72	23.6
381	Dumfries and Galloway		64.6	3.7	18.6	98.7	0.64	29.7
	PORTUGAL							
382	Viana do Castelo		51.0	2.9	12.0	45.3	0.95	6.0
383	Braga		67.0	4.1	17.0	48.4	1.14	6.3
384	Vila Real		42.0	2.5	9.0	28.6	1.02	5.5
385	Braganca		51.0	3.8	9.0	29.2	0.91	4.4
386	Guarda		31.0	3.9	16.0	33.0	0.80	7.1
387	Viseu		50.0	4.2	13.0	32.9	0.91	5.7
388	Porto		203.0	4.8	88.0	58.9	1.11	9.1
389	Aveiro		67.0	2.3	21.0	56.2	0.97	10.4
390	Coimbra		478.0	13.0	114.0	50.3	0.84	9.8
391	Castelo Branco		49.0	5.1	23.0	39.0	0.77	8.2
392	Portalegre		63.0	8.2	27.0	39.6	0.80	8.2

Table 7.3.1 cont

Area		Region	Indicators					
			GP	BED	CONS	BATH	ROOM	CAR
393	Santarem		55.0	2.9	22.0	52.4	0.85	8.3
394	Leiria		51.0	3.6	18.0	56.9	0.86	9.1
395	Lisboa		315.0	7.4	138.0	83.6	0.94	12.8
396	Setubal		94.0	1.9	23.0	79.4	1.00	8.6
397	Evora		68.0	7.4	18.0	44.2	0.85	9.1
398	Beja		63.0	4.1	18.0	27.6	0.87	5.9
399	Faro		53.0	3.5	31.0	52.7	0.87	10.1
400	Madeira		71.0	8.3	23.0	42.8	1.27	3.8
401	Azores		44.0	7.6	19.0	45.8	1.11	3.8
SPAIN								
402	La Coruña		69.9	3.6	50.3	78.7	0.75	20.8
403	Lugo		109.1	2.1	31.4	57.4	0.66	18.9
404	Orense		70.0	2.5	38.5	53.3	0.67	18.0
405	Pontevedra		65.8	3.0	39.0	78.7	0.84	22.1
406	Asturias		88.9	4.3	88.9	84.5	0.71	22.9
407	Cantabria		94.4	3.9	124.3	81.1	0.72	22.3
408	Alava		101.4	4.9	73.3	87.6	0.72	25.9
409	Guipuzcoa		81.0	4.3	60.2	84.0	0.84	23.7
410	Vizcaya		91.2	4.1	59.2	91.0	0.74	22.3
411	Navarra		92.2	4.9	44.7	91.5	0.70	25.6
412	Rioja		112.4	3.3	59.3	89.1	0.67	21.8
413	Huesca		114.3	4.6	41.5	86.0	0.57	24.5
414	Teruel		155.6	3.0	43.9	76.9	0.54	19.4
415	Zaragoza		85.9	5.2	73.6	86.8	0.71	22.2
416	Madrid Centro		105.7	4.3	77.3	92.1	0.78	27.3
417	Avila		136.0	2.1	46.6	72.0	0.70	17.2
418	Burgos		130.1	5.0	66.3	75.2	0.72	21.0
419	Leon		105.7	3.7	43.5	71.8	0.66	20.8
420	Palencia		136.2	2.7	52.8	75.5	0.68	20.4
421	Salamanca		120.8	4.1	59.3	70.7	0.70	19.1
422	Segovia		173.3	3.3	110.0	74.3	0.64	22.1
423	Soria		165.0	6.2	75.1	76.4	0.65	20.2
424	Valladolid		104.6	4.9	56.4	88.0	0.73	22.8
425	Zamora		122.3	3.3	41.9	54.2	0.63	17.1
426	Albacete		82.4	2.3	40.0	67.8	0.75	19.0
427	Ciudad Real		104.6	2.7	40.5	58.1	0.73	15.9
428	Cuenca		115.3	1.4	35.4	59.2	0.64	17.1
429	Guadalajara		174.3	5.9	92.0	79.2	0.60	21.4
430	Toledo		114.7	2.2	64.8	75.0	0.66	18.3
431	Badajoz		68.4	3.4	65.0	55.4	0.78	15.5
432	Caceres		119.2	2.6	47.6	56.4	0.64	15.9
433	Barcelona		99.8	4.0	47.0	94.2	0.74	27.4
434	Gerona		106.4	3.0	24.8	78.9	0.69	33.6
435	Lerida		94.4	3.4	44.5	89.3	0.61	26.5
436	Tarragona		118.7	3.7	62.7	83.0	0.69	26.2
437	Alicante		79.7	2.5	46.8	91.0	0.70	27.1
438	Castellon de la Plana		112.6	3.3	40.5	79.8	0.61	25.8
439	Valencia		95.4	3.5	67.8	89.6	0.73	25.3
440	Baleares		89.5	4.5	60.0	86.4	0.60	40.3
441	Almeria		76.4	2.2	28.6	70.1	0.66	18.3
442	Cadiz		57.8	3.8	51.6	77.4	0.95	18.3
443	Cordoba		81.2	3.0	69.9	75.9	0.77	16.6
444	Granada		83.3	4.1	72.3	72.1	0.72	16.1
445	Huelva		75.7	2.7	48.1	77.4	0.73	15.9
446	Jaen		71.9	3.4	51.8	58.4	0.70	13.8
447	Malaga		70.1	3.8	69.1	81.2	0.81	20.0
448	Sevilla		79.3	4.0	67.7	86.0	0.79	18.3
449	Murcia		77.5	3.5	72.0	85.4	0.75	23.0
450	Las Palmas		63.2	3.5	41.8	92.9	0.97	22.5
451	Sta Cruz de Tenerife		75.3	5.0	46.8	85.6	0.89	23.3

8. MAPS AND GRAPHS OF CHANGES BETWEEN 1974–78 AND 1980–84

These maps show SMRs (based on the EC standard) between 1974–78 and 1980–84). The SMRs used to describe mortality for 1974–78 are based on the EC standard used in the 1974–78 atlas. The SMRs used to describe mortality in 1980–84 are based on the EC 1980–84 standard calculated, excluding Spain and Portugal.

In each time period areas with SMRs in the top two sextiles were rated as high, those in the middle two sextiles as medium, and those in the bottom two sextiles as low. The shading scales for the maps of changes over time were defined as follows:

1. Improved: changed from high (top third) in 1974–78 to medium (middle third) or low (bottom third) in 1980–84 *or* changed from medium in 1974–78 to low in 1980–84.

2. Remained low: low in 1974–78, low in 1980–84.

3. Remained medium: medium in 1974–78, medium in 1980–84.

4. Remained high: high in 1974–78, high in 1980–84.

5. Deteriorated: changed from low in 1974–78 to medium or high in 1980–84 *or* changed from medium in 1974–78 to high in 1980–84.

The graphs plot the SMRs for small areas of the EC in 1980–84 against the SMRs for 1974–78. The SMRs are in both cases based on the EC standard for 1974–78. The Spearman rank correlation coefficient is given.

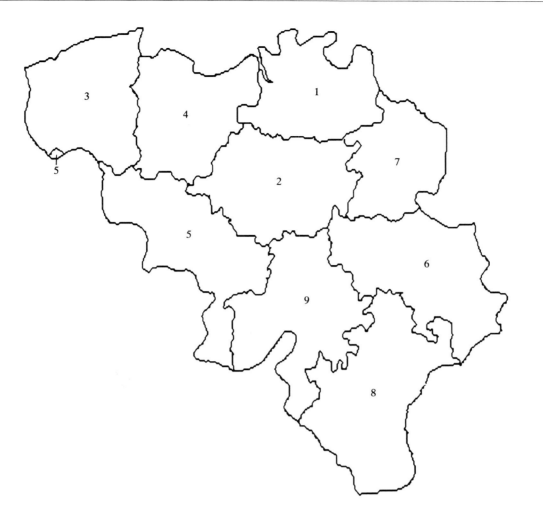

BELGIUM

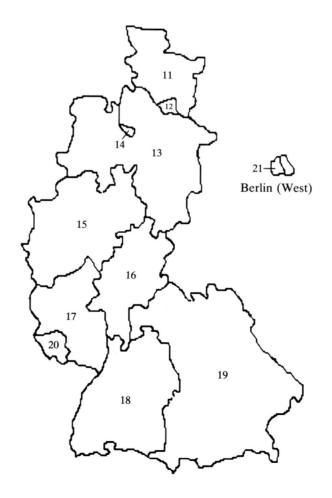

FEDERAL REPUBLIC
OF GERMANY

Berlin (West)

DENMARK

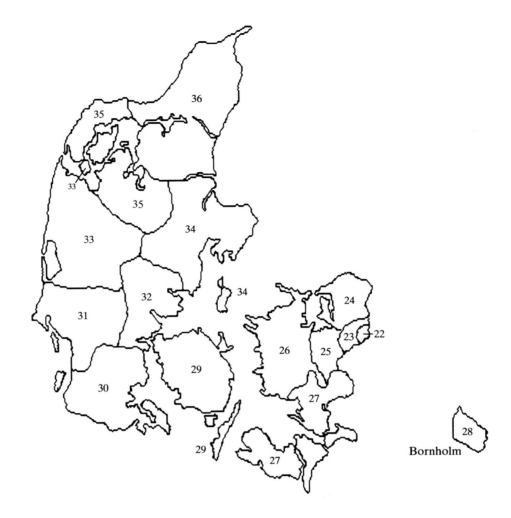

FRANCE

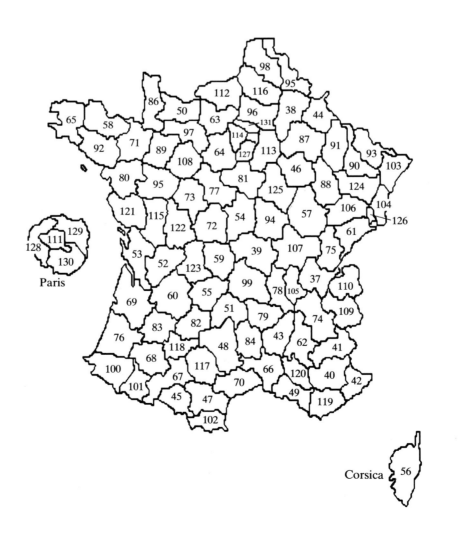

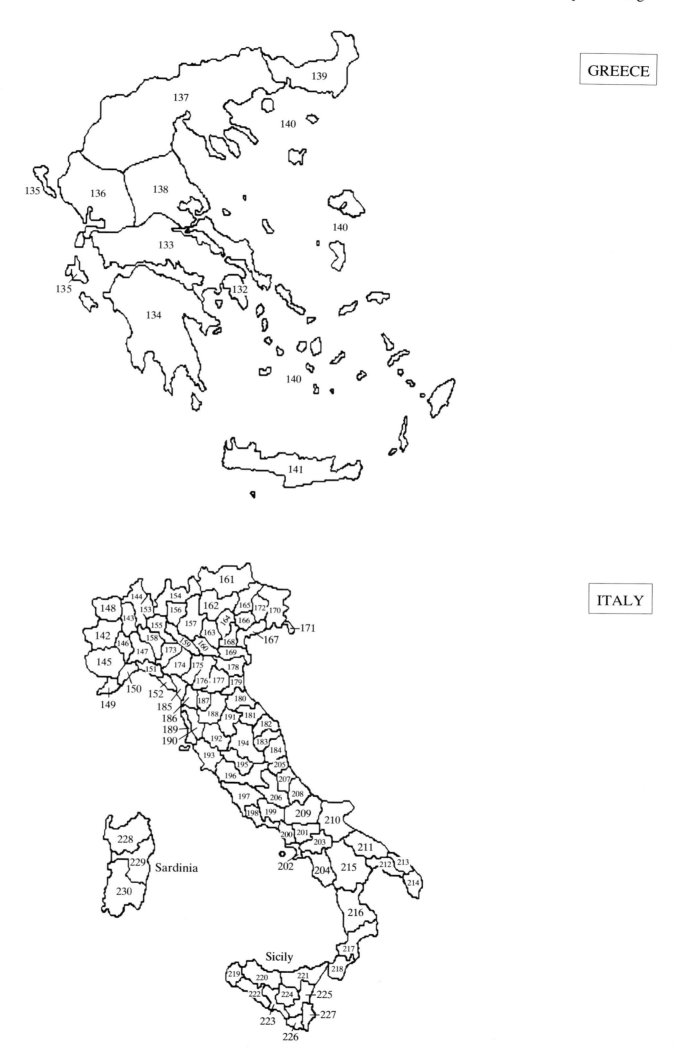

GREECE

ITALY

IRELAND

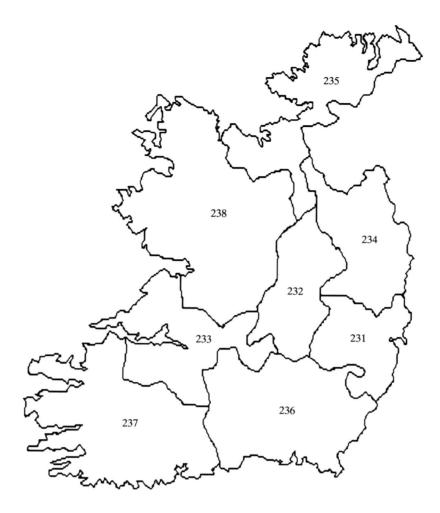

NETHERLANDS

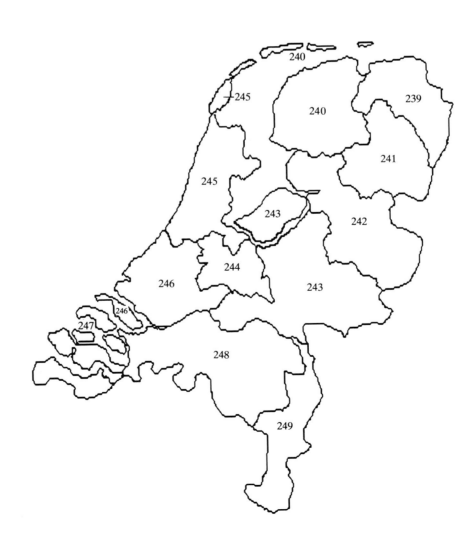

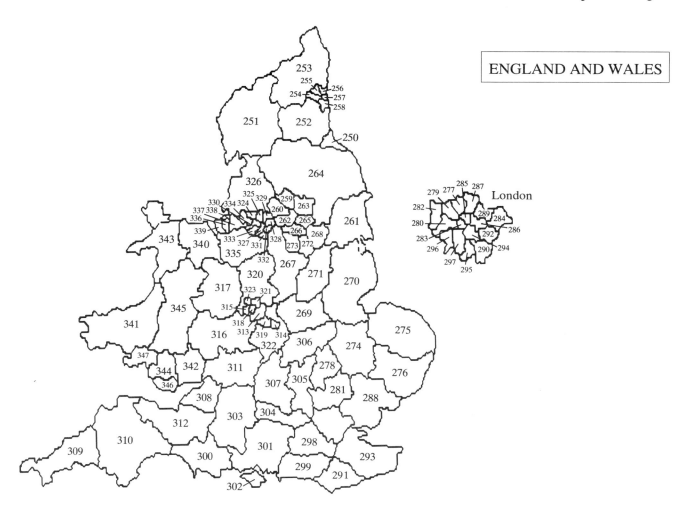

ENGLAND AND WALES

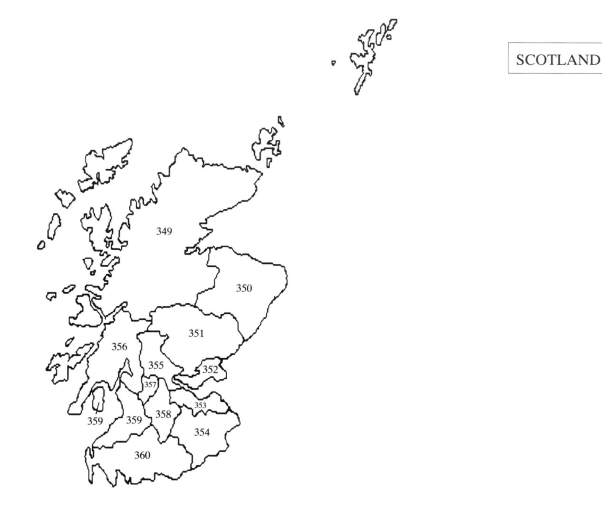

SCOTLAND

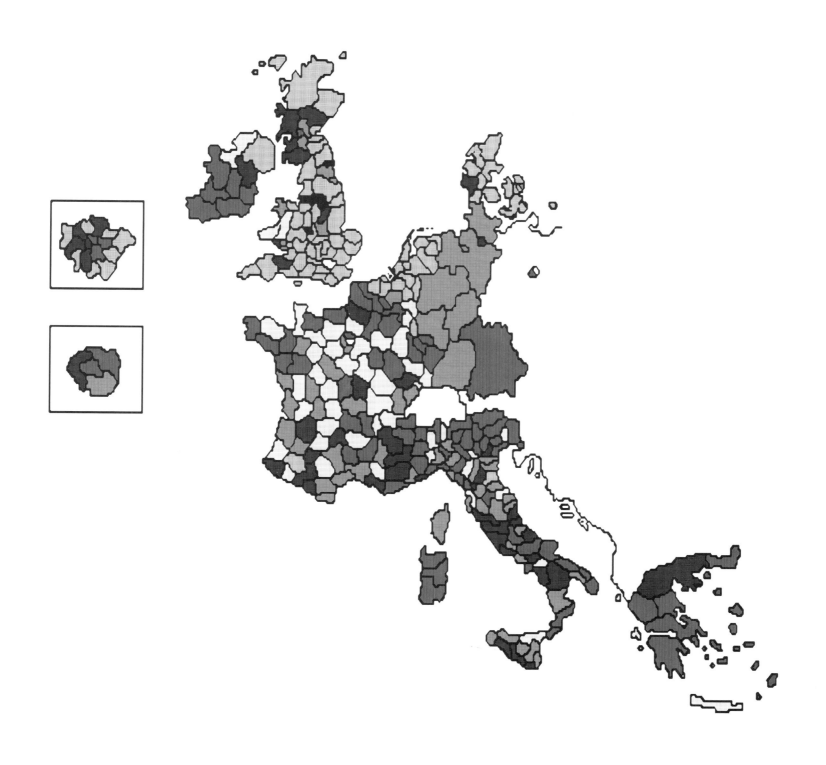

SMRS

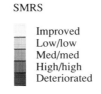

Improved
Low/low
Med/med
High/high
Deteriorated

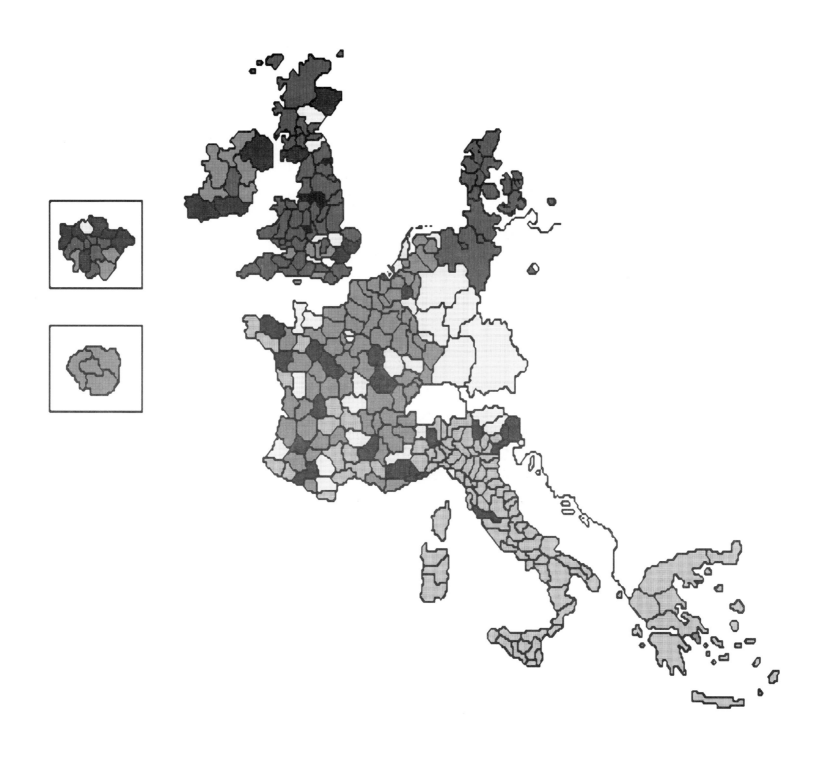

SMRS

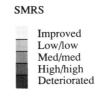

Improved
Low/low
Med/med
High/high
Deteriorated

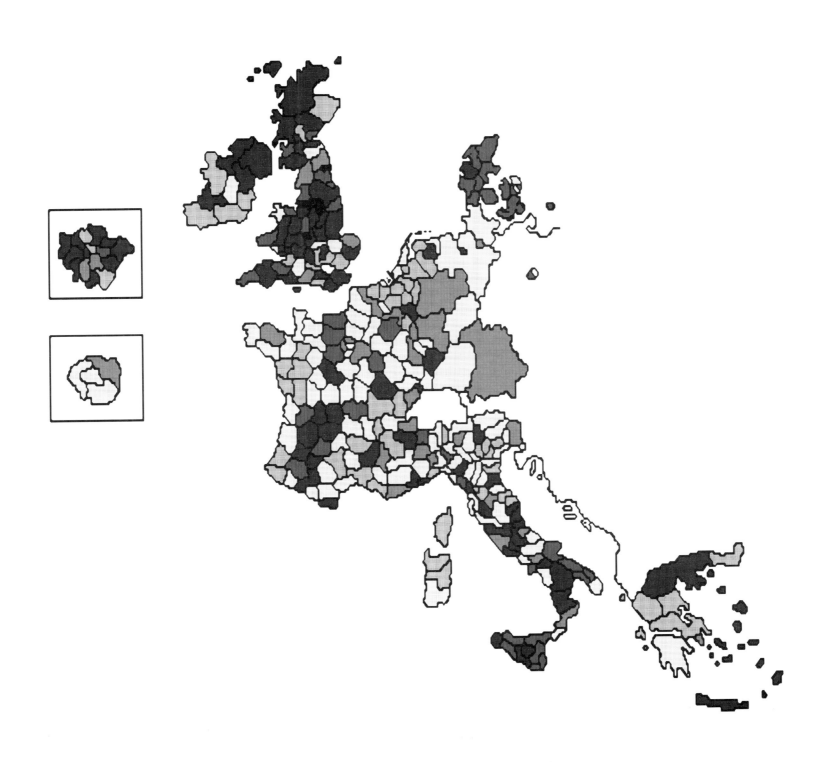

SMRS

Improved
Low/low
Med/med
High/high
Deteriorated

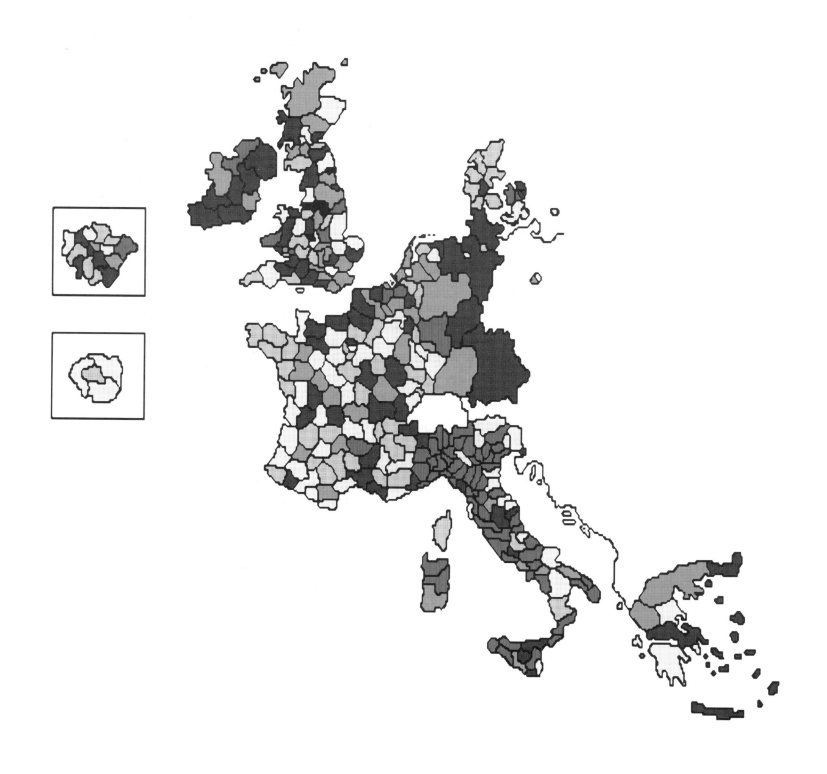

SMRS

Improved
Low/low
Med/med
High/high
Deteriorated

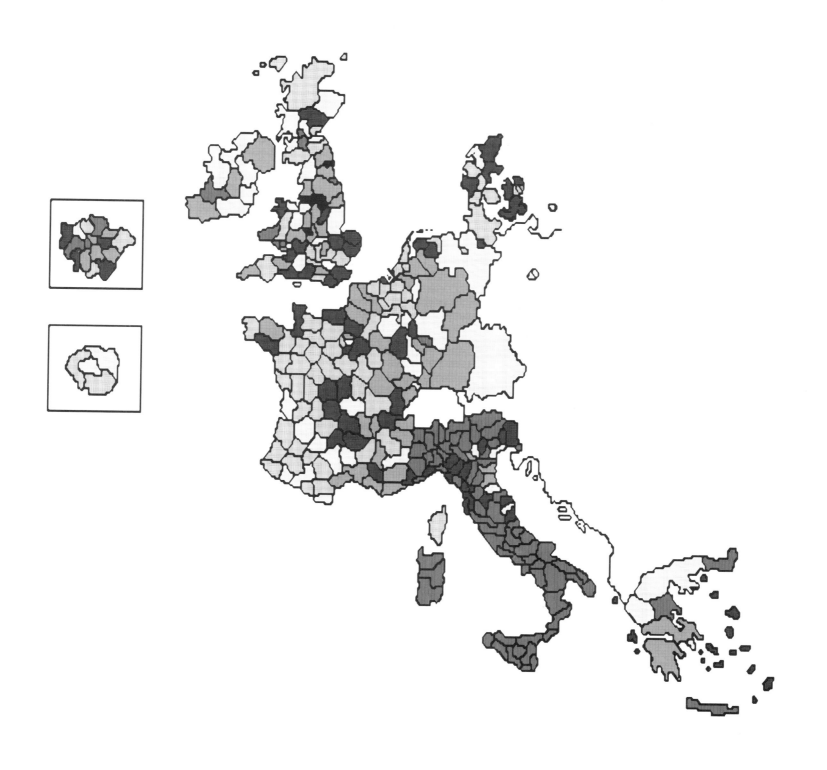

SMRS

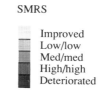

Improved
Low/low
Med/med
High/high
Deteriorated

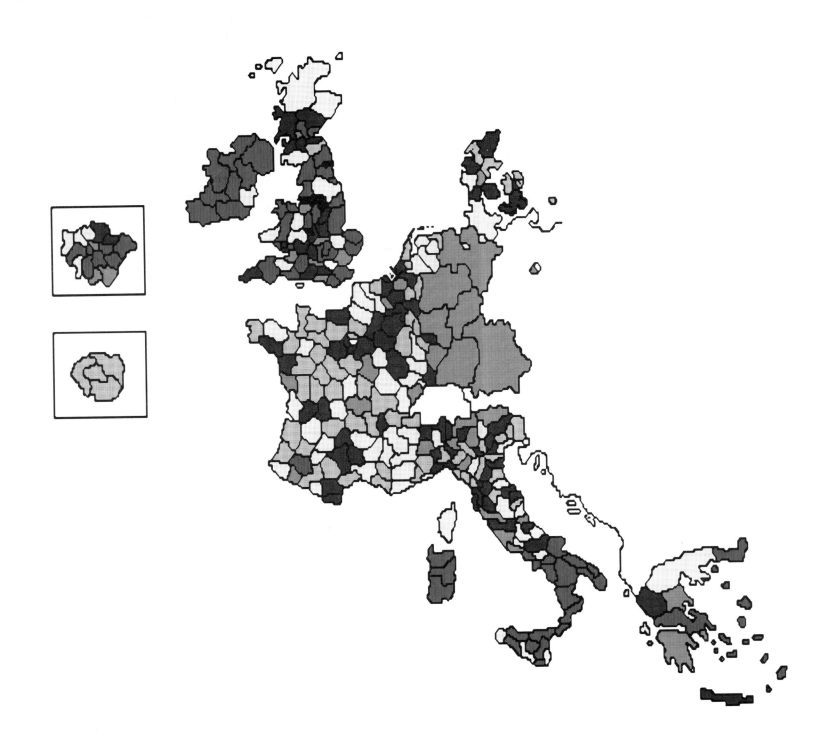

SMRS

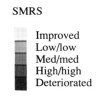

Improved
Low/low
Med/med
High/high
Deteriorated

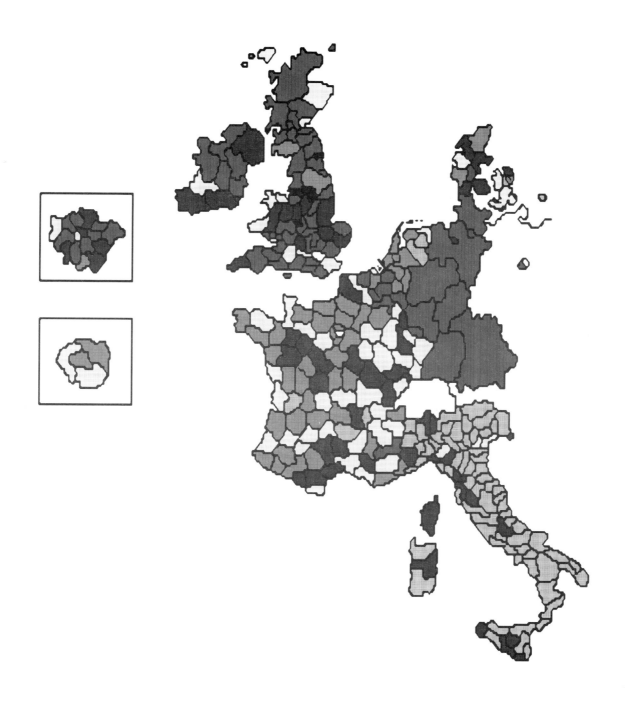

SMRS

Improved
Low/low
Med/med
High/high
Deteriorated

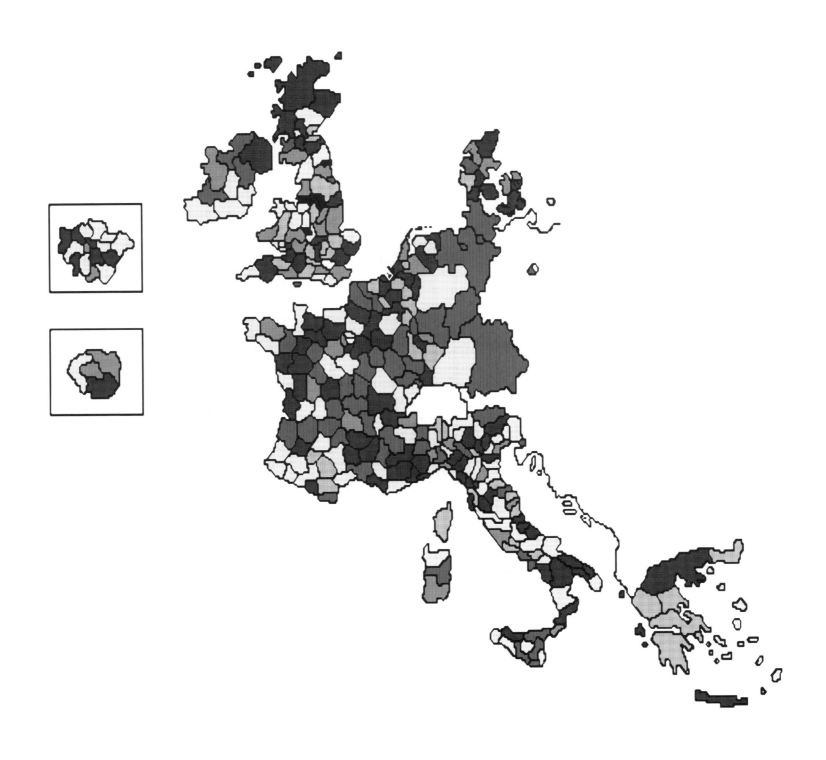

SMRS

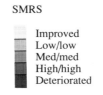

Improved
Low/low
Med/med
High/high
Deteriorated

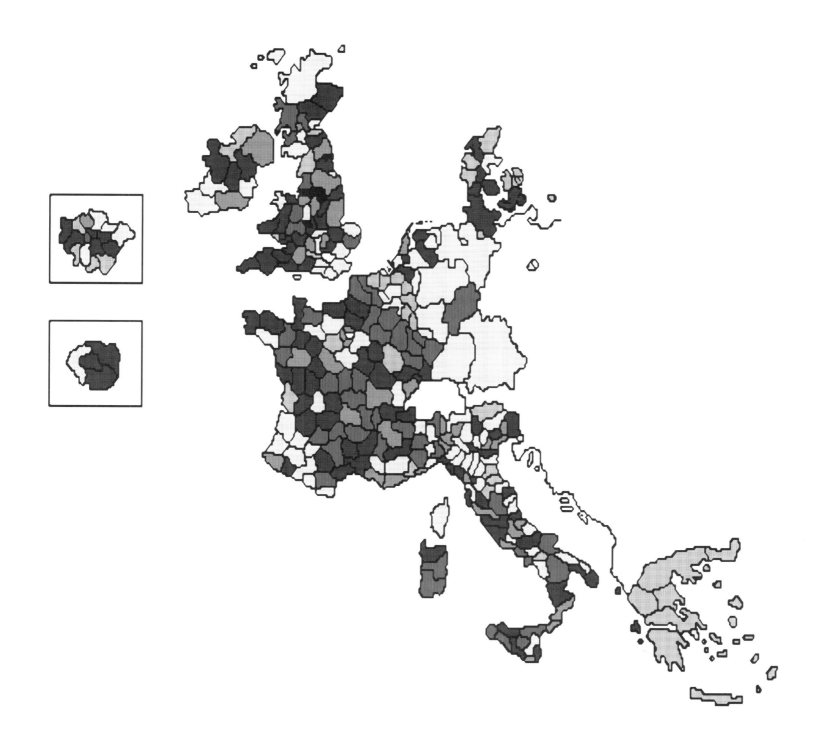

SMRS

Improved
Low/low
Med/med
High/high
Deteriorated

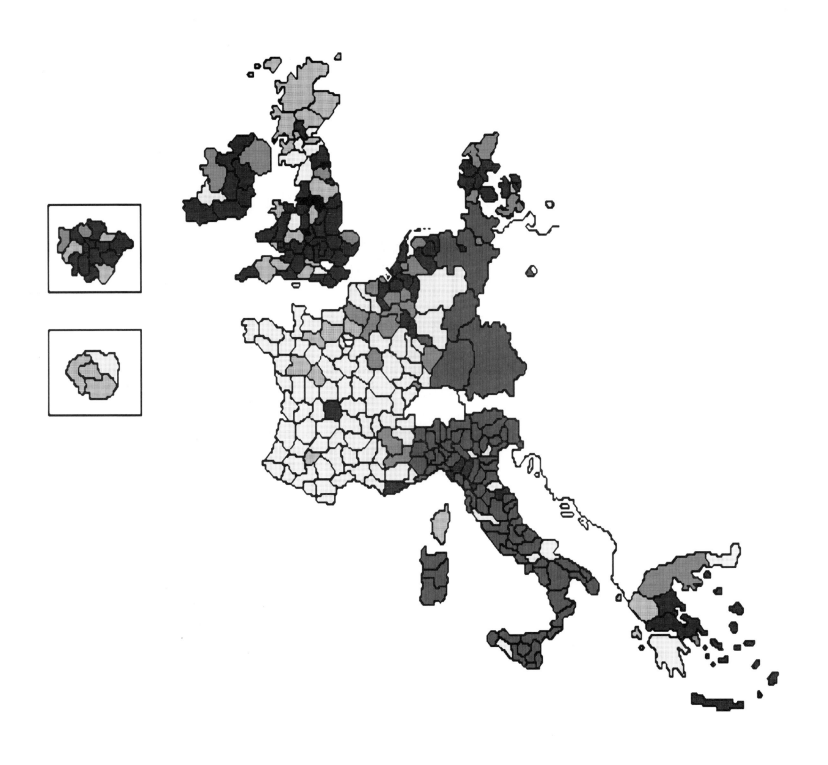

SMRS

Improved
Low/low
Med/med
High/high
Deteriorated

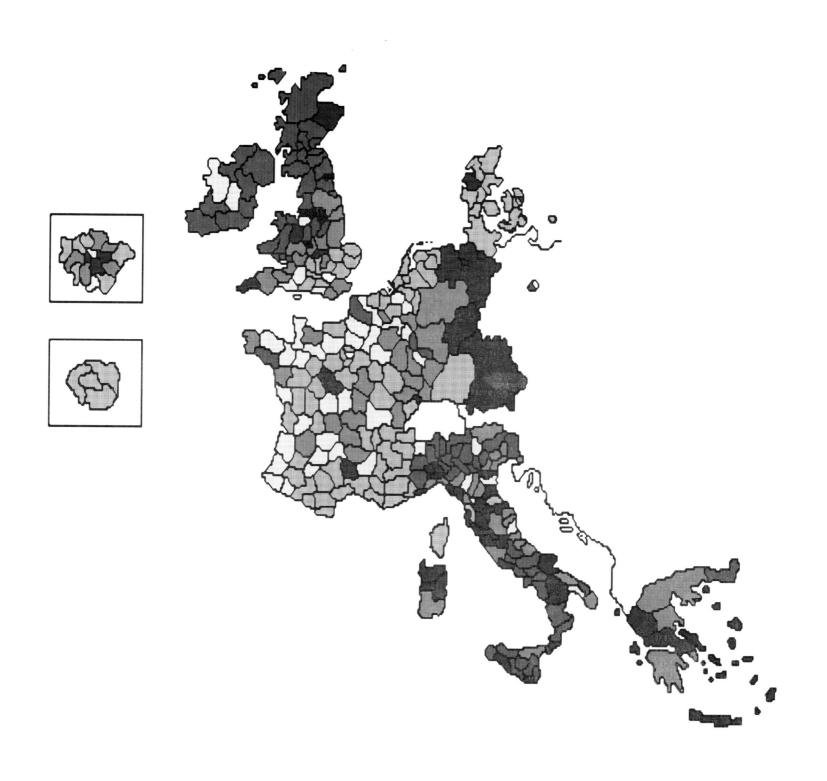

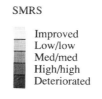

SMRS

Improved
Low/low
Med/med
High/high
Deteriorated

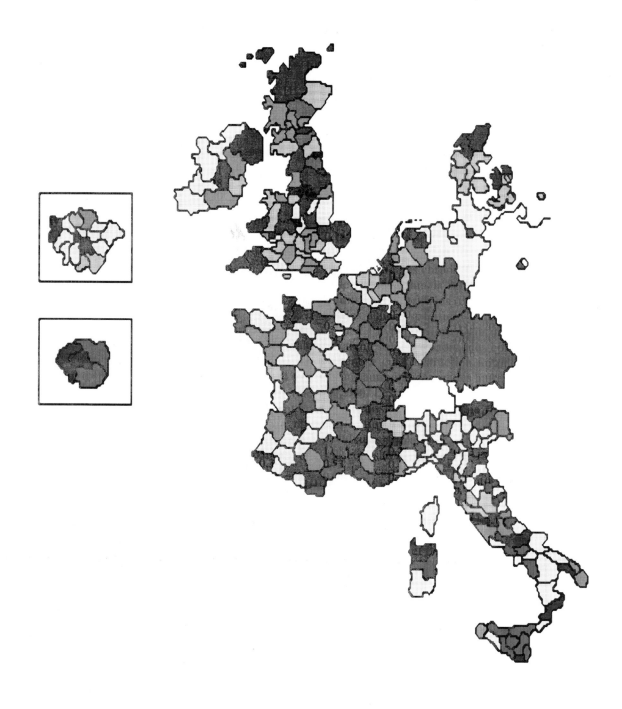

SMRS

Improved
Low/low
Med/med
High/high
Deteriorated

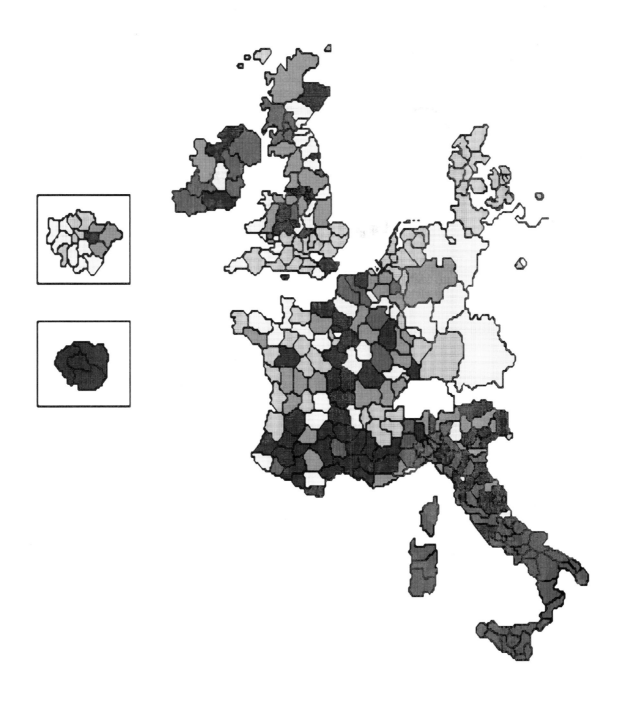

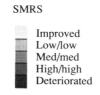

SMRS

Improved
Low/low
Med/med
High/high
Deteriorated

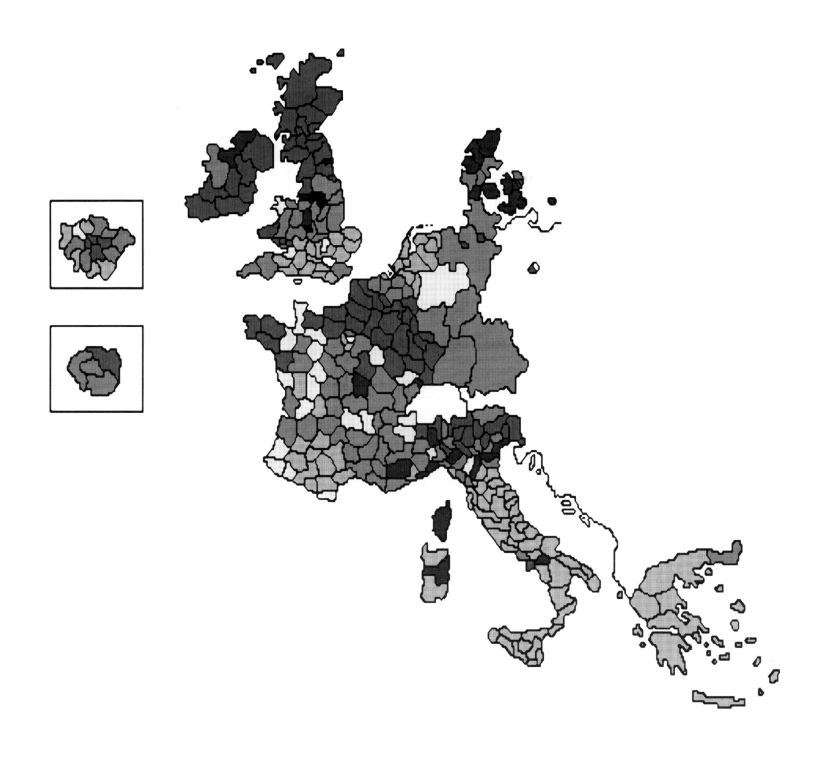

SMRS

Improved
Low/low
Med/med
High/high
Deteriorated

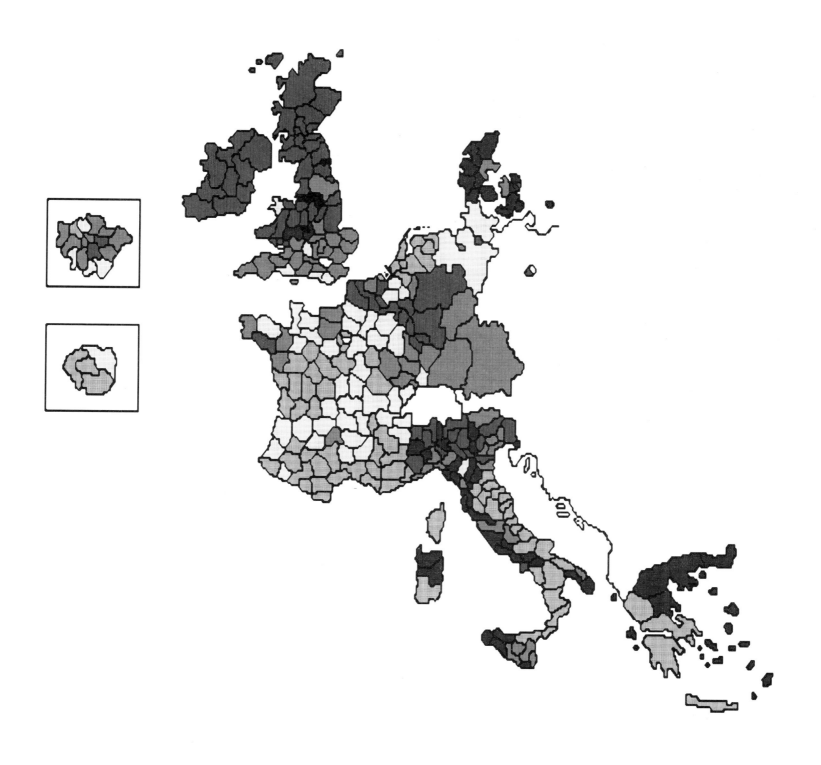

SMRS

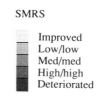

Improved
Low/low
Med/med
High/high
Deteriorated

Tuberculosis (ages 5–64): SMRs for 1974–78 and 1980–84 (based on the 1974–78 EC standard) for 360 health administration areas of the EC (1974 boundaries)

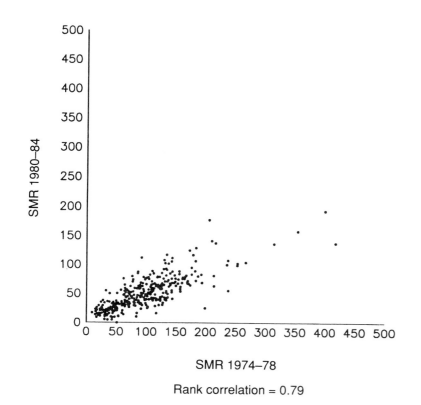

Rank correlation = 0.79

Malignant neoplasm of cervix uteri (ages 15–64): SMRs for 1974–78 and 1980–84 (based on the 1974–78 EC standard) for 360 health administration areas of the EC (1974 boundaries).

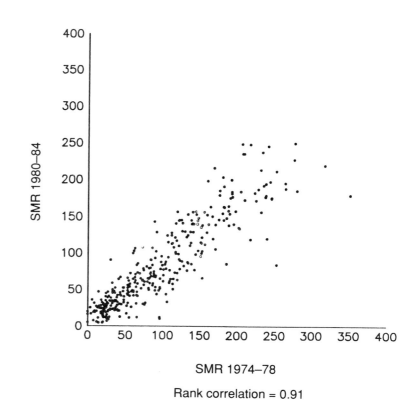

Rank correlation = 0.91

Malignant neoplasm of cervix and body of uterus (ages 15–54): SMRs for 1974–78 and 1980–84 (based on the 1974–78 EC standard) for 360 health administration areas of the EC (1974 boundaries).

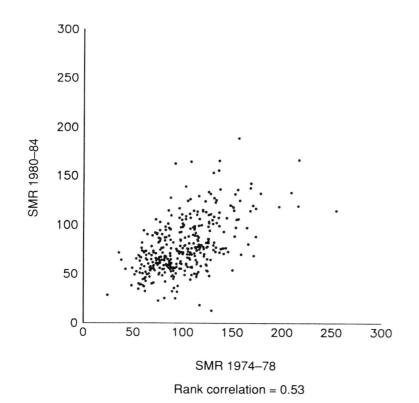

Rank correlation = 0.53

Hodgkin's disease (ages 5–64): SMRs for 1974–78 and 1980–84 (based on the 1974–78 EC standard) for 360 health administration areas of the EC (1974 boundaries)

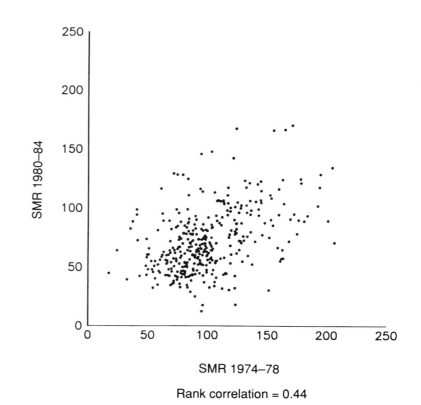

Rank correlation = 0.44

Chronic rheumatic heart disease (ages 5–44): SMRs for 1974–78 and 1980–84 (based on the 1974–78 EC standard) for 360 health administration areas of the EC (1974 boundaries)

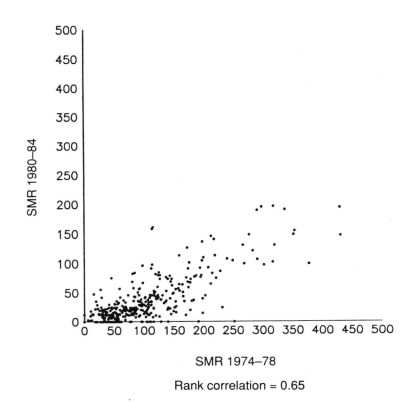

Rank correlation = 0.65

All respiratory diseases (ages 1–14): SMRs for 1974–78 and 1980–84 (based on the 1974–78 EC standard) for 360 health administration areas of the EC (1974 boundaries)

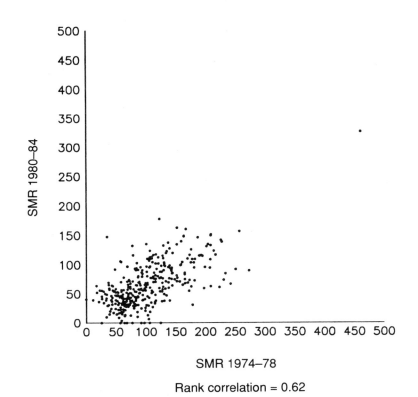

Rank correlation = 0.62

Asthma (ages 5–44): SMRs for 1974–1978 and 1980–84 (based on the 1974–78 EC standard) for 360 health administration areas of the EC (1974 boundaries)

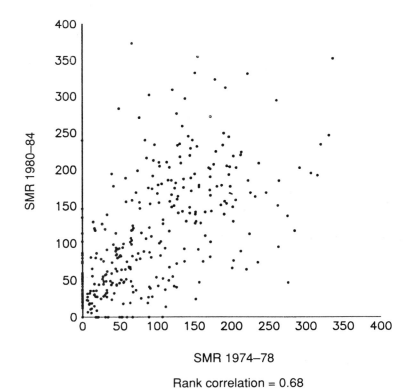

Rank correlation = 0.68

Appendicitis (ages 5–64): SMRs for 1974–78 and 1980–84 (based on the 1974–78 EC standard) for 360 health administration areas of the EC (1974 boundaries)

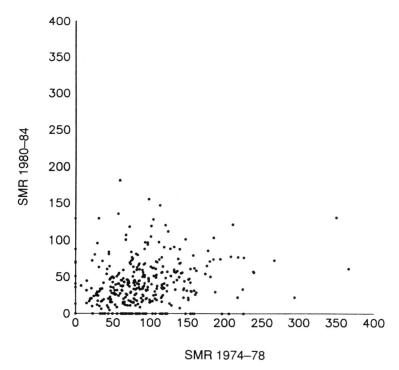

Rank correlation = 0.21

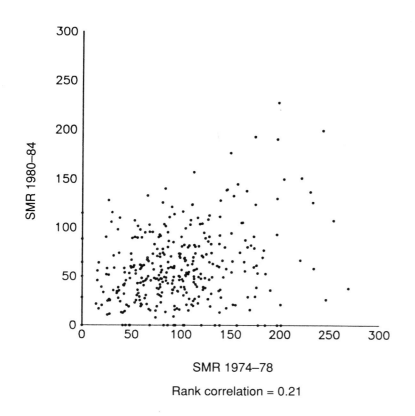

Abdominal hernia (ages 5–64): SMRs for 1974–78 and 1980–84 (based on the 1974–78 EC standard) for 360 health administration areas of the EC (1974 boundaries)

Rank correlation = 0.21

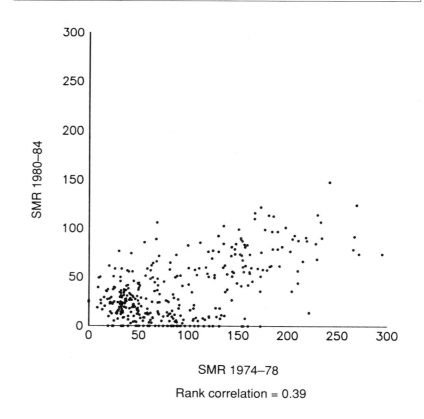

Cholelithiasis and cholecystitis (ages 5–64): SMRs for 1974–78 and 1980–84 (based on the 1974–78 EC standard) for 360 health administration areas of the EC (1974 boundaries)

Rank correlation = 0.39

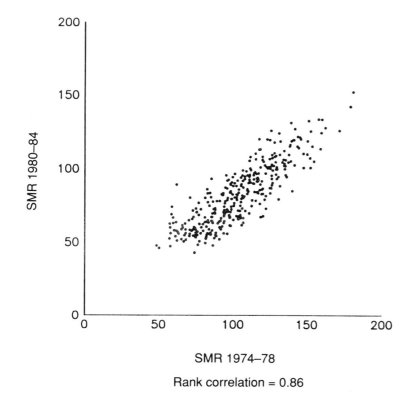

Hypertensive and cerebrovascular diseases (ages 35–64): SMRs for 1974–78 and 1980–84 (based on the 1974–78 EC standard) for 360 health administration areas of the EC (1974 boundaries)

Rank correlation = 0.86

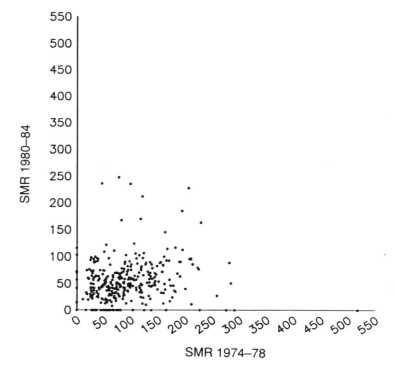

Maternal deaths (all ages): SMRs for 1974–78 and 1980–84 (based on the 1974–78 EC standard) for 360 health administration areas of the EC (1974 boundaries)

Rank correlation = 0.27

Perinatal deaths: SMRs for 1974–78 and 1980–84 (based on the 1974–78 EC standard) for 360 health administration areas of the EC (1974 boundaries)

All causes (ages 5–64): SMRs for 1974–78 and 1980–84 (based on the 1974–78 EC standard) for 360 health administration areas of the EC (1974 boundaries)

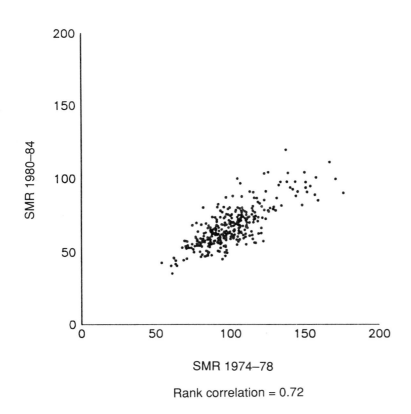

Rank correlation = 0.72

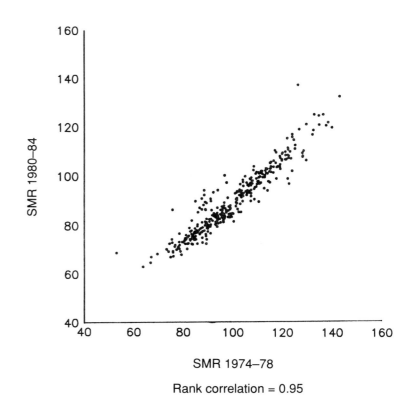

Rank correlation = 0.95

All causes (all ages): SMRs for 1974–78 and 1980–84 (based on the 1974–78 EC standard) for 360 health administration areas of the EC (1974 boundaries)

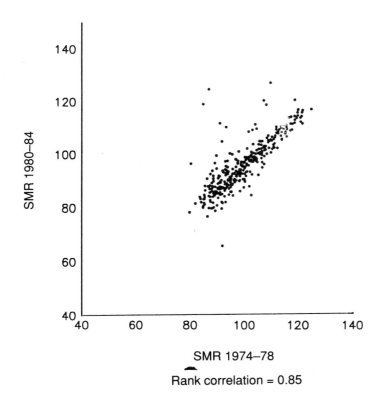

Rank correlation = 0.85

9. TABLES OF CHANGES BETWEEN 1974–78 AND 1980–84

Mortality data for the earlier time period are for 1974–78 except for France (1973–77); population data are for 1974–78 except for France (1975), Ireland (1976) and N. Ireland (1976)

Mortality data for the later time period are for 1980–84 except for Greece (1980–82) and Spain (1979–83); population data are for 1980–84 except for France (1982), Ireland (1981), Spain (1981), and Greece (1981). All data for Italy are for 1979–83

Table 9.1.1(a)–(o). Observed numbers of 'avoidable deaths', crude death rates (per 100 000), and age-standardized death rates (per 100 000) for 1974–78 and 1980–84, by disease and country

Table 9.1.2(a). Population of countries in 1974–78 and 1980–84, by sex and 10-year age groups

Table 9.1.2(b)–(l). Observed numbers of 'avoidable deaths' and age-specific death rates (per 100 000) for 1974–78 and 1980–84 and changes in age-specific death rates (per 100 000) between 1974–78 and 1980–84, by disease and country

Table 9.1.3(a)–(c). Age-standardized death rates (per 100 000) for 1974–78 and 1980–84 standardized to the EC standard, by disease and small area

Tables 9.1.1(a)–(o). Observed numbers of 'avoidable deaths', crude death rate (per 100 000), and age-standardized death rate (per 100 000) for 1974–78 and 1980–84, by disease and country

Notes on the use of these tables

1. These tables show the total number of 'avoidable deaths', the crude death rates (per 100 000), and age-standardized death rates (per 100 000) for 1974–78 and 1980–84. The age-standardized death rates are calculated by multiplying the small-area SMR based on the EC standard for that time period by the EC crude death rate for that time period.

2. The mortality data for the earlier time period are for 1974–78, except for France (1973–77). The population data for the earlier time period are for 1974–78, except for France (1975), Ireland (1976), and N. Ireland (1976).

3. The mortality data for the later time period are for 1980–84, except for Greece (1980–82). The population data are for 1980–84, except for France (1982), Ireland (1981), and Greece (1981). All data for Italy are for 1979–83.

Table 9.1.1(a). Tuberculosis (ICD8 010–019; ICD9 010–018,137), ages 5–64

Country	No. of deaths		Crude death rate (per 100 000)		Age-standardized death rate (per 100 000)	
	1974–78	1980–84	1974–78	1980–84	1974–78	1980–84
Belgium	731	331	1.87	0.84	1.85	0.81
Luxembourg	18	5	1.24	0.34	1.21	0.34
Federal Republic of Germany	5382	2828	2.18	1.15	2.16	1.12
Denmark	167	97	0.83	0.48	0.81	0.48
France	5317	2732	2.55	1.25	2.68	1.29
Greece	1066	367	2.90	1.58	2.86	1.60
Italy	5808	3132	2.58	1.37	2.56	1.37
Ireland	375	232	2.95	1.71	3.37	2.12
Netherlands	241	188	0.43	0.32	0.48	0.36
UK :England and Wales	2305	1417	1.18	0.73	1.11	0.70
:Northern Ireland	73	37	1.19	0.60	1.30	0.68
:Scotland	371	220	1.79	1.07	1.75	1.07
EC	21854	11586	2.05	1.08	2.05	1.08

Table 9.1.1(b). Malignant neoplasm of the cervix uteri (ICD8 180; ICD9 180), ages 15–64

Country	No. of deaths		Crude death rate (per 100 000)		Age-standardized death rate (per 100 000)	
	1974–78	1980–84	1974–78	1980–84	1974–78	1980–84
Belgium	571	524	3.63	3.21	3.67	3.17
Luxembourg	32	19	5.40	3.07	5.40	3.13
Federal Republic of Germany	7354	4980	7.26	4.74	6.97	4.59
Denmark	968	753	11.98	9.05	12.05	9.14
France	2553	2352	3.10	2.65	3.30	2.73
Greece	215	165	1.43	1.75	1.43	1.74
Italy	1238	1161	1.36	1.24	1.36	1.22
Ireland	167	167	3.60	3.35	3.95	3.83
Netherlands	1113	782	5.08	3.30	5.61	3.62
UK :England and Wales	6026	5333	7.73	6.63	7.42	6.57
:Northern Ireland	117	124	5.08	5.22	5.26	5.55
:Scotland	637	576	7.68	6.79	7.49	6.79
EC	20991	16936	4.89	3.83	4.89	3.83

Table 9.1.1(c). Malignant neoplasm of the cervix and body of the uterus (ICD8 180. 182; ICD9 179, 180, 182), ages 15–54

Country	No. of deaths		Crude death rate (per 100 000)		Age-standardized death rate (per 100 000)	
	1974–78	1980–84	1974–78	1980–84	1974–78	1980–84
Belgium	627	471	4.73	3.49	4.68	3.47
Luxembourg	31	23	6.23	4.42	6.15	4.31
Federal Republic of Germany	5898	3763	7.05	4.35	6.81	4.22
Denmark	625	462	9.38	6.68	9.96	6.91
France	4278	2882	6.06	3.89	6.21	4.02
Greece	603	323	4.80	4.03	4.75	3.66
Italy	5036	3588	6.58	4.58	6.39	4.37
Ireland	136	114	3.48	2.68	4.04	3.19
Netherlands	798	538	4.28	2.67	4.85	2.94
UK :England and Wales	3825	3455	6.03	5.23	6.08	5.37
:Northern Ireland	84	89	4.37	4.47	4.70	4.86
:Scotland	399	373	5.88	5.33	5.98	5.48
EC	22340	16081	6.23	4.38	6.23	4.38

Table 9.1.1(d). Hodgkin's disease (ICD8 201; ICD9 201), ages 5–64

Country	No. of deaths		Crude death rate (per 100 000)		Age-standardized death rate (per 100 000)	
	1974–78	1980–84	1974–78	1980–84	1974–78	1980–84
Belgium	504	428	1.29	1.09	1.28	1.06
Luxembourg	11	10	0.76	0.68	0.73	0.67
Federal Republic of Germany	2939	2617	1.19	1.06	1.18	1.03
Denmark	194	165	0.96	0.81	0.94	0.81
France	2113	1487	1.01	0.68	1.04	0.69
Greece	544	214	1.48	0.92	1.47	0.94
Italy	3802	2845	1.69	1.24	1.68	1.25
Ireland	136	149	1.07	1.10	1.19	1.27
Netherlands	566	428	1.00	0.73	1.06	0.76
UK :England and Wales	2264	1657	1.16	0.85	1.13	0.84
:Northern Ireland	64	67	1.04	1.09	1.12	1.20
:Scotland	227	170	1.09	0.83	1.10	0.83
EC	13364	10237	1.25	0.95	1.25	0.95

Table 9.1.1(e). Chronic rheumatic heart disease (ICD8 393–398; ICD9 393–398), ages 5–44

Country	No. of deaths		Crude death rate (per 100 000)		Age-standardized death rate (per 100 000)	
	1974–78	1980–84	1974–78	1980–84	1974–78	1980–84
Belgium	87	11	0.31	0.04	0.31	0.04
Luxembourg	7	5	0.67	0.48	0.63	0.46
Federal Republic of Germany	1574	314	0.88	0.18	0.82	0.16
Denmark	60	25	0.41	0.17	0.42	0.16
France	1015	263	0.66	0.17	0.69	0.18
Greece	338	51	1.27	0.31	1.21	0.31
Italy	3254	1515	2.01	0.92	1.96	0.93
Ireland	107	24	1.10	0.23	1.33	0.28
Netherlands	223	75	0.52	0.17	0.57	0.17
UK :England and Wales	1220	391	0.88	0.28	0.92	0.28
:Northern Ireland	45	11	0.97	0.24	1.13	0.27
:Scotland	195	49	1.31	0.33	1.40	0.35
EC	8125	2734	1.05	0.35	1.05	0.35

Table 9.1.1(f). All respiratory diseases (ICD8 460–519; ICD9 460–519), ages 1–14

Country	No. of deaths		Crude death rate (per 100 000)		Age-standardized death rate (per 100 000)	
	1974–78	1980–84	1974–78	1980–84	1974–78	1980–84
Belgium	212	159	2.10	1.77	2.11	1.74
Luxembourg	7	4	2.09	1.27	2.13	1.26
Federal Republic of Germany	1629	829	2.66	1.70	2.88	1.74
Denmark	80	62	1.50	1.30	1.47	1.32
France	1267	683	2.13	1.22	2.02	1.18
Greece	417	157	4.00	2.43	3.79	2.31
Italy	2277	1416	3.63	2.45	3.54	2.50
Ireland	258	130	5.57	2.69	5.30	2.56
Netherlands	306	177	1.90	1.24	1.93	1.26
UK :England and Wales	2059	1275	3.90	2.75	3.95	2.73
:Northern Ireland	82	59	3.97	3.09	3.94	3.01
:Scotland	181	121	3.06	2.41	3.12	2.42
EC	8775	5072	3.01	1.98	3.01	1.98

Table 9.1.1(g). Asthma (ICD8 493; ICD9 493), ages 5–44

Country	No. of deaths		Crude death rate (per 100 000)		Age-standardized death rate (per 100 000)	
	1974–78	1980–84	1974–78	1980–84	1974–78	1980–84
Belgium	244	261	0.87	0.94	0.87	0.94
Luxembourg	0	8	0.00	0.76	0.00	0.74
Federal Republic of Germany	1606	1886	0.90	1.08	0.86	1.02
Denmark	38	62	0.26	0.41	0.27	0.41
France	492	581	0.32	0.37	0.33	0.38
Greece	44	—	0.17	—	0.16	—
Italy	88	245	0.05	0.15	0.05	0.15
Ireland	65	95	0.67	0.89	0.75	0.99
Netherlands	117	151	0.27	0.34	0.29	0.34
UK :England and Wales	1012	1312	0.73	0.94	0.75	0.94
:Northern Ireland	22	45	0.48	0.97	0.52	1.03
:Scotland	129	119	0.87	0.80	0.90	0.82
EC	3857	4765	0.50	0.62	0.50	0.62

Table 9.1.1(h). Appendicitis (ICD8 540–543; ICD9 540–543), ages 5–64

Country	No. of deaths		Crude death rate (per 100 000)		Age-standardized death rate (per 100 000)	
	1974–78	1980–84	1974–78	1980–84	1974–78	1980–84
Belgium	71	29	0.18	0.07	0.18	0.07
Luxembourg	8	4	0.55	0.27	0.55	0.28
Federal Republic of Germany	1362	465	0.55	0.19	0.55	0.19
Denmark	42	31	0.21	0.15	0.21	0.15
France	688	353	0.33	0.16	0.34	0.16
Greece	47	14	0.13	0.06	0.13	0.06
Italy	762	324	0.34	0.14	0.34	0.14
Ireland	46	17	0.36	0.13	0.38	0.14
Netherlands	121	67	0.21	0.11	0.23	0.12
UK :England and Wales	485	201	0.25	0.10	0.24	0.10
:Northern Ireland	11	8	0.18	0.13	0.18	0.14
:Scotland	51	24	0.25	0.12	0.24	0.12
EC	3694	1537	0.35	0.14	0.35	0.14

Table 9.1.1(i). Abdominal hernia (ICD8 550–553; ICD9 550–553), ages 5–64

Country	No. of deaths		Crude death rate (per 100 000)		Age-standardized death rate (per 100 000)	
	1974–78	1980–84	1974–78	1980–84	1974–78	1980–84
Belgium	95	41	0.24	0.10	0.24	0.10
Luxembourg	1	2	0.07	0.14	0.07	0.14
Federal Republic of Germany	1001	398	0.41	0.16	0.40	0.16
Denmark	28	27	0.14	0.13	0.13	0.13
France	721	558	0.35	0.26	0.37	0.26
Greece	61	19	0.17	0.08	0.17	0.08
Italy	870	558	0.39	0.24	0.39	0.25
Ireland	33	14	0.26	0.10	0.29	0.13
Netherlands	137	78	0.24	0.13	0.27	0.15
UK :England and Wales	704	420	0.36	0.21	0.33	0.20
:Northern Ireland	21	13	0.34	0.21	0.37	0.24
:Scotland	75	41	0.36	0.20	0.35	0.19
EC	3747	2169	0.35	0.20	0.35	0.20

Table 9.1.1(j). Cholelithiasis and cholecystitis (ICD8 574–575; ICD9 574–575.1, 576.1), ages 5–64

Country	No. of deaths		Crude death rate (per 100 000)		Age-standardized death rate (per 100 000)	
	1974–78	1980–84	1974–78	1980–84	1974–78	1980–84
Belgium	195	139	0.50	0.35	0.50	0.34
Luxembourg	10	7	0.69	0.48	0.67	0.49
Federal Republic of Germany	2787	1080	1.13	0.44	1.12	0.43
Denmark	77	52	0.38	0.26	0.37	0.25
France	1369	152	0.66	0.07	0.70	0.07
Greece	134	40	0.36	0.17	0.36	0.18
Italy	3224	1476	1.43	0.64	1.43	0.65
Ireland	33	39	0.26	0.29	0.30	0.36
Netherlands	271	221	0.48	0.38	0.54	0.42
UK :England and Wales	646	498	0.33	0.25	0.30	0.24
:Northern Ireland	23	20	0.37	0.33	0.41	0.37
:Scotland	66	4	0.32	0.02	0.31	0.02
EC	8835	3728	0.83	0.35	0.83	0.35

Table 9.1.1(k). Hypertensive and cerebrovascular diseases (ICD8 400–404, 430–438; ICD9 401–405, 430–438), ages 35–64

Country	No. of deaths		Crude death rate (per 100 000)		Age-standardized death rate (per 100 000)	
	1974–78	1980–84	1974–78	1980–84	1974–78	1980–84
Belgium	8463	6385	49.70	36.45	49.55	35.09
Luxembourg	430	322	65.15	48.57	66.58	51.05
Federal Republic of Germany	50667	43928	45.03	38.09	47.01	39.49
Denmark	3182	2991	37.24	33.02	34.54	33.07
France	40567	31290	46.92	34.10	48.30	33.52
Greece	7992	4558	48.45	44.08	49.07	46.02
Italy	59761	50342	59.63	49.24	61.09	50.35
Ireland	3479	2406	74.88	50.90	70.43	50.12
Netherlands	7479	6518	34.45	27.41	34.24	28.37
UK :England and Wales	52715	40556	61.56	46.82	56.30	44.87
:Northern Ireland	1771	1287	75.12	54.45	70.96	53.59
:Scotland	7524	5713	85.50	64.87	79.30	61.70
EC	244030	196296	52.47	41.48	52.47	41.48

Table 9.1.1(l). Maternal deaths (ICD8 630–678; ICD9 630–676), all ages

Country	No. of deaths		Crude death rate (per 100 000)		Age-standardized death rate (per 100 000)	
	1974–78	1980–84	1974–78	1980–84	1974–78	1980–84
Belgium	72	44	11.79	7.27	—	—
Luxembourg	12	0	59.73	0.00	—	—
Federal Republic of Germany	1015	487	33.96	15.97	—	—
Denmark	19	15	5.68	5.62	—	—
France	772	545	20.38	13.85	—	—
Greece	—	58	—	8.40	—	—
Italy	906	355	22.77	11.39	—	—
Ireland	49	24	14.14	6.83	—	—
Netherlands	95	67	10.65	7.60	—	—
UK :England and Wales	370	271	12.26	8.52	—	—
:Northern Ireland	11	12	8.28	8.64	—	—
:Scotland	49	45	14.72	13.38	—	—
EC	3370	1865	20.49	11.74	—	—

Table 9.1.1(m). Perinatal mortality (all causes), aged under 1 week plus stillbirths

Country	No. of deaths		Crude death rate (per 100 000)		Age-standardized death rate (per 100 000)	
	1974–78	1980–84	1974–78	1980–84	1974–78	1980–84
Belgium	11472	7713	18.79	12.74	—	—
Luxembourg	286	236	14.24	11.04	—	—
Federal Republic of Germany	51602	30320	17.27	9.94	—	—
Denmark	4064	2357	12.14	8.83	—	—
France	63989	46876	16.89	11.92	—	—
Greece	—	12251	—	17.73	—	—
Italy	89598	49514	22.52	15.89	—	—
Ireland	6927	4857	20.00	13.83	—	—
Netherlands	12345	9159	13.83	10.39	—	—
UK :England and Wales	54417	36429	18.02	11.45	—	—
:Northern Ireland	2990	1895	22.50	13.64	—	—
:Scotland	6413	3897	19.26	11.59	—	—
EC	304103	193253	18.49	12.17	—	—

Table 9.1.1(n). All causes (all ICD8/ICD9 codes), ages 5–64

Country	No. of deaths		Crude death rate (per 100 000)		Age-standardized death rate (per 100 000)	
	1974–78	1980–84	1974–78	1980–84	1974–78	1980–84
Belgium	131663	123752	337.53	314.44	334.95	302.81
Luxembourg	5597	5096	384.33	346.55	377.03	350.80
Federal Republic of Germany	815758	753470	330.77	305.98	329.30	298.66
Denmark	63292	64659	314.08	317.26	304.31	317.76
France	655326	633730	314.43	290.48	330.64	297.59
Greece	87612	51676	238.58	223.07	236.22	227.99
Italy	663873	625425	295.32	272.76	294.72	274.87
Ireland	40264	37293	316.57	275.03	352.25	330.87
Netherlands	136603	131631	242.50	224.37	266.43	246.14
UK :England and Wales	671866	602565	343.73	308.36	320.90	298.23
:Northern Ireland	22400	19434	363.72	317.41	389.76	351.93
:Scotland	85278	77203	411.27	376.10	399.03	371.78
EC	3379532	3125934	316.26	291.50	316.26	291.50

Table 9.1.1(o). All causes (all ICD8/ICD9 codes), all ages 1+ years

Country	No. of deaths		Crude death rate (per 100 000)		Age-standardized death rate (per 100 000)	
	1974–78	1980–84	1974–78	1980–84	1974–78	1980–84
Belgium	573074	556370	1182.61	1142.90	1155.41	1136.25
Luxembourg	21176	20465	1193.69	1136.76	1218.14	1167.47
Federal Repubic of Germany	3584934	3532962	1174.72	1160.44	1107.34	1095.34
Denmark	255278	278511	1019.74	1099.99	1011.73	1065.79
France	2710066	2697770	1030.27	993.58	1018.78	1019.22
Greece	386198	251781	854.54	875.35	938.41	946.70
Italy	2638168	2675194	953.79	952.91	1020.51	1002.63
Ireland	163677	160310	1036.13	954.94	1249.68	1218.34
Netherlands	552676	578586	814.20	814.31	973.00	917.29
UK :England and Wales	2875097	2844578	1176.73	1160.46	1111.34	1089.88
:Northern Ireland	81499	79009	1077.89	1044.22	1260.04	1208.00
:Scotland	314746	314266	1225.42	1234.12	1229.62	1223.93
EC	14156590	13989803	1067.19	1054.03	1067.19	1054.03

Table 9.1.2(a). Population of countries in 1974–78 and 1980–84, by sex and 10-year age groups

Notes on the use of this table

1. This table shows average populations in 100s for countries in the two time periods 1974–78 and 1980–84 and 10-year age groups.

2. The earlier population data are for 1974–78 except for France (1975), Ireland (1976), and N. Ireland (1976). The later population data are for 1980–84 except for France (1982), Ireland (1981), Spain (1981), and Greece (1981). All data for Italy are for 1979–83.

Table 9.1.2(a). Population in 100s for the two time periods 1974–78 and 1980–84, by country and sex and 10-year age groups

Country	Sex	Age group (year)								
		<1	1–4	5–14	15–24	25–34	35–44	45–54	55–64	65+
1974–78										
Belgium	M	619	2646	7663	7906	6931	6010	6261	4459	5530
	F	588	2510	7331	7544	6583	5952	6418	4955	8215
	T	1207	5156	14994	15450	13514	11962	12679	9414	13745
Luxembourg	M	20	85	258	282	285	260	230	164	191
	F	19	80	248	272	248	236	239	191	279
	T	39	165	506	554	533	496	469	355	470
Fed. Rep. Germany	M	3045	13478	49275	45602	42749	46875	34951	24179	33725
	F	2894	12878	46908	43765	39927	43557	40100	35354	57023
	T	5939	26356	96183	89367	82676	90432	75051	59533	90748
Denmark	M	342	1463	3994	3827	4080	2979	2811	2651	2958
	F	327	1399	3804	3637	3869	2930	2888	2831	3945
	T	669	2862	7798	7464	7949	5909	5699	5482	6903
France	M	*	17532	43358	42911	38596	32125	32307	21209	29464
	F	*	16715	41502	41639	35921	30820	32856	23591	45541
	T	7896	34247	84860	84550	74517	62945	65163	44800	75005
Greece	M	921	3105	7592	6937	5869	6106	5429	4335	4784
	F	860	2936	7196	6671	6187	6500	5774	4849	6120
	T	1781	6041	14788	13608	12056	12606	11203	9184	10904
Italy	M	4134	17588	46700	41192	38741	37167	34900	24976	29030
	F	3916	16649	44372	39747	38399	37912	36976	28528	40337
	T	8050	34237	91072	80939	77140	75079	71876	53504	69367
Ireland	M	352	1361	3382	2788	2073	1657	1567	1457	1588
	F	339	1293	3229	2673	2001	1595	1552	1464	1916
	T	691	2654	6611	5461	4074	3252	3119	2921	3504
Netherlands	M	915	4119	12360	11900	11272	8296	7331	5896	6341
	F	871	3933	11803	11409	10498	7811	7552	6534	8702
	F	1786	8052	24163	23309	21770	16107	14883	12430	15043
UK : England & Wales	M	3042	13621	40647	36219	35125	28631	29452	26340	27741
	F	2882	12889	38526	34826	34314	27878	29930	29041	43494
	T	5924	26510	79173	71045	69439	56509	59382	55381	71235
: N. Ireland	M	134	564	1572	1340	1036	815	777	694	684
	F	125	520	1475	1212	967	823	840	766	1037
	T	259	1084	3047	2552	2003	1638	1617	1460	1721
: Scotland	M	337	1504	4575	4103	3448	2894	2960	2564	2644
	F	319	1422	4344	3982	3419	3003	3166	3013	4329
	T	656	2926	8919	8085	6867	5897	6126	5577	6973
EC	M	27721	154126	442750	410009	380405	347625	317948	237844	289355
	F	26278	146442	421471	394751	364662	338029	336581	282229	441874
	T	27001	150290	432114	402384	372538	342832	327267	260041	365618
1980–84										
Belgium	M	611	2487	6725	7982	7610	6087	5981	5226	5409
	F	579	2367	6420	7655	7281	5932	6100	5711	8386
	T	1190	4854	13145	15637	14891	12019	12081	10937	13795
Luxembourg	M	22	84	239	286	296	253	246	157	194
	F	22	81	227	285	282	236	238	196	301
	T	44	165	466	571	578	489	484	353	495

Table 9.1.2(a) cont

Country	Sex	Age group (year)								
		<1	1–4	5–14	15–24	25–34	35–44	45–54	55–64	65+
Fed. Rep. Germany	M	3102	12166	37840	52480	44169	44864	39929	26757	32674
	F	2948	11578	36116	49362	41903	42538	39191	37347	59989
	T	6050	23744	73956	101842	86072	87402	79120	64104	92663
Denmark	M	275	1208	3684	4004	3896	3688	2716	2609	3150
	F	264	1157	3518	3822	3721	3543	2753	2806	4363
	T	539	2365	7202	7826	7617	7231	5469	5415	7513
France	M	4053	16063	41502	43670	43229	33273	31443	26433	29317
	F	3843	15314	39504	42485	42418	31743	31483	29144	46020
	T	7896	31377	81006	86155	85647	65016	62926	55577	75337
Greece	M	791	3216	7853	7223	6527	5880	6566	4241	5498
	F	726	3048	7439	7081	6632	6261	6769	4749	6895
	T	1517	6264	15292	14304	13159	12141	13335	8990	12393
Italy	M	3274	14493	44860	44789	39427	36757	35078	27226	30724
	F	3096	13726	42636	43247	39173	37376	36735	31290	43941
	T	6370	28219	87496	88036	78600	74133	71813	58516	74665
Ireland	M	374	1432	3535	3063	2419	1837	1523	1405	1641
	F	353	1359	3355	2947	2346	1745	1477	1467	2024
	T	727	2791	6890	6010	4765	3582	3000	2872	3665
Netherlands	M	894	3620	10987	12675	12020	9821	7621	6389	6819
	F	853	3459	10498	12151	11454	9198	7543	7041	9938
	T	1747	7079	21485	24826	23474	19019	15164	13430	16757
UK: England & Wales	M	3215	12455	35218	40514	35017	31448	27607	26732	29557
	F	3058	11823	33351	38978	34492	30969	27603	28889	45594
	T	6273	24278	68569	79492	69509	62417	55210	55621	75151
: N. Ireland	M	139	537	1419	1418	1028	884	738	669	724
	F	133	518	1341	1316	996	891	784	762	1108
	T	272	1055	2760	2734	2024	1775	1522	1431	1832
: Scotland	M	339	1321	3836	4472	3622	3082	2817	2607	2772
	F	323	1253	3646	4299	3564	3131	2995	2984	4530
	T	662	2574	7482	8771	7186	6213	5812	5591	7302
Portugal	M	742	3100	8683	8415	6724	5469	5447	4656	4716
	F	698	2951	8341	8275	6865	6007	6102	5401	7362
	T	1440	6051	17024	16690	13589	11476	11549	10057	12078
Spain	M	3000	12762	33948	31511	25153	21323	22851	17127	17343
	F	2825	12007	32052	30638	24874	21439	23552	19294	25282
	T	5825	24769	66000	62149	50027	42762	46403	36421	42625
EC	M	33552	169885	480654	524997	462269	409331	381121	304463	341074
	F	31750	161277	456886	505077	452000	402013	386645	354158	531461
	T	32656	165585	468773	515043	457138	405675	383888	329315	436271

M, male; F, female; T, total.
* Separate male and female data not available.

Tables 9.1.2 (b)–(l). Observed numbers of 'avoidable deaths' and age-specific death rates (per 100 000) for 1974–78 and 1980–84, and changes in age-specific death rates (per 100 000) between 1974–78 and 1980–84, by disease and country

Table 9.1.2(b). Tuberculosis (ICD8 010–019; ICD9 010–018, 137)

	Age group (years)					
	5–14	15–24	25–34	35–44	45–54	55–64
Belgium						
Deaths 1974–78	3	4	28	83	246	367
Deaths 1980–84	3	5	13	34	111	165
Death rate 1974–78	0.04	0.05	0.41	1.39	3.88	7.80
Death rate 1980–84	0.05	0.06	0.17	0.57	1.84	3.02
Change in rate	0.01	0.01	-0.24	-0.82	-2.04	-4.78
Luxembourg						
Deaths 1974–78	0	0	2	3	6	7
Deaths 1980–84	0	0	0	0	3	2
Death rate 1974–78	0.00	0.00	0.75	1.21	2.56	3.94
Death rate 1980–84	0.00	0.00	0.00	0.00	1.24	1.13
Change in rate	0.00	0.00	-0.75	-1.21	-1.32	-2.81
Federal Republic of Germany						
Deaths 1974–78	20	100	285	857	1653	2467
Deaths 1980–84	8	37	126	410	864	1383
Death rate 1974–78	0.04	0.22	0.69	1.90	4.41	8.29
Death rate 1980–84	0.02	0.07	0.29	0.94	2.18	4.31
Change in rate	-0.02	-0.15	-0.40	-0.96	-2.22	-3.97
Denmark						
Deaths 1974–78	0	0	2	5	58	102
Deaths 1980–84	2	0	2	7	17	69
Death rate 1974–78	0.00	0.00	0.05	0.17	2.04	3.72
Death rate 1980–84	0.06	0.00	0.05	0.19	0.62	2.55
Change in rate	0.06	0.00	0.00	0.02	-1.41	-1.17
France						
Deaths 1974–78	31	79	223	755	1789	2440
Deaths 1980–84	10	28	120	290	843	1441
Death rate 1974–78	0.07	0.19	0.60	2.40	5.49	10.89
Death rate 1980–84	0.02	0.06	0.28	0.89	2.68	5.19
Change in rate	-0.05	-0.12	-0.32	-1.51	-2.81	-5.71

Table 9.1.2(b) cont

	Age group (years)					
	5–14	15–24	25–34	35–44	45–54	55–64
Greece						
Deaths 1974–78	7	28	35	133	310	553
Deaths 1980–84	6	11	16	25	124	185
Death rate 1974–78	0.09	0.41	0.58	2.11	5.53	12.04
Death rate 1980–84	0.13	0.26	0.41	0.69	3.10	6.86
Change in rate	0.04	-0.16	-0.18	-1.42	-2.43	-5.18
Italy						
Deaths 1974–78	40	104	262	756	1879	2767
Deaths 1980–84	9	63	133	328	949	1650
Death rate 1974–78	0.09	0.26	0.68	2.01	5.23	10.34
Death rate 1980–84	0.02	0.14	0.34	0.88	2.64	5.64
Change in rate	-0.07	-0.11	-0.34	-1.13	-2.59	-4.70
Ireland						
Deaths 1974–78	2	10	11	46	97	209
Deaths 1980–84	0	2	9	14	52	155
Death rate 1974–78	0.06	0.37	0.54	2.83	6.22	14.31
Death rate 1980–84	0.00	0.07	0.38	0.78	3.47	10.79
Change in rate	-0.06	-0.30	-0.16	-2.05	-2.75	-3.51
Netherlands						
Deaths 1974–78	4	7	11	8	66	145
Deaths 1980–84	2	2	12	13	34	125
Death rate 1974–78	0.03	0.06	0.10	0.10	0.89	2.33
Death rate 1980–84	0.02	0.02	0.10	0.14	0.45	1.86
Change in rate	-0.01	-0.04	0.00	0.04	-0.44	-0.47
UK: England and Wales						
Deaths 1974–78	20	60	76	198	763	1188
Deaths 1980–84	11	26	54	119	358	849
Death rate 1974–78	0.05	0.17	0.22	0.70	2.57	4.29
Death rate 1980–84	0.03	0.07	0.16	0.38	1.30	3.05
Change in rate	-0.02	-0.10	-0.06	-0.32	-1.27	-1.24
UK: N. Ireland						
Deaths 1974–78	0	0	2	5	31	35
Deaths 1980–84	0	0	2	2	11	22
Death rate 1974–78	0.00	0.00	0.20	0.61	3.83	4.79
Death rate 1980–84	0.00	0.00	0.20	0.23	1.45	3.08
Change in rate	0.00	0.00	0.00	-0.39	-2.39	-1.72

Table 9.1.2(b) cont

	Age group (years)					
	5–14	15–24	25–34	35–44	45–54	55–64
UK: Scotland						
Deaths 1974–78	0	3	18	41	122	187
Deaths 1980–84	0	2	2	18	74	124
Death rate 1974–78	0.00	0.07	0.52	1.39	3.98	6.71
Death rate 1980–84	0.00	0.05	0.06	0.58	2.55	4.44
Change in rate	0.00	-0.03	-0.47	-0.81	-1.44	-2.27
Portugal						
Deaths 1974–78	—	—	—	—	—	—
Deaths 1980–84	10	33	110	244	499	690
Death rate 1974–78	—	—	—	—	—	—
Death rate 1980–84	0.12	0.40	1.62	4.25	8.64	13.72
Change in rate	—	—	—	—	—	—
Spain						
Deaths 1974–78	—	—	—	—	—	—
Deaths 1980–84	37	63	204	474	1095	1569
Death rate 1974–78	—	—	—	—	—	—
Death rate 1980–84	0.11	0.20	0.82	2.22	4.72	8.62
Change in rate	—	—	—	—	—	—
EC						
Deaths 1974–78	127	395	955	2890	7020	10467
Deaths 1980–84	98	272	803	1978	5034	8429
Death rate 1974–78	0.06	0.19	0.49	1.63	4.14	7.72
Death rate 1980–84	0.04	0.11	0.36	0.99	2.66	5.18
Change in rate	-0.01	-0.08	-0.14	-0.64	-1.48	-2.54

Table 9.1.2(c). Malignant neoplasm of the cervix uteri (ICD8 180; ICD9 180)

	Age group (years)					
	5–14	15–24	25–34	35–44	45–54	55–64
Belgium						
Deaths 1974–78	0	2	6	75	219	269
Deaths 1980–84	0	2	24	68	173	257
Death rate 1974–78	0.00	0.05	0.18	2.52	6.82	10.86
Death rate 1980–84	0.00	0.05	0.66	2.29	5.67	9.00
Change in rate	0.00	0.00	0.48	-0.23	-1.15	-1.86
Luxembourg						
Deaths 1974–78	0	0	0	5	14	13
Deaths 1980–84	0	0	0	5	8	6
Death rate 1974–78	0.00	0.00	0.00	4.24	11.71	13.61
Death rate 1980–84	0.00	0.00	0.00	4.24	6.72	6.13
Change in rate	0.00	0.00	0.00	0.00	-4.99	-7.48
Federal Republic of Germany						
Deaths 1974–78	2	20	329	1185	2501	3319
Deaths 1980–84	0	13	277	886	1423	2381
Death rate 1974–78	0.01	0.09	1.65	5.44	12.47	18.78
Death rate 1980–84	0.00	0.05	1.32	4.17	7.26	12.75
Change in rate	-0.01	-0.04	-0.33	-1.28	-5.21	-6.03
Denmark						
Deaths 1974–78	0	4	63	129	341	431
Deaths 1980–84	0	6	58	120	214	355
Death rate 1974–78	0.00	0.22	3.26	8.80	23.61	30.45
Death rate 1980–84	0.00	0.31	3.12	6.77	15.55	25.30
Change in rate	0.00	0.09	-0.14	-2.03	-8.07	-5.15
France						
Deaths 1974–78	0	7	98	391	1041	1016
Deaths 1980–84	0	5	120	367	797	1063
Death rate 1974–78	0.00	0.03	0.55	2.54	6.34	8.61
Death rate 1980–84	0.00	0.02	0.57	2.31	5.06	7.29
Change in rate	0.00	-0.01	0.02	-0.23	-1.27	-1.32
Greece						
Deaths 1974–78	0	2	8	39	80	86
Deaths 1980–84	0	0	12	33	70	50
Death rate 1974–78	0.00	0.06	0.26	1.20	2.77	3.55
Death rate 1980–84	0.00	0.00	0.60	1.76	3.45	3.51
Change in rate	0.00	-0.06	0.34	0.56	0.68	-0.04

Table 9.1.2(c) cont

	Age group (years)					
	5–14	15–24	25–34	35–44	45–54	55–64
Italy						
Deaths 1974–78	1	1	33	154	442	608
Deaths 1980–84	1	2	44	155	359	601
Death rate 1974–78	0.00	0.01	0.17	0.81	2.39	4.26
Death rate 1980–84	0.00	0.01	0.22	0.83	1.95	3.84
Change in rate	0.00	0.00	0.05	0.02	-0.44	-0.42
Ireland						
Deaths 1974 –78	0	1	7	26	55	78
Deaths 1980–84	0	0	19	21	40	87
Death rate 1974–78	0.00	0.07	0.70	3.26	7.09	10.65
Death rate 1980–84	0.00	0.00	1.62	2.41	5.42	11.86
Change in rate	0.00	-0.07	0.92	-0.85	-1.67	1.21
Netherlands						
Deaths 1974–78	0	5	49	139	430	490
Deaths 1980–84	0	3	42	127	241	367
Death rate 1974–78	0.00	0.09	0.93	3.56	11.39	15.00
Death rate 1980–84	0.00	0.05	0.73	2.76	6.39	10.42
Change in rate	0.00	-0.04	-0.20	-0.80	-5.00	-4.57
UK: England and Wales						
Deaths 1974–78	0	26	338	707	2028	2927
Deaths 1980–84	0	32	539	963	1350	2449
Death rate 1974–78	0.00	0.15	1.97	5.07	13.55	20.16
Death rate 1980–4	0.00	0.16	3.13	6.22	9.78	16.95
Change in rate	0.00	0.01	1.16	1.15	-3.77	-3.20
UK: N. Ireland						
Deaths 1974–78	0	1	4	18	43	51
Deaths 1980–84	0	3	13	22	35	51
Death rate 1974–78	0.00	0.17	0.83	4.37	10.24	13.32
Death rate 1980–84	0.00	0.46	2.61	4.94	8.93	13.39
Change in rate	0.00	0.29	1.78	0.57	-1.31	0.07
UK: Scotland						
Deaths 1974–78	0	0	25	88	218	306
Deaths 1980–84	0	6	45	110	157	258
Death rate 1974–78	0.00	0.00	1.46	5.86	13.77	20.31
Death rate 1980–84	0.00	0.28	2.52	7.03	10.48	17.29
Change in rate	0.00	0.28	1.06	1.16	-3.29	-3.02

Table 9.1.2(c) cont

	Age group (years)					
	5–14	15–24	25–34	35–44	45–54	55–64
Portugal						
Deaths 1974–78	—	—	—	—	—	—
Deaths 1980–84	1	1	34	79	183	189
Death rate 1974–78	—	—	—	—	—	—
Death rate 1980–84	0.02	0.02	0.99	2.63	6.00	7.00
Change in rate	—	—	—	—	—	—
Spain						
Deaths 1974–78	—	—	—	—	—	—
Deaths 1980–84	0	6	43	145	303	411
Death rate 1974–78	—	—	—	—	—	—
Death rate 1980–84	0.00	0.04	0.35	1.35	2.57	4.26
Change in rate	—	—	—	—	—	—
EC						
Deaths 1974–78	3	69	960	2956	7412	9594
Deaths 1980–84	2	79	1270	3101	5353	8525
Death rate 1974–78	0.00	0.07	1.01	3.38	8.49	13.04
Death rate 1980–84	0.00	0.06	1.14	3.12	5.62	9.73
Change in rate	0.00	0.00	0.12	-0.25	-2.87	-3.31

Table 9.1.2(d). Malignant neoplasm of the cervix and body of the uterus (ICD8 180, 182; ICD9 179, 180, 182)

	Age group (years)					
	5–14	15–24	25–34	35–44	45–54	55–64
Belgium						
Deaths 1974–78	0	4	21	132	470	763
Deaths 1980–84	0	2	32	106	331	676
Death rate 1974–78	0.00	0.11	0.64	4.44	14.65	30.80
Death rate 1980–84	0.00	0.05	0.88	3.57	10.85	23.67
Change in rate	0.00	-0.05	0.24	-0.86	-3.79	-7.13
Luxembourg						
Deaths 1974–78	0	0	0	7	24	38
Deaths 1980–84	0	0	0	6	17	23
Death rate 1974–78	0.00	0.00	0.00	5.94	20.07	39.79
Death rate 1980–84	0.00	0.00	0.00	5.09	14.27	23.52
Change in rate	0.00	0.00	0.00	-0.84	-5.79	-16.27
Federal Republic of Germany						
Deaths 1974–78	4	29	412	1581	3876	6507
Deaths 1980–84	0	17	351	1164	2231	4850
Death rate 1974–78	0.02	0.13	2.06	7.26	19.33	36.81
Death rate 1980–84	0.00	0.07	1.68	5.47	11.39	25.97
Change in rate	-0.02	-0.06	-0.39	-1.79	-7.95	-10.84
Denmark						
Deaths 1974–78	0	4	64	143	414	627
Deaths 1980–84	0	6	59	133	264	548
Death rate 1974–78	0.00	0.22	3.31	9.76	28.67	44.30
Death rate 1980–84	0.00	0.31	3.17	7.51	19.18	39.06
Change in rate	0.00	0.09	-0.14	-2.25	-9.49	-5.24
France						
Deaths 1974–78	2	14	192	991	3081	4032
Deaths 1980–84	3	13	217	690	1962	3669
Death rate 1974–78	0.01	0.07	1.07	6.43	18.75	34.18
Death rate 1980–84	0.02	0.06	1.02	4.35	12.46	25.18
Change in rate	0.01	-0.01	-0.05	-2.08	-6.29	-9.00
Greece						
Deaths 1974–78	1	7	32	154	410	481
Deaths 1980–84	0	1	29	76	217	241
Death rate 1974–78	0.03	0.21	1.03	4.74	14.20	19.84
Death rate 1980–84	0.00	0.05	1.46	4.05	10.69	16.92
Change in rate	-0.03	-0.16	0.42	-0.69	-3.51	-2.92

Table 9.1.2(d) cont

	Age group (years)					
	5–14	15–24	25–34	35–44	45–54	55–64
Italy						
Deaths 1974–78	4	20	232	1136	3648	5275
Deaths 1980–84	5	21	227	882	2458	4518
Death rate 1974–78	0.02	0.10	1.21	5.99	19.73	36.98
Death rate 1980–84	0.02	0.10	1.16	4.72	13.38	28.88
Change in rate	0.01	0.00	-0.05	-1.27	-6.35	-8.10
Ireland						
Deaths 1974–78	0	1	9	36	90	166
Deaths 1980–84	0	1	19	25	69	190
Death rate 1974–78	0.00	0.07	0.90	4.52	11.60	22.67
Death rate 1980–84	0.00	0.07	1.62	2.87	9.34	25.90
Change in rate	0.00	-0.01	0.72	-1.65	-2.25	3.23
Netherlands						
Deaths 1974–78	0	8	52	170	568	875
Deaths 1980–84	0	4	45	142	347	691
Death rate 1974–78	0.00	0.14	0.99	4.35	15.04	26.78
Death rate 1980–84	0.00	0.07	0.79	3.09	9.20	19.63
Change in rate	0.00	-0.07	-0.20	-1.27	-5.84	-7.15
UK: England and Wales						
Deaths 1974–78	1	38	361	791	2635	4580
Deaths 1980–84	1	35	558	1049	1813	4020
Death rate 1974–78	0.01	0.22	2.10	5.67	17.61	31.54
Death rate 1980–84	0.01	0.18	3.24	6.77	13.14	27.83
Change in rate	0.00	-0.04	1.13	1.10	-4.47	-3.71
UK: N. Ireland						
Deaths 1974–78	0	1	7	22	54	99
Deaths 1980–84	0	3	14	25	47	95
Death rate 1974–78	0.00	0.17	1.45	5.35	12.86	25.85
Death rate 1980–84	0.00	0.46	2.81	5.61	11.99	24.94
Change in rate	0.00	0.29	1.36	0.27	-0.86	-0.91
UK: Scotland						
Deaths 1974–78	0	0	26	96	277	491
Deaths 1980–84	0	6	47	118	202	392
Death rate 1974–78	0.00	0.00	1.52	6.39	17.50	32.59
Death rate 1980–84	0.00	0.28	2.64	7.54	13.49	26.27
Change in rate	0.00	0.28	1.12	1.14	-4.01	-6.32

Table 9.1.2(d) cont

	Age group (years)					
	5–14	15–24	25–34	35–44	45–54	55–64
Portugal						
Deaths 1974–78	—	—	—	—	—	—
Deaths 1980–84	1	3	69	191	497	690
Death rate 1974–78	—	—	—	—	—	—
Death rate 1980–84	0.02	0.07	2.01	6.36	16.29	25.55
Change in rate	—	—	—	—	—	—
Spain						
Deaths 1974–78	—	—	—	—	—	—
Deaths 1980–84	2	20	109	461	1359	2294
Death rate 1974–78	—	—	—	—	—	—
Death rate 1980–84	0.01	0.13	0.88	4.30	11.54	23.78
Change in rate	—	—	—	—	—	—
EC						
Deaths 1974–78	12	126	1408	5259	15547	23934
Deaths 1980–84	12	132	1776	5068	11814	22897
Death rate 1974–78	0.01	0.12	1.49	6.01	17.81	32.53
Death rate 1980–84	0.01	0.11	1.59	5.11	12.40	26.14
Change in rate	0.00	-0.02	0.10	-0.90	-5.41	-6.39

Table 9.1.2(e). Hodgkin's disease (ICD8 201; ICD9 201)

	Age group (years)					
	5–14	15–24	25–34	35–44	45–54	55–64
Belgium						
Deaths 1974–78	4	48	105	107	105	135
Deaths 1980–84	6	40	87	78	92	125
Death rate 1974–78	0.05	0.62	1.55	1.79	1.66	2.87
Death rate 1980–84	0.09	0.51	1.17	1.30	1.52	2.29
Change in rate	0.04	-0.11	-0.39	-0.49	-0.13	-0.58
Luxembourg						
Deaths 1974–78	0	1	3	4	2	1
Deaths 1980–84	0	0	4	0	3	3
Death rate 1974–78	0.00	0.36	1.13	1.61	0.85	0.56
Death rate 1980–84	0.00	0.00	1.38	0.00	1.24	1.70
Change in rate	0.00	-0.36	0.26	-1.61	0.39	1.13
Federal Republic of Germany						
Deaths 1974–78	51	328	532	657	663	708
Deaths 1980–84	33	284	412	485	583	820
Death rate 1974–78	0.11	0.73	1.29	1.45	1.77	2.38
Death rate 1980–84	0.09	0.56	0.96	1.11	1.47	2.56
Change in rate	-0.02	-0.18	-0.33	-0.34	-0.29	0.18
Denmark						
Deaths 1974–78	2	15	45	37	41	54
Deaths 1980–84	4	21	33	33	31	43
Death rate 1974–78	0.05	0.40	1.13	1.25	1.44	1.97
Death rate 1980–84	0.11	0.54	0.87	0.91	1.13	1.59
Change in rate	0.06	0.13	-0.27	-0.34	-0.31	-0.38
France						
Deaths 1974–78	30	240	467	448	445	483
Deaths 1980–84	11	161	345	289	327	354
Death rate 1974–78	0.07	0.57	1.25	1.42	1.37	2.16
Death rate 1980–84	0.03	0.37	0.81	0.89	1.04	1.27
Change in rate	-0.04	-0.19	-0.45	-0.53	-0.33	-0.88
Greece						
Deaths 1974–78	17	45	75	88	134	185
Deaths 1980–84	2	21	30	32	55	74
Death rate 1974–78	0.23	0.66	1.24	1.40	2.39	4.03
Death rate 1980–84	0.04	0.49	0.76	0.88	1.37	2.74
Change in rate	-0.19	-0.17	-0.48	-0.52	-1.02	-1.29

Table 9.1.2(e) cont

	Age group (years)					
	5–14	15–24	25–34	35–44	45–54	55–64
Italy						
Deaths 1974–78	108	332	621	709	943	1089
Deaths 1980–84	50	261	459	536	688	851
Death rate 1974–78	0.24	0.82	1.61	1.89	2.62	4.07
Death rate 1980–84	0.11	0.59	1.17	1.45	1.92	2.91
Change in rate	-0.12	-0.23	-0.44	-0.44	-0.71	-1.16
Ireland						
Deaths 1974–78	2	13	26	24	27	44
Deaths 1980–84	5	21	26	23	29	45
Death rate 1974–78	0.06	0.48	1.28	1.48	1.73	3.01
Death rate 1980 –84	0.15	0.70	1.09	1.28	1.93	3.13
Change in rate	0.08	0.22	-0.18	-0.19	0.20	0.12
Netherlands						
Deaths 1974–78	6	51	149	109	94	157
Deaths 1980–84	1	45	98	86	85	113
Death rate 1974–78	0.05	0.44	1.37	1.35	1.26	2.53
Death rate 1980–84	0.01	0.36	0.83	0.90	1.12	1.68
Change in rate	-0.04	-0.08	-0.53	-0.45	-0.14	-0.84
UK: England and Wales						
Deaths 1974–78	28	258	458	387	466	667
Deaths 1980–84	12	204	348	319	287	487
Death rate 1974–78	0.07	0.73	1.32	1.37	1.57	2.41
Death rate 1980–84	0.04	0.51	1.00	1.02	1.04	1.75
Change in rate	-0.04	-0.21	-0.32	-0.35	-0.53	-0.66
UK: N. Ireland						
Deaths 1974–78	1	13	10	12	15	13
Deaths 1980–84	1	11	14	8	13	20
Death rate 1974–78	0.07	1.02	1.00	1.47	1.86	1.78
Death rate 1980–84	0.07	0.80	1.38	0.90	1.71	2.80
Change in rate	0.01	-0.21	0.38	-0.56	-0.15	1.01
UK: Scotland						
Deaths 1974–78	3	30	37	39	48	70
Deaths 1980–84	1	23	42	36	34	34
Death rate 1974–78	0.07	0.74	1.08	1.32	1.57	2.51
Death rate 1980–84	0.03	0.52	1.17	1.16	1.17	1.22
Change in rate	-0.04	-0.22	0.09	-0.16	-0.40	-1.29

Table 9.1.2(e) cont

	Age group (years)					
	5–14	15–24	25–34	35–44	45–54	55–64
Portugal						
Deaths 1974–78	—	—	—	—	—	—
Deaths 1980–84	7	25	55	46	61	75
Death rate 1974–78	—	—	—	—	—	—
Death rate 1980–84	0.08	0.30	0.81	0.80	1.06	1.49
Change in rate	—	—	—	—	—	—
Spain						
Deaths 1974–78	—	—	—	—	—	
Deaths 1980–84	39	121	218	178	265	307
Death rate 1974–78	—	—	—	—	—	—
Death rate 1980–84	0.12	0.39	0.87	0.83	1.14	1.69
Change in rate	—	—	—	—	—	—
EC						
Deaths 1974–78	252	1374	2528	2621	2983	3606
Deaths 1980–84	172	1238	2171	2149	2553	3351
Death rate 1974–78	0.11	0.66	1.31	1.48	1.76	2.66
Death rate 1980–84	0.07	0.49	0.96	1.07	1.35	2.06
Change in rate	-0.04	-0.17	-0.35	-0.41	-0.41	-0.60

Table 9.1.2(f). Chronic rheumatic heart disease (ICD8 393–398; ICD9 393–398)

	Age group (years)					
	5–14	15–24	25–34	35–44	45–54	55–64
Belgium						
Deaths 1974–78	0	11	26	50	200	336
Deaths 1980–84	1	1	4	5	35	103
Death rate 1974–78	0.00	0.14	0.38	0.84	3.15	7.14
Death rate 1980–84	0.02	0.01	0.05	0.08	0.58	1.88
Change in rate	0.02	-0.13	-0.33	-0.75	-2.57	-5.25
Luxembourg						
Deaths 1974–78	0	1	2	4	7	21
Deaths 1980–84	0	0	0	5	4	6
Death rate 1974–78	0.00	0.36	0.75	1.61	2.98	11.82
Death rate 1980–84	0.00	0.00	0.00	2.05	1.65	3.40
Change in rate	0.00	-0.36	-0.75	0.43	-1.33	-8.43
Federal Republic of Germany						
Deaths 1974–78	31	116	320	1107	3110	4638
Deaths 1980–84	2	22	60	230	718	1759
Death rate 1974--8	0.06	0.26	0.77	2.45	8.29	15.58
Death rate 1980–84	0.01	0.04	0.14	0.53	1.81	5.49
Change in rate	-0.06	-0.22	-0.63	-1.92	-6.47	-10.09
Denmark						
Deaths 1974–78	4	1	12	43	119	302
Deaths 1980–84	2	1	9	13	68	206
Death rate 1974–78	0.10	0.03	0.30	1.46	4.18	11.02
Death rate 1980–84	0.06	0.03	0.24	0.36	2.49	7.61
Change in rate	-0.05	0.00	-0.07	-1.10	-1.69	-3.41
France						
Deaths 1974–78	60	118	244	593	1312	2167
Deaths 1980–84	12	31	59	161	443	1069
Death rate 1974–78	0.14	0.28	0.65	1.88	4.03	9.67
Death rate 1980–84	0.03	0.07	0.14	0.50	1.41	3.85
Change in rate	-0.11	-0.21	-0.52	-1.39	-2.62	-5.83
Greece						
Deaths 1974–78	10	47	87	194	405	493
Deaths 1980–84	0	3	15	33	86	127
Death rate 1974–78	0.14	0.69	1.44	3.08	7.23	10.74
Death rate 1980--84	0.00					
Change in rate	-0.14	-0.62	-1.06	-2.17	-5.08	-6.03

Table 9.1.2(f) cont

	Age group (years)					
	5–14	15–24	25–34	35–44	45–54	55–64

Italy

Deaths 1974–78	145	418	846	1845	4395	5398
Deaths 1980–84	43	173	382	917	2360	4108
Death rate 1974–78	0.32	1.03	2.19	4.92	12.23	20.18
Death rate 1980–84	0.10	0.39	0.97	2.47	6.57	14.04
Change in rate	-0.22	-0.64	-1.22	-2.44	-5.66	-6.14

Ireland

Deaths 1974–78	0	13	30	64	192	337
Deaths 1980-84	0	1	6	17	66	135
Death rate 1974–78	0.00	0.48	1.47	3.94	12.31	23.07
Death rate 1980–84	0.00					
Change in rate	0.00	-0.44	-1.22	-2.99	-7.91	-13.67

Netherlands

Deaths 1974–78	3	26	56	138	429	794
Deaths 1980–84	0	7	19	49	139	293
Death rate 1974–78	0.02	0.22	0.51	1.71	5.76	12.78
Death rate 1980–84	0.00	0.06	0.16	0.52	1.83	4.36
Change in rate	-0.02	-0.17	-0.35	-1.20	-3.93	-8.41

UK: England and Wales

Deaths 1974–78	23	58	235	904	2948	6546
Deaths 1980–84	7	16	68	300	1161	3191
Death rate 1974–78	0.06	0.16	0.68	3.20	9.93	23.64
Death rate 1980–84	0.02	0.04	0.20	0.96	4.21	11.47
Change in rate	-0.04	-0.12	-0.48	-2.24	-5.72	-12.17

UK: N. Ireland

Deaths 1974–78	2	4	5	34	92	192
Deaths 1980–84	0	0	2	9	27	84
Death rate 1974–78	0.13	0.31	0.50	4.15	11.38	26.30
Death rate 1980–84	0.00	0.00	0.20	1.01	3.55	11.74
Change in rate	-0.13	-0.31	-0.30	-3.14	-7.83	-14.56

UK: Scotland

Deaths 1974–78	4	7	38	146	378	694
Deaths 1980–84	1	0	13	35	188	448
Death rate 1974–78	0.09	0.17	1.11	4.95	12.34	24.89
Death rate 1980–84	0.03	0.00	0.36	1.13	6.47	16.03
Change in rate	-0.06	-0.17	-0.74	-3.83	-5.87	-8.86

Table 9.1.2(f) cont

| | Age group (years) | | | | | |
	5–14	15–24	25–34	35–44	45–54	55–64
Portugal						
Deaths 1974–78	—	—	—	—	—	—
Deaths 1980-84	12	63	122	225	344	427
Death rate 1974–78	—	—	—	—	—	—
Death rate 1980–84	0.14	0.75	1.80	3.92	5.96	8.49
Change in rate	—	—	—	—	—	—
Spain						
Deaths 1974–78	—	—	—	—	—	—
Deaths 1980–84	33	108	271	580	1680	2591
Death rate 1974–78	—	—	—	—	—	—
Death rate 1980–84	0.10	0.35	1.08	2.71	7.24	14.23
Change in rate	—	—	—	—	—	—
EC						
Deaths 1974–78	282	820	1901	5122	13587	21918
Deaths 1980–84	113	426	1030	2579	7319	14547
Death rate 1974–78	0.13	0.39	0.98	2.89	8.00	16.16
Death rate 1980–84	0.05	0.17	0.46	1.29	3.87	8.93
Change in rate	-0.08	-0.22	-0.53	-1.60	-4.14	-7.23

Table 9.1.2(g). Asthma (ICD8 493; ICD9 493)

	Age group (years)					
	5–14	15–24	25–34	35–44	45–54	55–64
Belgium						
Deaths 1974–78	12	47	60	125	279	446
Deaths 1980–84	11	58	78	114	249	497
Death rate 1974–78	0.16	0.61	0.89	2.09	4.40	9.48
Death rate 1980–84	0.17	0.74	1.05	1.90	4.12	9.09
Change in rate	0.01	0.13	0.16	-0.19	-0.28	-0.39
Luxembourg						
Deaths 1974–78	0	0	0	0	0	0
Deaths 1980–84	0	3	3	2	12	17
Death rate 1974–78	0.00	0.00	0.00	0.00	0.00	0.00
Death rate 1980–84	0.00	1.05	1.04	0.82	4.96	9.62
Change in rate	0.00	1.05	1.04	0.82	4.96	9.62
Federal Republic of Germany						
Deaths 1974–78	198	296	303	809	1773	3389
Deaths 1980–84	137	524	428	797	2120	3893
Death rate 1974–78	0.41	0.66	0.73	1.79	4.72	11.39
Death rate 1980–84	0.37	1.03	0.99	1.82	5.36	12.15
Change in rate	-0.04	0.37	0.26	0.03	0.63	0.76
Denmark						
Deaths 1974–78	2	7	7	22	50	99
Deaths 1980–84	5	15	18	24	71	136
Death rate 1974–78	0.05	0.19	0.18	0.74	1.75	3.61
Death rate 1980–84	0.14	0.38	0.47	0.66	2.60	5.02
Change in rate	0.09	0.20	0.30	-0.08	0.84	1.41
France						
Deaths 1974–78	24	130	103	235	596	914
Deaths 1980–84	30	159	171	221	582	1065
Death rate 1974–80	0.06	0.31	0.28	0.75	1.83	4.08
Death rate 1980–84	0.07	0.37	0.40	0.68	1.85	3.83
Change in rate	0.02	0.06	0.12	-0.07	0.02	-0.25
Greece						
Deaths 1974–78	1	5	6	32	84	416
Deaths 1980–84	—	—	—	—	—	—
Death rate 1974–78	0.01	0.07	0.10	0.51	1.50	9.06
Death rate 1980–84	—	—	—	—	—	—
Change in rate	—	—	—	—	—	—

Table 9.1.2(g) cont

	Age group (years)					
	5–14	15–24	25–34	35–44	45–54	55–64

Italy

Deaths 1974–78	11	18	19	40	91	276
Deaths 1980–84	32	60	50	103	257	699
Death rate 1974–78	0.02	0.04	0.05	0.11	0.25	1.03
Death rate 1980–84	0.07	0.14	0.13	0.28	0.72	2.39
Change in rate	0.05	0.09	0.08	0.17	0.46	1.36

Ireland

Deaths 1974–78	9	14	17	25	76	143
Deaths 1980–84	10	25	19	41	72	128
Death rate 1974–78	0.27	0.51	0.83	1.54	4.87	9.79
Death rate 1980–84	0.29	0.83	0.80	2.29	4.80	8.91
Change in rate	0.02	0.32	-0.04	0.75	-0.07	-0.88

Netherlands

Deaths 1974–78	8	27	31	51	108	134
Deaths 1980–84	9	39	53	50	95	168
Death rate 1974–78	0.07	0.23	0.28	0.63	1.45	2.16
Death rate 1980–84	0.08	0.31	0.45	0.53	1.25	2.50
Change in rate	0.02	0.08	0.17	-0.11	-0.20	0.35

UK: England and Wales

Deaths 1974–78	134	234	268	376	714	1124
Deaths 1980–84	166	391	341	414	923	1582
Death rate 1974–78	0.34	0.66	0.77	1.33	2.40	4.06
Death rate 1980–84	0.48	0.98	0.98	1.33	3.34	5.69
Change in rate	0.15	0.33	0.21	0.00	0.94	1.63

UK: N. Ireland

Deaths 1974–78	4	4	6	8	24	36
Deaths 1980–84	5	14	9	17	38	50
Death rate 1974–78	0.26	0.31	0.60	0.98	2.97	4.93
Death rate 1980–84	0.36	1.02	0.89	1.92	5.00	6.99
Change in rate	0.10	0.71	0.29	0.94	2.03	2.06

UK: Scotland

Deaths 1974–78	20	39	19	51	87	134
Deaths 1980–84	16	35	22	46	113	165
Death rate 1974–78	0.45	0.96	0.55	1.73	2.84	4.81
Death rate 1980–84	0.43	0.80	0.61	1.48	3.89	5.90
Change in rate	-0.02	-0.17	0.06	-0.25	1.05	1.10

Table 9.1.2(g) cont

	Age group (years)					
	5–14	15–24	25–34	35–44	45–54	55–64
Portugal						
Deaths 1974–78	—	—	—	—	—	—
Deaths 1980–84	—	—	—	—	—	—
Death rate 1974–78	—	—	—	—	—	—
Death rate 1980–84	—	—	—	—	—	—
Change in rate	—	—	—	—	—	—
Spain						
Deaths 1974–78	—	—	—	—	—	—
Deaths 1980–84	21	45	48	119	339	841
Death rate 1974–78	—	—	—	—	—	—
Death rate 1980-84	0.06	0.14	0.19	0.56	1.46	4.62
Change in rate	—	—	—	—	—	—
EC						
Deaths 1974–78	423	821	839	1774	3882	7111
Deaths 1980–84	442	1368	1240	1948	4871	9241
Death rate 1974–78	0.19	0.39	0.43	1.00	2.29	5.24
Death rate 1980–84	0.19	0.54	0.55	0.97	2.57	5.67
Change in rate	0.00	0.14	0.11	-0.03	0.29	0.43

Table 9.1.2(h). Appendicitis (ICD8 540–543; ICD9 540–543)

	Age group (years)					
	5–14	15–24	25–34	35–44	45–54	55–64
Belgium						
Deaths 1974–78	6	4	11	13	15	22
Deaths 1980–84	2	3	2	2	4	16
Death rate 1974–78	0.08	0.05	0.16	0.22	0.24	0.47
Death rate 1980–84	0.03	0.04	0.03	0.03	0.07	0.29
Change in rate	-0.05	-0.01	-0.14	-0.18	-0.17	-0.17
Luxembourg						
Deaths 1974–78	1	0	3	1	1	2
Deaths 1980–84	0	1	1	0	1	1
Death rate 1974–78	0.39	0.00	1.13	0.40	0.43	1.13
Death rate 1980–84	0.00	0.35	0.35	0.00	0.41	0.57
Change in rate	-0.39	0.35	-0.78	-0.40	-0.01	-0.56
Federal Republic of Germany						
Deaths 1974–78	131	120	103	182	300	526
Deaths 1980–84	34	39	30	55	103	204
Death rate 1974–78	0.27	0.27	0.25	0.40	0.80	1.77
Death rate 1980–84	0.09	0.08	0.07	0.13	0.26	0.64
Change in rate	-0.18	-0.19	-0.18	-0.28	-0.54	-1.13
Denmark						
Deaths 1974–78	6	2	3	6	11	14
Deaths 1980–84	3	3	1	4	8	12
Death rate 1974–78	0.15	0.05	0.08	0.20	0.39	0.51
Death rate 1980–84	0.08	0.08	0.03	0.11	0.29	0.44
Change in rate	-0.07	0.02	-0.05	-0.09	-0.09	-0.07
France						
Deaths 1974–78	87	80	74	79	171	197
Deaths 1980–84	36	42	38	39	76	122
Death rate 1974–78	0.21	0.19	0.20	0.25	0.52	0.88
Death rate 1980 –84	0.09	0.10	0.09	0.12	0.24	0.44
Change in rate	-0.12	-0.09	-0.11	-0.13	-0.28	-0.44
Greece						
Deaths 1974–78	3	7	7	4	12	14
Deaths 1980–84	1	1	4	3	1	4
Death rate 1974–78	0.04	0.10	0.12	0.06	0.21	0.30
Death rate 1980–84	0.02	0.02	0.10	0.08	0.02	0.15
Change in rate	-0.02	-0.08	-0.01	0.02	-0.19	-0.16

Table 9.1.2(h) cont

	Age group (years)					
	5–14	15–24	25–34	35–44	45–54	55–64
Italy						
Deaths 1974–78	103	66	54	99	158	282
Deaths 1980–84	49	24	30	22	82	117
Death rate 1974–78	0.23	0.16	0.14	0.26	0.44	1.05
Death rate 1980–84	0.11	0.05	0.08	0.06	0.23	0.40
Change in rate	-0.11	-0.11	-0.06	-0.20	-0.21	-0.65
Ireland						
Deaths 1974–78	7	10	1	4	8	16
Deaths 1980–84	6	1	1	1	2	6
Death rate 1974–78	0.21	0.37	0.05	0.25	0.51	1.10
Death rate 1980–84	0.17	0.03	0.04	0.06	0.13	0.42
Change in rate	-0.04	-0.33	-0.01	-0.19	-0.38	-0.68
Netherlands						
Deaths 1974–78	13	22	9	15	24	38
Deaths 1980–84	8	6	8	7	13	25
Death rate 1974–78	0.19	0.08	0.19	0.32	0.61	
Death rate 1980–84	0.07	0.05	0.07	0.07	0.17	0.37
Change in rate	-0.03	-0.14	-0.01	-0.11	-0.15	-0.24
UK: England and Wales						
Deaths 1974–78	80	48	31	45	107	174
Deaths 1980–84	26	9	12	8	48	98
Death rate 1974–78	0.20	0.14	0.09	0.16	0.36	0.63
Death rate 1980–84	0.08	0.02	0.03	0.03	0.17	0.35
Change in rate	-0.13	-0.11	-0.05	-0.13	-0.19	-0.28
UK: N. Ireland						
Deaths 1974–78	2	1	0	1	3	4
Deaths 1980–84	1	1	0	0	1	5
Death rate 1974–78	0.13	0.08	0.00	0.12	0.37	0.55
Death rate 1980–84	0.07	0.07	0.00	0.00	0.13	0.70
Change in rate	-0.06	-0.01	0.00	-0.12	-0.24	0.15
UK: Scotland						
Deaths 1974 –78	9	2	4	3	11	22
Deaths 1980–84	2	4	1	4	3	10
Death rate 1974–78	0.20	0.05	0.12	0.10	0.36	0.79
Death rate 1980–84	0.05	0.09	0.03	0.13	0.10	0.36
Change in rate	-0.15	0.04	-0.09	0.03	-0.26	-0.43

Table 9.1.2(h) cont

	Age group (years)					
	5–14	15–24	25–34	35–44	45–54	55–64
Portugal						
Deaths 1974–78	—	—	—	—	—	—
Deaths 1980–84	20	7	4	8	17	23
Death rate 1974–78	—	—	—	—	—	—
Death rate 1980–84	0.23	0.08	0.06	0.14	0.29	0.46
Change in rate	—	—	—	—	—	—
Spain						
Deaths 1974–78	—	—	—	—	—	—
Deaths 1980–84	23	27	16	22	56	91
Death rate 1974–78	—	—	—	—	—	—
Death rate 1980–84	0.07	0.09	0.06	0.10	0.24	0.50
Change in rate	—	—	—	—	—	—
EC						
Deaths 1974–78	448	362	300	452	821	1311
Deaths 1980–84	211	168	148	175	415	734
Death rate 1974–78	0.20	0.17	0.16	0.25	0.48	0.97
Death rate 1980–84	0.09	0.07	0.07	0.09	0.22	0.45
Change in rate	-0.11	-0.11	-0.09	-0.17	-0.26	-0.52

Table 9.1.2(i). Abdominal hernia (ICD8 550–553; ICD9 550–553)

	Age group (years)					
	5–14	15–24	25–34	35–44	45–54	55–64
Belgium						
Deaths 1974–78	0	0	1	6	20	68
Deaths 1980–84	0	2	2	3	8	26
Death rate 1974–78	0.00	0.00	0.01	0.10	0.32	1.44
Death rate 1980–84	0.00	0.03	0.03	0.05	0.13	0.48
Change in rate	0.00	0.03	0.01	-0.05	-0.18	-0.97
Luxembourg						
Deaths 1974–78	0	0	0	1	0	0
Deaths 1980–84	0	0	0	0	1	1
Death rate 1974–78	0.00	0.00	0.00	0.40	0.00	0.00
Death rate 1980–84	0.00	0.00	0.00	0.00	0.41	0.57
Change in rate	0.00	0.00	0.00	-0.40	0.41	0.57
Federal Republic of Germany						
Deaths 1974–78	7	8	22	96	244	624
Deaths 1980–84	2	1	3	30	98	264
Death rate 1974–78	0.01	0.02	0.05	0.21	0.65	2.10
Death rate 1980–84	0.01	0.00	0.01	0.07	0.25	0.82
Change in rate	-0.01	-0.02	-0.05	-0.14	-0.40	-1.27
Denmark						
Deaths 1974–78	1	0	0	2	5	20
Deaths 1980–84	0	1	0	2	7	17
Death rate 1974–78	0.03	0.00	0.00	0.07	0.18	0.73
Death rate 1980–84	0.00	0.03	0.00	0.06	0.26	0.63
Change in rate	-0.03	0.03	0.00	-0.01	0.08	-0.10
France						
Deaths 1974–78	1	3	8	49	224	436
Deaths 1980–84	4	5	8	31	131	379
Death rate 1974–78	0.00	0.01	0.02	0.16	0.69	1.95
Death rate 1980–84	0.01	0.01	0.02	0.10	0.42	1.36
Change in rate	0.01	0.00	0.00	-0.06	-0.27	-0.58
Greece						
Deaths 1974–78	1	0	3	3	13	41
Deaths 1980–84	0	0	0	0	7	12
Death rate 1974–78	0.01	0.00	0.05	0.05	0.23	0.89
Death rate 1980–84	0.00	0.00	0.00	0.00	0.17	0.44
Change in rate	-0.01	0.00	-0.05	-0.05	-0.06	-0.45

Table 9.1.2(i) cont

	Age group (years)					
	5–14	15–24	25–34	35–44	45–54	55–64

Italy

Deaths 1974–78	7	7	17	61	207	571
Deaths 1980–84	2	6	12	32	130	376
Death rate 1974–78	0.02	0.02	0.04	0.16	0.58	2.13
Death rate 1980–84	0.00	0.01	0.03	0.09	0.36	1.29
Change in rate	-0.01	0.00	-0.01	-0.08	-0.21	-0.85

Ireland

Deaths 1974–78	0	0	2	3	7	21
Deaths 1980–84	0	0	0	1	2	11
Death rate 1974–78	0.00	0.00	0.10	0.18	0.45	1.44
Death rate 1980–84	0.00	0.00	0.00	0.06	0.13	0.77
Change in rate	0.00	0.00	-0.10	-0.13	-0.32	-0.67

Netherlands

Deaths 1974–78	4	6	4	5	30	88
Deaths 1980–84	2	4	4	4	12	52
Death rate 1974–78	0.03	0.05	0.04	0.06	0.40	1.42
Death rate 1980–84	0.02	0.03	0.03	0.04	0.16	0.77
Change in rate	-0.01	-0.02	0.00	-0.02	-0.24	-0.64

UK: England and Wales

Deaths 1974–78	12	13	17	44	169	449
Deaths 1980–84	6	11	12	14	100	277
Death rate 1974–78	0.03	0.04	0.05	0.16	0.57	1.62
Death rate 1980–84	0.02	0.03	0.03	0.04	0.36	1.00
Change in rate	-0.01	-0.01	-0.01	-0.11	-0.21	-0.63

UK: N. Ireland

Deaths 1974–78	1	1	1	2	3	13
Deaths 1980–84	0	0	1	1	3	8
Death rate 1974–78	0.07	0.08	0.10	0.24	0.37	1.78
Death rate 1980–84	0.00	0.00	0.10	0.11	0.39	1.12
Change in rate	-0.07	-0.08	0.00	-0.13	0.02	-0.66

UK: Scotland

Deaths 1974–78	3	4	0	7	14	47
Deaths 1980–84	0	1	2	4	11	23
Death rate 1974–78	0.07	0.10	0.00	0.24	0.46	1.69
Death rate 1980–84	0.00	0.02	0.06	0.13	0.38	0.82
Change in rate	-0.07	-0.08	0.06	-0.11	-0.08	-0.86

Table 9.1.2(i) cont

	Age group (years)					
	5–14	15–24	25–34	35–44	45–54	55–64

Portugal

	5–14	15–24	25–34	35–44	45–54	55–64
Deaths 1974–78	—	—	—	—	—	—
Deaths 1980–84	2	0	3	1	17	47
Death rate 1974–78	—	—	—	—	—	—
Death rate 1980–84	0.02	0.00	0.04	0.02	0.29	0.93
Change in rate	—	—	—	—	—	—

Spain

	5–14	15–24	25–34	35–44	45–54	55–64
Deaths 1974–78	—	—	—	—	—	—
Deaths 1980–84	3	2	6	16	63	200
Death rate 1974–78	—	—	—	—	—	—
Death rate 1980–84	0.01	0.01	0.02	0.07	0.27	1.10
Change in rate	—	—	—	—	—	—

EC

	5–14	15–24	25–34	35–44	45–54	55–64
Deaths 1974–78	37	42	75	279	936	2378
Deaths 1980–84	21	33	53	139	590	1693
Death rate 1974–78	0.02	0.02	0.04	0.16	0.55	1.75
Death rate 1980–84	0.01	0.01	0.02	0.07	0.31	1.04
Change in rate	-0.01	-0.01	-0.02	-0.09	-0.24	-0.71

Table 9.1.2(j). Cholelithiasis and cholecystitis (ICD8 574–575; ICD9 574–575.1, 576.1)

	Age group (years)					
	5–14	15–24	25–34	35–44	45–54	55–64
Belgium						
Deaths 1974–78	0	0	4	20	48	123
Deaths 1980–84	0	1	3	7	25	103
Death rate 1974–78	0.00	0.00	0.06	0.33	0.76	2.61
Death rate 1980–84	0.00	0.01	0.04	0.12	0.41	1.88
Change in rate	0.00	0.01	-0.02	-0.22	-0.34	-0.73
Luxembourg						
Deaths 1974–78	0	0	0	0	4	6
Deaths 1980–84	0	0	1	1	0	5
Death rate 1974–78	0.00	0.00	0.00	0.00	1.70	3.38
Death rate 1980–84	0.00	0.00	0.35	0.41	0.00	2.83
Change in rate	0.00	0.00	0.35	0.41	-1.70	-0.55
Federal Republic of Germany						
Deaths 1974–78	1	23	73	265	720	1705
Deaths 1980–84	0	10	18	75	229	748
Death rate 1974–78	0.00	0.05	0.18	0.59	1.92	5.73
Death rate 1980–84	0.00	0.02	0.04	0.17	0.58	2.33
Change in rate	0.00	-0.03	-0.13	-0.41	-1.34	-3.39
Denmark						
Deaths 1974-78	0	0	0	4	10	63
Deaths 1980-84	0	0	0	2	16	34
Death rate 1974-78	0.00	0.00	0.00	0.14	0.35	2.30
Death rate 1980-84	0.00	0.00	0.00	0.06	0.59	1.26
Change in rate	0.00	0.00	0.00	-0.08	0.23	-1.04
France						
Deaths 1974–78	1	17	51	123	358	819
Deaths 1980–84	0	2	5	10	34	101
Death rate 1974–78	0.00	0.04	0.14	0.39	1.10	3.66
Death rate 1980–84	0.00	0.00	0.01	0.03	0.11	0.36
Change in rate	0.00	-0.04	-0.13	-0.36	-0.99	-3.29
Greece						
Deaths 1974–78	0	0	5	11	39	79
Deaths 1980–84	0	2	2	4	6	26
Death rate 1974–78	0.00	0.00	0.08	0.17	0.70	1.72
Death rate 1980–84	0.00	0.05	0.05	0.11	0.15	0.96
Change in rate	0.00	0.05	-0.03	-0.06	-0.55	-0.76

Table 9.1.2(j) cont

	Age group (years)					
	5–14	15–24	25–34	35–44	45–54	55–64

Italy

Deaths 1974–78	6	33	123	345	947	1770
Deaths 1980–84	1	10	46	128	386	905
Death rate 1974–78	0.01	0.08	0.32	0.92	2.64	6.62
Death rate 1980–84	0.00	0.02	0.12	0.35	1.08	3.09
Change in rate	-0.01	-0.06	-0.20	-0.57	-1.56	-3.52

Ireland

Deaths 1974–78	0	0	2	2	10	19
Deaths 1980–84	0	0	1	2	13	23
Death rate 1974–78	0.00	0.00	0.10	0.12	0.64	1.30
Death rate 1980–84	0.00	0.00	0.04	0.11	0.87	1.60
Change in rate	0.00	0.00	-0.06	-0.01	0.23	0.30

Netherlands

Deaths 1974–78	0	1	8	15	68	179
Deaths 1980–84	0	1	6	11	53	149
Death rate 1974–78	0.00	0.01	0.07	0.19	0.91	2.88
Death rate 1980–84	0.00	0.01	0.05	0.12	0.70	2.22
Change in rate	0.00	0.00	-0.02	-0.07	-0.21	-0.66

UK: England and Wales

Deaths 1974–78	0	7	25	49	173	392
Deaths 1980–84	0	2	19	26	122	329
Death rate 1974–78	0.00	0.02	0.07	0.17	0.58	1.42
Death rate 1980–84	0.00	0.01	0.05	0.08	0.44	1.18
Change in rate	0.00	-0.01	-0.02	-0.09	-0.14	-0.23

UK: N. Ireland

Deaths 1974–78	0	0	0	4	3	16
Deaths 1980–84	0	0	0	3	1	16
Death rate 1974–78	0.00	0.00	0.00	0.49	0.37	2.19
Death rate 1980–84	0.00	0.00	0.00	0.34	0.13	2.24
Change in rate	0.00	0.00	0.00	-0.15	-0.24	0.04

UK: Scotland

Deaths 1974–78	0	0	1	7	14	44
Deaths 1980–84	0	0	0	0	0	4
Death rate 1974–78	0.00	0.00	0.03	0.24	0.46	1.58
Death rate 1980–84	0.00	0.00	0.00	0.00	0.00	0.14
Change in rate	0.00	0.00	-0.03	-0.24	-0.46	-1.43

Table 9.1.2(j) cont

	Age group (years)					
	5–14	15–24	25–34	35–44	45–54	55–64
Portugal						
Deaths 1974–78	—	—	—	—	—	—
Deaths 1980–84	0	0	2	13	29	79
Death rate 1974–78	—	—	—	—	—	—
Death rate 1980–84	0.00	0.00	0.03	0.23	0.50	1.57
Change in rate	—	—	—	—	—	—
Spain						
Deaths 1974–78	—	—	—	—	—	—
Deaths 1980–84	0	4	19	41	146	302
Death rate 1974–78	—	—	—	—	—	—
Death rate 1980–84	0.00	0.01	0.08	0.19	0.63	1.66
Change in rate	—	—	—	—	—	—
EC						
Deaths 1974–78	8	81	292	845	2394	5215
Deaths 1980–84	1	32	122	323	1060	2824
Death rate 1974–78	0.00	0.04	0.15	0.48	1.41	3.85
Death rate 1980–84	0.00	0.01	0.05	0.16	0.56	1.73
Change in rate	0.00	-0.03	-0.10	-0.32	-0.85	-2.11

Table 9.1.2(k). Hypertensive and cerebrovascular diseases (ICD8 400–404, 430–438; ICD9 401–405, 430–438)

	Age group (years)					
	5–14	15–24	25–34	35–44	45–54	55–64
Belgium						
Deaths 1974–78	43	132	212	635	2190	5638
Deaths 1980–84	36	105	237	482	1573	4330
Death rate 1974–78	0.57	1.71	3.14	10.62	34.54	119.78
Death rate 1980–84	0.55	1.34	3.18	8.02	26.04	79.17
Change in rate	-0.03	-0.37	0.05	-2.60	-8.50	-40.60
Luxembourg						
Deaths 1974–78	1	3	8	35	96	299
Deaths 1980–84	1	4	11	17	88	217
Death rate 1974–78	0.39	1.08	3.01	14.13	40.90	168.36
Death rate 1980–84	0.43	1.40	3.80	6.96	36.36	122.81
Change in rate	0.03	0.32	0.80	-7.17	-4.54	-45.55
Federal Republic of Germany						
Deaths 1974–78	158	459	1200	4303	11712	34652
Deaths 1980–84	115	465	1211	3952	11383	28593
Death rate 1974–78	0.33	1.03	2.90	9.52	31.21	116.41
Death rate 1980–84	0.31	0.91	2.81	9.04	28.77	89.21
Change in rate	-0.02	-0.11	-0.09	-0.47	-2.44	-27.20
Denmark						
Deaths 1974–78	9	30	102	291	812	2079
Deaths 1980–84	15	25	111	293	702	1996
Death rate 1974–78	0.23	0.80	2.57	9.85	28.49	75.85
Death rate 1980–84	0.42	0.64	2.91	8.10	25.67	73.73
Change in rate	0.19	-0.16	0.35	-1.74	-2.82	-2.12
France						
Deaths 1974–78	241	610	1194	3535	11819	25213
Deaths 1980–84	135	503	1293	2671	8453	20166
Death rate 1974–78	0.57	1.44	3.20	11.23	36.28	112.56
Death rate 1980–84	0.33	1.17	3.02	8.22	26.87	72.57
Change in rate	-0.23	-0.28	-0.19	-3.02	-9.41	-39.99
Greece						
Deaths 1974–78	59	119	214	512	1737	5743
Deaths 1980–84	32	84	115	315	1081	3162
Death rate 1974–78	0.80	1.75	3.55	8.12	31.01	125.07
Death rate 1980–84	0.70	1.96	2.91	8.65	27.02	117.24
Change in rate	-0.10	0.21	-0.64	0.52	-3.99	-7.83

Table 9.1.2(k) cont

	Age group (years)					
	5–14	15–24	25–34	35–44	45–54	55–64

Italy

Deaths 1974–78	252	580	1261	4219	15746	39796
Deaths 1980–84	245	549	1150	3630	12785	33927
Death rate 1974–78	0.55	1.43	3.27	11.24	43.82	148.77
Death rate 1980–84	0.56	1.25	2.93	9.79	35.61	115.96
Change in rate	0.01	-0.19	-0.34	-1.45	-8.21	-32.81

Ireland

Deaths 1974–78	24	75	96	238	860	2381
Deaths 1980–84	16	49	79	207	517	1682
Death rate 1974–78	0.73	2.75	4.71	14.64	55.14	163.00
Death rate 1980–84	0.46	1.63	3.32	11.56	34.47	117.13
Change in rate	-0.26	-1.12	-1.40	-3.08	-20.67	-45.87

Netherlands

Deaths 1974–78	49	153	300	681	1872	4926
Deaths 1980–84	29	126	289	610	1629	4270
Death rate 1974–78	0.41	1.31	2.76	8.46	25.16	79.26
Death rate 1980–84	0.27	1.02	2.46	6.41	21.48	63.59
Change in rate	-0.14	-0.30	-0.29	-2.04	-3.67	-15.67

UK: England and Wales

Deaths 1974–78	131	396	1076	3120	11432	33330
Deaths 1980–84	113	427	1053	2780	8906	28870
Death rate 1974–78	0.33	1.11	3.10	11.04	38.50	120.37
Death rate 1980–84	0.33	1.07	3.03	8.91	32.26	103.80
Change in rate	0.00	-0.04	-0.07	-2.13	-6.24	-16.56

UK: N. Ireland

Deaths 1974–78	9	21	42	105	415	1251
Deaths 1980–84	6	24	41	83	291	913
Death rate 1974–78	0.59	1.65	4.19	12.82	51.33	171.37
Death rate 1980–84	0.43	1.76	4.05	9.35	38.26	127.62
Change in rate	-0.16	0.11	-0.14	-3.47	-13.07	-43.75

UK: Scotland

Deaths 1974–78	19	79	209	511	1759	5254
Deaths 1980–84	13	64	166	434	1266	4013
Death rate 1974–78	0.43	1.95	6.09	17.33	57.43	188.41
Death rate 1980–84	0.35	1.46	4.62	13.97	43.56	143.56
Change in rate	-0.08	-0.49	-1.47	-3.36	-13.87	-44.85

Table 9.1.2(k) cont

	Age group (years)					
	5–14	15–24	25–34	35–44	45–54	55–64
Portugal						
Deaths 1974–78	—	—	—	—	—	—
Deaths 1980–84	72	137	278	777	3312	10402
Death rate 1974–78	—	—	—	—	—	—
Death rate 1980–84	0.85	1.64	4.09	13.54	57.36	206.86
Change in rate	—	—	—	—	—	—
Spain						
Deaths 1974–78	—	—	—	—	—	—
Deaths 1980–84	325	588	962	2022	6783	17923
Death rate 1974–78	—	—	—	—	—	—
Death rate 1980–84	0.98	1.89	3.85	9.46	29.24	98.42
Change in rate	—	—	—	—	—	—
EC						
Deaths 1974–78	995	2657	5914	18185	60450	160562
Deaths 1980–84	1153	3150	6996	18273	58769	160464
Death rate 1974–78	0.44	1.27	3.06	10.26	35.61	118.41
Death rate 1980–84	0.50	1.24	3.10	9.12	31.05	98.53
Change in rate	0.06	-0.03	0.03	-1.14	-4.56	-19.88

Table 9.1.2(l). All causes (all ICD8/ICD9 codes)

	Age group (years)					
	5–14	15–24	25–34	35–44	45–54	55–64
Belgium						
Deaths 1974–78	2532	7101	6900	12303	34906	67921
Deaths 1980–84	1816	6366	7666	11457	30059	66388
Death rate 1974–78	33.78	91.92	102.11	205.69	550.54	1442.98
Death rate 1980–84	27.63	81.42	102.96	190.64	497.63	1213.92
Change in rate	-6.15	-10.50	0.86	-15.05	-52.91	-229.06
Luxembourg						
Deaths 1974–78	71	307	305	631	1413	2870
Deaths 1980–84	66	276	344	566	1357	2487
Death rate 1974–78	28.04	110.83	114.62	254.74	602.05	1615.99
Death rate 1980–84	28.30	96.77	118.99	231.68	560.74	1407.47
Change in rate	0.26	-14.06	4.37	-23.06	-41.30	-208.52
Federal Republic of Germany						
Deaths 1974–78	16867	45829	47353	102146	208294	395269
Deaths 1980–84	9638	42337	41620	90294	199955	369626
Death rate 1974–78	35.07	102.56	114.55	225.91	555.07	1327.91
Death rate 1980–84	26.06	83.14	96.71	206.62	505.45	1153.22
Change in rate	-9.01	-19.42	-17.84	-19.29	-49.62	-174.69
Denmark						
Deaths 1974–78	1168	2651	3289	5726	15329	35129
Deaths 1980–84	802	2578	3855	6874	14558	35992
Death rate 1974–78	29.96	71.03	82.75	193.78	537.92	1281.57
Death rate 1980–84	22.27	65.89	101.21	190.11	532.36	1329.44
Change in rate	-7.68	-5.14	18.46	-3.67	-5.55	47.88
France						
Deaths 1974–78	13601	43793	42578	77368	189545	288441
Deaths 1980–84	10482	39820	47940	66241	167659	301588
Death rate 1974–78	32.06	103.59	114.28	245.83	581.76	1287.68
Death rate 1980–84	25.88	92.44	111.95	203.77	532.88	1085.29
Change in rate	-6.18	-11.15	-2.33	-42.06	-48.87	-202.39
Greece						
Deaths 1974–78	2417	4487	4764	8836	21238	45870
Deaths 1980–84	1213	2800	2934	4843	13647	26239
Death rate 1974–78	32.69	65.95	79.03	140.20	379.16	998.93
Death rate 1980–84	26.44	65.25	74.32	132.97	341.13	972.90
Change in rate	-6.25	-0.70	-4.7	-1.24	-38.03	-26.04

Table 9.1.2(l) cont

	Age group (years)					
	5–14	15–24	25–34	35–44	45–54	55–64

Italy

Deaths 1974–78	14722	27508	30690	67180	182831	340942
Deaths 1980–84	11846	29320	29674	58735	165447	330403
Death rate 1974–78	32.33	67.97	79.57	178.97	508.75	1274.51
Death rate 1980–84	27.08	66.61	75.51	158.46	460.77	1129.29
Change in rate	-5.25	-1.37	-4.07	-20.51	-47.98	-145.23

Ireland

Deaths 1974–78	1068	1902	1827	3180	9296	22991
Deaths 1980–84	922	2122	1907	3100	7964	21278
Death rate 1974–78	32.31	69.67	89.68	195.58	596.01	1573.97
Death rate 1980–84	26.76	70.62	80.04	173.09	530.93	1481.75
Change in rate	-5.55	0.95	-9.64	-22.50	-65.08	-92.22

Netherlands

Deaths 1974–78	3777	7686	7651	12424	33218	71847
Deaths 1980–84	2572	6626	7844	12889	30299	71197
Death rate 1974–78	31.26	65.95	70.29	154.26	446.38	1156.01
Death rate 1980–84	23.94	53.38	66.83	135.53	399.60	1060.24
Change in rate	-7.32	-12.57	-3.46	-18.72	-46.77	-95.77

UK: England and Wales

Deaths 1974–78	10467	22771	25298	49270	165321	398739
Deaths 1980–84	7704	22305	23903	45802	130763	372088
Death rate 1974–78	26.44	64.10	72.87	174.38	556.83	1439.97
Death rate 1980–84	22.47	56.12	68.78	146.76	473.73	1337.88
Change in rate	-3.97	-7.98	-4.09	-27.62	-83.10	-102.10

UK: N. Ireland

Deaths 1974–78	538	1341	1206	1852	5233	12230
Deaths 1980–84	370	1026	994	1638	4162	11244
Death rate 1974–78	35.31	105.09	120.42	226.13	647.25	1675.34
Death rate 1980–84	26.81	75.07	98.22	184.54	547.20	1571.71
Change in rate	-8.51	-30.02	-22.20	-41.59	-100.05	-103.63

UK: Scotland

Deaths 1974–78	1350	2907	3302	7186	21293	49240
Deaths 1980–84	995	2788	3149	6245	17995	46031
Death rate 1974–78	30.27	71.91	96.17	243.73	695.21	1765.76
Death rate 1980–84	26.60	63.58	87.64	201.06	619.21	1646.73
Change in rate	-3.68	-8.33	-8.53	-42.68	-76.00	-119.03

Table 9.1.2(l) cont

	Age group (years)					
	5–14	15–24	25–34	35–44	45–54	55–64
Portugal						
Deaths 1974–78	—	—	—	—	—	—
Deaths 1980–84	4165	8813	9075	13602	31218	58852
Death rate 1974–78	—	—	—	—	—	—
Death rate 1980–84	48.93	105.61	133.56	237.05	540.67	1170.37
Change in rate	—	—	—	—	—	—
Spain						
Deaths 1974–78	—	—	—	—	—	—
Deaths 1980–84	9886	20107	21825	35246	93792	179247
Death rate 1974–78	—	—	—	—	—	—
Death rate 1980–84	29.96	64.71	87.25	164.85	404.25	984.31
Change in rate	—	—	—	—	—	—
EC						
Deaths 1974–78	68578	168283	175163	348102	887917	1731489
Deaths 1980–84	62477	187284	202730	357532	908875	1892660
Death rate 1974–78	30.48	80.41	90.69	196.32	523.05	1276.94
Death rate 1980–84	27.01	73.54	89.73	178.40	480.19	1162.14
Change in rate	-3.48	-6.87	-0.97	-17.92	-42.86	-114.80

Table 9.1.3(a). Age-standardized death rates (per 100 000) for 1974–78 and 1980–84 by small area standardized to the EC standard, for tuberculosis, malignant neoplasm of the cervix uteri, malignant neoplasm of the cervix and body of the uterus, Hodgkin's disease, and chronic rheumatic heart disease

Notes on the use of this table

1. This table shows the mortality rates for small areas standardized to the EC standard for 1974–78 and 1980–84. The rates are in deaths per 100 000 population. The age-standardized death rates are calculated by multiplying the small-area SMR based on the EC standard for that time period by the EC crude death rate for that time period.

2. Key for the abbreviations used for columns of the table:
   TUB   — tuberculosis (ICD8 010–019; ICD9 101–018, 137), ages 5–64;
   CERV — malignant neoplasm of the cervix uteri (ICD8 180; ICD9 180), ages 15–64;
   UTER — malignant neoplasm of the cervix and body of the uterus (ICD8 180, 182; ICD9 179, 180, 182), ages 15–64;
   HODG — Hodgkin's disease (ICD8 201; ICD9 201), ages 5–64;
   CRHD — chronic rheumatic heart disease (ICD8 393–398; ICD9 393–398), ages 5–44.

3. The small area numbers are as in the key maps (pp. 241–5).

4. The indicators have been tested for indicating significant excess mortality relative to EC rates. The *p*-values achieved for one-tail tests are indicated as follows: *$p<0.05$; **$p<0.01$; ***$p<0.001$.

5. The mortality data for the earlier time period are for 1974–78, except for France (1973–77). The population data are for 1974–78, except for France (1975), Ireland (1976), and N. Ireland (1976).

6. The mortality data for the later time period are for 1980–84, except for Greece (1980–82). The population data are for 1980–84 except for France (1982), Ireland (1981), and Greece (1981). All data for Italy are for 1979–83.

Table 9.1.3(a)

Area	Age-standardized death rates (per 100 000)									
	TUB		CERV		UTER		HODG		CRHD	
	1974–78	1980–84	1974–78	1980–84	1974–78	1980–84	1974–78	1980–84	1974–78	1980–84
BELGIUM	1.85	0.81	3.67	3.17	4.68	3.47	1.28	1.06*	0.31	0.04
1 Antwerpen	0.73	0.29	2.77	3.51	3.89	3.10	1.46	1.42***	0.11	0.02
2 Brabant	2.31*	1.22	3.96	2.51	4.71	3.61	1.20	0.77	0.60	0.05
3 West-Vlaanderen	0.89	0.52	4.04	3.22	5.10	3.07	1.00	1.01	0.06	0.03
4 Oost-Vlaanderen	0.78	0.33	3.25	3.56	3.58	3.31	1.47	1.51***	0.13	0.03
5 Hainaut	3.55***	1.33*	4.39	4.52*	6.14	3.58	1.29	0.96	0.32	0.09
6 Liège	2.59**	0.93	4.50	2.12	5.16	4.04	1.22	0.90	0.36	0.07
7 Limburg	0.93	0.60	2.00	3.10	3.64	3.51	1.25	1.04	0.19	0.00
8 Luxembourg (province)	2.39	0.34	3.49	2.51	4.20	3.19	1.05	1.03	1.21	0.00
9 Namur	3.07**	1.31	3.69	2.94	5.89	3.91	1.56	0.79	0.48	0.00
LUXEMBOURG										
10 Luxembourg	1.21	0.34	5.40	3.13	6.13	4.31	0.73	0.67	0.63	0.46
FEDERAL REPUBLIC OF GERMANY	2.16***	1.12*	6.97***	4.59***	6.81***	4.22	1.18	1.03***	0.82	0.16
11 Schleswig–Holstein	1.47	0.86	8.37***	5.10***	7.74***	4.58	1.03	1.01	0.58	0.04
12 Hamburg	1.36	0.93	7.23***	5.01***	6.37	4.72	0.98	0.60	0.32	0.19
13 Neidersachsen	1.87	0.95	7.49***	4.98***	7.33***	4.59	1.20	1.47***	0.71	0.10
14 Bremen	1.72	0.91	7.67***	5.43**	6.97	5.32	1.15	0.67	0.51	0.09
15 Nordrhein–Westfalen	1.89	1.03	7.06***	4.77***	6.66**	4.17	1.23	0.90	0.88	0.18
16 Hessen	1.63	1.00	6.49***	3.69	6.44	3.59	1.20	1.04	0.96	0.31
17 Rheinland–Pfalz	2.09	0.94	5.96***	4.45**	6.78	4.18	1.36	1.37***	1.22*	0.25
18 Baden Wurttemberg	2.23**	1.20*	6.01***	3.78	5.83	3.57	1.15	0.85	0.85	0.23
19 Bayern	3.01***	1.43***	6.16***	4.29***	6.50	4.16	1.11	1.10***	0.72	0.04
20 Saarland	2.82***	1.30	6.52***	4.27	7.14	3.71	1.09	1.00	1.35*	0.41
21 Berlin(West)	3.75***	1.53***	13.71***	8.92***	13.02***	7.87***	1.14	1.00	0.62	0.13

Table 9.1.3(a) cont

Area		Age-standardized death rates (per 100 000)									
		TUB		CERV		UTER		HODG		CRHD	
		1974–78	1980–84	1974–78	1980–84	1974–78	1980–84	1974–78	1980–84	1974–78	1980–84
DENMARK		0.81	0.48	12.05***	9.14***	9.96***	6.91***	0.94	0.81	0.42	0.16
22	Kobenhavn and Frederiksberg (M)	2.12	1.07	13.57***	11.98***	13.50***	9.74***	0.99	0.89	0.81	0.20
23	Kobenhavns County	0.46	0.48	9.56***	6.73***	7.05	4.50	1.01	1.09	0.25	0.15
24	Frederiksborg County	0.72	0.41	11.73***	5.69*	8.76*	4.44	0.97	0.75	0.39	0.17
25	Roskilde County	0.46	0.27	11.15***	8.81***	7.15	6.57*	1.47	1.35	0.16	0.13
26	Vestsjaellands County	0.37	0.45	17.20***	8.59***	15.88***	6.73*	1.39	1.36	0.41	0.24
27	Storstroms County	0.63	0.28	8.95***	7.85***	8.35	7.41**	1.72	0.67	0.30	0.27
28	Bornholms County	0.99	0.52	15.53***	10.58**	10.45	6.75	1.05	0.54	0.82	0.00
29	Fyns County	0.49	0.50	12.34***	10.16***	9.66***	8.01***	0.61	0.56	0.33	0.08
30	Sonderjyllands County	0.84	0.21	12.95***	9.06***	12.26***	7.01*	0.63	0.61	0.29	0.14
31	Ribe County	0.50	0.74	11.32***	10.23***	13.46***	7.02*	0.74	0.60	0.86	0.63
32	Vejle County	0.32	0.39	13.52***	10.90***	9.79**	7.34**	0.63	0.78	0.23	0.00
33	Ringkobing County	0.73	0.10	8.83***	7.41***	4.71	5.11	1.01	0.69	0.28	0.00
34	Arhus County	0.61	0.37	11.65***	9.26***	9.50***	7.66***	0.67	0.62	0.38	0.17
35	Viborg County	0.44	0.33	11.43***	11.43***	9.59*	6.23	1.01	0.56	1.17	0.00
36	Nordjyllands County	0.93	0.42	12.93***	9.38***	10.49***	8.40***	0.89	0.73	0.31	0.22
FRANCE		2.68***	1.29***	3.30	2.73	6.21	4.02	1.04	0.69	0.69	0.18
37	Ain	1.87	0.69	2.66	2.21	6.70	2.61	0.97	0.43	0.56	0.16
38	Aisne	3.36***	1.57*	5.56	2.45	8.80**	4.19	1.02	0.53	0.56	0.15
39	Allier	2.14	0.83	3.17	2.07	7.04	5.52	1.30	0.82	0.62	0.00
40	Alpes-de-Haute-Provence	1.29	1.00	2.30	2.53	5.56	1.92	0.68	0.42	0.66	0.30
41	Hautes-Alpes	2.26	1.84	4.69	0.58	8.06	0.75	1.55	0.23	1.10	0.00
42	Alpes-Maritimes	1.39	1.18	1.32	2.26	3.53	3.79	0.30	0.82	0.51	0.17
43	Ardèche	3.15**	1.54	1.78	2.53	3.93	4.12	0.61	0.94	0.60	0.14
44	Ardennes	3.42***	1.69*	5.11	3.80	8.36*	6.07	1.14	0.61	0.82	0.13
45	Ariège	1.18	1.15	4.00	3.86	5.45	3.45	2.05	0.73	0.59	0.00
46	Aube	3.61***	1.73*	3.00	4.97	7.29	6.28*	1.04	0.45	0.39	0.00
47	Aude	1.62	0.73	3.70	1.43	5.87	1.92	1.23	0.98	0.46	0.00
48	Aveyron	1.88	0.93	1.78	1.73	3.80	2.23	0.92	0.73	0.84	0.15
49	Bouches-du-Rhne	2.20	1.30*	2.97	2.32	4.55	3.61	0.96	0.86	1.11	0.24
50	Calvados	2.81**	1.53*	5.84	3.49	8.17*	4.41	0.86	0.92	0.58	0.13
51	Cantal	2.24	1.46	3.57	3.02	6.72	3.40	1.10	0.93	0.24	0.25
52	Charente	2.74*	0.87	4.13	4.40	7.50	6.78**	0.86	0.82	0.45	0.12
53	Charente-Maritime	1.96	0.89	4.41	2.59	8.93**	4.56	1.54	0.54	0.86	0.15
54	Cher	3.46***	1.40	4.71	3.14	9.88**	4.17	1.42	0.56	0.36	0.24
55	Corrèze	2.73	1.12	1.01	1.42	3.6	4.43	0.84	0.61	0.49	0.00
56	Corse	2.13	1.18	1.84	1.27	2.63	3.26	0.41	0.51	0.15	0.14
57	Côte-d'Or	1.90	0.63	4.46	4.91	4.99	4.53	1.16	0.82	0.86	0.23
58	Côtes-du-Nord	4.86***	1.14	2.30	2.31	6.70	4.29	1.04	0.42	0.75	0.23
59	Creuse	2.53	0.80	2.52	0.85	6.97	5.86	0.89	1.65*	0.59	0.34
60	Dordogne	1.87	1.42	2.59	2.73	6.59	5.30	0.88	0.46	0.65	0.00
61	Doubs	1.75	0.99	2.59	3.17	6.67	3.81	1.12	0.33	0.72	0.37
62	Drôme	1.89	0.98	3.19	4.04	5.99	4.28	1.30	0.72	0.70	0.28
63	Eure	3.22***	1.13	4.10	3.83	7.93	5.55	1.09	0.56	0.51	0.15
64	Eure-et-Loir	2.68	0.90	3.11	3.00	7.89	6.01	1.44	0.58	0.55	0.00
65	Finistère	3.96***	1.42*	2.35	1.97	5.61	3.38	0.90	0.49	0.62	0.14
66	Gard	2.27	1.16	2.53	1.34	4.28	2.39	0.61	0.74	0.83	0.21
67	Haute-Garonne	1.27	0.99	1.61	2.41	4.33	5.28	1.33	0.48	0.90	0.09
68	Gers	0.95	0.39	4.38	2.38	7.24	5.24	1.17	0.57	0.22	0.00
69	Gironde	1.96	1.16	3.98	2.39	7.34*	4.24	1.21	0.66	0.35	0.13
70	Hérault	1.78	0.79	1.57	1.68	5.47	3.12	1.62	0.70	0.88	0.26
71	Ille-et-Vilaine	3.47***	1.49*	3.06	2.86	5.63	3.14	0.86	0.45	0.42	0.05
72	Indre	2.73	0.80	3.20	2.28	7.90	2.88	1.18	0.85	0.32	0.17
73	Indre-et-Loire	2.53	0.79	2.94	3.11	7.37	3.44	1.23	0.87	0.31	0.15
74	Isère	1.92	1.31	3.65	3.67	4.78	3.30	0.99	0.57	0.51	0.11
75	Jura	1.76	0.72	4.04	2.84	5.04	3.26	0.44	1.06	0.62	0.62
76	Landes	2.10	0.56	2.72	2.01	5.08	1.52	1.27	0.42	0.26	0.13
77	Loir-et-Cher	1.52	0.95	1.49	4.38	5.36	5.76	1.34	0.71	0.00	0.13
78	Loire	2.55*	1.32	3.15	2.59	5.25	3.51	1.07	0.55	0.72	0.20
79	Haute-Loire	2.47	0.82	3.21	0.60	3.74	2.29	1.42	1.36	0.57	0.39

Table 9.1.3(a) cont

Area | Age-standardized death rates (per 100 000)

		TUB		CERV		UTER		HODG		CRHD	
		1974–78	1980–84	1974–78	1980–84	1974–78	1980–84	1974–78	1980–84	1974–78	1980–84
80	Loire-Atlantique	2.94***	1.83***	2.11	2.21	4.47	3.17	0.85	0.55	0.35	0.04
81	Loiret	1.87	0.50	3.08	3.20	7.76	3.84	0.75	0.72	0.44	0.13
82	Lot	2.35	0.58	5.34	2.99	8.81	5.57	1.19	0.16	0.80	0.00
83	Lot-et-Garonne	2.24	0.84	1.71	2.31	4.54	3.96	1.13	0.82	0.26	0.13
84	Lozère	3.61*	1.96	0.89	1.73	7.74	3.48	1.04	0.69	2.64*	0.00
85	Maine-et-Loire	2.93**	1.42	2.57	2.14	4.29	3.27	1.09	1.00	0.53	0.06
86	Manche	2.94**	0.85	3.24	2.01	7.73	3.20	1.17	0.72	0.17	0.52
87	Marne	2.78*	1.03	3.89	2.93	6.79	3.37	1.67*	0.77	0.80	0.26
88	Haute-Marne	3.14*	1.40	5.19	1.61	9.07*	4.31	0.76	1.50	1.07	0.18
89	Mayenne	2.25	1.24	1.31	1.91	3.61	2.34	1.12	0.77	0.14	0.15
90	Meurthe-et-Moselle	2.65*	1.92***	4.11	4.39	5.90	4.34	1.12	0.56	0.68	0.10
91	Meuse	4.07***	0.52	2.84	2.30	5.48	3.60	1.06	0.91	0.94	0.39
92	Morbihan	3.76***	2.67***	1.85	1.69	5.68	2.13	0.69	0.65	0.53	0.27
93	Moselle	3.50***	1.40*	5.68	3.56	8.29**	4.31	1.17	0.69	0.81	0.25
94	Nivre	1.96	1.62	2.97	2.03	7.39	4.74	0.54	0.54	0.32	0.00
95	Nord	4.85***	2.23***	4.30	3.47	6.32	4.68	1.29	0.87	0.90	0.21
96	Oise	3.21***	1.22	3.84	3.90	7.83*	4.87	0.81	0.55	0.46	0.21
97	Orne	2.39	0.85	4.70	2.58	8.54*	4.28	0.73	1.04	0.38	0.00
98	Pas-de-Calais	5.46***	2.16***	4.33	3.38	7.12	4.41	0.95	0.94	0.99	0.31
99	Puy-de-Dôme	2.47	1.26	2.34	1.57	6.77	2.89	1.54	1.00	0.56	0.24
100	Pyrénées-Atlantiques	1.78	1.31	1.92	1.40	4.38	3.47	0.92	0.54	0.48	0.07
101	Hautes-Pyrénées	2.62	0.71	2.17	2.02	7.04	3.83	0.77	0.75	0.64	0.00
102	Pyrénées-Orientales	2.23	0.88	1.32	1.50	4.54	4.26	1.07	0.37	0.78	0.12
103	Bas-Rhin	2.51*	1.65***	4.82	4.62	6.08	5.03	1.25	0.72	0.90	0.23
104	Haut-Rhin	2.58*	1.21	4.92	2.97	6.99	4.58	0.87	0.70	0.91	0.27
105	Rhône	2.53**	0.92	4.25	2.82	4.76	3.02	0.84	0.55	0.93	0.24
106	Haute-Saône	2.25	1.37	3.92	3.14	7.31	1.08	1.11	0.68	1.02	0.33
107	Saône-et-Loire	2.35	0.87	3.59	3.06	4.34	3.69	0.79	0.81	0.47	0.07
108	Sarthe	2.48	0.63	1.59	2.86	6.11	3.27	1.10	0.62	0.46	0.08
109	Savoie	3.05**	1.58*	4.11	3.53	4.77	3.75	0.92	0.54	1.12	0.33
110	Haute-Savoie	2.88**	1.36	4.21	3.99	5.47	3.80	0.97	0.81	0.87	0.26
111	Paris	3.02***	1.70***	2.67	2.98	7.15*	5.00*	0.99	0.64	1.57***	0.20
112	Seine-Maritime	3.66***	2.43***	4.78	4.23	7.42*	5.90**	0.79	1.15	0.49	0.27
113	Seine-et-Marne	2.32	1.24	2.97	2.22	6.55	4.43	1.09	0.56	0.39	0.18
114	Yvelines	1.63	0.87	4.22	2.67	5.44	4.02	1.00	0.60	0.56	0.08
115	Deux-Sèvres	1.83	0.67	2.70	0.57	3.55	2.33	1.20	0.23	0.57	0.12
116	Somme	2.01	1.55*	4.63	2.36	10.32***	4.76	0.51	1.21	0.64	0.21
117	Tarn	1.73	0.34	2.60	1.55	5.67	2.82	0.68	0.58	0.11	0.12
118	Tarn-et-Garonne	1.32	0.75	3.09	3.46	3.62	4.01	0.98	0.53	0.43	0.00
119	Var	2.57*	1.28	2.72	2.60	6.24	4.21	1.54	0.41	0.69	0.26
120	Vaucluse	2.60	0.64	2.34	1.73	7.13	2.96	1.04	0.64	0.54	0.33
121	Vendée	1.70	0.81	1.89	1.90	3.81	3.42	0.61	0.65	0.43	0.08
122	Vienne	1.87	1.06	4.72	2.48	7.71	4.85	0.82	0.77	0.22	0.00
123	Haute-Vienne	1.99	0.81	1.78	2.20	4.38	4.29	1.08	0.49	0.33	0.00
124	Vosges	2.63	1.06	5.11	2.12	7.58	4.17	0.88	0.59	1.32	0.10
125	Yonne	2.78*	0.90	4.94	3.75	8.20	4.87	0.64	0.84	0.40	0.13
126	Territoire-de-Belfort	2.39	0.80	3.39	3.49	6.18	6.24	1.01	0.58	1.58	0.27
127	Essonne	2.04	1.00	3.65	2.69	7.10	2.75	0.93	0.51	0.49	0.25
128	Hauts-de-Seine	2.20	1.27	2.59	2.35	5.37	3.72	1.06	0.72	0.58	0.14
129	Seine-Saint-Denis	3.04***	1.47**	2.89	2.35	6.55	4.30	1.24	0.61	0.68	0.10
130	Val-de-Marne	2.17	1.03	3.25	2.81	7.10	4.36	1.30	0.56	0.50	0.14
131	Val-d'Oise	2.46	1.30	2.59	2.05	6.21	4.12	1.01	0.79	0.70	0.24
GREECE		2.86***	1.60***	1.43	1.74	4.75	3.66	1.47***	0.94	1.21**	0.31
132	Greater Athens	2.44**	1.66***	2.59	2.53	5.27	3.89	1.75***	0.92	1.14	0.13
133	Rest of Central Greece and Eubea	2.38	1.32	0.75	1.35	3.47	2.42	1.31	1.08	0.89	0.23
134	Peloponnisos	2.66**	1.36	1.52	1.36	5.42	3.31	1.43	0.74	0.88	0.26
135	Ionian Islands	2.04	0.63	0.43	1.55	4.39	2.48	2.01*	0.71	0.21	0.38
136	Epirus	3.27**	1.43	0.39	0.94	4.69	1.38	1.15	0.94	1.35	0.00
137	Thessaly	1.76	1.79**	0.46	1.01	4.38	4.42	1.26	0.80	1.21	0.08
138	Macedonia	3.83***	1.69***	1.04	1.40	4.79	3.69	1.49*	0.88	1.37**	0.49

Table 9.1.3(a) cont

Area		TUB 1974–78	TUB 1980–84	CERV 1974–78	CERV 1980–84	UTER 1974–78	UTER 1980–84	HODG 1974–78	HODG 1980–84	CRHD 1974–78	CRHD 1980–84
		\multicolumn{11}{l}{Age-standardized death rates (per 100 000)}									
139	Thrace	8.18***	4.08***	0.40	0.95	3.02	2.30	0.93	1.65*	1.97**	0.85*
140	Aegean Islands	2.73*	1.69*	0.29	1.75	5.13	5.89	0.85	1.14	0.98	0.62
141	Crete	1.45	0.60	1.43	1.69	4.62	5.50	1.30	1.07	2.25***	0.90**
ITALY		2.56***	1.37***	1.36	1.22	6.39*	4.37	1.68***	1.25***	1.96***	0.93***
142	Torino	3.28***	1.59***	1.94	2.05	5.86	4.40	2.05***	1.33***	2.04***	0.83***
143	Vercelli	2.73*	1.07	1.62	2.32	7.27	4.69	1.52	1.82***	1.18	0.98***
144	Novara	4.37***	1.69**	1.60	1.13	7.78*	4.66	2.04***	1.59**	1.82**	0.74**
145	Cuneo	3.94***	1.73**	2.11	2.10	8.62**	4.53	1.78*	1.20	1.94***	0.83***
146	Asti	2.92*	1.15	2.05	1.04	6.98	4.11	1.54	1.03	1.67	1.22***
147	Alessandria	1.74	1.22	1.46	1.15	7.56	4.10	2.27***	1.14	1.33	0.86**
148	Aosta	8.54***	2.87***	4.70	0.50	10.80**	5.27	1.23	1.05	1.67	0.57
149	Imperia	2.30	1.76*	2.13	3.27	5.45	7.69**	2.06*	2.13***	1.33	0.79*
150	Savona	2.56	1.35	0.86	1.38	4.71	2.96	1.81*	1.34	0.87	0.47
151	Genova	2.69***	1.47**	2.18	1.45	6.53	3.44	2.43***	1.64***	1.60**	0.60*
152	La Spezia	2.29	0.87	3.60	1.48	7.04	4.60	1.69	1.55*	0.29	0.60
153	Varese	2.35	1.02	0.95	0.98	5.12	2.51	2.23***	1.56***	1.50*	0.85***
154	Como/Sondrio	3.30***	1.63***	0.80	1.20	5.24	3.43	1.40	1.10	1.72***	0.69**
155	Milano	2.29*	1.15	1.31	0.97	5.32	3.34	1.75***	1.35***	1.52***	0.74***
156	Bergamo	3.53***	2.62***	1.36	0.56	6.50	4.51	2.43***	1.51***	1.44*	0.83***
157	Brescia	6.43***	2.86***	1.19	1.35	5.52	2.81	1.77**	1.55***	1.87***	0.79***
158	Pavia	2.60*	1.37	1.65	1.15	7.19	5.06	2.14***	2.18***	1.34	0.41
159	Cremona	3.18**	1.84**	1.18	1.99	5.35	3.56	2.19***	1.00	1.79*	0.82**
160	Mantova	2.53	1.20	1.19	0.58	6.80	3.38	2.56***	1.72***	0.72	0.28
161	Bolzano	5.18***	2.15***	3.16	1.50	6.07	3.60	1.34	0.90	1.44	0.39
162	Trento	4.29***	2.94***	1.72	2.32	5.09	4.06	1.61	0.90	1.84**	1.09***
163	Verona	2.47*	1.29	1.20	1.22	4.15	3.38	2.00***	1.21	1.40	0.35
164	Vicenza	2.65*	1.35	1.17	1.44	3.21	2.93	2.51***	1.15	0.94	0.55
165	Belluno	7.25***	3.28***	2.82	1.28	7.23	4.77	2.16**	1.21	1.73*	0.47
166	Treviso	4.37***	1.32	1.74	1.63	4.39	3.29	1.65*	1.51**	1.27	0.47
167	Venezia	3.22***	1.29	1.20	2.18	5.83	3.40	1.80**	1.58***	1.18	0.31
168	Padova	2.15	1.57**	1.76	1.05	3.72	2.65	2.23***	1.60***	1.29	0.50
169	Rovigo	2.02	1.01	1.38	2.01	5.64	2.70	1.53	1.15	2.08**	0.43
170	Udine/Gorizia	3.72***	1.85***	2.34	2.55	6.51	3.96	1.48	0.96	0.96	0.49
171	Trieste	5.18***	2.04***	3.76	1.55	10.66***	4.11	0.99	1.64**	1.30	0.86**
172	Pordenone	2.92*	1.09	1.61	2.20	6.36	3.15	2.58***	0.91	1.03	0.73*
173	Piacenza	2.07	1.00	0.56	1.33	5.79	3.04	1.78*	1.26	0.85	0.89**
174	Parma	2.34	1.40	1.18	0.92	5.08	3.96	2.41***	1.30	0.60	0.35
175	Reggio Emilia	2.02	0.70	1.35	1.06	7.22	3.11	1.94***	2.12***	0.50	0.25
176	Modena	1.84	0.94	0.87	0.93	5.72	3.33	1.64*	1.58***	1.30	0.45
177	Bologna	1.31	1.12	1.93	1.09	6.02	3.32	1.56*	1.05	1.29	0.65**
178	Ferrara	2.05	0.84	1.24	1.36	4.14	2.84	1.66	0.97	1.13	0.28
179	Ravenna	1.23	0.43	1.25	0.76	4.95	4.31	1.24	0.66	1.01	0.29
180	Forli	1.55	0.93	1.11	1.24	6.34	2.92	1.46	1.21	1.46*	0.22
181	Pesaro	1.46	0.55	1.25	0.35	3.83	2.70	1.24	0.58	1.27	0.43
182	Ancona	2.28	0.88	1.04	1.51	3.71	3.03	2.04**	0.83	1.11	0.41
183	Macerata	1.43	1.14	0.38	0.37	4.57	3.84	1.13	1.06	1.18	0.37
184	Ascoli Piceno	1.32	1.35	0.00	0.80	3.46	4.13	1.91*	1.15	0.77	0.50
185	Massa-Carrara	2.75	2.43***	1.93	1.62	7.24	5.97	1.05	1.42	1.19	1.06**
186	Lucca	2.76*	1.89***	0.58	1.00	4.90	3.86	2.30***	1.20	0.54	0.18
187	Pistoia	2.05	1.38	0.87	0.84	4.95	3.27	1.80	1.37	1.03	1.04***
188	Firenze	2.15	0.84	1.12	0.99	4.66	3.60	1.38	1.36**	1.23	0.53*
189	Livorno	2.04	0.83	2.09	0.62	7.09	2.86	1.90*	0.96	0.69	0.40
190	Pisa	2.08	0.52	1.17	1.70	7.10	3.58	1.90**	1.42*	1.15	0.45
191	Arezzo	2.59	1.40	1.26	1.58	5.82	4.53	1.27	0.91	0.89	0.91**
192	Siena	1.74	1.21	1.41	0.61	5.20	4.82	1.93*	1.09	1.22	0.57
193	Grosseto	2.02	0.96	1.48	1.67	9.35*	3.23	1.34	0.53	1.53	0.79*
194	Perugia	1.41	0.94	0.68	0.56	5.92	2.26	1.18	1.86***	1.31	0.91***
195	Terni	1.20	0.74	0.71	2.30	7.55	4.54	1.70	1.02	1.19	1.70***
196	Viterbo/Rieti	1.86	1.31	0.98	0.68	3.84	4.39	1.81*	1.47*	1.82**	0.98***
197	Roma	2.22	1.37***	1.63	1.67	6.06	4.68	1.66***	1.31***	1.93***	0.84***
198	Latina	1.75	1.26	0.17	1.22	6.92	6.77**	1.69	1.37*	2.08***	1.47***

Table 9.1.3(a) cont

Area

Age-standardized death rates (per 100 000)

		TUB		CERV		UTER		HODG		CRHD	
		1974–78	1980–84	1974–78	1980–84	1974–78	1980–84	1974–78	1980–84	1974–78	1980–84
199	Frosinone	2.24	1.09	0.71	1.21	4.92	5.41	1.29	1.10	2.29***	1.52***
200	Caserta	2.27	0.80	0.99	0.27	7.12	4.61	1.29	0.83	4.50***	2.10***
201	Benevento	2.12	1.62*	0.21	0.83	6.01	4.27	2.12**	1.16	2.30***	1.23***
202	Napoli	3.18***	1.76***	0.99	0.98	9.43***	6.78***	1.58**	1.24**	3.71***	1.68***
203	Avellino	1.82	0.70	0.59	0.29	4.11	4.25	1.25	0.78	3.35***	1.41***
204	Salerno	2.05	1.61***	1.03	0.58	8.66***	4.54	1.70**	1.21	3.04***	2.05***
205	L'Aquila	2.92*	2.18***	1.52	1.89	6.35	5.24	0.73	0.67	2.23***	1.58***
206	Teramo	1.76	1.83**	0.71	0.23	6.09	5.03	1.61	1.12	1.56	0.54
207	Pescara	2.19	1.10	1.97	1.02	6.95	4.25	1.50	0.78	1.81*	1.36***
208	Chieti	2.31	1.39	0.48	0.93	7.69	3.59	1.34	1.20	2.04**	1.00***
209	Isernia/Campobasso	2.78*	1.47	1.46	1.08	6.96	3.03	1.60	1.31	3.33***	2.12***
210	Foggia	2.43	1.63**	1.61	1.52	7.86*	5.09	1.59	0.93	2.52***	1.17***
211	Bari	2.92***	1.59***	2.07	1.46	8.09**	6.22***	1.16	0.95	3.69***	1.61***
212	Taranto	2.10	1.05	1.19	0.59	9.4***	5.24	1.56	1.12	3.05***	1.16***
213	Brindisi	3.45***	1.46	1.75	1.15	7.6	7.37***	1.57	1.35	3.12***	2.11***
214	Lecce	2.64*	1.59**	0.63	1.25	7.5	4.62	1.42	1.35*	2.09***	1.19***
215	Potenza/Matera	1.59	1.47*	1.12	1.17	4.9	4.60	1.34	0.91	2.97***	1.31***
216	Cosenza	1.60	1.12	0.88	1.18	6.1	6.61***	1.01	0.65	2.80***	1.42***
217	Catanzaro	2.56*	1.33	1.01	0.85	5.4	4.54	1.40	1.19	3.53***	2.07***
218	Reggio Calabria	2.39	1.36	1.03	1.14	7.2	4.49	1.46	1.26	3.96***	1.08***
219	Trapani	1.97	1.12	0.93	1.20	6.7	9.79***	1.49	1.25	2.07***	1.13***
220	Palermo	1.46	0.73	0.92	0.81	8.5***	6.70***	1.49	1.29*	2.18***	1.01***
221	Messina	1.65	0.70	1.35	0.44	9.7***	6.34**	1.21	1.10	2.62***	1.13***
222	Agrigento	1.32	0.81	1.01	0.69	9.5***	5.82*	1.35	1.36*	2.90***	1.60***
223	Caltanisetta	0.67	1.15	0.95	0.23	6.0	5.53	1.31	0.84	3.16***	1.05***
224	Enna	1.82	1.22	0.00	0.97	5.3	6.87*	0.78	1.22	4.51***	1.58***
225	Catania	1.56	0.89	1.81	1.10	10.6***	7.12***	1.70**	1.26*	3.32***	1.11***
226	Ragusa	1.51	1.30	0.94	1.57	10.4***	8.21***	1.05	1.13	1.21	1.74***
227	Siracusa	1.83	0.96	1.25	0.50	10.2***	5.76	1.63	0.93	2.82***	1.08***
228	Sassari	2.70*	2.15***	1.20	0.63	3.8	1.93	1.54	1.30	1.86**	0.73*
229	Nuoro	2.46	1.36	0.00	0.25	1.5	1.70	1.92*	1.39	2.40***	0.94**
230	Cagliari/Oristano	3.38***	1.65**	1.15	1.19	5.5	3.61	1.28	0.73	1.46*	0.80***
IRELAND		3.37***	2.12***	3.95	3.83	4.04	3.19	1.19	1.27***	1.33**	0.28
231	Eastern	2.87***	1.79***	3.99	3.08	3.90	2.49	1.23	0.95	1.22	0.25
232	Midland	2.67	2.24**	7.44*	4.80	7.72	3.47	1.05	1.61*	1.10	0.21
233	Mid-Western	4.21***	3.71***	3.46	3.11	4.71	3.84	0.97	0.96	1.55	0.53
234	North Eastern	1.93	1.41	5.25	4.50	2.20	4.20	0.95	1.23	1.52	0.14
235	North Western	2.54	0.86	4.08	3.43	5.10	4.02	1.55	2.16***	1.10	0.00
236	South Eastern	2.94*	2.33***	3.07	5.12	4.17	3.18	1.29	1.90***	1.86*	0.22
237	Southern	4.82***	2.09***	3.57	5.17*	3.64	3.50	1.18	1.50**	0.98	0.39
238	Western	4.43***	2.86***	2.74	2.77	3.06	3.30	1.20	0.95	1.60	0.38
NETHERLANDS		0.48	0.36	5.61***	3.62	4.85	2.94	1.06	0.76	0.57	0.17
239	Groningen	0.45	0.30	7.50***	3.14	5.76	1.48	0.91	0.83	0.47	0.06
240	Friesland	0.30	0.29	5.04	4.03	5.02	3.45	0.82	0.68	0.40	0.18
241	Drenthe	0.93	0.56	5.35	3.67	3.91	3.87	1.22	0.48	0.44	0.32
242	Overijssel	0.42	0.62	5.31	2.84	3.90	2.74	1.20	0.96	0.69	0.27
243	Gelderland	0.71	0.25	4.43	3.28	3.85	2.68	1.11	0.77	0.62	0.22
244	Utrecht	0.35	0.55	5.60	3.08	4.94	2.83	1.28	0.69	0.48	0.11
245	Noord Holland	0.41	0.27	6.57***	4.12	5.58	2.84	1.08	0.87	0.50	0.14
246	Zuid Holland	0.45	0.28	6.27***	3.94	5.57	3.25	1.09	0.77	0.49	0.15
247	Zeeland	0.63	0.23	5.49	5.41*	6.44	3.48	1.17	0.88	0.11	0.20
248	Noord Brabant	0.37	0.32	4.93	3.32	4.10	2.95	0.94	0.59	0.65	0.20
249	Limburg	0.56	0.62	4.14	3.27	3.98	2.92	0.81	0.72	0.91	0.15
UK: ENGLAND AND WALES		1.11	0.70	7.42***	6.57***	6.08	5.37***	1.13	0.84	0.92	0.28
250	Cleveland	1.85	0.92	12.03***	8.49***	8.98**	6.35**	1.33	1.46**	1.26	0.44
251	Cumbria	0.53	0.34	6.56*	7.43***	6.24	4.28	0.97	1.13	1.10	0.15
252	Durham	1.53	1.10	9.69***	7.64***	7.84*	5.84*	1.24	0.81	1.08	0.29
253	Northumberland	0.62	0.72	7.25**	7.17***	6.01	4.31	1.82*	0.99	1.01	0.36
254	Gateshead	1.35	1.09	6.87*	6.8**	5.42	4.24	0.22	0.58	2.00*	0.00

Table 9.1.3(a) cont

Area — Age-standardized death rates (per 100 000)

		TUB		CERV		UTER		HODG		CRHD	
		1974–78	1980–84	1974–78	1980–84	1974–78	1980–84	1974–78	1980–84	1974–78	1980–84
255	Newcastle upon Tyne	1.48	1.03	9.22***	7.6***	6.90	4.83	0.91	0.80	1.47	0.00
256	Northern Tyneside	0.87	0.68	11.50***	9.3***	8.49	6.40	0.95	0.86	0.37	0.00
257	Southern Tyneside	2.69	0.83	9.22***	8.04***	4.27	4.70	1.15	0.75	0.90	0.24
258	Sunderland	1.33	1.24	7.83**	7.40***	6.22	5.82	1.19	0.67	2.13**	0.49
259	Bradford	1.60	1.56*	11.65***	8.65***	7.84	5.09	0.94	0.84	1.16	0.49
260	Calderdale	1.57	1.67	11.92***	9.55***	7.86	7.91**	1.43	1.33	1.44	0.57
261	Humberside	0.93	0.69	11.01***	8.34***	8.53**	5.88**	1.38	1.12	0.78	0.21
262	Kirklees	1.67	0.61	10.02***	8.89***	7.12	6.52*	0.94	1.09	1.61*	0.28
263	Leeds	1.42	0.65	9.35***	8.51***	6.53	7.39***	0.87	1.06	1.07	0.46
264	North Yorkshire	0.47	0.43	6.68**	5.35**	5.09	5.19	1.28	0.89	1.03	0.21
265	Wakefield	0.62	0.39	12.02***	8.44***	11.08***	7.80***	1.04	1.27	1.06	0.44
266	Barnsley	1.04	0.00	9.48***	8.57***	8.58	8.09**	1.21	0.55	0.99	0.32
267	Derbyshire	0.62	0.45	6.55**	6.02***	4.80	5.61*	1.19	0.90	0.86	0.39
268	Doncaster	1.17	0.67	10.24***	11.40***	7.98	7.82***	1.98*	0.86	1.65	0.62
269	Leicestershire	1.38	0.74	7.92***	6.73***	6.96	5.82*	1.35	1.15	1.17	0.16
270	Lincolnshire	0.31	0.48	5.76	6.81***	4.49	5.45	1.48	1.00	0.76	0.13
271	Nottinghamshire	1.02	0.79	8.60***	7.0***	6.87	5.79**	0.88	0.63	1.15	0.50
272	Rotherham	1.27	0.29	11.34***	7.5***	9.39*	6.96*	1.89*	0.39	0.73	0.27
273	Sheffield	1.00	0.44	5.54	5.5**	5.10	5.00	1.34	0.69	0.96	0.61*
274	Cambridgeshire	0.56	0.44	6.78**	4.0	5.38	3.58	1.49	0.69	0.32	0.23
275	Norfolk	0.52	0.55	8.20***	5.8***	6.77	4.52	1.48	0.40	0.23	0.31
276	Suffolk	0.34	0.42	5.20	6.0***	4.27	4.08	0.96	0.97	0.19	0.23
277	Barnet	0.90	0.33	5.86	3.0	3.33	3.09	1.58	0.93	0.49	0.00
278	Bedfordshire	0.63	0.41	5.85	7.52***	3.64	4.50	1.13	0.89	0.84	0.26
279	Brent and Harrow	0.80	1.06	2.93	4.80	2.36	3.79	0.52	0.93	0.83	0.15
280	Ealing/Hammersmith/Hounslow	1.27	1.59**	5.81	5.63**	4.82	4.38	0.75	0.58	1.28	0.43
281	Hertfordshire	0.55	0.49	4.42	3.24	3.53	3.03	0.84	0.78	0.59	0.07
282	Hillingdon	0.87	0.10	5.48	6.20**	6.11	5.79	2.02*	0.74	0.30	0.45
283	Kensington/Chelsea/Westminster	1.89	2.36***	7.20**	6.90***	4.53	6.14*	1.06	1.17	1.19	0.49
284	Barking and Havering	0.99	0.63	4.49	6.27***	4.00	5.41	1.60	1.28	0.56	0.00
285	Camden and Islington	2.87*	1.41	6.18	6.23**	4.64	3.46	1.09	0.78	0.77	0.20
286	City and East London	2.82**	2.13***	8.17***	7.27***	8.00*	6.55**	1.10	0.60	1.00	0.42
287	Enfield and Haringey	0.57	0.81	4.36	6.90***	5.17	5.17	0.94	0.53	1.25	0.88***
288	Essex	0.89	0.55	5.73*	4.89**	4.61	3.60	1.19	0.84	0.58	0.09
289	Redbridge and Waltham Forest	1.12	0.66	4.21	5.16*	4.25	3.83	0.73	0.45	0.74	0.24
290	Bromley	1.03	0.45	5.55	2.80	4.22	3.31	1.10	1.04	0.48	0.23
291	East Sussex	0.88	0.44	6.00*	7.07***	5.50	6.52**	1.22	0.84	0.40	0.24
292	Greenwich and Bexley	1.22	0.68	4.31	3.61	3.32	3.87	1.06	0.86	1.01	0.32
293	Kent	0.76	0.51	6.37***	6.27***	5.36	5.27*	1.14	0.81	0.57	0.26
294	Lambeth/Southwark/Lewisham	2.58*	1.79***	6.75**	5.52**	6.62	4.81	0.89	0.85	1.05	0.32
295	Croydon	1.22	0.62	5.95	5.31*	4.82	5.08	0.96	0.46	0.32	0.11
296	Kingston and Richmond	0.65	0.32	3.27	4.12	3.98	3.79	0.92	1.08	0.36	0.23
297	Merton/Sutton/Wandsworth	1.36	0.91	5.71	5.86***	5.45	5.00	0.92	0.71	0.89	0.23
298	Surrey	0.54	0.51	5.92*	4.79*	5.06	3.79	1.07	0.82	0.68	0.21
299	West Sussex	0.68	0.48	4.86	4.05	4.06	3.60	0.78	0.77	0.39	0.11
300	Dorset	0.83	0.56	5.74	4.84*	3.92	4.38	0.83	0.69	0.43	0.26
301	Hampshire	0.71	0.47	6.47***	5.89***	5.62	4.86	0.98	0.77	0.27	0.21
302	Isle of Wight	0.97	0.60	4.75	3.81	3.55	4.03	1.33	0.44	1.15	0.00
303	Wiltshire	1.09	0.24	10.64***	5.74**	7.80	3.11	1.19	1.06	1.13	0.13
304	Berkshire	0.92	0.67	6.98**	3.70	4.41	3.47	1.12	0.75	0.61	0.14
305	Buckinghamshire	0.20	0.36	4.30	3.25	3.44	2.05	1.15	0.74	0.32	0.11
306	Northamptonshire	1.04	0.53	7.38***	4.58	6.10	3.69	1.24	0.77	0.86	0.13
307	Oxfordshire	0.35	0.20	3.62	3.78	4.75	3.95	0.90	0.65	0.46	0.12
308	Avon	0.65	0.40	5.09	4.25	4.19	3.41	0.62	0.78	0.36	0.19
309	Cornwall and Scilly Isles	1.04	0.44	9.89***	6.56***	8.14*	6.01*	0.90	0.47	0.87	0.17
310	Devon	1.00	0.48	6.90***	6.27***	6.26	5.90**	1.10	0.61	0.56	0.04
311	Gloucestershire	0.83	0.48	6.20*	6.84***	6.11	5.50	1.02	0.60	0.31	0.21
312	Somerset	0.92	0.74	7.39**	5.57**	7.15	5.27	1.04	0.83	0.66	0.17
313	Birmingham	1.95	1.21	7.47***	5.90***	6.87	5.34	1.04	0.95	1.23	0.48
314	Coventry	1.84	1.30	7.63**	7.50***	4.80	6.11	2.00**	1.49*	1.26	0.12
315	Dudley	1.02	0.70	7.50**	6.69***	6.22	6.02	1.85*	1.12	1.24	0.55
316	Hereford and Worcester	0.77	0.51	7.17***	6.76***	6.42	6.43**	0.70	0.71	1.08	0.37

Table 9.1.3(a) cont

Area

Age-standardized death rates (per 100 000)

		TUB		CERV		UTER		HODG		CRHD	
		1974–78	1980–84	1974–78	1980–84	1974–78	1980–84	1974–78	1980–84	1974–78	1980–84
317	Salop	0.97	0.20	6.78*	6.99***	6.70	6.32*	1.39	0.74	1.08	0.09
318	Sandwell	1.93	1.05	9.30***	7.50***	6.66	6.63*	1.50	1.04	1.78*	0.12
319	Solihull	0.62	0.12	5.05	4.13	3.68	4.87	1.24	0.85	0.51	0.00
320	Staffordshire	1.02	0.55	8.91***	7.89***	7.69*	6.67***	1.13	1.16	1.13	0.36
321	Walsall	1.84	1.24	9.09***	7.19***	7.50	6.85*	0.99	0.64	2.43***	0.26
322	Warwickshire	1.08	0.71	6.81**	6.76***	5.15	5.62	1.62	0.98	0.68	0.21
323	Wolverhampton	2.20	1.02	8.93***	9.30***	6.01	6.40*	0.92	1.27	0.84	0.74*
324	Bolton	1.65	1.25	8.85***	9.81***	9.21*	7.06*	0.96	0.68	2.32***	0.81*
325	Bury	0.94	0.58	7.17*	6.73**	6.63	3.91	0.97	0.58	1.01	0.00
326	Lancashire	1.32	0.59	10.26***	8.38***	8.19***	6.43***	1.31	0.61	0.96	0.37
327	Manchester	2.73*	1.94***	10.63***	12.04***	8.48*	9.22***	1.17	0.79	1.67*	0.70*
328	Oldham	1.48	0.68	11.62***	8.52***	10.79**	6.87*	2.11*	0.93	1.83*	0.64
329	Rochdale	1.05	0.49	10.11***	12.01***	6.01	6.90*	0.96	0.87	1.61	0.17
330	Salford	1.40	0.78	10.92***	8.86***	8.20	7.58**	1.41	0.41	0.89	0.47
331	Stockport	0.98	0.50	9.10***	4.13	6.22	4.53	1.19	0.94	0.98	0.12
332	Tameside	1.04	0.67	9.25***	6.68**	8.16	4.69	2.21**	1.15	1.02	0.00
333	Trafford	0.72	0.77	7.81**	6.23**	4.61	5.39	1.18	0.68	0.48	0.81*
334	Wigan	0.48	0.49	8.05***	7.87***	7.87	6.07	1.45	0.57	1.50	0.43
335	Cheshire	0.80	0.53	8.65***	8.96***	6.68	7.47***	1.03	0.67	1.05	0.15
336	Liverpool	1.83	1.35	10.14***	11.45***	8.52**	9.84***	0.86	0.80	1.89**	0.39
337	St Helens and Knowsley	1.01	0.70	11.80***	11.91***	9.73**	11.19***	1.01	0.70	0.96	0.10
338	Sefton	1.63	0.72	9.42***	9.73***	6.41	8.31***	1.07	1.00	0.72	0.25
339	Wirral	1.34	0.93	7.86***	9.63***	5.74	9.64***	1.29	0.75	1.00	0.22
340	Clwyd	0.88	0.19	9.44***	8.89***	8.29*	7.26**	1.26	1.18	1.43	0.37
341	Dyfed	1.63	0.62	8.64***	8.72***	7.24	7.70***	1.55	1.11	1.54	0.67
342	Gwent	1.32	0.64	7.45***	5.52**	6.70	5.72	1.66	1.23	1.50	0.24
343	Gwynedd	1.44	1.07	6.94*	6.82**	7.85	4.87	1.55	1.01	0.53	0.33
344	Mid Glamorgan	1.65	0.81	7.07**	7.61***	6.41	6.26**	1.09	0.93	2.06***	0.86***
345	Powys	1.71	0.21	6.12	7.06*	3.80	4.28	0.46	1.14	0.00	0.00
346	South Glamorgan	1.42	0.95	6.87*	7.58***	5.40	5.71	0.83	0.71	1.08	0.19
347	West Glamorgan	1.20	0.76	9.94***	6.50***	8.32*	4.58	1.03	1.07	1.92**	0.40
UK:NORTHERN IRELAND											
348	Northern Ireland	1.30	0.68	5.26	5.55***	4.70	4.86	1.12	1.20*	1.12	0.27
UK: SCOTLAND		1.75	1.07	7.49***	6.79***	5.98	5.48***	1.10	0.83	1.40***	0.35
349	Highlands and Islands	0.91	0.39	8.91***	7.01***	6.29	5.91	1.24	0.97	0.60	0.13
350	Grampian	0.88	0.70	5.61	5.20*	5.19	3.48	1.12	0.68	0.73	0.15
351	Tayside	0.79	0.74	6.02	4.35	4.85	4.01	1.07	0.90	0.38	0.19
352	Fife	1.10	0.22	8.28***	10.42***	8.16	9.07***	1.04	1.12	0.11	0.11
353	Lothian	0.78	0.44	7.42***	6.54***	5.29	6.01**	0.66	0.70	1.76***	0.38
354	Borders	0.47	0.24	12.36***	4.08	7.99	3.84	0.51	1.26	0.40	0.00
355	Forth Valley	1.47	1.10	6.71*	6.25**	5.17	3.55	1.58	0.83	1.47	0.26
356	Argyll and Clyde	2.18	1.73**	5.96	7.01***	4.79	4.97	1.00	1.01	2.08***	0.16
357	Greater Glasgow	3.74***	2.20***	8.37***	6.77***	6.95	5.72*	1.35	0.71	2.23***	0.71**
358	Lanarkshire	1.79	0.77	7.11**	7.40***	5.46	5.68*	1.22	0.98	1.73**	0.55
359	Ayrshire and Arran	1.05	1.06	9.45***	8.77***	7.86	6.54*	1.21	0.81	1.17	0.38
360	Dumfries and Galloway	1.34	1.14	5.48	6.04*	3.78	5.65	0.70	0.52	0.53	0.00
EC		2.05	1.08	4.89	3.83	6.23	4.38	1.25	0.95	1.05	0.35

Table 9.1.3(b). Age-standardized death rates (per 100 000) for 1974–78 and 1980–84 by small area standardized to the EC standard, for all respiratory diseases, asthma, appendicitis, abdominal hernia, and cholelithiasis/cholecystitis

Notes on the use of this table

1. This table shows the mortality rates for small areas standardized to the EC standard for 1974–78 and 1980–84. The rates are in deaths per 100 000 population. The age-standardized death rates are calculated by multiplying the small-area SMR based on the EC standard for that time period by the EC crude death rate for that time period.

2. Key for the abbreviations used for columns of the table:
   RESP — all respiratory diseases (ICD8 460–519; ICD9 460–519), ages 1–14;
   ASTH — asthma (ICD8 493; ICD9 493), ages 5–44;
   APP — appendicitis (ICD8 540–543; ICD9 540–543), ages 5–64;
   HERN — abdominal hernia (ICD8 550–553; ICD9 550–553), ages 5–64;
   CHOLY— cholelithiasis and cholecystitis (ICD8 574–575; ICD9 574–575.1,576.1), ages 5–64.

3. The small area numbers are as in the key maps (pp. 241–5).

4. The indicators have been tested for indicating significant excess mortality relative to EC rates. The *p*-values achieved for one-tail tests are indicated as follows:
   *p<0.05; **p<0.01; ***p<0.001.

5. The mortality data for the earlier time period are for 1974–78, except for France (1973–77). The population data are for 1974–78, except for France (1975), Ireland (1976), and N. Ireland (1976).

6. The mortality data for the later time period are for 1980–84, except for Greece (1980–82). The population data are for 1980–84 except for France (1982), Ireland (1981), and Greece (1981). All data for Italy are for 1979–83.

Table 9.1.3(b)

Area — Age-standardized death rates (per 100 000)

Area		RESP 1974–78	RESP 1980–84	ASTH 1974–78	ASTH 1980–84	APP 1974–78	APP 1980–84	HERN 1974–78	HERN 1980–84	CHOLY 1974–78	CHOLY 1980–84
BELGIUM		2.11	1.74	0.87***	0.94***	0.18	0.07	0.24	0.10	0.50	0.34
1	Antwerpen	2.85	1.46	0.97***	0.78	0.19	0.03	0.14	0.05	0.27	0.24
2	Brabant	1.15	1.98	0.73**	0.87**	0.18	0.10	0.34	0.13	0.58	0.34
3	West-Vlaanderen	1.93	1.27	1.06***	1.11***	0.12	0.02	0.10	0.09	0.41	0.37
4	Oost-Vlaanderen	3.29	2.34	0.45	0.61	0.17	0.15	0.19	0.09	0.27	0.17
5	Hainaut	2.35	1.43	1.30***	1.49***	0.23	0.06	0.46	0.17	0.83	0.49*
6	Liège	1.89	2.36	0.89**	1.13***	0.22	0.05	0.17	0.07	0.42	0.34
7	Limburg	1.82	1.28	0.41	0.44	0.08	0.04	0.09	0.04	0.57	0.31
8	Luxembourg (province)	2.11	0.89	0.00*	0.33	0.11	0.00	0.23	0.11	0.57	0.88**
9	Namur	1.18	1.74	1.68***	1.77***	0.32	0.18	0.32	0.12	0.83	0.35
LUXEMBOURG											
10	Luxembourg	2.13	1.26	0.00	0.74	0.55	0.28	0.07	0.14	0.67	0.49
FEDERAL REPUBLIC OF GERMANY		2.88	1.74	0.86***	1.02***	0.55***	0.19***	0.40***	0.16	1.12***	0.43***
11	Schleswig–Holstein	2.61	1.34	0.97***	1.05***	0.56***	0.20	0.22	0.15	0.90	0.44
12	Hamburg	3.49	2.10	0.86***	1.04***	0.37	0.21	0.15	0.12	0.78	0.34
13	Neidersachsen	2.96	1.93	1.01***	1.11***	0.67***	0.26***	0.40	0.16	1.20***	0.46***
14	Bremen	3.18	1.29	0.38	1.39***	0.92***	0.25	0.33	0.14	0.72	0.42
15	Nordrhein–Westfalen	2.86	1.66	0.88***	1.06***	0.52***	0.16	0.37	0.12	1.23***	0.37
16	Hessen	2.66	1.52	0.98***	1.25***	0.53***	0.21**	0.43*	0.25*	0.88	0.48***
17	Rheinland–Pfalz	2.45	1.61	0.94***	1.18***	0.47**	0.20*	0.40	0.17	1.13***	0.29
18	Baden Wurttemberg	2.76	1.76	0.64***	0.83***	0.46***	0.15	0.44**	0.17	1.05***	0.44**
19	Bayern	3.21	1.82	0.85***	0.88***	0.60***	0.19**	0.50***	0.18	1.19***	0.47***
20	Saarland	2.82	2.69	0.72*	1.16***	0.33	0.11	0.49	0.13	1.13*	0.52*
21	Berlin(West)	2.56	1.95	0.93***	0.93**	0.82***	0.20	0.48*	0.13	1.22***	0.72***

Table 9.1.3(b) cont

Area		Age-standardized death rates (per 100 000)									
		RESP		ASTH		APP		HERN		CHOLY	
		1974–78	1980–84	1974–78	1980–84	1974–78	1980–84	1974–78	1980–84	1974–78	1980–84
DENMARK		1.47	1.32	0.27	0.41	0.21	0.15	0.13	0.13	0.37	0.25
22	Kobenhavn and Frederiksberg (M)	1.20	0.61	0.33	0.59	0.22	0.13	0.12	0.12	0.34	0.23
23	Kobenhavns County	1.02	6.28	0.26	0.26	0.12	0.11	0.16	0.07	0.35	0.22
24	Frederiksborg County	1.03	0.30	0.00	0.28	0.34	0.16	0.19	0.08	0.18	0.25
25	Roskilde County	1.61	1.42	0.16	0.15	0.00	0.13	0.00	0.00	0.16	0.00
26	Vestsjaellands County	2.03	1.15	0.53	0.00	0.28	0.09	0.09	0.09	0.27	0.18
27	Storstroms County	2.33	3.97*	0.44	0.14	0.28	0.28	0.00	0.18	0.70	0.27
28	Bornholms County	2.04	0.00	0.00	0.00	0.51	0.00	0.00	0.00	0.96	0.00
29	Fyns County	1.47	1.44	0.08	0.62	0.22	0.17	0.05	0.16	0.21	0.49
30	Sonderjyllands County	2.53	2.83	0.00	0.69	0.00	0.31	0.10	0.41	0.53	0.21
31	Ribe County	2.46	1.35	0.34	0.63	0.00	0.00	0.13	0.12	0.13	0.25
32	Vejle County	2.20	1.56	0.67	0.74	0.32	0.23	0.23	0.23	0.16	0.31
33	Ringkobing County	1.58	1.41	0.68	0.38	0.40	0.20	0.00	0.10	0.73	0.61
34	Arhus County	1.09	0.90	0.12	0.40	0.27	0.14	0.28	0.14	0.37	0.19
35	Viborg County	0.78	0.00	0.16	0.47	0.33	0.11	0.21	0.22	0.64	0.22
36	Nordjyllands County	0.97	1.51	0.23	0.43	0.05	0.16	0.15	0.05	0.41	0.15
FRANCE		2.02	1.18	0.33	0.38	0.34	0.16**	0.37	0.26***	0.70	0.07
37	Ain	1.96	0.42	0.28	0.25	0.35	0.37**	0.29	0.50**	1.09	0.06
38	Aisne	1.56	1.45	0.27	0.47	0.10	0.33*	0.60*	0.29	0.49	0.15
39	Allier	2.23	1.79	0.61	0.21	0.40	0.26	0.64*	0.25	0.70	0.06
40	Alpes-de-Haute-Provence	2.62	0.94	0.33	0.00	0.22	0.21	0.42	0.00	1.27	0.00
41	Hautes-Alpes	2.77	0.00	1.10	1.68*	0.26	0.23	0.25	0.23	0.74	0.23
42	Alpes-Maritimes	1.47	1.00	0.33	0.53	0.18	0.11	0.11	0.13	0.52	0.03
43	Ardèche	3.82	1.13	0.44	0.00	0.20	0.18	0.39	0.44*	0.88	0.18
44	Ardennes	2.15	2.24	0.22	0.47	0.78**	0.00	0.85**	0.71***	0.75	0.18
45	Ariège	2.37	0.89	0.00	1.21	0.00	0.17	0.32	0.00	0.49	0.00
46	Aube	2.58	0.32	0.76	0.12	0.75*	0.27	0.20	0.36	0.59	0.27
47	Aude	0.79	1.68	0.15	0.29	0.00	0.00	0.58	0.31	0.91	0.00
48	Aveyron	2.10	1.99	0.00	0.57	0.71*	0.00	0.58	0.49*	1.00	0.08
49	Bouches-du-Rhône	1.73	0.81	0.27	0.24	0.22	0.13	0.28	0.20	0.53	0.07
50	Calvados	2.12	0.86	0.55	0.47	0.19	0.18	0.42	0.37*	0.73	0.05
51	Cantal	0.53	1.93	1.38**	0.24	1.21***	0.45*	0.58	0.28	1.32	0.00
52	Charente	1.04	1.48	0.11	0.22	0.53	0.15	0.30	0.29	0.45	0.07
53	Charente-Maritime	2.98	0.79	0.23	0.22	0.21	0.10	0.20	0.09	0.87	0.05
54	Cher	2.18	1.29	0.24	0.47	0.41	0.00	0.89.***	0.38	1.06	0.15
55	Corrèze	2.10	0.97	0.33	0.50	0.62	0.29	0.28	0.45*	1.43*	0.00
56	Corse	3.04	0.93	0.16	0.30	0.21	0.00	0.38	0.10	0.28	0.00
57	Côte-d'Or	2.50	1.16	0.00	0.44	0.53	0.17	0.37	0.28	0.87	0.06
58	Côtes-du-Nord	2.39	1.07	0.51	0.21	0.24	0.09	0.19	0.38*	0.60	0.04
59	Creuse	2.32	0.00	0.29	0.00	0.51	0.34	0.31	0.31	0.31	0.15
60	Dordogne	4.17	1.82	0.42	0.54	0.46	0.31*	0.30	0.34	1.03	0.00
61	Doubs	2.60	1.40	0.56	0.07	0.52	0.11	0.32	0.18	0.71	0.00
62	Drôme	2.84	1.19	0.49	0.27	0.43	0.39**	0.44	0.26	0.95	0.06
63	Eure	2.11	0.90	0.33	0.60	0.19	0.11	0.77**	0.24	0.35	0.12
64	Eure-et-Loir	1.39	1.65	0.32	0.10	0.32	0.14	0.17	0.00	0.84	0.00
65	Finistère	1.78	0.11	0.46	0.41	0.37	0.09	0.27	0.26	0.76	0.09
66	Gard	3.15	0.20	0.45	0.21	0.35	0.41***	0.34	0.26	1.13	0.09
67	Haute-Garonne	1.32	1.31	0.22	0.45	0.30	0.03	0.34	0.12	0.57	0.12
68	Gers	5.75*	3.45	0.22	0.45	0.43	0.00	0.67	0.13	0.80	0.00
69	Gironde	1.95	0.97	0.27	0.50	0.36	0.18	0.41	0.18	0.53	0.07
70	Hérault	1.65	1.04	0.06	0.41	0.35	0.14	0.38	0.37*	0.84	0.13
71	Ille-et-Vilaine	1.62	0.68	0.25	0.42	0.37	0.17	0.39	0.25	0.47	0.11
72	Indre	1.55	0.45	0.47	0.97	0.31	0.20	0.69*	0.68***	0.49	0.10
73	Indre-et-Loire	1.86	1.14	0.22	0.42	0.39	0.26	0.35	0.26	0.23	0.10
74	Isère	2.23	1.04	0.47	0.14	0.49	0.19	0.30	0.17	0.59	0.20
75	Jura	2.41	0.77	0.15	0.61	0.65	0.10	0.33	0.00	0.66	0.00
76	Landes	0.65	1.10	0.39	0.13	0.53	0.00	0.69*	0.00	0.69	0.08
77	Loir-et-Cher	2.10	1.33	0.13	0.64	0.28	0.00	0.28	0.17	0.66	0.08
78	Loire	2.10	0.88	0.09	0.44	0.48	0.24	0.43	0.37*	0.67	0.10
79	Haute-Loire	3.20	0.00	0.00	0.19	0.25	0.24	0.49	0.46*	1.83***	0.11

Table 9.1.3(b) cont

Area		Age-standardized death rates (per 100 000)									
		RESP		ASTH		APP		HERN		CHOLY	
		1974–78	1980–84	1974–78	1980–84	1974–78	1980–84	1974–78	1980–84	1974–78	1980–84
80	Loire-Atlantique	1.62	1.59	0.52	0.42	0.28	0.21	0.48	0.30	1.09	0.00
81	Loiret	1.80	1.33	0.28	0.33	0.44	0.05	0.40	0.15	0.51	0.05
82	Lot	2.78	0.76	0.26	0.00	0.33	0.00	0.61	0.28	0.76	0.00
83	Lot-et-Garonne	1.94	0.36	0.26	0.26	0.00	0.24	0.49	0.00	0.73	0.00
84	Lozère	1.26	1.41	0.51	1.06	0.34	0.33	0.00	0.31	1.28	0.00
85	Maine-et-Loire	1.57	1.15	0.00	0.42	0.21	0.16	0.32	0.21	0.32	0.08
86	Manche	1.77	0.57	0.32	0.24	0.68**	0.00	0.17	0.21	0.40	0.11
87	Marne	2.11	1.42	0.58	0.25	0.26	0.29*	0.40	0.26	0.74	0.00
88	Haute-Marne	1.40	1.64	0.34	0.17	0.37	0.25	0.13	0.13	0.65	0.00
89	Mayenne	2.87	1.22	0.14	0.27	0.20	0.47**	0.10	0.38	0.71	0.09
90	Meurthe-et-Moselle	2.45	1.00	0.14	0.38	0.11	0.04	0.56*	0.38*	0.72	0.04
91	Meuse	1.18	0.45	0.36	0.18	0.39	0.51**	0.55	0.52*	0.68	0.00
92	Morbihan	2.12	1.51	0.45	0.44	0.40	0.13	0.45	0.17	0.45	0.04
93	Moselle	2.07	1.32	0.68	0.46	0.16	0.22	0.41	0.29	0.79	0.05
94	Nivre	1.14	0.92	0.31	0.34	0.73*	0.42*	0.81**	0.49*	0.40	0.00
95	Nord	2.55	1.37	0.58	0.58	0.39	0.34***	0.61***	0.44***	1.09**	0.15
96	Oise	2.01	0.86	0.38	0.40	0.50	0.12	0.37	0.36	0.21	0.04
97	Orne	2.10	0.90	0.24	0.00	0.18	0.17	0.28	0.08	0.37	0.08
98	Pas-de-Calais	2.22	1.15	0.45	0.77	0.43	0.20	0.51*	0.50***	1.10*	0.09
99	Puy-de-Dôme	1.96	0.67	0.24	0.41	0.31	0.13	0.32	0.21	0.91	0.04
100	Pyrénées-Atlantiques	2.25	0.38	0.34	0.61	0.24	0.00	0.28	0.21	0.74	0.00
101	Hautes-Pyrénées	2.99	1.97	0.32	0.33	0.54	0.10	0.31	0.39	0.62	0.00
102	Pyrénées-Orientales	0.69	1.68	0.78	0.24	0.55	0.21	0.43	0.13	1.30*	0.06
103	Bas-Rhin	3.30	1.56	0.19	0.22	0.21	0.00	0.49	0.33	0.87	0.15
104	Haut-Rhin	2.81	2.41	0.63	0.36	0.30	0.24	0.23	0.25	0.96	0.00
105	Rhne	2.03	1.59	0.16	0.19	0.40	0.09	0.40	0.29	1.00	0.07
106	Haute-Saône	3.94	1.50	0.16	0.31	0.36	0.44**	0.25	0.23	0.62	0.00
107	Saône-et-Loire	1.49	1.18	0.45	0.20	0.32	0.30*	0.28	0.17	0.69	0.13
108	Sarthe	1.38	0.53	0.07	0.65	0.48	0.30*	0.11	0.21	0.68	0.10
109	Savoie	3.21	0.58	0.33	0.21	1.02***	0.08	0.54	0.48*	1.06	0.08
110	Haute-Savoie	1.91	1.07	0.29	0.26	0.30	0.16	0.39	0.45*	0.51	0.11
111	Paris	1.80	1.05	0.31	0.34	0.26	0.10	0.27	0.25	0.39	0.03
112	Seine-Maritime	1.16	1.80	0.23	0.40	0.36	0.09	0.20	0.32*	0.78	0.02
113	Seine-et-Marne	1.75	2.14	0.26	0.33	0.15	0.21	0.50	0.24	0.49	0.10
114	Yvelines	1.83	1.37	0.26	0.42	0.28	0.15	0.35	0.17	0.46	0.07
115	Deux-Sèvres	1.65	0.27	0.22	0.33	0.23	0.37*	0.24	0.37	1.19	0.22
116	Somme	2.51	1.27	0.54	0.26	0.20	0.14	0.05	0.20	0.75	0.15
117	Tarn	2.01	1.26	0.22	0.58	0.22	0.07	0.29	0.26	0.43	0.07
118	Tarn-et-Garonne	2.58	0.57	0.63	0.21	0.14	0.00	0.65	0.00	0.39	0.00
119	Var	3.27	1.06	0.52	0.52	0.27	0.07	0.37	0.19	0.30	0.19
120	Vaucluse	1.81	0.46	0.09	0.41	0.78**	0.12	0.46	0.12	0.65	0.12
121	Vendée	2.69	1.74	0.25	0.23	0.47	0.16	0.18	0.21	0.97	0.05
122	Vienne	1.93	0.00	0.21	0.49	0.29	0.14	0.15	0.21	0.89	0.07
123	Haute-Vienne	0.89	1.63	0.32	0.54	0.36	0.00	0.27	0.13	0.88	0.00
124	Vosges	2.62	1.35	0.27	0.09	0.47	0.19	0.49	0.40*	0.69	0.00
125	Yonne	2.26	1.55	0.38	0.74	0.62	0.25	0.18	0.32	0.62	0.08
126	Territoire-de-Belfort	3.75	0.00	0.00	0.52	0.83*	0.19	0.00	0.41	0.66	0.21
127	Essonne	1.77	1.72	0.20	0.38	0.21	0.16	0.37	0.18	0.50	0.03
128	Hauts-de-Seine	0.80	1.27	0.23	0.22	0.40	0.12	0.26	0.07	0.37	0.03
129	Seine-Saint-Denis	1.69	1.35	0.33	0.42	0.28	0.12	0.35	0.29	0.67	0.04
130	Val-de-Marne	1.26	1.20	0.18	0.25	0.13	0.15	0.21	0.17	0.34	0.02
131	Val-d'Oise	1.86	0.71	0.30	0.38	0.26	0.06	0.37	0.22	0.73	0.03
GREECE		3.79***	2.31*	0.16	-	0.13	0.06	0.17	0.08	0.36	0.18
132	Greater Athens	2.77	1.75	0.07	-	0.16	0.06	0.27	0.11	0.44	0.17
133	Rest of Central Greece and Eubea	3.87*	2.34	0.10	-	0.15	0.04	0.05	0.08	0.17	0.24
134	Peloponnisos	2.99	1.70	0.26	-	0.10	0.04	0.10	0.04	0.41	0.12
135	Ionian Islands	3.35	0.84	0.64	-	0.11	0.44*	0.09	0.21	0.27	0.00
136	Epirus	3.21	3.42	0.34	-	0.08	0.00	0.24	0.00	0.24	0.13
137	Thessaly	4.02*	2.18	0.10	-	0.07	0.12	0.07	0.12	0.41	0.36
138	Macedonia	3.02	1.87	0.13	-	0.10	0.06	0.13	0.09	0.33	0.15

Table 9.1.3(b) cont

Area   Age-standardized death rates (per 100 000)

		RESP		ASTH		APP		HERN		CHOLY	
		1974–78	1980–84	1974–78	1980–84	1974–78	1980–84	1974–78	1980–84	1974–78	1980–84
139	Thrace	13.90***	9.89***	0.49	-	0.00	0.00	0.17	0.00	0.58	0.00
140	Aegean Islands	8.23***	2.74	0.54	-	0.29	0.00	0.22	0.10	0.28	0.20
141	Crete	2.79	2.64	0.08	-	0.11	0.09	0.15	0.00	0.36	0.26
ITALY		3.54***	2.50***	0.05	0.15	0.34	0.14	0.39**	0.25***	1.43***	0.65***
142	Torino	2.23	2.04	0.05	0.18	0.46*	0.21*	0.57***	0.38***	2.23***	1.06***
143	Vercelli	3.47	1.01	0.09	0.00	0.41	0.12	0.59*	0.06	1.19*	0.68**
144	Novara	3.25	2.33	0.14	0.28	0.19	0.00	0.50	0.29	1.74***	0.47
145	Cuneo	1.98	1.11	0.07	0.34	0.35	0.22	0.52	0.63***	1.94***	0.76***
146	Asti	1.06	4.41*	0.00	0.18	0.33	0.11	0.59	0.10	1.28	0.73*
147	Alessandria	1.31	0.95	0.16	0.25	0.44	0.30*	0.61*	0.32	1.26*	0.74**
148	Aosta	1.76	3.15	0.00	0.00	1.27***	0.21	0.82*	0.21	2.25***	0.62
149	Imperia	2.98	0.63	0.16	0.17	0.21	0.63***	0.38	0.19	1.61**	0.68*
150	Savona	3.03	2.88	0.00	0.00	0.75**	0.08	0.41	0.14	1.43**	0.42
151	Genova	1.74	1.39	0.07	0.29	0.32	0.13	0.27	0.28	1.90***	0.95***
152	La Spezia	1.86	0.57	0.15	0.00	0.37	0.00	0.25	0.34	0.58	0.60
153	Varese	2.06	2.14	0.00	0.30	0.16	0.06	0.30	0.16	1.08	0.78***
154	Como/Sondrio	2.19	2.18	0.14	0.25	0.48	0.03	0.44	0.14	1.81***	0.74***
155	Milano	2.22	1.86	0.06	0.10	0.31	0.12	0.30	0.21	1.48***	0.49**
156	Bergamo	2.08	1.73	0.07	0.18	0.50	0.11	0.31	0.21	1.21**	0.67***
157	Brescia	2.94	1.79	0.03	0.16	0.18	0.17	0.39	0.08	1.34***	0.46
158	Pavia	1.58	1.60	0.00	0.15	0.40	0.14	0.33	0.22	1.30**	0.52
159	Cremona	1.27	0.73	0.00	0.22	0.36	0.21	0.41	0.21	1.21	0.62*
160	Mantova	1.35	1.90	0.00	0.19	0.12	0.06	0.17	0.24	1.69***	0.30
161	Bolzano	2.38	1.74	0.08	0.15	0.49	0.24	0.20	0.13	2.21***	0.78**
162	Trento	2.96	1.23	0.08	0.16	0.29	0.00	0.06	0.23	1.38**	0.97***
163	Verona	2.00	0.96	0.04	0.09	0.16	0.13	0.32	0.03	1.29**	0.70***
164	Vicenza	1.30	1.93	0.09	0.05	0.32	0.17	0.48	0.22	1.46***	0.84***
165	Belluno	1.78	1.61	0.00	0.16	0.22	0.11	0.61	0.11	1.43*	0.63
166	Treviso	1.85	1.00	0.10	0.14	0.25	0.00	0.11	0.25	1.03	0.58*
167	Venezia	2.48	0.90	0.20	0.24	0.27	0.12	0.28	0.15	1.28**	0.51
168	Padova	3.08	3.29**	0.21	0.17	0.28	0.06	0.39	0.22	1.36***	0.38
169	Rovigo	1.54	0.44	0.14	0.14	0.10	0.09	0.09	0.46*	1.74***	0.73*
170	Udine/Gorizia	2.15	0.92	0.00	0.16	0.42	0.11	0.23	0.24	0.93	0.72***
171	Trieste	3.51	1.14	0.00	0.27	0.38	0.24	0.39	0.07	1.12	0.85***
172	Pordenone	1.71	0.00	0.00	0.00	0.56	0.09	0.27	0.18	0.99	0.64
173	Piacenza	1.66	0.51	0.26	0.00	0.16	0.16	0.29	0.00	1.81***	0.76**
174	Parma	2.64	1.73	0.00	0.28	0.17	0.17	0.61*	0.21	0.56	0.74**
175	Reggio Emilia	3.14	0.90	0.00	0.00	0.40	0.06	0.47	0.00	0.73	0.42
176	Modena	0.90	1.04	0.06	0.06	0.45	0.04	0.65**	0.19	1.18*	0.60*
177	Bologna	1.49	1.57	0.04	0.12	0.24	0.14	0.40	0.18	1.03	0.65***
178	Ferrara	1.13	2.08	0.00	0.00	0.36	0.06	0.27	0.11	1.15	0.44
179	Ravenna	1.48	0.73	0.00	0.10	0.52	0.06	0.12	0.12	0.92	0.49
180	Forli	2.25	1.31	0.00	0.00	0.00	0.00	0.20	0.12	1.15*	0.31
181	Pesaro	3.24	3.32	0.00	0.11	0.36	0.21	0.62*	0.14	0.82	0.69*
182	Ancona	2.62	2.37	0.00	0.08	0.22	0.05	0.21	0.21	1.29*	0.46
183	Macerata	0.00	1.23	0.00	0.13	0.24	0.16	0.37	0.08	1.19	0.68*
184	Ascoli Piceno	2.53	0.94	0.10	0.00	0.07	0.07	0.53	0.19	1.52**	0.52
185	Massa-Carrara	1.00	1.18	0.00	0.18	0.23	0.35	0.22	0.22	1.53**	0.66
186	Lucca	1.61	0.94	0.00	0.38	0.12	0.25	0.29	0.18	1.05	0.41
187	Pistoia	0.80	1.37	0.00	0.41	0.18	0.09	0.17	0.17	0.76	0.43
188	Firenze	1.88	1.70	0.06	0.03	0.24	0.04	0.32	0.13	0.98	0.50*
189	Livorno	1.49	1.76	0.00	0.11	0.34	0.54***	0.19	0.19	1.26*	0.75**
190	Pisa	0.55	1.57	0.00	0.28	0.12	0.06	0.34	0.06	1.38**	0.92***
191	Arezzo	0.35	1.19	0.00	0.00	0.23	0.15	0.21	0.07	1.32*	0.69*
192	Siena	1.45	2.77	0.00	0.31	0.00	0.44**	0.23	0.47*	1.08	0.63*
193	Grosseto	2.93	0.00	0.00	0.17	0.31	0.00	0.09	0.10	1.90***	0.57
194	Perugia	3.69	1.81	0.00	0.06	0.25	0.00	0.46	0.30	0.99	0.45
195	Terni	2.34	2.16	0.00	0.16	0.40	0.00	0.37	0.18	1.74***	0.37
196	Viterbo/Rieti	1.72	3.19*	0.00	0.18	0.46	0.11	0.27	0.32	1.57***	0.81***
197	Roma	2.64	2.09	0.09	0.14	0.24	0.14	0.29	0.26	1.27***	0.61***

Table 9.1.3(b) cont

Area   Age-standardized death rates (per 100 000)

		RESP		ASTH		APP		HERN		CHOLY	
		1974–78	1980–84	1974–78	1980–84	1974–78	1980–84	1974–78	1980–84	1974–78	1980–84
198	Latina	3.38	2.13	0.08	0.08	0.06	0.06	0.28	0.19	1.24*	0.84***
199	Frosinone	3.10	0.40	0.00	0.08	0.17	0.05	0.62*	0.22	1.40**	0.49
200	Caserta	6.28***	3.29**	0.00	0.18	0.63**	0.17	0.69**	0.82***	2.20***	0.66**
201	Benevento	6.30***	1.91	0.00	0.13	0.17	0.00	0.42	0.17	1.27*	0.34
202	Napoli	4.94***	4.48***	0.00	0.23	0.61***	0.23*	0.71***	0.54***	1.93***	0.91***
203	Avellino	6.86***	4.18***	0.16	0.17	0.35	0.06	0.24	0.06	1.12	0.71**
204	Salerno	4.85***	3.16**	0.03	0.14	0.29	0.28*	0.42	0.19	1.26**	0.62**
205	L'Aquila	4.58	2.17	0.00	0.26	0.40	0.08	0.30	0.23	2.44***	0.61
206	Teramo	2.34	1.45	0.00	0.13	0.19	0.09	0.09	0.18	1.68**	0.64*
207	Pescara	2.45	2.79	0.00	0.25	0.26	0.25	0.27	0.17	1.50**	0.51
208	Chieti	3.83	1.64	0.00	0.10	0.27	0.26	0.51	0.06	1.53**	0.94***
209	Isernia/Campobasso	2.50	2.74	0.00	0.11	0.52	0.07	0.36	0.29	1.52**	0.81**
210	Foggia	6.17***	4.07***	0.10	0.00	0.28	0.04	0.43	0.34	1.42***	0.30
211	Bari	6.01***	2.90**	0.05	0.16	0.28	0.22	0.40	0.20	1.28***	0.57**
212	Taranto	5.51***	3.32**	0.06	0.06	0.29	0.23	0.33	0.41*	1.89***	0.72**
213	Brindisi	3.90	4.01***	0.00	0.00	0.34	0.33*	0.43	0.14	1.00	0.42
214	Lecce	4.79***	3.03*	0.09	0.18	0.56*	0.10	0.19	0.32	1.12*	0.50
215	Potenza/Matera	6.54***	3.52**	0.00	0.18	0.30	0.21	0.45	0.31	1.34**	0.62*
216	Cosenza	4.37**	3.62***	0.05	0.09	0.37	0.11	0.24	0.34	1.43***	1.03***
217	Catanzaro	5.88***	3.47***	0.00	0.19	0.26	0.25	0.28	0.16	1.59***	0.52
218	Reggio Calabria	3.48	2.48	0.12	0.13	0.31	0.09	0.36	0.23	1.19*	0.42
219	Trapani	4.99**	2.29	0.09	0.60	0.55	0.00	0.43	0.25	1.35*	0.50
220	Palermo	7.76***	4.74***	0.03	0.12	0.31	0.20	0.35	0.32*	1.33***	0.46
221	Messina	4.59**	4.05***	0.05	0.05	0.41	0.22	0.69**	0.33	1.71***	0.78***
222	Agrigento	6.30***	4.01***	0.15	0.15	0.55	0.11	0.69**	0.47**	1.32*	0.35
223	Caltanisetta	6.95***	2.24	0.00	0.37	0.72*	0.27	0.38	0.39	1.45*	0.48
224	Enna	5.45*	3.12	0.00	0.37	0.38	0.13	0.78*	0.54*	1.30	0.68
225	Catania	6.81***	4.30***	0.04	0.03	0.64**	0.26*	0.62**	0.19	1.49***	0.96***
226	Ragusa	5.65**	4.43**	0.13	0.26	0.38	0.18	0.38	0.19	1.69***	0.75*
227	Siracusa	5.20**	1.67	0.09	0.00	0.40	0.00	0.36	0.42*	1.78***	0.56
228	Sassari	5.29***	3.14*	0.00	0.00	0.32	0.00	0.27	0.33	1.57***	0.67*
229	Nuoro	5.12**	3.33*	0.00	0.38	0.50	0.19	0.44	0.32	1.64**	0.85**
230	Cagliari/Oristano	5.82***	3.50***	0.08	0.23	0.28	0.12	0.53	0.34	2.00***	1.26***
IRELAND		5.30***	2.56**	0.75***	0.99***	0.38	0.14	0.29	0.13	0.30	0.36
231	Eastern	5.31***	1.91	0.72*	1.09***	0.38	0.12	0.26	0.03	0.29	0.31
232	Midland	7.04***	2.60	1.01	0.75	0.28	0.00	0.15	0.15	0.15	0.30
233	Mid-Western	4.76*	3.03	1.31***	0.48	0.64*	0.36*	0.58	0.20	0.58	0.10
234	North Eastern	6.45***	3.78**	0.85	1.02	0.40	0.19	0.21	0.32	0.53	0.54
235	North Western	3.51	2.32	0.61	0.76	0.78*	0.26	0.13	0.14	0.26	0.42
236	South Eastern	4.37*	2.62	0.43	1.09*	0.30	0.07	0.32	0.16	0.08	0.41
237	Southern	6.26***	2.89*	0.53	0.91	0.26	0.05	0.33	0.06	0.17	0.52
238	Western	4.32	2.89	0.86	1.37**	0.24	0.16	0.31	0.25	0.40	0.25
NETHERLANDS		1.93	1.26	0.29	0.34	0.23	0.12	0.27	0.15	0.54	0.42**
239	Groningen	1.80	0.94	0.19	0.12	0.14	0.19	0.30	0.05	0.40	0.15
240	Friesland	3.46	1.08	0.32	0.52	0.43	0.14	0.15	0.19	0.86	0.29
241	Drenthe	2.19	0.93	0.17	0.00	0.25	0.06	0.34	0.06	0.27	0.49
242	Overijssel	2.31	1.16	0.14	0.23	0.27	0.18	0.17	0.22	0.57	0.41
243	Gelderland	2.23	1.16	0.32	0.34	0.30	0.12	0.36	0.11	0.55	0.38
244	Utrecht	1.30	1.11	0.23	0.31	0.15	0.03	0.20	0.15	0.65	0.22
245	Noord Holland	1.92	0.88	0.37	0.44	0.25	0.10	0.26	0.17	0.52	0.52**
246	Zuid Holland	1.84	1.48	0.36	0.39	0.17	0.10	0.26	0.14	0.53	0.42
247	Zeeland	1.54	1.40	0.44	0.10	0.15	0.29	0.54	0.07	0.55	0.30
248	Noord Brabant	1.35	1.68	0.19	0.30	0.18	0.13	0.18	0.22	0.56	0.56***
249	Limburg	2.13	1.31	0.24	0.47	0.31	0.19	0.45	0.10	0.47	0.43
UK: ENGLAND AND WAL ES		3.95***	2.73***	0.75***	0.94***	0.24	0.10	0.33	0.20	0.30	0.24
250	Cleveland	4.26*	2.83	0.98**	0.98*	0.48	0.26	0.48	0.22	0.31	0.35
251	Cumbria	4.22	2.97	0.78	0.91	0.30	0.00	0.14	0.05	0.42	0.10
252	Durham	5.72***	3.48**	0.89*	1.64***	0.27	0.16	0.15	0.15	0.42	0.19

Table 9.1.3(b) cont

Area		Age-standardized death rates (per 100 000)									
		RESP		ASTH		APP		HERN		CHOLY	
		1974–78	1980–84	1974–78	1980–84	1974–78	1980–84	1974–78	1980–84	1974–78	1980–84
253	Northumberland	3.61	2.44	0.76	0.72	0.32	0.00	0.30	0.16	0.31	0.23
254	Gateshead	2.99	2.07	0.33	1.89***	0.21	0.11	0.20	0.11	0.31	0.21
255	Newcastle upon Tyne	1.43	1.65	0.38	0.77	0.48	0.17	0.22	0.17	0.08	0.33
256	Northern Tyneside	3.89	3.36	0.55	0.19	0.11	0.12	0.21	0.22	0.21	0.33
257	Southern Tyneside	1.73	0.70	1.31**	0.93	0.42	0.00	0.13	0.40	0.40	0.13
258	Sunderland	4.48	2.27	0.86	0.83	0.25	0.41**	0.41	0.08	0.25	0.66*
259	Bradford	6.09***	3.97***	1.45***	1.02*	0.27	0.05	0.26	0.05	0.58	0.11
260	Calderdale	3.36	1.61	0.81	0.38	0.25	0.13	0.35	0.25	0.23	0.13
261	Humberside	3.86	3.48**	0.64	0.71	0.20	0.09	0.28	0.25	0.33	0.23
262	Kirklees	4.19	2.33	0.60	0.94	0.26	0.27	0.25	0.27	0.19	0.20
263	Leeds	3.49	2.29	0.95**	0.70	0.16	0.07	0.34	0.17	0.35	0.27
264	North Yorkshire	5.48***	2.21	0.39	0.58	0.07	0.07	0.35	0.14	0.28	0.07
265	Wakefield	4.59*	4.91***	0.47	0.88	0.39	0.00	0.53	0.08	0.15	0.23
266	Barnsley	4.32	2.29	0.65	1.11	0.21	0.00	0.51	0.21	0.41	0.31
267	Derbyshire	4.14*	2.90*	0.16	0.70	0.16	0.08	0.35	0.21	0.28	0.13
268	Doncaster	3.08	1.39	1.12**	0.85	0.08	0.08	0.08	0.33	0.25	0.16
269	Leicestershire	3.34	3.16**	0.60	0.84	0.27	0.15	0.15	0.15	0.24	0.21
270	Lincolnshire	3.50	3.09*	0.21	0.91	0.27	0.09	0.26	0.17	0.13	0.17
271	Nottinghamshire	3.05	2.66	0.66	1.06**	0.27	0.15	0.17	0.19	0.29	0.27
272	Rotherham	3.41	2.31	0.29	0.96	0.10	0.10	0.87**	0.10	0.29	0.29
273	Sheffield	4.87**	1.98	0.54	0.66	0.13	0.00	0.34	0.26	0.31	0.21
274	Cambridgeshire	4.22*	1.17	0.50	0.85	0.18	0.04	0.32	0.31	0.00	0.22
275	Norfolk	4.03	3.61**	1.53***	1.00*	0.33	0.07	0.57*	0.24	0.48	0.24
276	Suffolk	4.30*	2.72	0.45	1.54***	0.00	0.13	0.45	0.41*	0.37	0.16
277	Barnet	3.95	1.16	0.86	0.96	0.31	0.09	0.36	0.16	0.43	0.25
278	Bedfordshire	4.98**	2.54	0.77	1.17**	0.05	0.05	0.32	0.16	0.27	0.31
279	Brent and Harrow	4.73*	2.17	0.83*	1.52***	0.05	0.11	0.24	0.06	0.29	0.17
280	Ealing/Hammersmith/Hounslow	4.22*	3.87***	0.64	1.17**	0.25	0.04	0.21	0.36*	0.38	0.04
281	Hertfordshire	3.76	2.37	0.62	0.93*	0.15	0.00	0.17	0.27	0.17	0.19
282	Hillingdon	3.88	1.89	1.06*	0.45	0.10	0.10	0.19	0.20	0.57	0.20
283	Kensington/Chelsea/Westminster	4.31	2.82	1.37***	0.68	0.27	0.16	0.45	0.39	0.38	0.24
284	Barking and Havering	4.14	4.15**	0.74	1.22**	0.40	0.12	0.38	0.06	0.38	0.17
285	Camden and Islington	2.53	1.64	0.48	1.05*	0.27	0.22	0.32	0.44*	0.26	0.29
286	City and East London	6.30***	4.55***	0.77	1.77***	0.29	0.05	0.23	0.18	0.51	0.41
287	Enfield and Haringey	3.13	3.34*	0.44	0.89	0.34	0.05	0.41	0.11	0.09	0.43
288	Essex	3.10	2.00	0.76*	0.71	0.21	0.13	0.32	0.13	0.29	0.30
289	Redbridge and Waltham Forest	3.29	3.44*	1.06**	1.14*	0.31	0.06	0.28	0.11	0.19	0.11
290	Bromley	2.73	1.96	0.24	1.45**	0.23	0.08	0.14	0.00	0.29	0.07
291	East Sussex	7.57***	2.78	0.99**	1.03*	0.26	0.00	0.36	0.14	0.30	0.21
292	Greenwich and Bexley	3.81	2.67	0.42	1.21**	0.16	0.17	0.15	0.17	0.26	0.39
293	Kent	4.98***	2.60*	0.79**	0.65	0.31	0.12	0.36	0.13	0.20	0.32
294	Lambeth/Southwark/Lewisham	4.57**	2.48	1.15***	0.81	0.15	0.28*	0.29	0.38*	0.18	0.21
295	Croydon	2.95	1.99	0.54	0.64	0.29	0.16	0.21	0.08	0.14	0.31
296	Kingston and Richmond	4.16	2.12	0.48	1.20*	0.08	0.25	0.21	0.08	0.07	0.16
297	Merton/Sutton/Wandsworth	3.91	2.75	0.71	1.24***	0.23	0.04	0.28	0.12	0.36	0.16
298	Surrey	3.22	2.93*	1.11***	0.95*	0.23	0.09	0.40	0.20	0.49	0.11
299	West Sussex	3.09	2.09	1.03**	0.81	0.40	0.08	0.33	0.07	0.11	0.14
300	Dorset	3.52	3.55**	1.65***	1.25**	0.29	0.12	0.22	0.34	0.30	0.23
301	Hampshire	3.21	3.73***	0.68	0.89*	0.16	0.02	0.23	0.17	0.26	0.10
302	Isle of Wight	3.84	2.09	0.75	1.70*	0.42	0.42	0.36	0.00	0.55	0.00
303	Wiltshire	3.95	3.10*	0.76	0.65	0.20	0.14	0.39	0.24	0.25	0.14
304	Berkshire	2.70	1.58	0.86*	0.52	0.15	0.07	0.19	0.11	0.23	0.11
305	Buckinghamshire	3.64	3.09*	0.58	0.80	0.10	0.09	0.39	0.09	0.10	0.23
306	Northamptonshire	2.51	1.98	0.78	0.90	0.00	0.14	0.49	0.05	0.20	0.19
307	Oxfordshire	2.83	2.57	0.51	0.90	0.00	0.05	0.30	0.20	0.10	0.20
308	Avon	3.31	1.68	0.68	0.95*	0.03	0.13	0.25	0.21	0.31	0.31
309	Cornwall and Scilly Isles	3.42	2.61	0.29	0.80	0.23	0.00	0.21	0.21	0.32	0.48
310	Devon	3.55	2.81*	1.18***	1.06**	0.10	0.10	0.38	0.30	0.26	0.12
311	Gloucestershire	3.03	4.07***	0.75	0.99*	0.25	0.15	0.28	0.28	0.34	0.28
312	Somerset	4.00	1.78	0.65	1.19**	0.12	0.06	0.28	0.33	0.22	0.11
313	Birmingham	3.19	2.89*	0.63	1.39***	0.27	0.07	0.42	0.26	0.32	0.35

Table 9.1.3(b) cont

Area		RESP		ASTH		APP		HERN		CHOLY	
		1974–78	1980–84	1974–78	1980–84	1974–78	1980–84	1974–78	1980–84	1974–78	1980–84
314	Coventry	4.81*	4.21**	0.99*	0.89	0.50	0.08	0.07	0.07	0.42	0.37
315	Dudley	5.14*	2.10	0.58	0.35	0.32	0.24	0.70*	0.08	0.63	0.39
316	Hereford and Worcester	4.99**	2.07	0.60	0.76	0.25	0.16	0.56*	0.27	0.28	0.12
317	Salop	6.74***	1.86	0.20	0.99	0.34	0.07	0.41	0.40*	0.41	0.13
318	Sandwell	3.70	5.35***	0.82	0.72	0.50	0.15	0.40	0.29	0.27	0.15
319	Solihull	7.30***	2.02	0.69	1.53**	0.12	0.12	0.13	0.36	1.00	0.00
320	Staffordshire	3.63	3.40***	0.56	1.07**	0.37	0.07	0.53*	0.24	0.48	0.50*
321	Walsall	6.32***	4.55**	0.51	0.79	0.44	0.18	0.61	0.70***	0.26	0.26
322	Warwickshire	3.39	3.50*	0.60	1.58***	0.26	0.00	0.25	0.30	0.26	0.25
323	Wolverhampton	5.23*	3.52*	0.96*	1.57***	0.09	0.28	0.34	0.18	0.35	0.63
324	Bolton	5.04*	4.84***	0.57	0.95	0.28	0.10	0.62	0.00	0.36	0.47
325	Bury	5.46*	2.87	1.42**	0.60	0.41	0.14	0.40	0.57*	0.27	0.29
326	Lancashire	4.34**	2.59	0.73*	0.96**	0.34	0.13	0.51*	0.51***	0.32	0.26
327	Manchester	3.07	2.44	0.62	0.86	0.34	0.16	0.46	0.27	0.33	0.32
328	Oldham	2.37	3.51	0.33	0.80	0.54	0.00	0.21	0.22	0.21	0.34
329	Rochdale	3.72	2.67	1.23**	0.85	0.23	0.00	0.23	0.24	0.46	0.73*
330	Salford	3.94	3.12	0.72	0.74	0.27	0.20	0.08	0.19	0.26	0.19
331	Stockport	4.06	1.43	0.86	0.73	0.42	0.17	0.24	0.17	0.16	0.08
332	Tameside	5.32*	3.80*	1.01*	0.66	0.32	0.34	0.70*	0.00	0.41	0.22
333	Trafford	2.07	2.92	0.63	0.81	0.42	0.00	0.30	0.00	0.20	0.43
334	Wigan	5.38**	0.95	0.93*	0.77	0.32	0.00	0.55	0.00	0.71	0.24
335	Cheshire	2.70	2.06	0.58	1.04**	0.27	0.05	0.34	0.18	0.37	0.39
336	Liverpool	4.35*	1.95	1.03**	1.01*	0.17	0.10	0.45	0.23	0.42	0.33
337	St Helens and Knowsley	5.96***	1.81	1.01**	0.38	0.13	0.07	0.94***	0.14	0.68	0.55
338	Sefton	2.74	2.89	0.36	0.86	0.16	0.16	0.23	0.08	0.31	0.24
339	Wirral	2.68	2.14	1.09**	0.33	0.07	0.07	0.45	0.07	0.26	0.21
340	Clwyd	4.07	3.70**	0.60	0.28	0.26	0.00	0.36	0.25	0.37	0.25
341	Dyfed	3.72	1.65	0.82	0.56	0.29	0.14	0.13	0.27	0.33	0.47
342	Gwent	5.36**	3.30*	1.57***	0.98	0.16	0.11	0.21	0.16	0.21	0.21
343	Gwynedd	4.61	2.35	0.69	0.66	0.54	0.11	0.49	0.10	0.40	0.10
344	Mid Glamorgan	2.62	2.77	0.82*	1.72***	0.40	0.14	0.25	0.18	0.51	0.48
345	Powys	3.78	2.96	0.37	1.01	0.22	0.00	0.21	0.21	0.00	0.21
346	South Glamorgan	3.17	3.24*	0.75	0.64	0.31	0.06	0.36	0.25	0.37	0.19
347	West Glamorgan	3.70	2.34	0.90*	0.90	0.38	0.07	0.06	0.06	0.18	0.12
	UK:NORTHERN IRELAND										
348	Northern Ireland	3.94**	3.01***	0.52	1.03***	0.18	0.14	0.37	0.24	0.41	0.37
	UK: SCOTLAND	3.12	2.42*	0.90***	0.82**	0.24	0.12	0.35	0.19	0.31	0.02
349	Highlands and Islands	3.85	1.74	1.59***	1.19*	0.20	0.19	0.40	0.10	0.20	0.00
350	Grampian	3.49	1.46	1.12***	0.57	0.11	0.11	0.22	0.16	0.27	0.00
351	Tayside	3.31	3.31*	0.46	0.55	0.25	0.06	0.30	0.36	0.24	0.06
352	Fife	3.98	2.94	0.85	0.41	0.22	0.00	0.36	0.00	0.51	0.00
353	Lothian	3.38	2.39	0.95**	0.79	0.16	0.07	0.13	0.10	0.19	0.00
354	Borders	2.02	1.11	1.17	0.38	0.00	0.24	0.00	0.23	0.46	0.00
355	Forth Valley	4.94*	4.45**	1.31***	0.77	0.18	0.09	0.82**	0.45*	0.27	0.18
356	Argyll and Clyde	2.62	2.41	0.77	0.46	0.11	0.22	0.64*	0.27	0.32	0.05
357	Greater Glasgow	2.55	1.95	0.95***	1.25***	0.33	0.07	0.27	0.16	0.27	0.00
358	Lanarkshire	2.55	3.08*	0.72	0.71	0.31	0.17	0.46	0.22	0.42	0.00
359	Ayrshire and Arran	2.12	1.86	0.67	1.32**	0.46	0.20	0.45	0.32	0.32	0.00
360	Dumfries and Galloway	5.22	2.20	0.51	0.51	0.34	0.17	0.33	0.00	0.66	0.00
EC		3.01	1.98	0.50	0.63	0.35	0.14	0.35	0.20	0.83	0.35

324 Tables of changes

Table 9.1.3(c). Age-standardized death rates (per 100 000) for 1974–78 and 1980–84 by small area standardized to the EC standard, for hypertensive/cerebrovascular diseases, maternal deaths, perinatal deaths, all causes (ages 5–64), and all causes (all ages)

Notes on the use of this table

1. This table shows the mortality rates for small areas standardized to the EC standard for 1974–78 and 1980–84. The rates are in deaths per 100 000 population. The age-standardized death rates are calculated by multiplying the small-area SMR based on the EC standard for that time period by the EC crude death rate for that time period.

2. Key for the abbreviations used for columns of the table:
   HYP/S — hypertensive and cerebrovascular diseases (ICD8 400–404, 430–438; ICD9 401–405, 430–438), ages 35–64;
   MAT — maternal deaths (ICD8 630–678; ICD9 630–676), all ages;
   PER — perinatal mortality (all causes), deaths aged under 1 week plus stillbirths;
   ALL — mortality from all causes (all ICD8/ICD9 codes), ages 5–64;
   ALL — mortality from all causes (all ICD8/ICD9 codes), all ages 1+ years

3. The small area numbers are as in the key maps (pp. 241–5).

4. The indicators have been tested for indicating significant excess mortality relative to EC rates. The *p*-values achieved for one-tail tests are indicated as follows: *p<0.05; **p<0.01; ***p<0.001.

5. The mortality data for the earlier time period are for 1974–78, except for France (1973–77). The population data are for 1974–78, except for France (1975), Ireland (1976), and N. Ireland (1976).

6. The mortality data for the later time period are for 1980–84, except for Greece (1980–82). The population data are for 1980–84 except for France (1982), Ireland (1981), and Greece (1981). All data for Italy are for 1979–83.

Table 9.1.3(c)

Area	HYP/S 1974–78	HYP/S 1980–84	MAT 1974–78	MAT 1980–84	PER 1974–78	PER 1980–84	ALL (5–64) 1974–78	ALL (5–64) 1980–84	ALL (all ages) 1974–78	ALL (all ages) 1980–84
BELGIUM	49.6	35.1	12	7	19*	13**	335***	303***	1155***	1136***
1 Antwerpen	51.1	35.1	10	9	19	13*	306	271	1103***	1073***
2 Brabant	45.3	32.7	12	8	17	12	313	286	1102***	1091***
3 West-Vlaanderen	32.7	26.5	6	4	19	14**	303	276	1077*	1062*
4 Oost-Vlaanderen	47.7	31.1	11	4	19	13	321*	289	1149***	1132***
5 Hainaut	55.7*	42.4	11	4	20***	12	387***	360***	1246***	1258***
6 Liège	55.2	40.0	18	9	18	12	384***	346***	1277***	1256***
7 Limburg	56.0	32.6	13	12	20*	14***	312	271	1099***	1027
8 Luxembourg (province)	65.7***	43.1	14	13	21**	13	383***	346***	1217***	1163***
9 Namur	62.2***	46.3*	19	8	20	13	396***	365***	1269***	1263***
LUXEMBOURG										
10 Luxembourg	66.6***	51.0***	60***	0	14	11	376***	351***	1218***	1167***
FEDERAL REPUBLIC OF GERMANY	47.0	39.5	34***	16***	17	10	329***	299***	1107***	1095***
11 Schleswig–Holstein	43.7	33.5	21	12	15	9	322**	296**	1113***	1104***
12 Hamburg	39.7	36.4	27	14	15	9	350***	323***	1135***	1139***
13 Neidersachsen	44.2	38.6	30***	10	18	10	334***	300***	1108***	1092***
14 Bremen	43.4	44.5*	35*	3	18	9	350***	328***	1091***	1090***
15 Nordrhein–Westfalen	49.7	40.2	43***	20***	19**	11	340***	307***	1128***	1110***
16 Hessen	45.7	37.4	31***	18***	17	9	307	282	1066	106***
17 Rheinland–Pfalz	59.8***	48.0***	43***	20***	18	10	333***	304***	1117***	1119***
18 Baden Wurttemberg	45.2	35.9	25*	13	15	9	299	269	1037	1013
19 Bayern	39.5	37.6	33***	17***	17	9	320***	291	1095***	1080***
20 Saarland	66.9***	52.8***	25	10	21***	11	365***	334***	1178***	1177***
21 Berlin(West)	63.0***	54.9***	39***	13	15	11	426***	405***	1270***	1322***

Table 9.1.3(c) cont

Area	Age-standardized death rates (per 100 000)									
	HYP/S		MAT		PER		ALL (5–64)		ALL (all ages)	
	1974–78	1980–84	1974–78	1980–84	1974–78	1980–84	1974–78	1980–84	1974–78	1980–84
DENMARK	34.5	33.1	6	6	12	9	304	318***	1012	1066***
22 Kobenhavn and Frederiksberg (M)	44.7	42.0	12	8	12	8	400***	444***	1101***	1197***
23 Kobenhavns County	34.8	31.0	8	7	11	7	280	306***	947	996
24 Frederiksborg County	31.7	30.0	5	12	10	8	288	293	995	1031
25 Roskilde County	30.3	30.9	7	0	12	9	281	292	982	1042
26 Vestsjaellands County	34.3	30.5	6	14	13	10	308	316***	1036	1080**
27 Storstroms County	32.4	33.0	7	0	11	8	306	326***	1046	1112***
28 Bornholms County	30.0	27.3	0	0	16	10	269	292	993	1071
29 Fyns County	30.5	29.1	3	0	12	8	277	295	995	1053
30 Sonderjyllands County	30.2	32.4	6	0	14	10	274	283	942	1035
31 Ribe County	35.6	32.4	0	0	13	8	288	295	971	1013
32 Vejle County	31.3	34.5	9	0	12	8	291	304**	998	1038
33 Ringkobing County	30.9	38.3	5	6	13	10	283	290	968	1015
34 Arhus County	32.5	29.9	0	3	13	11	297	306***	1002	1050
35 Viborg County	30.8	35.7	6	8	13	10	277	281	995	1016
36 Nordjyllands County	34.6	31.9	6	15	13	10	280	300*	985	1029
FRANCE	48.3	33.5	20	14***	17	12	331***	298***	1019	1019
37 Ain	44.6	29.2	8	20	15	11	315	276	1011	996
38 Aisne	62.0***	39.4	34*	19	19	13	385***	347***	1128***	1158***
39 Allier	54.2	37.0	32	15	18	13	323	304**	1055	1058
40 Alpes-de-Haute-Provence	41.4	31.1	17	14	18	14	281	280	928	877
41 Hautes-Alpes	46.6	28.2	16	14	14	13	310	271	964	959
42 Alpes-Maritimes	26.4	23.9	19	10	18	13	284	258	875	894
43 Ardcèhe	51.4	34.8	7	18	16	14	324	278	1038	1010
44 Ardennes	59.0*	38.5	16	13	22***	14*	405***	350***	1150***	1133***
45 Ariège	45.4	24.9	106***	0	17	15	265	247	946	998
46 Aube	44.9	34.7	0	15	20	12	344***	308***	1001	1032
47 Aude	35.1	26.3	7	13	20	11	257	242	932	955
48 Aveyron	43.1	27.8	6	20	17	13	258	228	961	937
49 Bouches-du-Rhône	43.2	31.4	23	20**	17	13	308	280	975	993
50 Calvados	54.9	36.9	7	9	16	10	364***	316***	1053	1033
51 Cantal	63.1**	43.0	58**	10	17	15**	328*	299	1044	1073*
52 Charente	49.2	29.0	32	18	19	13	294	264	973	986
53 Charente-Maritime	46.3	28.5	16	6	16	11	304	269	981	959
54 Cher	52.6	33.8	20	10	16	12	327*	302*	1041	1027
55 Corrèze	56.0	34.5	47*	0	17	11	302	270	1003	1017
56 Corse	31.3	32.6	24	7	20	14*	279	287	925	968
57 Côte-d'Or	46.5	29.2	20	17	14	13	320	285	1000	980
58 Côtes-du-Nord	66.0***	45.0*	23	9	18	9	410***	345***	1096***	1099***
59 Creuse	55.9	47.7	0	3	22*	10	333*	304*	1042	1057
60 Dordogne	55.7	37.9	20	48**	17	12	305	270	1017	998
61 Doubs	43.8	32.7	25	20	18	12	303	280	1002	973
62 Drôme	47.7	27.0	33	3	16	13	306	269	988	963
63 Eure	55.1	34.3	15	14	18	13	368***	330***	1060	1054
64 Eure-et-Loir	42.0	29.8	19	7	17	11	322	282	1006	975
65 Finistère	60.0***	43.6	38**	14	16	10	407***	358***	1094***	1095***
66 Gard	40.7	26.3	7	20	18	14**	294	272	974	985
67 Haute-Garonne	42.8	25.7	16	14	17	11	268	241	944	927
68 Gers	43.3	28.6	35	12	16	12	271	250	963	960
69 Gironde	48.6	31.5	19	9	16	11	313	275	1017	1013
70 Hérault	37.3	28.9	23	18	18	14*	270	250	913	952
71 Ille-et-Vilaine	68.6***	41.0	18	11	17	11	361***	306***	1069	1072***
72 Indre	55.0	35.4	34	0	19	13	311	284	986	1024
73 Indre-et-Loire	39.0	22.2	18	9	13	10	294	261	951	930
74 Isère	39.5	27.6	6	10	15	11	306	273	999	985
75 Jura	50.8	36.6	6	12	19	13	316	275	1031	997
76 Landes	55.5	31.9	12	0	17	12	317	265	1011	994
77 Loir-et-Cher	46.0	37.7	5	5	15	9	308	279	930	956
78 Loire	48.5	31.3	36**	10	18	11	340***	298*	1049	1040
79 Haute-Loire	50.6	37.0	24	16	16	12	327*	298	1036	1048

Table 9.1.3(c)

Area		Age-standardized death rates (per 100 000)									
		HYP/S		MAT		PER		ALL (5–64)		ALL (all ages)	
		1974–78	1980–84	1974–78	1980–84	1974–78	1980–84	1974–78	1980–84	1974–78	1980–84
80	Loire-Atlantique	56.7*	36.8	18	8	16	11	392***	331***	1085***	1059
81	Loiret	44.6	28.6	25	3	15	12	301	274	996	962
82	Lot	62.3*	34.8	13	0	19	12	282	235	1020	973
83	Lot-et-Garonne	38.8	31.3	30	11	16	12	277	243	981	964
84	Lozère	38.4	37.1	22	22	20	15	315	271	1048	1029
85	Maine-et-Loire	48.2	30.4	16	5	16	11	308	277	992	979
86	Manche	58.1*	36.1	6	9	17	10	344***	294	1022	1023
87	Marne	51.6	31.6	28	18	18	11	362***	318***	1052	1034
88	Haute-Marne	44.9	33.3	25	43***	20	13	346***	321***	1056	1070
89	Mayenne	54.2	34.2	14	5	16	11	327*	278	1049	994
90	Meurthe-et-Moselle	50.3	37.3	31*	11	19	11	354***	331***	1077*	1093***
91	Meuse	56.4	41.9	47*	34**	18	15**	388***	348***	1124***	1123***
92	Morbihan	77.6***	52.2***	12	9	19	11	443***	389***	1177***	1160***
93	Moselle	61.4***	43.0	24	35***	19	13	377***	334***	1143***	1136***
94	Nivre	52.7	38.7	28	14	17	12	332**	324***	1034	1078**
95	Nord	66.5***	46.7***	23	12	20***	14***	435***	391***	1214***	1222***
96	Oise	55.2	34.5	24	8	16	12	388***	315***	1112***	1080***
97	Orne	51.3	34.5	27	9	18	9	337***	303*	1048	1030
98	Pas-de-Calais	66.2***	48.2***	24	14	21***	15***	438***	395***	1203***	1192***
99	Puy-de-Dôme	51.6	36.4	18	10	18	14***	344***	310***	1078*	1064
100	Pyrénées-Atlantiques	50.5	28.9	19	21	18	11	296	266	964	980
101	Hautes-Pyrénées	54.6	35.1	33	8	20	14	304	264	1028	992
102	Pyrénées-Orientales	38.6	28.3	42*	47***	17	13	287	258	948	944
103	Bas-Rhin	59.2***	40.5	8	6	16	9	372***	321***	1096***	1113***
104	Haut-Rhin	55.4	41.0	39**	19	16	12	387***	321***	1125***	1146***
105	Rhône	43.0	27.1	19	15	15	11	313	273	1000	970
106	Haute-Saône	52.0	41.1	37	24	20	12	338***	303*	1056	1070*
107	Saône-et-Loire	54.3	34.0	29	16	17	13	322	293	1028	1021
108	Sarthe	40.2	25.0	8	20	16	11	294	263	956	943
109	Savoie	47.1	32.5	9	4	14	9	350***	291	1070	997
110	Haute-Savoie	45.2	29.9	18	11	15	10	339***	292	1021	979
111	Paris	37.2	28.1	18	19**	16	12	320**	294	895	915
112	Seine-Maritime	46.0	36.2	15	9	17	12	364***	342***	1042	1070***
113	Seine-et-Marne	44.1	28.7	32*	15	15	11	329***	292	1062	1060
114	Yvelines	35.9	26.6	14	23***	14	11	284	252	966	948
115	Deux-Sèvres	41.1	29.1	21	18	18	12	271	235	956	946
116	Somme	53.6	35.1	30	17	20**	13	365***	343***	1103***	1145***
117	Tarn	43.1	27.6	15	10	18	12	265	234	939	958
118	Tarn-et-Garonne	51.3	31.8	57**	0	19	14	282	245	970	956
119	Var	40.0	29.6	5	9	19	13	304	274	954	942
120	Vaucluse	43.5	29.1	16	10	17	14*	305	275	968	984
121	Vendée	63.2***	35.1	5	0	16	10	304	266	994	980
122	Vienne	45.9	27.4	41*	8	18	12	288	249	934	910
123	Haute-Vienne	48.1	33.5	46**	16	16	9	284	255	953	964
124	Vosges	55.6	41.4	17	34***	18	12	372***	336***	1075	1086***
125	Yonne	49.1	36.5	10	10	18	11	353***	328***	1065	1066
126	Territoire-de-Belfort	46.3	37.1	10	10	14	11	337**	312**	1071	1093**
127	Essonne	39.4	30.1	12	20*	14	10	286	265	956	956
128	Hauts-de-Seine	35.4	28.3	5	16	14	12	292	271	932	946
129	Seine-Saint-Denis	40.7	32.1	21	15	15	13	339***	315***	1018	1019
130	Val-de-Marne	39.1	28.1	26	18*	14	11	310	279	990	994
131	Val-d'Oise	40.0	28.3	19	12	15	12	301	281	999	1034
GREECE		49.1	46.0***	-	8	-	18***	236	346	938	938
132	Greater Athens	52.0	46.9***	-	5	-	19***	246	231	947	943
133	Rest of Central Greece and Eubea	44.9	48.1***	-	12	-	15***	220	222	912	927
134	Peloponnisos	49.0	43.1	-	4	-	19***	211	210	911	916
135	Ionian Islands	32.6	46.2	-	9	-	14*	168	222	858	1061
136	Epirus	40.4	39.6	-	18	-	18***	232	228	906	889
137	Thessaly	50.9	47.8**	-	0	-	15***	239	241	932	976
138	Macedonia	49.8	44.9**	-	7	-	19***	247	232	972	972

Table 9.1.3(c) cont

Area | Age-standardized death rates (per 100 000)

		HYP/S		MAT		PER		ALL (5–64)		ALL (all ages)	
		1974–78	1980–84	1974–78	1980–84	1974–78	1980–84	1974–78	1980–84	1974–78	1980–84
139	Thrace	73.2***	61.1***	-	42***	-	18***	309	280	1091**	1034
140	Aegean Islands	43.6	43.1	-	21	-	15***	212	218	942	968
141	Crete	37.4	41.5	-	8	-	14***	202	205	852	863
ITALY		61.1***	50.4***	23***	11	23***	16***	295	275	1021	1003
142	Torino	62.2***	52.1***	30**	14	26***	17***	313	283	1096***	938
143	Vercelli	74.5***	65.6***	15	7	19	19***	330***	311***	1145***	1317***
144	Novara	74.2***	61.6***	28	9	20	13	351***	315***	1148***	1094***
145	Cuneo	71.1***	54.8***	28	12	21***	15**	334***	303***	1139***	1069**
146	Asti	60.5**	55.1***	40	38*	24***	15*	290	266	1085*	1190***
147	Alessandria	57.1*	50.9***	14	7	22***	15***	302	277	1070	988
148	Aosta	69.1***	45.5	17	0	23**	15	406***	351***	1172***	1390***
149	Imperia	48.5	42.8	28	0	22**	12	272	277	1013	946
150	Savona	53.7	45.7	21	0	21**	15*	287	268	1051	994
151	Genova	51.6	43.8*	21	12	20*	13	296	283	1067	966
152	La Spezia	44.4	43.2	17	12	18	13	261	256	972	1224***
153	Varese	66.2***	53.1***	16	8	15	15***	313	281	1088***	974
154	Como/Sondrio	77.5***	56.8***	26	2	19	12	346***	311***	1139***	1051
155	Milano	68.0***	51.8***	13	7	20***	13***	327***	297***	1052	956
156	Bergamo	83.8***	64.0***	12	8	20**	14***	379***	347***	1155***	1306***
157	Brescia	78.9***	61.2***	16	6	20*	13	380***	355***	1173***	1115***
158	Pavia	73.1***	67.7***	11	11	22***	13	343***	337***	1140***	1154***
159	Cremona	84.0***	68.9***	30	14	23***	13	396***	360***	1247***	1254***
160	Mantova	69.3***	61.2***	32	7	19	13	325*	299*	1119***	1070*
161	Bolzano	50.4	44.6	7	19	16	12	321	303**	1023	1044
162	Trento	65.5***	44.8	15	5	18	13	357***	323***	1076	1031
163	Verona	72.3***	56.5***	28	13	18	15***	325**	304***	1068	1003
164	Vicenza	70.6***	57.8***	28	11	17	12	347***	314***	1118***	1076***
165	Belluno	65.6***	61.7***	24	21	17	12	393***	379***	1112***	1223***
166	Treviso	56.1*	45.0*	12	6	16	12	327***	299**	1024	934
167	Venezia	57.5**	42.7	14	0	18	14**	335***	313***	1015	997
168	Padova	58.3**	46.9***	18	8	20*	14*	325**	307***	1050	1017
169	Rovigo	59.9*	50.1**	13	17	19	12	335***	312***	1117***	1206***
170	Udine/Gorizia	64.4***	52.3***	19	8	18	13	405***	355***	1124***	1019
171	Trieste	55.0	38.7	16	13	13	8	340***	322***	1079*	1121***
172	Pordenone	54.5	44.4	15	8	19	12	360***	334***	1072	1087***
173	Piacenza	63.8***	53.0***	29	10	17	13	326*	314***	1063	998
174	Parma	57.9*	46.7**	14	14	19	16***	294	270	991	950
175	Reggio Emilia	64.1***	42.1	14	0	20	14	296	258	1017	945
176	Modena	53.0	41.6	24	8	19	14*	283	268	991	930
177	Bologna	48.9	42.4	33*	17	22***	14*	271	258	979	905
178	Ferrara	61.9***	44.2	18	16	21***	14	305	286	1021	1099***
179	Ravenna	39.8	36.4	16	0	18	13	255	239	934	906
180	Forli	46.1	35.9	8	19	17	12	264	242	961	893
181	Pesaro	43.7	39.9	35	19	19	13	252	237	930	969
182	Ancona	51.9	41.0	24	5	15	13	249	225	944	881
183	Macerata	53.7	41.5	24	15	18	16***	240	225	935	944
184	Ascoli Piceno	61.0**	43.4	18	6	17	15**	241	219	944	903
185	Massa-Carrara	55.2	48.6*	10	11	22**	15*	289	280	993	1038
186	Lucca	51.7	43.2	4	6	17	14	292	276	1015	967
187	Pistoia	49.2	35.0	0	0	21*	12	248	249	934	1019
188	Firenze	41.2	37.4	17	4	19	14***	249	233	923	848
189	Livorno	42.7	41.4	10	22	20	15**	268	256	980	1150***
190	Pisa	42.6	32.9	39*	19	18	14*	256	241	982	966
191	Arezzo	45.4	40.1	37	8	20	15**	253	237	944	965
192	Siena	47.8	40.3	7	0	22**	16***	232	227	928	927
193	Grosseto	53.0	46.6*	9	48***	23***	15*	271	261	978	995
194	Perugia	57.5**	44.5	6	7	16	11	256	242	954	871
195	Terni	46.8	40.3	0	0	20	18***	240	224	951	1064
196	Viterbo/Rieti	55.8	49.4***	19	14	24***	15***	264	266	1008	961
197	Roma	50.6	41.3	15	11	18	15***	264	253	979	885

Table 9.1.3(c) cont

Area	Age-standardized death rates (per 100 000)									
	HYP/S		MAT		PER		ALL (5–64)		ALL (all ages)	
	1974–78	1980–84	1974–78	1980–84	1974–78	1980–84	1974–78	1980–84	1974–78	1980–84
198 Latina	55.9	51.0***	25	7	23***	16***	267	251	928	1364***
199 Frosinone	62.2***	58.4***	23	13	22***	16***	264	248	965	923
200 Caserta	94.8***	78.4***	25	17	32***	18***	321	295	1077	1063
201 Benevento	63.4***	54.2***	33	30**	29***	16***	259	235	946	1013
202 Napoli	79.4***	68.3***	27**	11	29***	19***	338***	322***	1147***	1072***
203 Avellino	61.2***	48.5**	33	7	27***	15***	239	280	905	1305***
204 Salerno	66.3***	56.4***	26	18*	28***	18***	262	252	905	886
205 L'Aquila	64.1***	50.1***	20	12	21**	16***	286	267	1011	1103***
206 Teramo	51.6	46.4*	18	12	21*	13	236	235	913	972
207 Pescara	55.4	46.2*	22	25	20	15**	237	218	909	902
208 Chieti	53.8	40.7	25	5	20	16***	234	225	938	880
209 Isernia/Campobasso	63.0***	55.9***	19	15	24***	16***	256	243	940	948
210 Foggia	59.7***	49.4***	37**	9	26***	18***	255	239	912	898
211 Bari	56.6**	48.0***	27*	5	27***	18***	267	241	947	888
212 Taranto	63.0***	44.6	11	25**	25***	18***	262	240	958	1099***
213 Brindisi	61.5**	50.0***	17	9	25***	18***	278	253	1004	1002
214 Lecce	55.3	45.6*	20	9	26***	17***	260	236	994	910
215 Potenza/Matera	58.3**	54.5***	37**	7	28***	17***	243	234	910	935
216 Cosenza	61.8***	58.3***	24	9	28***	17***	239	237	897	906
217 Catanzaro	60.9***	48.3***	19	17	27***	17***	248	238	907	919
218 Reggio Calabria	52.3	48.8***	43***	2	28***	19***	268	249	892	925
219 Trapani	61.7***	62.0***	20	10	24***	15***	255	240	965	1003
220 Palermo	67.1***	57.1***	28*	18	25***	22***	270	253	981	940
221 Messina	58.3**	47.8***	46***	16	26***	19***	251	221	940	983
222 Agrigento	58.8**	51.2***	53***	6	29***	16***	245	227	921	1002
223 Caltanisetta	73.0***	54.3***	58***	18	31***	21***	271	253	1002	1076**
224 Enna	66.0***	65.0***	33	20	33***	17***	259	244	1006	1031
225 Catania	75.4***	59.4***	43***	20*	23***	19***	280	253	1008	940
226 Ragusa	58.6*	55.8***	16	51***	21***	17***	242	232	997	1213***
227 Siracusa	70.6***	52.8***	44**	18	28***	18***	264	235	1017	951
228 Sassari	58.2*	49.0**	10	15	21***	17***	285	261	994	960
229 Nuoro	53.1	49.9**	25	22	27***	16***	281	281	959	1044
230 Cagliari/Oristano	51.6	46.0**	22	12	23***	19***	277	264	982	905
IRELAND	70.4***	50.1***	14	7	20***	14***	352***	331***	1250***	1218***
231 Eastern	65.2***	51.9***	10	4	20***	14***	343***	333***	1185***	1172***
232 Midland	73.5***	44.0	10	14	20*	11	363***	331***	1297***	1282***
233 Mid-Western	79.8***	55.6***	12	6	21**	13*	368***	345***	1334***	1294***
234 North Eastern	81.2***	54.5***	14	10	20*	14**	376***	337***	1299***	1236***
235 North Western	68.0***	52.6**	36	5	19	14*	329*	320***	1224***	1207***
236 South Eastern	71.1***	49.6**	13	10	19	15***	353***	330***	1296***	1265***
237 Southern	71.5***	49.0***	12	4	21***	14***	364***	342***	1293***	1241***
238 Western	63.7***	41.0	29	12	18	11	310	297	1173***	1162***
NETHERLANDS	34.2	28.4	11	8	14	10	266	246	973	917
239 Groningen	33.3	28.9	12	3	14	10	275	255	975	967
240 Friesland	35.8	29.1	10	10	15	10	267	245	1000	977
241 Drenthe	34.3	27.0	11	12	14	10	282	248	959	949
242 Overijssel	35.8	30.4	14	8	14	10	277	251	974	961
243 Gelderland	38.0	29.9	11	3	14	10	268	252	982	726
244 Utrecht	32.9	29.5	12	9	13	11	256	236	973	947
245 Noord Holland	30.4	24.5	16	10	13	11	257	247	971	959
246 Zuid Holland	32.2	27.9	9	9	13	10	256	242	953	937
247 Zeeland	25.5	24.7	14	0	14	11	248	229	932	926
248 Noord Brabant	37.4	30.1	5	9	15	11	269	242	970	948
249 Limburg	39.2	30.9	8	5	15	11	284	261	1014	979
UK: ENGLAND AND WALES	56.3***	44.9***	12	9	18	11	321***	298***	1111***	1090***
250 Cleveland	65.4***	56.6***	10	10	20**	13	387***	366***	1216***	1222***
251 Cumbria	63.3***	55.6***	18	18	19	13	341***	322***	1153***	1138***
252 Durham	66.4***	56.9***	22	13	20*	12	379***	349***	1232***	1193***

Table 9.1.3(c) cont

Area		Age-standardized death rates (per 100 000)									
		HYP/S		MAT		PER		ALL (5–64)		ALL (all ages)	
		1974–78	1980–84	1974–78	1980–84	1974–78	1980–84	1974–78	1980–84	1974–78	1980–84
253	Northumberland	68.0***	49.4**	11	0	19	10	349***	322***	1201***	1195***
254	Gateshead	64.6***	63.6***	238	22**	13	393***	380***	1217***	1224***	
255	Newcastle upon Tyne	65.7***	53.2***	1	6	17	12	390***	361***	1191***	1182***
256	Northern Tyneside	66.2***	47.1*	0	9	19	11	377***	344***	1214***	1184***
257	Southern Tyneside	67.7***	57.8***	11	10	19	13	394***	376***	1227***	1230***
258	Sunderland	67.3***	57.4***	21	10	21*	13	384***	356***	1238***	1214***
259	Bradford	75.9***	60.5***	30	8	20**	14**	365***	341***	1208***	1210***
260	Calderdale	60.5*	58.5***	0	24	20	14*	368***	341***	1218***	1196***
261	Humberside	52.5	46.8***	17	9	20*	13	328***	309***	1129***	1114***
262	Kirklees	66.1***	54.0***	8	11	20*	14*	358***	336***	1195***	1220***
263	Leeds	59.8***	47.7***	11	9	19	12	351***	332***	1126***	1127***
264	North Yorkshire	53.7	43.7	8	8	17	13	295	276	1074	1080***
265	Wakefield	57.5*	45.2	0	14	21*	14	360***	338***	1196***	1212***
266	Barnsley	62.6**	43.9	8	7	20*	10	354***	331***	1200***	1133***
267	Derbyshire	61.4***	48.8***	11	12	18	12	327***	304***	1136***	1116***
268	Doncaster	56.6	50.3***	5	20	17	11	352***	320***	1153***	1128***
269	Leicestershire	52.3	43.6	5	10	20*	11	296	279	1069	1049
270	Lincolnshire	54.4	44.4	21	9	19	11	305	293	1114***	1091***
271	Nottinghamshire	62.7***	48.5***	13	2	17	11	330***	306***	1130***	1107***
272	Rotherham	58.3*	50.9***	6	12	17	14**	339***	324***	1148***	1126***
273	Sheffield	61.5***	49.3***	3	7	17	12	339***	319***	1138***	1116***
274	Cambridgeshire	45.1	35.6	5	8	15	10	275	253	1011	1012
275	Norfolk	43.3	33.9	18	15	15	11	260	249	1032	998
276	Suffolk	43.3	33.9	8	13	14	10	264	247	1030	1001
277	Barnet	39.4	29.9	6	5	16	9	277	240	1031	988
278	Bedfordshire	52.9	40.5	14	13	17	11	297	266	1069	1029
279	Brent and Harrow	42.6	35.4	13	3	17	10	287	261	991	957
280	Ealing/Hammersmith/Hounslow	50.4	41.6	28	4	17	10	322*	308***	1086***	1084***
281	Hertfordshire	45.2	33.9	5	5	16	9	274	251	1048	997
282	Hillingdon	44.0	31.2	7	13	17	11	281	268	1014	990
283	Kensington/Chelsea/Westminster	50.1	50.6***	5	10	15	10	353***	334***	1036	1035
284	Barking and Havering	48.2	35.2	29	13	17	11	303	285	1067	1056
285	Camden and Islington	61.2***	44.6	15	4	15	11	359***	338***	1095***	1082***
286	City and East London	60.2***	51.9***	33*	10	19	13*	379***	358***	1163***	1156***
287	Enfield and Haringey	49.4	38.0	20	13	16	11	295	278	1056	1059
288	Essex	43.9	33.5	14	5	16	10	276	259	1049	1031
289	Redbridge and Waltham Forest	49.3	39.3	24	10	19	11	297	274	1075	1015
290	Bromley	38.7	35.6	6	0	17	8	262	244	1013	991
291	East Sussex	49.4	38.1	0	12	18	10	283	267	1072	1045
292	Greenwich and Bexley	49.9	37.2	15	7	18	11	297	276	1079*	1035
293	Kent	51.8	39.2	11	4	16	12	296	271	1095***	1074***
294	Lambeth/Southwark/Lewisham	57.5**	50.8***	11	12	20*	12	347***	333***	1122***	1109***
295	Croydon	60.5**	41.4	10	0	18	10	282	266	1102***	1075**
296	Kingston and Richmond	40.5	36.3	18	6	15	9	273	256	1028	997
297	Merton/Sutton/Wandsworth	49.6	40.5	19	3	17	10	305	289	1088***	1076***
298	Surrey	38.5	31.1	13	11	15	10	268	245	1036	999
299	West Sussex	49.2	33.5	15	8	15	11	269	248	1038	1016
300	Dorset	49.5	34.1	18	7	16	9	278	260	1023	977
301	Hampshire	47.6	33.9	8	5	16	10	286	261	1051	1023
302	Isle of Wight	64.2**	38.7	0	0	17	12	301	267	1052	1009
303	Wiltshire	51.1	36.2	15	9	16	10	281	263	1043	1026
304	Berkshire	37.0	34.3	2	4	15	9	271	254	1029	1030
305	Buckinghamshire	38.2	34.7	11	8	16	11	257	244	1004	1000
306	Northamptonshire	48.6	43.5	14	8	16	12	294	276	1064	1056
307	Oxfordshire	41.9	32.9	9	3	12	8	264	248	1016	981
308	Avon	49.4	36.5	6	7	17	11	288	264	1060	1025
309	Cornwall and Scilly Isles	46.2	38.8	9	12	17	10	300	278	1068	1048
310	Devon	51.9	38.3	12	13	16	10	290	276	1054	1038
311	Gloucestershire	51.3	44.4	7	0	16	10	282	267	1045	1028
312	Somerset	56.0	42.4	4	4	17	10	283	259	1065	1036
313	Birmingham	70.3***	56.4***	14	7	21***	13**	359***	332***	1174***	1165***

Table 9.1.3(c) cont

Area		Age-standardized death rates (per 100 000)									
		HYP/S		MAT		PER		ALL (5–64)		ALL (all ages)	
		1974–78	1980–84	1974–78	1980–84	1974–78	1980–84	1974–78	1980–84	1974–78	1980–84
314	Coventry	58.5*	53.3***	10	9	21*	14**	329**	320***	1087**	1081***
315	Dudley	60.8**	51.2***	11	0	23***	11	322	293	1106***	1090***
316	Hereford and Worcester	57.9**	44.8*	5	15	17	12	288	271	1065	1074***
317	Salop	58.2*	50.1***	0	21	19	15**	311	278	1101***	1078***
318	Sandwell	73.9***	63.4***	5	19	23***	17***	374***	341***	1188***	1135***
319	Solihull	40.6	33.1	16	9	17	12	283	244	973	942
320	Staffordshire	61.1***	48.4***	13	6	21***	14**	334***	320***	1150***	1142***
321	Walsall	65.2***	53.7***	13	6	23***	15**	349***	333***	1146***	1144***
322	Warwickshire	54.0	43.5	21	3	20	12	304	286	1086**	1097***
323	Wolverhampton	67.7***	51.0***	34	23	25***	15***	351***	328***	1157***	1110***
324	Bolton	71.1***	54.1***	17	16	22***	12	370***	363***	1253***	1234***
325	Bury	59.6*	47.7*	26	0	18	13	339***	316***	1163***	1183***
326	Lancashire	67.7***	52.9***	12	9	19*	13	365***	334***	1196***	1193***
327	Manchester	76.3***	64.4***	10	15	21**	14*	420***	410***	1255***	1262***
328	Oldham	68.8***	65.7***	20	19	19	13	371***	346***	1235***	1220***
329	Rochdale	67.6***	55.5***	7	13	23***	14*	372***	360***	1202***	1201***
330	Salford	76.6***	63.7***	6	6	22**	10	427***	397***	1291***	1259***
331	Stockport	54.0	48.7**	11	0	20	11	326*	292	1138***	1111***
332	Tameside	72.8***	61.6***	0	0	20*	12	377***	353***	1236***	1181***
333	Trafford	58.6*	48.0*	15	0	18	12	319	305**	1114***	1089***
334	Wigan	74.3***	54.3***	29	10	20	11	387***	356***	1261***	1235***
335	Cheshire	62.0***	45.3**	4	7	19	11	335***	309***	1135***	1130***
336	Liverpool	72.6***	61.1***	15	14	21***	11	419***	389***	1269***	1237***
337	St Helens and Knowsley	67.1***	62.4***	4	15	21***	11	386***	379***	1234***	1233***
338	Sefton	64.8***	53.2***	6	6	19	11	348***	321***	1166***	1131***
339	Wirral	50.5	48.8**	19	14	18	11	346***	331***	1188***	1149***
340	Clwyd	68.5***	50.1***	17	12	18	13	337***	309***	1138***	1100***
341	Dyfed	69.0***	58.2***	11	10	19	11	356***	312***	1179***	1127***
342	Gwent	66.1***	50.6***	15	4	20	12	355***	327***	1183***	1147***
343	Gwynedd	68.1***	52.9***	7	7	17	11	340***	306**	1136***	1086***
344	Mid Glamorgan	83.5***	60.2***	6	13	20**	14*	391***	352***	1252***	1207***
345	Powys	60.9*	48.5	0	0	18	12	302	288	1105**	1109***
346	South Glamorgan	62.8***	45.5*	13	4	18	11	329**	302**	1118***	1087***
347	West Glamorgan	70.8***	53.0***	13	9	20*	12	361***	332***	1185***	1136***
UK:NORTHERN IRELAND											
348	Northern Ireland	70.8***	53.6***	8	9	22***	14***	388***	352***	1258***	1208***
UK: SCOTLAND		79.3***	61.7***	15	13	19***	12	399***	372***	1230***	1224***
349	Highlands and Islands	78.8***	56.9***	11	11	17	11	418***	379***	1270***	1246***
350	Grampian	58.3*	49.3***	7	19	16	10	341***	315***	1133***	1156***
351	Tayside	69.9***	54.2***	4	12	16	9	357***	326***	1158***	1169***
352	Fife	80.0***	65.0***	9	9	17	12	365***	343***	1190***	1174***
353	Lothian	72.1***	54.1***	9	15	18	12	364***	334***	1167***	1158***
354	Borders	75.5***	63.2***	0	0	17	12	338**	314**	1164***	1158***
355	Forth Valley	80.6***	59.6***	40*	23	21*	13	383***	357***	1232***	1199***
356	Argyll and Clyde	85.2***	66.2***	16	10	21***	12	432***	406***	1300***	1288***
357	Greater Glasgow	82.8***	69.3***	16	14	20***	11	453***	430***	1283***	1289***
358	Lanarkshire	90.0***	65.1***	27	15	22***	12	411***	393***	1281***	1270***
359	Ayrshire and Arran	93.8***	73.7***	16	12	22***	14**	401***	386***	1280***	1279***
360	Dumfries and Galloway	80.0***	52.3**	0	0	19	11	387***	360***	1230***	1185***
EC		52.5	41.5	20	12	18	12	316	291	1067	1054

Appendix A   Selection of diseases

Disease	Tuberculosis	Age group — 5–64 years	ICD codes from 8th and 9th revisions

ICD8 : 010–019

Interventions

Screening, early dectection of cases, immunization
Contact tracing
Antibiotics

010	Silicotuberculosis
011	Pulmonary tuberculosis
012	Other respiratory tuberculosis
013	Tuberculosis of meninges and central nervous system
014	Tuberculosis of intestines, peritoneum, and mesenteric glands
015	Tuberculosis of bones and joints
016	Tuberculosis of genito-urinary system
017	Tuberculosis of other organs
018	Disseminated tuberculosis
019	Late effects of tuberculosis

Health care providers

Public health programme *
Primary care
Hospital

Other potential contributory factors to excess mortality

ICD9 : 010–018, 137

Incidence – social class
       – ethnic group
Non-compliance with treatment

010	Primary tuberculous infection
011	Pulmonary tuberculosis
012	Other respiratory tuberculosis
013	Tuberculosis of meninges and central nervous system
014	Tuberculosis of intestines, peritoneum, and mesenteric glands
015	Tuberculosis of bones and joints
016	Tuberculosis of genito-urinary system
017	Tuberculosis of other organs
018	Miliary tuberculosis
137	Late effects of tuberculosis

* Most important provider(s).

References

British Thoracic and Tuberculosis Association (1971). A survey of tuberculosis mortality in England and Wales in 1968. *Tubercle*, **52**, 1–18.

Johnston, R.F. and Wildnick, K.H. (1974). State of the art. Review of the impact of chemotherapy on the care of patients with tuberculosis. *American Review of Respiratory Disease*, **109**, 636–64.

Disease	Malignant neoplasm of cervix uteri	Age group — 15–64 years	ICD code from 8th and 9th revisions

Interventions

Screening, cytology
Surgery
Radiation therapy

180   Malignant neoplasm of cervix uteri

Health care providers

Community health services *
Primary care
Hospital

Other potential contributory factors to excess mortality

Incidence — social class
        — sexual habits

* Most important provider(s).

References

Clark, B.A. and Anderson, T.W. (1979). Does screening by 'PAP' smears help prevent cervical cancer? *Lancet*, **ii**, 1–4.

Editorial (whole issue on cancer of the cervix) (1976). Screening for carcinoma of the cervix. *Canadian Medical Association Journal*, **114**, 1013–26.

Macgregor, J.E. and Teper, S. (1978). Mortality from carcinoma of the cervix uteri in Britain. *Lancet*, **ii**, 774–6.

Disease	Malignant neoplasm of cervix uteri and body of uterus	Age group — 15–54 years	ICD codes from 8th and 9th revisions

Interventions

Screening, cytology
Surgery
Radiation therapy

Health care providers

Community health services *
Primary care
Hospital

Other potential contributory factors to excess mortality

Incidence — social class
           — sexual habits

Due to variation in coding practices between countries and
possible inclusion of malignant neoplasm of the body of the
uterus with that of the cervix uteri, the two have been combined for
between country comparisons. (Age limit 54 years for combined SMR,
to exclude the bulk of malignant neoplasm body uterus deaths which are
not avoidable.)

ICD8 : 180, 182

180   Malignant neoplasm of cervix uteri
182   Other malignant neoplasm of uterus

ICD9 : 179, 180, 182

179   Malignant neoplasm of uterus, part unspecified
180   Malignant neoplasm of cervix uteri
182   Other malignant neoplasm of uterus

* Most important provider(s).

References

Clark, B.A. and Anderson, T.W. (1979). Does screening by 'PAP' smears help prevent cervical cancer? *Lancet*, **ii**, 1–4.

Editorial (whole issue on cancer of the cervix) (1976). Screening for carcinoma of the cervix. *Canadian Medical Association Journal*, **114**, 1013–26.

Macgregor, J.E. and Teper, S. (1978). Mortality from carcinoma of the cervix uteri in Britain. *Lancet*, **ii**, 774–6.

Disease	Hodgkin's disease	Age group — 5–64 years	ICD code from 8th and 9th revisions

Interventions

Case dectection
Chemotherapy
Radiation therapy

Health care providers

Hospital *
Primary care
Pathology services

Other potential contributory factors to excess mortality

Social class
Radiation therapy services may not be available in each small area. Excess
mortality may reflect non referral or delayed referral of cases to regional
treatment centres

201   Hodgkin's disease

* Most important provider(s).

References

Aisenberg, A.C. (1978). The staging and treatment of Hodgkin's disease. *New England Journal of Medicine*, **299**, 1228–32.

Kaplan, H.S. (1980). *Hodgkin's Disease* (2nd edn). Harvard University Press, Cambridge, Massachusetts.

Disease	Chronic rheumatic heart disease	Age group — 5–44 years	ICD codes from 8th and 9th revisions

Interventions

| | | | 393 | Chronic rheumatic pericarditis |

Case detection of streptococci
Antibiotics

| | | | 394 | Diseases of mitral valve |

Prophylaxis
Valve replacement surgery

| | | | 395 | Diseases of aortic valve |

| | | | 396 | Diseases of mitral and aortic valves |

Health care providers

| | | | 397 | Diseases of other endocardial structures |

Hospital *
Primary care

| | | | 398 | Other rheumatic heart disease |

Other potential contributory factors to excess mortality

Social class

Long lag period between acute rheumatic fever and mortality.
Cardiothoracic surgery services may not be available at small area level
in all areas

* Most important provider(s).

References

Feinstein, A.R., Stern , E.K., and Spagnuola, M. (1966). The prognosis of acute rheumatic fever. *American Heart Journal*, **68**, 817–34.

Gordis, L. (1973). Effectiveness of comprehensive-care programs in preventing rheumatic fever. *New England Journal of Medicine*, **289**, 331–5.

Rammelkamp, C.H. (1952). Studies in the epidemiology of rheumatic fever in the armed services. *In Rheumatic fever* (ed. L. Thomas). University of Minneapolis Press, Minneapolis.

Disease	All respiratory diseases	Age group — 1–14 years	ICD codes from 8th and 9th revisions

Interventions

ICD8 : 460–519

Early detection of complications

Acute respiratory infections (460–466)
Influenza (470–474)
Pneumonia (480–486)

Health care providers

Bronchitis, emphysema and asthma (490–493)
Other diseases of upper respiratory tract (500–508)

Primary care
Hospital

Other diseases of respiratory system (510–519)

ICD9 : 460–519

Other potential contributory factors to excess mortality

Acute respiratory infections (460–466)

Social class
Urban pollution

Other diseases of upper respiratory tract (470–478)
Pneumonia and influenza (480–487)
Chronic obstructive pulmonary disease and allied conditions (490–496)
Pneumoconiosis and other lung diseases due to external agents (500–508)
Other diseases of respiratory system (510–519)

References

Editorial (1985). Acute respiratory infections in under-fives: 15 million deaths a year. *Lancet*, **ii**, 699–701.

Disease	Asthma	Age group — 5–44 years	ICD codes from 8th and 9th revisions

Interventions

Casualty department care   493   Asthma
Treatment
Early referral of status asthmaticus

Health care providers

Primary care *
Hospital

Other potential contributory factors to excess mortality

Social class
Prevalence
Inappropriate drug treatment

There is a potential coding error with chronic obstructive airways disease.
Not all asthma deaths are avoidable and therefore variation in prevalence
between areas is an important consideration

* Most important provider(s).

References

Johnston, A.J., Nunn, A.J., Somner, A.R., Stableforth, D.E., and Stewart, C.J. (1984). Circumstances of death from asthma. *British Medical Journal*, **288**, 1870–2.

Speizer, F.E., Doll, R., and Heaf, P. (1968). Observations on recent increase in mortality from asthma. *British Medical Journal*, **1**, 335–9.

Stableforth, D.E. (1983). Death from asthma (editorial). *Thorax*, **38**, 801–5.

Disease	Appendicitis	Age group — 5–64 years	ICD codes from 8th and 9th revisions

Interventions   540   Acute appendicitis

Case detection   541   Appendicitis, unqualified
Surgery
                                                           542   Other appendicitis
Health care providers
                                                           543   Other diseases of appendix
Hospital *
Primary care

Other potential contributory factors to excess mortality

Coding error — acute abdominal pain with no positive diagnosis

* Most important provider(s).

References

Editorial (1985). Perioperative deaths. *Lancet*, **ii**, 1049.

Disease	Abdominal hernia	Age group — 5–64 years	ICD codes from 8th and 9th revisions

Interventions

ICD8 : 550–553

Case detection
Surgery prior to complications

550   Inguinal hernia without mention of obstruction
551   Other hernia of abdominal cavity without mention of obstruction
552   Inguinal hernia with obstruction
553   Other hernia of abdominal cavity with obstruction

Health care providers

Hospital *
Primary care

ICD9 : 550–553

550   Inguinal hernia
551   Other hernia of abdominal cavity, with gangrene
552   Other hernia of abdominal cavity with obstruction, without mention of gangrene
553   Other hernia of abdominal cavity without mention of obstruction or gangrene

Other potential contributory factors to excess mortality

Coding error — acute abdominal pain with no positive diagnosis
Incidence of strangulated abdominal hernia

* Most important provider(s).

References

Editorial (1985). Perioperative deaths. *Lancet,* **ii**, 1049.

Disease	Cholelithiasis and cholecystitis	Age group — 5–64 years	ICD codes from 8th and 9th revisions

Interventions

ICD8 : 574–575

Case detection
Surgery prior to complications

574   Cholelithiasis
575   Other disorders of gallbladder

Health care providers

ICD9 : 574–575.1, 576.1

Hospital *
Primary care

574   Cholelithiasis
575.0 Acute cholecystitis
575.1 Other cholecystitis
576.1 Cholangitis

Other potential contributory factors to excess mortality

Coding error — acute abdominal pain with no positive diagnosis

* Most important provider(s).

References

Editorial (1985). Perioperative deaths. *Lancet,* **ii**, 1049.

Fitzpatrick,.G., Neutra, R., and Gilbert, J.P. (1977). Cost benefits of cholecystectomy for silent gallstones. In *Cost, risks and effectiveness of surgery* (ed. J.P. Bunker, B.A. Barnes, and F. Mosteller), pp. 246–76. Oxford University Press, New York.

Ransohoff,D.F., Gracie, W.A., Wolfenson,L.B., and Neuhauser, D. (1983). Prophylactic cholecystectomy or expectant management for silent gallstones. A decision analysis to assess survival. *Annals of Internal Medicine,* **99**, 199–204.

Disease	Hypertensive and cerebrovascular diseases	Age group — 35–64 years	ICD codes from 8th and 9th revisions

Interventions

Case detection
Antihypertensive medication
Treatment of complications of cerebrovascular disease

Health care providers

Primary care *
Hospital

Other potential contributory factors to excess mortality

Coding error—ischaemic heart disease
Lack of screening/case finding
Social factors
Non-compliance with treatment
Nutrition
Weight
Smoking (cerebrovascular disease)
Malignant hypertension

Due to potential case transfer (coding) between hypertension and cerebrovascular disease, the two diseases have been combined. The lower age limit has been raised to 35 years to exclude cerebrovascular disease which is not considered avoidable, for example, Berry aneurysms.

ICD8 : 400–404, 430–438

400 Malignant hypertension
401 Essential benign hypertension
402 Hypertensive heart disease
403 Hypertensive renal disease
404 Hypertensive heart and renal disease

430 Subarachnoid haemorrhage
431 Cerebral haemorrhage
432 Occlusion of precerebral arteries
433 Cerebral thrombosis
434 Cerebral embolism
435 Transient cerebral ischaemia
436 Acute but ill-defined cerebrovascular disease
437 Generalized ischaemic cerebrovascular disease
438 Other and ill-defined cerebrovascular disease

ICD9 : 401–405, 430–438

401 Essential hypertension
402 Hypertensive heart disease
403 Hypertensive renal disease
404 Hypertensive heart and renal disease
405 Secondary hypertension

430 Subarachnoid haemorrhage
431 Intracerebral haemorrhage
432 Other and unspecified intracranial heamorrhage
433 Occlusion and stenosis of precerebral arteries
434 Occlusion of cerebral arteries
435 Transient cerebral ischaemia
436 Acute but ill-defined cerebrovascular disease
437 Other and ill-defined cerebrovascular disease
438 Late effects of cerebrovascular disease

* Most important provider(s).

References

Hypertension Detection and Follow-Up Program Cooperative Group (1979). Five-year findings of the hypertension detection and follow-up program. I. Reduction in mortality in persons with high blood pressure, including mild hypertension. *Journal of the American Medical Association*, **242**, 2562–71.

Hypertension Detection and Follow-Up Program Cooperative Group (1982). Five year findings of the hypertension detection and follow-up programme. II. Reduction in stroke incidence among persons with high blood pressure. *Journal of the American Medical Association*, **247**, 633–8.

Veteran's Administration Cooperative Study Group on Antihypertensive Agents (1972). Effects of treatment on morbidity in hypertension. *Circulation*, **45**, 991–1004.

Disease	Maternal deaths (all causes)	Age group — all years	ICD codes from 8th and 9th revisions

Interventions

ICD8 : 630–678

Antenatal care
Obstetric care

630–634 Complications of pregnancy
635–639 Urinary infections and toxaemias of pregnancy and the puerperium
640–645 Abortion

Health care providers

650–662 Delivery
670–678 Complications of the puerperium

Hospital *
Primary care

ICD9 : 630–676

Other potential contributory factors to excess mortality

630–639 Pregnancy with abortive outcome
640–648 Complications mainly related to pregnancy

None

650–659 Normal delivery and other indications for care in pregnancy, labour and delivery
660–669 Complications occuring mainly in the course of labour and delivery
670–676 Complications of the puerperium

* Most important provider(s).

References

Department of Health and Social Security (1982). Report on confidential enquiries into maternal deaths in England and Wales 1976–8. *Report on Health and Social Subjects, 26.* HMSO, London.

Dambrosio, F. and Buscaglia, M. (1976). La mortalilita in Lombardia e le sue cause. Risultati di un'indagine condotta nelgi ospedali della Lombardia per gli anni 1966–73. *Annali di Ostetricia, Ginecologia, Medicina Perinatale,* **97,** 302–25.

Rumeau-Rouquette, C., du Mazaubrun, C., and Rabarison, Y. (1984). *Naître en France. Dix ans d'évolution.* INSERM-Doin, Paris.

Disease	Perinatal mortality	All causes, aged under 1 week, plus stillbirths

Interventions

Antenatal care
Obstetric care
Paediatric neonatal care

Health care providers

Hospital *
Primary care

Other potential contributory factors to excess mortality

Incidence — low birth weight
           — social class

* Most important provider(s).

References

Alberman, E. (1982). Perinatal audit (editorial). *Community Medicine,* **4,** 95–6.

Mersey Regional Health Authority (1982). Report of Working Party. Confidential Enquiry into perinatal deaths in the Mersey Region. *Lancet,* **i,** 491–4.

Donzelli, G. and Assenza., G. (1984). L'audit perinatale. *Salute e Territorio,* **34–35,** 71–4.

Rumeau-Rouquette, C., du Mazaubrun, C. and Rabarison, Y. (1984). *Naître en France. Dix ans d'évolution.* INSERM-Doin, Paris.

Disease	Infectious diseases	Age group :		ICD codes from 8th and 9th revisions
		Typhoid	5–64 years	
		Whooping cough	0–14 years	
		Tetanus	0–64 years	
		Measles	1–14 years	
		Osteomyelitis	1–64 years	

Interventions

ICD8 : 001, 033, 035, 055, 720

Case detection
Immunization
Contact tracing
Antibiotic treatment
Treatment of complications

001   Typhoid fever
033   Whooping cough
037   Tetanus
055   Measles
720   Osteomyelitis and periostitis

Health care providers

ICD9 : 002.0, 033, 037, 055, 730

Public health programme *
Primary care
Hospital

002.0 Typhoid fever
033   Whooping cough
037   Tetanus
055   Measles
730   Osteomyelitis, periostitis and other infections involving the bone

Other potential contributory factors to excess mortality

Incidence — social class

Usually small numbers at the small area level

* Most important provider(s).

References

Bouvier-Colle, M.H., Magescas, J.B., and Hatton, F. (1985). Causes de décès et jeunes étrangers en France. *Revue d'Epidémiologie et de Santé Publique,* **33**, 409–16.

Disease	Malignant neoplasm of trachea, bronchus, and lung	Age group — 5–64 years	ICD codes from 8th and 9th revisions

Interventions

162   Malignant neoplasm of trachea, bronchus, and lung

Primary prevention

Health care providers

Health education

Other potential contributory factors to excess mortality

Smoking
Asbestos

Long lag period between exposure and mortality. Apart from health education, intervention is usually outside the direct control of the health services

References

Doll, R. and Hill, A. B. (1964). Mortality in relation to smoking: ten years' observations of British doctors. *British Medical Journal,* **1**, 1399–1410 and 1460–7.

Disease	Cirrhosis of liver	Age group — 15-64 years	ICD codes from 8th and 9th Revisions

Interventions

Primary prevention
Treatment for alcoholism

Health care providers

Health education

Other potential contributory factors to excess mortality

Alcohol consumption

Intervention is usually outside the direct control of the health services

ICD8 : 571

571   Cirrhosis of liver

ICD9 : 571

571   Chronic liver disease and cirrhosis

References

Robine, J.M., Moine, C., Lion, J. B., and Hatton, F. (1984). Taux comparatif des disparités régionales de la mortalité par cirrhose du foie, alcoolisme et psychose alcoolique. In *Les Colloquès et Congrès du Haut-Comité d'Etude et d'Information sur l'Alcoolisme.* La Documentation Française, Paris.

Disease	Motor vehicle accidents	Age group — 5-64 years	ICD codes from 8th and 9th revisions

Interventions

Primary prevention
Emergency treatment

Health care providers

Hospital accident and emergency department
Health education

Other potential contributory factors to excess mortality

Lack of legislation
Road maintenance poor
Number of cars on roads

Mortality difficult to interpret as numerator and denominator
are not well established:

? per 1000 miles of road;
? per number of cars;
? accidents outside area of residence.

Intervention is usually outside the direct control of the
health services

ICD8 : E810–E823

Motor vehicle traffic accidents (E810–E819)
Motor vehicle non-traffic accidents (E820–E823)

ICD9 : E810–E825

Motor vehicle traffic accidents (E810–E819)
Motor vehicle non-traffic accidents (E820–E825)

References

Hatton, F., Bouvier-Colle, M.H., and Maujol, L. (1981). Evaluation chronologique des mesures préventives des accidents de la circulation routière en France. *Revue d–Epidémiologie et de Santé Publique,* **29**, 341–53.

Appendix B   Data sources

Belgium

National Institute for Statistics, Ministry of Economic Affairs and Ministry of Public Health and Family.

Luxembourg

Statistiques des causes de décès 1974–78, 1980–84
Direction de la Santé
Service des Statistiques Sanitaires
22, rue Goethe
1637 Luxembourg

Federal Republic of Germany

Mortality and population data 1974–78 and 1980–84

Fachserie 12, Gesundheitswesen — Reihe 4. "Todesursachen" (1975,...1978, 1980,...1984), Statistisches Bundesamt.

Gestorbene nach Todesursachen — Bericht A IV/3 (1974,...1978, 1980,...1984) Berichte der Statistischen Landesämter.

Fachserie A, Bevölkerung und Kultur, Reihe 7, II (1974), Statistisches Bundesamt.

Fachserie 1, Bevölkerung und Erwerbstätigkeit, Reihe 1.3.

Bevölkerung nach Alter und Familienstand (1975,...1980), Statistisches Bundesamt.

Fachserie 1, Bevölkerung und Erwerbstätigkeit, Reihe 1 Gebiet und Bevölkerung (1981,....1984).

Socio-economic and health service data 1974–78 and 1980–84

Fachserie 12, Gesundheitswesen — Reihe 5, Berufe des Gesundheitswesens (1976, 1980,...1984), Statistisches Bundesamt.

Fachserie 12, Gesundheitswesen — Reihe 6, Krankenhäuser (1976,1980,...1984), Statistisches Bundesamt.

Denmark

Mortality data

The National Board of Health and the Danish Institute for Clinical Epidemiology.

Population data

The Central Bureau of Statistics.

Socio-economic and health service data

Praksisoplysninger pr. 31.XII.1976. Ugeskrift for Laeger 1977, Statistisk tabelvaerk 1977: iv. Bevolkningen i de enkelte kommuner pr. 1. januar 1977. Danmarks Statistik 1977.

Sundhedsstyrelsen, Medicinalstatistiske meddelser 1976:6 og 1978:1.

Danmarks Statistik, Statistisk Årborg 1978.

Danmarks Statistik, Statistisk Årborg 1984.

Danmarks Statistik, Statistisk Tabelvaerk 1982: II.

Sundhedsstyrelsen, Sygehusstatistik II: 7: 1982.

Praksisoplysninger pr. 31. XII 1983. Ugeskrift for Laeger 1983, 2973.

France

Mortality and population data 1973–77 and 1980–84

Unité 164 de Recherche sur l'Evaluation de l'Etat de Santé et des Systèmes de Soins et de Prévention – INSERM
16 Av. P. Vaillant-Couturier
94807 Villejuif.

Socio-economic and health service data 1974–78.

P.A. Audirac. *Recensement Général de la Population 1975.*
Les Collections de l'INSEE, 1979, 474–475.

Santé Securité Sociale Statistiques et Commentaires 1977, 3, 17–19.

Santé Securité Sociale Statistiques et Commentaires 1978, 3B, 71–82.

Santé Securité Sociale Statistiques et Commentaires 1977, 6A, 25–27.

Socio-economic and health service data 1980–84

B. Faur. *La situation démographique en 1982.*
Les Collections de l'INSEE, Séries D, No 106.

P.A. Audirac. *Recensement Général de la Population 1982: Principaux resultats.*
Les Collections de l'INSEE, Séries D, No 97.

Annuaires des Statistiques Sanitaires et Sociales 1984.
SESI. Ministère des Affaires Sociales et de la Solidarité Nationale.

Greece

Mortality and population data

Published and unpublished material (census, vital registration) compiled and offered by the National Statistical Service of Greece.

Socio-economic and health service data

Statistical Department
Ministry of Social Services
"Social Welfare and Health Statistics" (Annual publication).

Italy

Mortality and population data 1974–79 and 1979–83

Mortality records 1975–83 were made available to the Istituto Superiore di Sanita by the ISTAT in the original form. We would like to thank M.L. Panichelli Fucci from ISTAT for her courtesy and the Department of Epidemiological Data Analysis of the Laboratorio di Epidemiologia e Biostatistica whose program of data extraction we have used (1–3). Intercensual Provinicial Population estimates were developed by Riccardo Capocaccia and Riccardo Scipione (4).

1) Capocaccia, R., Farchi, G., Mariotti, S., Verdecchia, A., Angeli, A., Morganti, P., and Panichelli Fucci, M.L. La mortalitá in Italia nel periodo 1970–79. *Rapporto ISTISAN*, 84/10.
2) Capocaccia, R., Farchi, G., Mariotti, S., Verdecchia, A., Angeli, A., Morganti, P., and Panichelli Fucci, M.L. La mortalitá in Italia nel l'anno 80. *Rapporto ISTISAN*, 85/10.
3) Capocaccia, R., Farchi, G., Mariotti, S., Verdecchia, A., Angeli, A., Morganti, P., Panichelli Fucci, M.L. La mortalitá in Italia nel l'anno 85. *Rapporto ISTISAN* 89/6.
4) Capocaccia, R. and Scipione, R. (1984) Stima della popolazione italiana per eta', sesso e provincia di residenza negli anni 1971–79 *Epidimiologie e prevenzione*, **21–22**: 57–61.

Perinatal data were extracted from *Booettino Mensile di Statistica* (ISTAT).

Socio-economic and health service data 1974–78 and 1979–83

Annuario di Statistiche Sanitarie, ISTAT, Roma.

Annuario Statistico Italiano, ISTAT, Roma.

Ireland

Mr John Stevens of the Central Statistics Office, Ardee Road, Dublin 6.

Netherlands

Mortality and population data 1974–78

Central Bureau of Statistics.

Socio–economic and health service data 1974–78

Regionaal statistisch zakboek 1976,1977,1980.

Mortality data 1980–84

Data from the Central Bureau of Statistics, processed by the Department of Public Health and Social Medicine, Erasmus University, Rotterdam.

Population data 1980–84

Central Bureau of Statistics.

Socio–economic data 1980–84

Woningbehoefte-onderzoek 1981 and *Statistiek Motorvoertuigen 1980*, both published by the Central Bureau of Statistics.

Health service data 1980–84

National Institute for Primary Health Care Research, Central Bureau of Statistics and Landelijk Informatie Systeem Ziekenfondsen.

United Kingdom: England, Wales, and Northern Ireland

Mortality and population data

Office of Population Censuses and Surveys (1974–78). *Mortality statistics series DH2 1–5*. HMSO, London.

Socio-economic and health service data

National dwelling and housing survey (1979). HMSO, London.

National dwelling and housing survey, phases II and III (1980). HMSO, London.

Department of Health and Social Security,
Statistics and Research Division,
Department of Health and Social Security,
Euston Tower,
286 Euston Road,
London NW1 3DN

Scotland

Mortality, population, and socio-economic data

Registrar General for Scotland,
Ladywell House,
Ladywell Road,
Edinburgh EH12 7TF

Health services data

Information and Statistics Division of Common Services Agency for the NHS Scotland,
Trinity Park House,
Edinburgh EH5 3SQ

Portugal

Mortality and population data 1980–84

Institudo Nacional de Estatistica, Lisboa.

Socio-economic and health service data 1980–84

Divisao Geral de Estatistica do Departamendo de Estúdos e Planeamendo da Saúde, Ministerio de Saúde, Lisboa.

Spain

All data were supplied by the National Statistics Institute and were collected and prepared by the 'Subdireccion General de Informacion Sanitaria y Epidemiologia' of the Spanish Ministry of Health.

Mortality 1980–84

'Movimiento Natural de la Poblacion Española'
Instituto Nacional de Estadistica
Paseo de la Castellana, 176
28071 Madrid
Spain

Population, socio-economic and health service data 1980–84

1981 Census of the Spanish population
Instituto Nacional de Estadistica

Appendix C   Further reading

REFERENCES TO RELATED WORK IN PARTICIPANT COUNTRIES

Belgium

Humblet, P., Lagasse, R., Moens, G.F.G., van de Voorde, H., and Wollast, E. (ed) (1986). *Atlas de la mortalité évitable en Belgique, 1974–1978 — Atlas van de vermijdbare sterfte in België*. Ecole de Santé Publique, Université Libre de Bruxelles/School voor Maatschappelijke Gezondheidszorg, Katholieke Universiteit Leuven.

Humblet, P.C., Lagasse, R., and Moens, G.F.G. (1988). Fiabilité du processus de codage des décès en Belgique communautarisée. *Archives Belges de Medecine Sociale, Hygiène, Medecine du Travail et Medecine Légale*, **46** (1–2), 42.

Humblet, P.C., Lagasse, R., Moens, G.F.G, Wollast, E., and van de Voorde, H. (1987). La mortalité évitable en Belgique. *Social Science and Medicine*, **25** (5), 485.

Mackenbach, J.P., Moens, G.F.G., and Lagasse, R. (1985). Verchillen in door gezondheidszorg vermijdbare sterfte tussen Nederland en Belgie. *Gezondheid en Samenleving*, **6** (4), 265.

Moens, G.F.G. (1985). Vermijdbare sterfte door Tuberculose. *Tijdschrift voor Sociale Gezondheidszorg*, **63**, 981.

Moens, G.F.G. (1987). Evaluation of the effect of a health service using an ecological method. *Tijdschrift voor Sociale Gezondheidszorg*, **65**, 764.

Moens, G.F.G., van de Voorde, M., Humblet, P., Lagasse, R., and Wollast, E. (1985*a*). Vermijdbare sterfte door tuberculose: een evaluatieinstrument van de effectiviteit van tuberculosebestrijdingsprogramm's in België. *Tijdschrift voor Sociale Gezonheidszorg*, **63**, 981.

Moens, G., Lagasse, R., Humblet, P., van de Voorde, M., and Wollast, E. (1985*b*). Evaluatie van de medische zorg in Belgie via monitoring van vermijdbare sterfte. *Tijdschrift voor Sociale Gezonheidszorg*, **63**, 880.

Moens, G.F.G., Lagasse, R., Humblet, P., van de Voorde, M., and Wollast, E. (1986). 'Vermijdbare sterfte': een evaluatie instrument van de gezondheidszorg in Belgie? *Tijdschrift voor Geneeskunde*, **42** (13), 921.

van den Bussche, P., Du Jardin, B., Wollast, E., *et al.* (1987). *Atlas de la Santé Périnatale et Infantile en Belgique— Atlas van Perinatale en Infantiele Gezondheid in België*. Société Royale Belge de Gynécologie et d'Obstétrique, Bruxelles.

Federal Republic of Germany

Borgers, D. and Huckauf, H. (1982). Respiratorische Erkrankungen bei Landarbeitern im europäischen Vergleich. Bericht über die 21. *Tagung der Deutschen Gesellschaft für Arbeitsmedizin*, Stuttgart.

Borgers, D., Kern, K., Leibing, C., and Müller-Späth, D. (1981). Mortalitäts-und Frühberentungsdaten als Grundlage der Ressourcenverteilung im Gesundheitswesen. *Öffenliche Gesundheitswesen*, **43**, 163.

Frenzel-Beyme, R., Leutner, R., Wagner, G., and Weibelt, H. (1979). *Krebs Atlas*. Springer Verlag, Berlin.

Denmark

Bjerregaard, P. (1988). Alcohol related death in Greenland. *Arctic Medical Research*, **47**, Supplement 1, 596.

Bjerregaard, P. (1988). Causes of Death in Greenland 1968–85. *Arctic Medical Research*, **47**, (3), 105.

Bjerregaard, P. and Juel, K. (1990). 'Avoidable' deaths in Greenland 1968–1985: Variations by region and period. *Arctic Medical Research*, **49**, 119.

Johansen, L.G. and Bjerregaard, P. (1988). Lost years of life in Greenland in the period 1968 to 1983. *Arctic Medical Research*, **47**, Supplement 1, 596.

Juel, K. (1984). Dødelighedsindeks for kommuner og amter 1971–80. Dansk Institut for Klinisk Epidemiologi. Sundhedsstyrelsen. *Vitalstatistik*, **1** (7), 1.

Juel, K. and Kamper-Jørgensen, F. (1986). 'Avoidable' deaths in Denmark during the period 1970–83. Variations with Hospital district and periods. *Ugeskrift For Laeger*, **148**, 1981.

Kamper-Jørgensen, F. and Juel, K. (1982). Aspects of preventable deaths in Denmark. Presented at EC-Workshop Health Status Asessment, Paris, 1–3 December 1982.

Knudsen, L. (1988). Fodsler og sociale forhold 1982–83. Dansk Institut for Klinisk Epidemiologi. Sundhedsstyrelsen. *Vitalstatistik*, **1** (22), 141.

France

Annuaire des Statistiques Sanitaires et Sociales (SESI) (1989). Ministère des Affaires Sociales et de la Solidarité Nationale, Paris.

Audirac, P.A. *Recensement général de la Population 1982: Principaux Résultats*. Les Collections de l'Insee, Paris. Séries D, no. 97.

Bouvier-Colle, M.H. (1987). Géographie de la mortalité en France, In: Données Sociales, Paris INSEE, 445.

Faur, B. *La situation démographique en 1982*. Les Collections de l'Insee, Paris, Séries D, no. 106.

Garros, B. and Bouvier-Colle, M.H. (1990). Les variations géographiques de la mortalité. In *Mortalité en France*, (ed. M.H. Bouvier-Colle and F. Hatton). INSERM-Doin, Paris.

Hatton, F., Tiret, L., Maujol, L., *et al.* (1983). Protocole de l'enquête épidémiologique sur les anesthésies. *Annales Françaises d'Anésthesie et de Réanimation*, **2**, 335.

Jougla, E. (1987). Analyse géographique de la relation entre le niveau du système de soins et le niveau de la mortalité en France. Université de Paris-Sud, DERBH.

Jougla, E., Goldberg, M., and Hatton, F. (1988). Relation entre l'évolution de l'état de santé et l'activité du système de santé dans les pays développés. *Revue d' Epidémiologie et de Santé Publique*, **36**, 464.

Jougla, E., Ducimetière, P., Bouvier-Colle, M.H., and Hatton, F. (1987). Relation entre le niveau de développement du système de soins et le niveau de la mortalité 'évitable' selon les départements français. *Revue d'Epidémiologie et de Santé Publique*, **35**, 365.

Noin, D., Thumerelle, P.J., and Kostrubiec, B. (1986). Analyse Géographique des causes de décès en France. *Espace, Population et Sociétés*, 269.

Rumeau-Rouquette, C., Breart, G, and Padieu, R. (1985). *Méthodes en épidémiologie*. Flammarion médecine sciences, Paris.

Italy

Baldi, P. and Morosini, P.L. (1984). *I dati di mortalitá per la programmazione sanitaria*. Atti del 2° Convegno Nazionale sugli Studi di Mortalitá Regione Toscana — CSPO, Firenze.

Buiatti, E., Barchielli, A., and Vannucchi, G. (1988). Eventi sentinella: esperienze, problemi aperti e prospettive. 4° Convegno nazionale sugli Studi di Mortalitá, Firenze.

Dambrosio, F. and Buscaglia, M. (1976). La mortalitá materna in Lombardia e le sue cause. Risultati di un'indagine condotta negli ospedali della Lombardia per gli anni 1966–73. *Annali di Ostetricia, Ginecologia, Medecina Perinatale*, **97**, 302.

Donzelli, G. and Assenza, G. (1984). L'audit perinatale. *Salute e Territorio*, **34–35**, 71.

Lauriola, P. and Goldoni, C.A. (1989). Osservazioni, commenti e proposte su una indagine condotta nella Regione Emilia Romagna nel 1987, su alcuni eventi sentinella. *Epidemiologia e Prevenzione*, **39**, 22.

Morosini, P.L. and Taroni, F. (1986). Valutazione di qualite dei servici sanitari. *Salute e Territorio*, **49**, 48.

Repetto, F. and Morosini, P.L. (1986). Sistema informativo, ricerca epidemiologica e valutazione dei servizi in Italia. *Epidemiologia e Prevenzione*, **26**, 1.

Taroni, F. (1985). *Il sistema informativo e la valutazione di qualitá*. Atti del Convegno Internazionale di studio sulla Verifica e Revisione della Qualitá della Assistenza Sanitaria e delle cure mediche. Giugno, Firenze.

The Netherlands

Kunst, A.E., Looman, C.W.N., and Mackenbach, J.P. (1988). Medical care and regional mortality differences within the countries of the European community. *European Journal of Population*, **4**, 223.

Mackenbach, J.P. (1984). Gezondheidszorg en vermijdbare sterfte. *Tijdschrift voor Sociale Gezondheidszorg*, **62**, 433.

Mackenbach, J.P. (1985). Het effect van antibiotica op de sterfte aan infectieziekten in Nederland. *Tijdschrift voor Sociale Gezondheidszorg*, **63**, 518.

Mackenbach, J.P. (1987a). Internationale en regionale verschillen in sterfte aan enkele door medische zorg (gedeeltelijk) voorkoombare of behandelbare aandoeningen. *Nederlands Tijdschrift voor Geneeskunde*, **131** (37), 1612.

Mackenbach, J.P. (1987b). Verbeteringen in de overleving van kankerpatienten sinds de jaren 1950. *Tijdschrift voor Sociale Gezondheidszorg*, **65** (2), 30.

Mackenbach, J.P. (1987c). Health care policy and regional epidemiology; International comparisons and a case-study from the Netherlands. *Social Science and Medicine*, **23** (3), 247.

Mackenbach, J.P. and Looman, C.W.N. (1988) Secular trends of infectious disease mortality in the Netherlands 1911–78: quantitative estimates of changes coinciding with the introduction of antibiotics. *International Journal of Epidemiology*, **17** (3), 618.

Mackenbach, J.P., Moens, G., and Lagasse, R. (1985). Verschillen tussen Nederland en België in door gezondheidszorg vermijdbare sterfte. *Gezondheid en samenleving*, **6** (4), 265.

Mackenbach, J.P., Van Duyne, W.M.J., and Kelson, M.C. (1987). Certification and coding of two underlying causes of death in the Netherlands and other countries of the European Community. *Journal of Epidemiology and Community Health*, **41**, 156.

Mackenbach, J.P., Looman, C.W.N., and Kunst, A.E. (1988a). De ontwikkeling van de sterfte aan aandoeningen die (gedeeltelijk) door medische zorg voorkoombaar of behandelbaar zijn geworden, 1950–84. *Nederlands Tijdschrift voor Geneeskunde*, **132** (36), 1665.

Mackenbach, J.P., Kunst, A.E., Looman, C.W.N., Habbema, J.D.F., and van der Maas, P.J. (1988b). Regional differences in mortality from conditions amenable to medical intervention in the Netherlands: a comparison of four time periods. *Journal of Epidemiology and Community Health*, **42** (4), 325.

Mackenbach, J.P., Looman, C.W.N., Kunst, A.E., Habbema, J.D.F., and van der Maas, P.J. (1988c). Post-1950 mortality trends and medical care: gains in life expectancy due to declines in mortality from conditions amenable to medical intervention in the Netherlands. *Social Science and Medicine*, **27** (9), 889.

Mackenbach, J.P., Looman, C.W.N., Kunst, A.E., Habbema, J.D.F., and van der Maas, P.J. (1988d). Regional differences in decline of mortality from conditions amenable to medical intervention in the Netherlands. *International Journal of Epidemiology*, **17** (4), 821.

Mackenbach, J.P., Stronks, K., and Kunst, A.E. (1989). The contribution of medical care to inequalities in health: differences between socio-economic groups in decline of mortality from conditions amenable to medical intervention. *Social Science and Medicine*, **29** (3), 369.

UK: England and Wales

Bauer, R.L. and Charlton, J.R.H. (1986). Area variation in mortality from diseases amenable to medical intervention: the contribution of differences in morbidity. *International Journal of Epidemiology*, **15**, 408.

Buck N., Devlin, H.B., and Lunn, J.N. (1987). Report of the confidential enquiry into perioperative deaths. London, Nuffield Provincial Hospitals Trust and the King's Fund for Hospitals.

Charlton, J.R.H. and Lakhani, A. (1985). Is the Jarman underprivileged area score valid? *British Medical Journal*, **290**, 1714.

Charlton, J.R.H. and Velez, R. (1986). Some international comparisons of mortality amenable to medical intervention. *British Medical Journal*, **292**.

Charlton, J.R.H., Hartley, R.M., Silver, R., and Holland, W.W. (1983). Geographical variation in mortality from conditions amenable to medical intervention in England and Wales. *Lancet* i, 691.

Charlton, J.R.H., Bauer, R., and Lakhani, A. (1984a). Outcome measures for district and regional health care planners. *Community Medicine*, **6**, 306.

Charlton, J.R.H., Prochazka, A., and Lakhani, A. (1984b). Death from appendicitis outside hospital? *Lancet*, **ii**, 399.

Charlton, J.R.H., Lakhani, A., and Aristidou, M. (1986). How have 'avoidable' death indices for England and Wales changed? 1974–78 compared with 1979–83. *Community Medicine*, **8**, 304.

Charlton, J.R.H., Holland, W.W., Lakhani, A., and Paul, E.A. (1987). Variations in 'avoidable' mortality and variations in health care. Committee of Public Accounts. (1989). *Quality of clinical care in National Health Service Hospitals*. London, HMSO.

Devlin, H.B. and Lunn, J.N. (1986). Confidential enquiry into perioperative deaths. *British Medical Journal*, **292**, 1622.

Holland, W.W. (1986). The 'avoidable' death guide to Europe. *Health Policy*, **6**, 115.

Holland, W.W. (1988). *European Community Atlas of Avoidable Death*. CEC Health Services Research Series No. 3. OUP/Council of the European Communities, Oxford.

Holland, W.W. and Breeze, E. (1988). The performance of health services. In *The political economy of health and welfare*. (ed. M. Keynes, D.A. Coleman, N.H. Dimsdale). Macmillan, Basingstoke.

Howard, J. (1987). 'Avoidable' mortality from cervical cancer: exploring the concept. *Social Science and Medicine*, **24**, 507.

Lunn, J.N. and Devlin, H.B. (1987). Lessons from the confidential enquiry into perioperative deaths in three NHS regions. *Lancet*, **ii**, 1384.

Mason, J.O., Koplan, J.P., and Layde, P.M. (1987). The prevention and control of chronic diseases: reducing unnecessary deaths and disability — a conference report. *Public Health Reports*, **102**, 17.

Moore, A. (1986). Preventable childhood deaths in Wolverhampton. British Medical Journal, **293**, 656.

O'Mahoney, M. and Holland, W.W. (1983). Review of the services for the control of Authority. In *Annual Report (1983) of the Department of Community Medicine, UMDS*, p.35. St Thomas' Campus, London SE1.

Paul, E.A., Evans, J., Barry, J., *et al.* (1989). Variations géographiques de la mortalité due a des maladies justiciables d'unes communautés européennes: atlas des décès 'évitables'. *World Health Statistics Quarterly*, **42**, 42.

Pledger, H.G., Fahy, L.T., van Mourik, G.A., and Bush, G.H. (1987). Deaths in children with a diagnosis of acute appendicitis in England and Wales 1980–4. *British Medical Journal*, **295**, 1233.

Reynolds, F. (1986). Obstetric anaesthetic services. *British Medical Journal*, **293**, 403.

Scrivens, E. and Charlton, J.R.H. (1983). Performance indicators: warning lights? *Health and Social Services Journal*, **15**, 1501.

Singal, G.M., Stilwell, P.J., Chambers, J., and Clews, B. (1985). *A confidential enquiry into premature preventable deaths*. Report to Walsall Health Authority, Walsall, England.

Smith, B.A. (1984). *Cost containment in health care: a study of twelve european countries 1977–83*. Bedford Square Press of the National Council for Voluntary Organisations, London. (Occasional Papers on Social Administration No. 73/ Social Administration Research Trust, London School of Economics).

Smith, B.A. and Maynard, A. (1979). *The organisation, financing and cost of health care in the European Community*. Collection Studies,

Social Policy Series, no. 36. Office for Official Publications of the European Community, Luxembourg.

Sunderland, R., Gardner, A., and Gordon, R.R. (1986). Why did postperinatal mortality rates fall in the 1970s. *Journal of Epidemiology and Community Health,* **40**, 228.

Valman, B. (1985). Preventing infant deaths. *British Medical Journal,* **290**, 339.

UK: Scotland

Carstairs, V. (1981). Multiple deprivation and health state. *Community Medicine,* **3**, 4.

Carstairs, V. (1989). Avoidable Mortality in European Countries — 1974–78. *Scottish Medical Journal,* Feb., 391.

Carstairs, V. and Morris, R. (1989). Deprivation: explaining differences in mortality between Scotland and England and Wales. *British Medical Journal,* **299**, 886.

Cole, S.K. (1989). Accuracy of death certificates in neonatal deaths. *Community Medicine,* **11**, 1.

Elbourne, D. and Mutch, L. (1987). Do locally based enquiries into perinatal mortality reduce the risk of perinatal death? In *Recent Advances in Community Medicine,* Vol 3 (ed. A. Smith), pp. 221. Churchill Livingstone, Edinburgh.

Information and Statistics Division, Common Services Agency Scotland (1988). Scottish neonatal and perinatal report for 1987.

Information and Statistics Division of Common Services Agency Scotland (1989). Scottish neonatal and perinatal report for 1988.

Scottish Home and Health Department (1989). Report on Maternal and Perinatal deaths in Scotland 1981–85. HMSO.

Portugal

Araújo, M.P. (1990). *Evolcão da Mortalidade Materna em Portugal: 1979–87.* Saúde en Números, Direcção-Geral Cuidos de Saúde Primários, 5 (1), Lisbon.

Cayolla da Motta, L. (1988). *Mortes 'evitáveis' na Europa: diferenças nacionais e regionais.* Saúde en Números, Direcção-Geral Cuidados de Saúde Primarios 4 (2), Lisbon.

Cayolla da Motta, L. and Marinho Falcão, J. (1987). *Atlas do Cancro em Portugal 1980–82.* Ministério da Saúde, Lisbon.

Cayolla da Motta, L., Sequeira, M.L., and Castanheira, J.L. (1989). *Anos da vida potenciais perdidos: mortalidade prematura (1–69 anos) por causas e distritos em Portugale sua evolução de 1976 a 1986 (Nota Prévia).* Saúde en Numeros, Direcao-Geral Cuidados de Saúde Primários 4 (2).

Spain

Gil, L.M.B. and Rathwell, T. (1989). The effect of Health Services on Mortality: amenable and non-amenable causes in Spain. *International Journal of Epidemiology,* **18** (3), 652.

Portugal and Spain

Cayolla da Motta, L. and Rodriguez, L.A.G. (1988). Anos potenciais de vida perdidos: Estudio comparativo de 'mortalidade evitauel' por causas entre Portugal e Espnha. *Revisita Portugesa de Saúde Pública,* **3** (4), 39.

Cayolla da Motta, L. and Rodriguez, L.A. (1989). Years of potential life lost: application of an indicator for assessing premature mortality in Spain and Portugal. *WHO Rapport Trimestriel de Statistiques Sanitaires Mondiales,* **42**, 1.

Further References

Aisenberg, A.C. (1978). The staging and treatment of Hodgkin's disease. *New England Journal of Medicine,* **299**, 1228.

Alberman, E. (1982). Perinatal audit (Editorial). *Community Medicine,* **4**, 95.

Bouvier-Colle, M.H., Magescas, J.B., and Hatton, F. (1985). Causes de décès et jeunes étrangers en France. *Revue d'Epidémiologie et de Santé Publique,* **33**, 409.

British Thoracic and Tuberculosis Association. (1971). A survey of tuberculosis mortality in England and Wales in 1968. *Tubercle,* **52**, 1.

Clark, B.A. and Anderson, T.W. (1979). Does screening by 'PAP' smears help prevent cervical cancer? *Lancet,* **ii**, 1.

Dambrosio, F. and Buscaglia, M. (1976). La mortalilitá in Lombardia e le sue cause. Risultati di un'indagine condotta negli ospedali della Lombardia per gli anni 1966–73. *Annali di Ostetricia, Ginecologia, Medicina Perinatale,* **97**, 302.

Department of Health and Social Security (1982). Report on confidential enquiries into maternal deaths in England and Wales 1976–8. *Report on Health and Social Subjects,* No. 26. HMSO, London.

Doll, R. and Hill, A.B. (1964). Mortality in relation to smoking: ten years' observations of British doctors. *British Medical Journal,* **1**, 1399 and 1460.

Donzelli, G. and Assenza., G. (1984). L'audit perinatale. *Salute e Territorio,* **34–35**, 71.

Editorial (whole issue on cancer of the cervix) (1976). Screening for carcinoma of the cervix. *Canadian Medical Association Journal*, **114**, 1013.

Editorial (1985*a*). Acute respiratory infections in under-fives: 15 million deaths a year. *Lancet, ii*, 699·

Editorial (1985*b*). Perioperative deaths. *Lancet, ii*, 1049.

Feinstein, A.R., Stern ,E.K., and Spagnuola, M. (1966). The prognosis of acute rheumatic fever. *American Heart Journal*, **68**, 817·

Fitzpatrick, G., Neutra, R., and Gilbert, J.P. (1977). Cost effectiveness of cholecystectomy for silent gallstones. In *Cost, risks and effectiveness of surgery* (ed. J.P. Bunker, B.A. Barnes, and F. Mostellen), pp.246 Oxford University Press, New York.

Gordis, L. (1973). Effectiveness of comprehensive programs in preventing rheumatic fever. *New England Journal of Medicine*, **289**, 331.

Hatton, F., Bouvier-Colle, M.H., and Maujol, L. (1981). Evaluation chronologique des mesures préventives des accidents de la circulation routière en France. *Revue d'Epidémiologie et de Santé Publique*, **29**, 341.

Hypertension Detection and Follow-Up Program Cooperative Group. (1979). Five year findings of the hypertension detection and follow-up programme. I. Reduction in mortality in persons with high blood pressure, including mild hypertension. *Journal of the American Medical Association*, **242**, 2562·

Hypertension Detection and Follow-Up Program Cooperative Group. (1982). Five year findings of the hypertension detection and follow-up programme. II. Reduction in stroke incidence among persons with high blood pressure. *Journal of the American Medical Association*, **247**, 633.

Johnston, R.F. and Wildnick, K.H. (1974). State of the art. Review of the impact of chemotherapy on the care of patients with tuberculosis. *American Review of Respiratory Disease*, **109**, 636.

Johnston, A.J., Nunn, A.J., Somner, A.R., Stableforth, D.E., and Stewart, C.J. (1984). Circumstances of death from asthma. *British Medical Journal*, **288**, 1870.

Kaplan, H.S. (1980). *Hodgkin's disease*, (2nd edn). Harvard University Press, Cambridge, Massachusetts.

Macgregor, J.E. and Temper, S. (1978). Mortality from carcinoma of the cervix uteri in Britain. *Lancet, ii*, 774.

Mersey Regional Health Authority (1982). Report of working party. Confidential Enquiry into perinatal deaths in the Mersey Region. *Lancet, i*, 491.

Poikolainen, K. and Eskola, J. (1986). Mortality from causes amenable to health services intervention (letter). *Lancet, i*, 1387.

Rammelkamp, C.H. (1952). Studies in the epidemiology of rheumatic fever in the armed services. In *Rheumatic Fever*. (ed. L. Thomas). University of Minneapolis Press, Minneapolis.

Ranshoff, D.F., Gracie, W.A., Wolfenson, L.B., and Newhamser, D. (1983). Prophylactic cholecystectomy or expedient management of silent gallstones. A decision analysis to assess survival. *Annals of Internal Medicine*, **99**, 199.

Robine, J.M., Moine, C., Lion, J., and Hatton, F. (1984). Taux comparatif des disparités régionales de la mortalité par cirrhose du foie, alcoolisme et psychose alcoolique in *Les Colloques et Congrès du Haut-Comité d'Etude et d'Information sur l'alcoolisme*. La Documentation Française, Paris.

Rumeau-Rouquette, C., du Mazaubrun, C., and Rabarison, Y. (1984). *Naître en France*. Dix ans d'évolution. INSERM-Doin, Paris.

Rutstein, D.D., Berenberg, W., Chalmers, T.C., *et al.* (1976). Measuring the quality of medical care. *New England Journal of Medicicne*, **294**, 582.

Rutstein, D.D., Berenberg, W., Chalmers, T.C., *et al.* (1980). Measuring the quality of medical care: second revision of tables of indexes. *New England Journal of Medicine*, **302**, 1146.

Speizer, F.E., Doll, R., and Heaf, P. (1968). Observations on recent increase in mortality from asthma. *British Medical Journal*, **1**, 335.

Stableforth, D.E. (1983). Death from asthma (editorial). *Thorax*, **38**, 801.

Veteran's Administration Cooperative Study Group on Antihypertensive Agents. (1972). Effects of treatment on morbidity in hypertension. *Circulation*, **45**, 991.

Wigle, D.T., *et al.* (1987). Declining risk of death in Canada: achievement and a challenge. *Journal of Chronic Diseases Canada*, **8**, 4.

Woolsey, T.D. (1981). *Toward an index of 'preventable' mortality*. United States Department of Health and Human Services. Hyattsville.